Chronic Lymphoid Leukemias

With compliments of

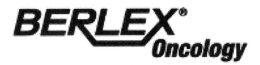

BASIC AND CLINICAL ONCOLOGY

Editor

Bruce D. Cheson, M.D.

National Cancer Institute
National Institutes of Health
Bethesda, Maryland

ADDITIONAL VOLUMES IN PREPARATION

Chronic Lymphoid Leukemias

Second Edition, Revised and Expanded

edited by
Bruce D. Cheson

National Cancer Institute
National Institutes of Health
Bethesda, Maryland

MARCEL DEKKER, INC.

NEW YORK • BASEL

The first edition of this book was published as *Chronic Lymphocytic Leukemia: Scientific Advances and Clinical Developments*, B. D. Cheson, ed., Marcel Dekker, Inc., 1993.

ISBN: 0-8247-0543-2

This book is printed on acid-free paper.

Headquarters
Marcel Dekker, Inc.
270 Madison Avenue, New York, NY 10016
tel: 212-696-9000; fax: 212-685-4540

Eastern Hemisphere Distribution
Marcel Dekker AG
Hutgasse 4, Postfach 812, CH-4001 Basel, Switzerland
tel: 41-61-261-8482; fax: 41-61-261-8896

World Wide Web
http://www.dekker.com

The publisher offers discounts on this book when ordered in bulk quantities. For more information, write to Special Sales/Professional Marketing at the headquarters address above.

Current printing (last digit):
10 9 8 7 6 5 4 3 2 1

PRINTED IN THE UNITED STATES OF AMERICA

Series Introduction

The current volume, *Chronic Lymphoid Leukemias: Second Edition, Revised and Expanded*, is the twenty-sixth in the Basic and Clinical Oncology series. Many of the advances in oncology have resulted from close interaction between the basic scientist and the clinical researcher. The current volume illustrates the success of this relationship as demonstrated by new insights into clinical drug resistance and means of circumventing this potential obstacle to effective cancer treatment.

As editor of the series, my goal is to recruit volume editors who not only have established reputations based on their outstanding contributions to oncology, but who also have an appreciation for the dynamic interface between the laboratory and the clinic. To date, the series has consisted of monographs on topics that are of a high level of current interest. *Chronic Lymphoid Leukemias* certainly fits into this category and is a most important addition to the series.

Volumes in progress focus on lung cancer, infections, myeloproliferative disorders, and myelodyoplastic syndromes. I anticipate that these books will provide a valuable contribution to the oncology literature.

Bruce D. Cheson

Preface

It has now been eight years since the publication of the first edition of this book. I am certain that the following pages will show that more than sufficient progress has taken place since then to warrant this updated and expanded text.

To present a comprehensive, state-of-the-art picture of the disease, I have once again assembled many of the leading experts in chronic lymphocytic leukemia (CLL). Their various chapters begin with a historical perspective of the disease, give its epidemiology, and even include the psychosocial aspects involving patient management. The diagnosis of this disease can now be made with increased precision. Recent improvements in molecular and genetic technology permit us to identify patients within clinical stage with markedly differing outcomes. Several lines of data now suggest that B-cell chronic lymphocytic leukemia (B-CLL) may actually be two diseases, reflecting the unmutated or a mutated state of the immunoglobulin heavy-chain genes. The current use of fluorescent in situ hybridization permits a more accurate evaluation of the cytogenetics of the malignant cells, identifying distinct subsets of patients with excellent correlations between the chromosome abnormality, clinical course, response to therapy, and outcome. As we explore this disease with newer technologies such as DNA microarray analysis, even more clinically meaningful insights should become available.

There have been important therapeutic advances as well. Several recently reported randomized trials have helped to transform our paradigms for the treatment of CLL. Based on these results, fludarabine is now commonly used as the preferred initial treatment for the disease. Nevertheless, the failure to cure patients has led to the development of a series of fludarabine-based chemotherapy and antibody combination regimens.

An increasing number of interesting new biological agents are being evaluated, including CAMPATH-1H, recently approved in the United States for the treatment of fludarabine-resistant CLL. There has been a proliferation in the use of submyeloablative transplants, offering a more immunology-based therapy than standard bone marrow transplantation, potentially with less toxicity. Other newer approaches are discussed in this text, including gene therapy.

Perhaps one of the most important events in the last few years has been the evolution of the CLL Research Consortium (CRC), a highly interactive collaboration among some of the foremost basic and clinical CLL researchers in the United States, many of whom have contributed chapters to this book. This new integrated research model is likely to result in major progress.

I hope that this book will not only be highly informative for the readers, but also stimulate a new generation of young investigators to study this fascinating disease and to make the contributions in biology, immunology, and therapy that will finally lead to its cure.

My deepest love and gratitude to my family, who continue to stick by me in spite of myself; to those colleagues whose friendship reminds me that it is not where you are but who you are that matters; and, finally, to all the patients who continue to look to us for hope—let us not disappoint them.

Bruce D. Cheson

Contents

Contents

Contributors

Vasantha Brito-Babapulle   Academic Department of Hematology and Cytogenetics, Institute of Cancer Research, Royal Marsden Hospital, London, England

Florencia Bullrich, M.D.   Kimmel Cancer Center, Thomas Jefferson University, Philadelphia, Pennsylvania

John C. Byrd, M.D.   Department of Internal Medicine, The Ohio State University, Columbus, Ohio

Federico Caligaris-Cappio, M.D.   Dipartimento di Scienze Biomediche e Oncologia Umana, University of Torino, Torino, Italy

Janine Campbell, M.B., B.S., Ph.D.   Department of Hematology and Medical Oncology, Peter MacCallum Cancer Institute, East Melbourne, Victoria, Australia

Daniel Catovsky, M.D.   Academic Department of Hematology and Cytogenetics, Institute of Cancer Research, Royal Marsden Hospital, London, England

Bruce D. Cheson, M.D., FACP   Medicine Section, Clinical Investigations Branch, Cancer Therapy Evaluation Program, Division of Cancer Treatment, National Cancer Institute, National Institutes of Health, Bethesda, Maryland

Nicholas Chiorazzi, M.D.   North Shore–Long Island Jewish Research Institute, Department of Medicine, North Shore University Hospital, and Departments of Medicine and Pathology, New York University School of Medicine, Manhasset, New York

Carlo M. Croce, M.D.   Kimmel Cancer Center, Thomas Jefferson University, Philadelphia, Pennsylvania

Claire Dearden, M.D. Department of Hematology, St. George's Hospital Medical School, London, England

Susan S. Devesa, Ph.D. National Cancer Institute, National Institutes of Health, Bethesda, Maryland

G. Dighiero, M.D. Institut Pasteur, Paris, France

Hartmut Döhner, M.D. Department of Internal Medicine III, University of Ulm, Ulm, Germany

Martin J. S. Dyer, M.D.* Academic Department of Hematology and Cytogenetics, Institute of Cancer Research, Royal Marsden Hospital, London, England

Manlio Ferrarini, M.D. The Division of Clinical Immunology, Istituto Nazionale per la Ricerca sul Cancro, and Dipartimento di Oncologia Clinica e Sperimentale, Università di Genova, Genova, Italy

Robin Foa, M.D. Dipartimento di Biotecnologie Cellulari ed Ematologia, University "La Sapienza," Rome, Italy

Varsha Gandhi, Ph.D. Departments of Experimental Therapeutics and Leukemia, The University of Texas M. D. Anderson Cancer Center, Houston, Texas

Randy D. Gascoyne, M.D. Department of Pathology, British Columbia Cancer Agency, Vancouver, British Columbia, Canada

Paolo Ghia, M.D. Dipartimento di Scienze Biomediche e Oncologia Umana, University of Torino, Torino, Italy

Michael R. Grever, M.D. Department of Internal Medicine, The Ohio State University, Columbus, Ohio

John G. Gribben, M.D., D.Sc. Dana-Farber Cancer Institute, Department of Medicine, Harvard Medical School, Boston, Massachusetts

Terry Hamblin, M.D. Department of Hematology, Royal Bournemouth Hospital, Bournemouth, England

Mark A. Hoffman, M.D. Long Island Jewish Medical Center, New Hyde Park, New York

Jimmie C. Holland, M.D. Department of Psychiatry and Behavioral Sciences, Memorial Sloan-Kettering Cancer Center, New York, New York

---

**Current affiliation*: Department of Hematology, University of Leicester, Leicester, England.

Michael J. Keating, M.D. Department of Leukemia, The University of Texas M. D. Anderson Cancer Center, Houston, Texas

Thomas J. Kipps, M.D., Ph.D. School of Medicine, University of California San Diego, San Diego, California

Shinichi Kitada, M.D. The Burnham Institute, La Jolla, California

Angela M. Krackhardt, M.D. Dana-Farber Cancer Institute, Department of Medicine, Harvard Medical School, Boston, Massachusetts

Peter Lichter, M.D. Deutsches Krebsforschungszentrum, Heidelberg, Germany

Martha S. Linet, M.D. National Cancer Institute, National Institutes of Health, Bethesda, Maryland

Thomas P. Loughran, Jr., M.D. Departments of Oncology, Medicine, and Microbiology/Immunology, H. Lee Moffitt Cancer Center and Research Institute, Tampa, Florida

Estella Matutes, M.D. Academic Department of Hematology and Cytogenetics, Institute of Cancer Research, Royal Marsden Hospital, London, England

Edgar G. Miranda, M.D. Departments of Oncology, Medicine, and Microbiology/Immunology, H. Lee Moffitt Cancer Center and Research Institute, Tampa, Florida

Stefano Molica, M.D. Department of Hematology/Oncology, Azienda Ospedaliera "Pugliese-Ciaccio," Catanzaro, Italy

Emilio Montserrat, M.D. Institute of Hematology and Oncology, Hospital Clinic, University of Barcelona, Barcelona, Spain

Vicki A. Morrison, M.D. Sections of Hematology/Oncology and Infectious Disease, Veterans Affairs Medical Center, Minneapolis, Minnesota

Susan M. O'Brien, M.D. Department of Leukemia, The University of Texas M. D. Anderson Cancer Center, Houston, Texas

Enrica Orsini, M.D. Dipartimento di Biotecnologie Cellulari ed Ematologia, University "La Sapienza," Rome, Italy

Anders Österborg, M.D. Department of Oncology and Hematology, Karolinska Hospital, Stockholm, Sweden

LoAnn C. Peterson, M.D. Department of Pathology, Northwestern University Medical School, Chicago, Illinois

William Plunkett, Ph.D. Departments of Experimental Therapeutics and Leukemia, The University of Texas M. D. Anderson Cancer Center, Houston, Texas

Kanti R. Rai, M.D.   Division of Hematology–Oncology, Long Island Jewish Medical Center, New Hyde Park, New York, and Albert Einstein College of Medicine, Bronx, New York

Farhad Ravandi, M.D.   Department of Leukemia, The University of Texas M. D. Anderson Cancer Center, Houston, Texas

John C. Reed, M.D.   The Burnham Institute, La Jolla, California

Andrew J. Roth, M.D.   Department of Psychiatry and Behavioral Sciences, Memorial Sloan-Kettering Cancer Center, New York, New York

Marjaneh Rouhani, M.D.   Department of Psychiatry and Behavioral Sciences, Memorial Sloan-Kettering Cancer Center, New York, New York

Jahandar Saifollahi, M.D.   Department of Psychiatry and Behavioral Sciences, Memorial Sloan-Kettering Cancer Center, New York, New York

John Seymour, M.B., B.S.   Department of Hematology and Medical Oncology, Peter MacCallum Cancer Institute, East Melbourne, Victoria, Australia

Maria T. Sgambati, M.D.   National Cancer Institute, National Institutes of Health, Bethesda, Maryland

Stephan Stilgenbauer, M.D.   Department of Internal Medicine III, University of Ulm, Ulm, Germany

Martin S. Tallman, M.D.   Division of Hematology–Oncology, Department of Medicine, Northwestern University Medical School, and Robert H. Lurie Comprehensive Cancer Center, Chicago, Illinois

Deborah A. Thomas, M.D.   Department of Leukemia, The University of Texas M. D. Anderson Cancer Center, Houston, Texas

Tarun Wasil, M.D.   Department of Medical Oncology, Dr. H. Bliss Murphy Cancer Center, St. John's, Newfoundland, Canada

M. R. Yullie   Academic Department of Hematology and Cytogenetics, Institute of Cancer Research, Royal Marsden Hospital, London, England

Chronic Lymphoid Leukemias

1

History of Chronic Lymphocytic Leukemia

KANTI R. RAI

Long Island Jewish Medical Center, New Hyde Park, New York, and Albert Einstein College of Medicine, Bronx, New York

TARUN WASIL

Dr. H. Bliss Murphy Cancer Center, St. John's, Newfoundland, Canada

The identification of chronic lymphocytic leukemia (CLL) came about several decades after leukemia as a separate clinical entity was first described. Therefore, a historical survey of CLL must start with the review of those early years of hematology that followed the discovery and applications of microscopy and the development of methods of staining blood cells to distinguish the lymphoid from the myeloid hematopoiesis. Understandably, the numerous subtypes of all leukemias we recognize today share a common historical period when clinicians and pathologists battled with the question of whether leukemia was indeed a recognizable disease.

I. THE EARLY PERIOD

The modern era perhaps started with the invention of microscopy by Anton van Leeuvanhock (1632–1723), description of thymus and the lymphatic system by William Hewson (1739–1774), and development of methods of performing blood counts by Gabriel Andral (1797–1876). Barth (1), with the help of Donne, in 1839, used a microscope to study the blood of a leukemia patient while the patient was still alive. Bennett, a physiologist, and Virchow, a pathologist, almost simultaneously, described leukemia as a separate entity (2,3). After their descriptions, many other cases were reported by others in rapid succession (4,5). Virchow, in 1847, was the first to use the word ''leukemia'' and also stated that the first case of leukemia was described in 1827 by Velpeau (6). Bennett published a series of 37 cases of leukemia in 1852, 17 of them diagnosed during life (7). Virchow published several studies on the nature of the disease in 1856 (8). He stated that the colorless corpuscles are always present in normal blood and increase after digestion, during pregnancy, and with inflammation, but leukemia was a separate and definite entity and must be differentiated from other conditions. Virchow was able to describe two different forms of leukemias—"splenic" or "lineal," associated with swelling of the spleen, and "lymphatic," in which lymph nodes swell and blood contains the colorless corpuscles mimicking those seen in the lymph nodes. Friedreich, in 1857, was able to classify leukemias into the acute and chronic forms and tabulated their respective clinical and pathological features (9). While several physicians were busy studying and understanding leukemias, others criticized this work by commenting that "Leukemia has no special causes, special symptoms, particular anatomic lesions or specific treatment and I thus conclude that it does not exist as a distinct malady" (Cahen, 1855) (10), and "There are enough diseases without inventing new ones" (Barthez, 1855) (11).

It was Neumann (12), in 1870, who proposed that bone marrow was an important site for the formation of blood corpuscles as indicated from autopsy studies on a patient with "splenic" leukemia. Gowers (13), in 1879, pointed out that anemia in patients with leukemia may either be due to decreased formation of the red cells or by their excessive destruction.

Approximately 100 years ago, Ehrlich (14) devised methods of staining blood cells that led to classification of leukemias into myeloid and lymphoid and the correlation of clinical features with characteristic morphological findings. In 1893, Kundrat (15) used the term "lymphosarcoma" to describe a condition affecting the lymph nodes or mucous membranes and later spread to other neighboring structures. He was able to point out a difference between lymphosarcoma and leukemia by features such as greater local invasiveness, less widespread generalized manifestations, and absence of a leukemic blood picture in lymphosarcoma. In 1903, Turk (16) coined the term lymphomatoses to include chronic lymphocytic leukemias (a benign form), acute leukemia or chloroma (acute but either benign or malignant), and lymphosarcoma (chronic malignant form). Sir William Osler reported his experience with CLL at the Johns Hopkins University in the early part of 20th century (17). Osler observed that CLL constituted approximately 22% of all leukemias and described the disease to be associated with generalized lymphadenopathy and long survival times of 3 to 11 years. In 1924, Minot and Isaacs published their series of 80 patients with CLL and reported the average survival time of approximately 40 months with no improvement with radiation therapy compared with no treatment (18).

A. Progress in Understanding the Clinical History of Chronic Lymphocytic Leukemia

The half-century period between 1924 and 1973 was noted for the developments in precise diagnostic criteria of CLL, identification of various treatment options, and improved understanding of the natural history of this disease.

CLL was recognized as the most common familial form among all leukemias. In 1929 (19), Dameshek described CLL in two patients who were identical twins and had the disease develop at approximately the same age; interestingly, the son of one of the twins also had CLL develop at about the same age as the parent. Leavell (20), in 1938, reviewed the incidence of CLL and the various factors that influenced the duration of survival with this disease. Wintrobe and Hasenbush (21), in 1939, provided detailed clinical data on 86 patients with CLL.

Boggs et al. (22) in (1966) published a comprehensive review on the diagnostic criteria, clinical features and response to treatment, and survival data in a large number of CLL patients seen in Wintrobe's department at Salt Lake City, Utah. Their experience was similar to others as far as wide range of survival times in this disease was concerned. They also observed that those patients surviving <5 years had more disease at diagnosis compared with those who survived for longer periods. In the same year (1966), Galton observed that the rapidity of increase in lymphocyte count in the blood predicted the clinical outcome (23). He also suggested that the basic pathological findings in CLL were accumulation of lymphocytes and not the abnormal proliferation. These observations were also made independently by Dameshek at almost the same time (1967). Dameshek (24) proposed a method of stratifying the extent of disease in CLL patients on the basis of certain clinical features such as disease-related symptoms, lymph node enlargement, presence or absence of splenomegaly and/or hepatomegaly, and blood count. The observations of Boggs et al. Galton, and Dameshek were further strengthened by Hansen in 1973, who published his experience on a large number of CLL patients followed in Denmark (25).

B. Development of Clinical Staging Systems and Other Prognostic Factors

Although prior investigators had recognized the importance of clinical findings in predicting outcome of patients with CLL, it was not until 1975 that a simple, reproducible and clinically applicable staging system was described by Rai et al. (26). The original system consisted of five stages (0 to IV), but it was modified to a three-stage method in 1987, because the survival curves of a large population of patients indicated three distinct categories—the low risk, intermediate risk, and the high risk (27). Binet et al., in France, in 1981, described a three-stage system in which the stage A is the low-risk, stage B the intermediate-risk, and stage C the high-risk category (28). Both the Rai and the Binet systems are used widely by clinicians everywhere, although several other staging systems were also described during this period (29–33).

Because of a well-recognized clinical heterogeneity within each clinical stage, additional prognostic markers were also developed. The initial observations of Galton in 1966 that the pattern of increase in blood lymphocyte count was predictive of the clinical course were corroborated almost two decades later by others (34,35). Patients with rapid lymphocyte doubling time ($\leq$ 12 months) were shown to have a worse outcome than those with a slow lymphocyte doubling time (> 12 months). The pattern of bone marrow (36–39) involvement by the leukemic cells (nodular vs. diffuse) was also shown by several investigators as a predictor of outcome. Within the past decade, several other prognostic markers such as soluble CD23 (40,41), serum β_2-microglobulin (42), karyotypic abnormalities (43,44), immunoglobulin variable region mutation status (45,46), and CD38 have been proposed (45).

C. Influence of Technological Developments on the Understanding of Chronic Lymphocytic Leukemia

The knowledge that CLL is a disorder of B-lymphocytes came from the observation of two groups of investigators almost at the same time, in 1972 (47,48). Soon followed the understanding of the phenotypic profile of CLL lymphocytes and recognition of CLL as a monoclonal disorder in which the leukemic cells are arrested at the intermediate stage of differentiation (49).

Further advances in immunology and flow cytometry resulted in establishing a phenotypic profile of monoclonal B-lymphocytes, which today is considered characteristic and, therefore, diagnostic of CLL (50). These advances include recognition of co-expression of CD5 and CD23 on leukemic B-cells expressing CD20 and CD19.

One of the most important recent advances in the understanding of immunopathology of CLL were the reports in 1999 simultaneously from two different laboratories, one led by Chiorazzi (45) in the United States and the other by Hamblin (46) in the United Kingdom. CLL lymphocytes have been previously considered to originate from immunologically naïve B-cells, but these two reports demonstrate that there are perhaps two types of CLL, one with somatic mutations of IgV genes of leukemic cells, suggesting that these cells were transformed at the postgerminal center stage, and the second, without such mutations, suggesting that the leukemic cells in those patients originated from the pregerminal center stage. These workers found that patients with somatic mutations had a significantly better overall survival and clinical course than their counterparts without mutations. Chiorazzi's group also demonstrated that patients with significant IgV gene mutations had a small percentage of CD5+/CD19+ B-CLL cells expressing CD38 and vice versa (45). It was not until 1978 that chromosomal studies in CLL became possible when cells were stimulated with various mitogens. Before that, it was difficult to obtain adequate metaphases in CLL. The development of techniques to study chromosomes with fluorescent in-situ hybridization (FISH) has broadened our knowledge of cytogenetics in CLL. It has also been possible to correlate prognosis with cytogenetic abnormalities (44).

II. PROGRESS IN THERAPY

Chlorambucil has been in use for almost 40 years for CLL (51). The historical review of advances in CLL ends on an optimistic note with the recent surge in development of newer drugs such as fludarabine and other nucleoside analogues (52–54) and anti-CD52 (55) and anti-CD20 (56,57) monoclonal antibodies such as Campath 1-H and rituximab, respectively. These developments hold new promise for improved treatment and improved overall outlook for patients with this disease. Thus, the story of CLL forms a somewhat unique chapter in the history of medicine in which in a relatively short span of about 150 years a single disease not only was discovered but also reached a point at which significant progress was made in its long-term control.

REFERENCES

1. F Barth. Altération du sang remarquable par la prédominance des globules blancs ou muquex; hypertrophy considérable de la rate. Bull Soc Méd Hôp Paris 3:39, 1856.
2. JH Bennett. Case of hypertrophy of the spleen and liver in which death took place from suppuration of the blood. Edinburgh M & S J 64:413, 1845.
3. R Virchow, Weisses Blut N, Notiz. a. d. Geb d. Nat. u. Heilk 36:151, 1845.
4. J Craigie. Case of the disease of the spleen, in which death took place in consequence of the presence of purulent matter in the blood. Edinburgh M & SJ 64:400, 1845.
5. HW Fuller. Particulars of a case in which enormous enlargement of the spleen and liver,

together with dilatation of all the blood vessels of the body were found coincident with a peculiarly altered condition of the blood. Lancet 2:43, 1846.

6. R Virchow, Weisses Blut. und Milztumoren 2. Med Ztg 16:15, 1847.

7. JH Bennett. Leucocythaemia, or White Cell Blood, in Relation to the Physiology and Pathology of the Lymphatic Glandular System. Edinburgh: Sutherland and Knox, 1852.

8. R Virchow. Die Leukämie. In: Gesammelte Abhandlungen zur weissenschaftlichen Medizin. Frankfurt: Meidinger Sohn & Comp, 1856, 190.

9. N Friedreich. Ein neuer Fall von Leukäemie. Arch Pathol Anat 12:37, 1857.

10. Cahen. Discussion on leucocythemia. Bull Soc Méd Hôp Paris 3:55, 1856.

11. F Barthez. Procès—verbal de la séance du 9 Janvier (Discussion on leukocythemia). Bull Soc Méd, Hôp Paris 3:59, 1856.

12. E Neumann. Ein Fall von Leukämie mit Erkankung des Knochenmarks. Arch Heilk, 11:1, 1870.

13. WR Gowers. Splenic Leucocythaemia. In: JR Reynolds, ed. System of Medicine Vol. 5. London: Lippincott, 1879, p. 216.

14. P Ehrlich. Farbenanalytische Untersuchungen zur Histologie und klinik des Blutes. Berlin: A. Hirschwald, 1891.

15. H Kundrat. Ueber Lympho-Sarkomatosis. Wien Klin Wchnschr 211:234, 1893.

16. W Türk. Elin System der Lymphomatosen. Wein Klin Wchnschr 16:1073, 1903.

17. W Osler. Leukaemia. In: The Principles and Practice of Medicine 7th ed. New York: D. Appleton 1909, pp. 731–738.

18. BG Minot, R Isaacs. Lymphatic leukemia: age, incidence, duration and benefit derived from irradiation. Boston Med Surg J 191:1–9, 1924.

19. W Dameshek, HA Savitz, B Arbor. Chronic lymphatic leukemia in twin brothers aged fifty-six. JAMA 92:1348, 1929.

20. BS Leavell. Chronic leukemia: a study of incidence and factors influencing the duration of life. Am J Med Sci 196:329–340, 1938.

21. MM Wintrobe, LL Hasenbush. Chronic leukemia: the early phase of chronic leukemia, the results of treatment and the effects of complicating infections; a study of eighty six adults. Arch Intern Med 64:701–718, 1939.

22. DR Boggs, SA Sofferman, MM Wintrobe, et al. Factors influencing the duration of survival of patients with chronic lymphocytic leukemia. Am J Med 40:243–254, 1966.

23. DAG Galton. The pathogenesis of chronic lymphocytic leukemia. Can Med Assoc J 94:1005–1010, 1966.

24. W Dameshek. Chronic lymphocytic leukemia—an accumulative disease of immunologically incompetent lymphocytes. Blood 29:566–584, 1967.

25. MM Hansen. Chronic lymphocytic leukemia: Clinical studies based on 189 cases followed for a long time. Scand Haematol 18(suppl):1–286, 1973.

26. KR Rai, A Sawistky, EP Cronkite, et al. Clinical staging of chronic lymphocytic leukemia. Blood 46:219–234, 1975.

27. KR Rai. A critical analysis of staging of CLL. In: RP Gale, KR Rai, eds. Chronic Lymphocytic Leukemia: Recent Progress and Future Directions. New York: Alan R. Liss, 1987, pp 253–264.

28. JL Binet, A Auquier, G Dighiero, et al. A new prognostic classification of chronic lymphocytic leukemia derived from a multivariate survival analysis. Cancer 48:198–206, 1981.

29. B Jaksic, B Vitale. A new parameter in chronic lymphocytic leukaemia. Br J Haematol 49:405–413, 1981.

30. M Baccarini, M Cavo, M Gobbi, et al. Staging of chronic lymphocytic leukemia. Blood 59:1191–1196, 1982.

31. C Rozman, E Montserrat, D Feliu, et al. Prognosis of chronic lymphocytic leukemia: a multivariate survival analysis of 150 cases. Blood 59:1001–1007, 1982.

32. F Mandelli, G De Rossi, P Mancini, et al. Prognosis in chronic lymphocytic leukemia: a retrospective multicentric study from the GIMEMA group. J Clin Oncol 5:398–406, 1987.

33. JS Lee, DO Dixon, HM Kantarjian, et al. Prognosis in chronic lymphocytic leukemia: A multivariate regression analysis of 325 untreated patients. Blood 69:929–936, 1987.
34. E Montserrat, J Sanchez-Bisono, N Viñolas, et al. Lymphocyte doubling time in chronic lymphocytic leukaemia: Analysis of its prognostic significance. Br J Haematol 62:567–575, 1986.
35. S Molica, A Alberti. Prognostic value of lymphocyte doubling time in chronic lymphocytic leukemia. Cancer 60:2712–2716, 1987.
36. C Rozman, E Montserrat, JM Rodriguez-Fernández, et al. Bone marrow histologic pattern—The best single prognostic parameter in chronic lymphocytic leukemia: A multivariate survival analysis of 329 cases. Blood 64:642–648, 1984.
37. GA Pangalis, PA Roussou, C Kittas, et al. Patterns of bone marrow involvement in chronic lymphocytic leukemia and small lymphocytic (well differentiated) non-Hodgkin's lymphomas. Cancer 54:702–708, 1984.
38. T Han, M Barcos, L Emrich, et al. Bone marrow infiltration patterns and their prognostic significance in chronic lymphocytic leukemia: Correlation with clinical, immunological, phenotypic, and cytogenetic data. J Clin Oncol 2:562–570, 1984.
39. GA Pangalis, PA Roussou, C Kittas, et al. B-chronic lymphocytic leukemias. Prognostic implication of bone marrow histology in 120 cases. Cancer 59:767–771, 1987.
40. W Reinisch, M Willheim, M Hilgarth, et al. Soluble CD23 reliably reflects disease activity in B-cell chronic lymphocytic leukemia. J Clin Oncol 12:2146–2152, 1994.
41. M Sarfati, S Chevret, C Chastang, et al. Prognostic significance of soluble CD23 level in chronic lymphocytic leukemia. Blood 88:4259–4264, 1996.
42. M Keating, S Lerner, H Kantarjian, et al. The serum beta2-microglobulin is more powerful than stage in predicting response and survival in chronic lymphocytic leukemia, (abstr). Blood 86(Suppl 1):606a, 1995.
43. G Juliusson, DG Oscier, M Fitchett, et al. Prognostic subgroups in B-cell chronic lymphocytic leukemia defined by specific chromosomal abnormalities. N Engl J Med 323:720, 1990.
44. H Dohner, S Stilgenbauer, K Dohner, et al. Chromosome aberrations in B-cell chronic lymphocytic leukemia: reassessment based on molecular cytogenetic analysis. J Mol Med 77:266–281, 1999.
45. RN Damle, T Wasil, F Fais, et al. IgV gene mutation status and CD38 expression as novel prognostic indicators in chronic lymphocytic leukemia. Blood 94:1840–1847, 1999.
46. TJ Hamblin, Z Davis, A Gardiner, DG Oscier, FK Stevenson. Unmutated IgV (H) genes are associated with a more aggressive form of chronic lymphocytic leukemia. Blood 94:1848–1854, 1999.
47. AC Aisenberg, KJ Bloch. Immunoglobulins on the surface of neoplastic lymphocytes. N Engl J Med 287:272–276, 1972.
48. JL Preud'homme, M Seligmann. Surface bound immunoglobulins as a cell marker in human lymphoproliferative disease. Blood 40:777–794, 1972.
49. C Geisler, JK Larsen, MM Hansen, et al. Prognostic importance of flow cytometric immunophenotyping of 540 consecutive patients with B-cell chronic lymphocytic leukemia. Blood 78:1795–1802, 1991.
50. BD Cheson, JM Bennett, M Grever, et al. National Cancer Institute-Sponsored Working Group guidelines for chronic lymphocytic leukemia: Revised guidelines for diagnosis and treatment. Blood 87:4990–4997, 1996.
51. DAG Galton, E Wiltshaw, I Szur, et al. The use of chlorambucil and steroids in the treatment of chronic lymphocytic leukaemia. Br J Haematol 7:73–81, 1961.
52. MR Grever, KJ Kopecky, CA Coltman, et al. Fludarabine monophosphate: A potentially useful agent in chronic lymphocytic leukemia. Nouv Rev Fr Hematol 30:457–459, 1988.
53. MJ Keating. Fludarabine phosphate in the treatment of chronic lymphocytic leukemia. Semin Oncol 17:49–62, 1990.

54. MJ Keating, H Kantarjian, S O'Brien, et al. Fludarabine: A new agent with marked cytoreductive activity in untreated chronic lymphocytic leukemia. J Clin Oncol 9:44–49, 1991.
55. A Osterborg, AS Fassas, A Anagnostopoulos, et al. Humanized CD52 antibody Campath-1H as first-line treatment in chronic lymphocytic leukaemia. Br J Haematol 93:151–153, 1996.
56. ME Reff, K Carner, S Chambers, et al. Depletion of B cells in vivo by a chimeric mouse human monoclonal antibody to CD20. Blood 83:435–445, 1994.
57. DG Maloney. Advance in immunotherapy of hematologic malignancies. Curr Opin Hematol 5:237–43, 1998.

2

Molecular Biology of Chronic Lymphocytic Leukemia

FLORENCIA BULLRICH and CARLO M. CROCE

Thomas Jefferson University, Philadelphia, Pennsylvania

I. INTRODUCTION

A. Role and Significance of Genetic Abnormalities

The Philadelphia (Ph) chromosome found in chronic myelogenous leukemia (CML) was the first chromosomal abnormality to be recognized as a specific, nonrandom rearrangement associated with cancer (1). Evidence that such chromosomal abnormalities play a direct role in the malignant process came from the molecular characterization of the t(8;14) translocation associated with Burkitt's lymphomas (2). This translocation juxtaposes the *myc* gene on chromosome 8q24 with immunoglobulin gene enhancer elements at 14q32 and results in deregulation of *MYC* expression (2). Myc, a member of the basic domain, helix-loop-helix (bHLH) family of transcription factors, binds DNA and activates transcription as a heterodimer with Max (for review see Ref. 4). Myc/Max heterodimerization was shown to be required for transformation by Myc (for review see [3]). Mice overexpressing the *MYC* gene under control of the Cμ enhancer develop B-cell lymphoma, indicating that in Burkitt s lymphomas the initiating event in the process that will lead to malignant transformation is transcriptional activation of the *MYC* oncogene (for review see Refs. 3 and 4). Since the time of these initial studies, many other chromosomal rearrangements have been characterized, and the genes involved have been cloned and in some instances their function has been extensively studied. Indeed, oncogene deregulation through juxtaposition to enhancer elements of the immunoglobulins or T-cell receptor (*TCR*) genes is now known to be a major mechanism of oncogene activation and to be an initiating event in many leukemias and lymphomas (3). Translocations involving the immunoglobulins or *TCR* loci are thought to occur during the physiological rearrangement steps that give rise to functional antigen receptor genes (5). The clone carrying the translocation, can, in most instances, differentiate further and will accumulate additional genetic changes giving rise to the phenotype and morphology of the neoplasm (6).

Another mechanism of oncogene activation through translocation involves the formation of oncogenic fusion genes. In CML, the Ph chromosome was found to result in the fusion of breakpoint cluster region (*BCR*) and *ABL* coding sequences, derived from chromosomes 22 and 9, respectively, and thus in the formation of a chimeric gene with oncogenic potential (7). The transforming activity of fusion proteins results from the abnormal function of the individual fusion partners and from the activity of the fusion protein itself. Oncogenic transformation by the Bcr-Abl protein depends on the constitutive activation of Abl tyrosine kinase (8). The Bcr portion of the fusion protein is required for constitutive kinase activation and results in abnormal substrate selection by the Abl kinase, thus contributing to the oncogenic potential of the fusion protein (9). Other fusion proteins, such as the E2a-Pbx1 protein derived from the t(1;19) translocation associated with pre-B-ALL, result in the formation of chimeric transcription factors with one protein contributing the DNA-binding domain and the other contributing the transactivation domain (10,11).

In solid tumors translocations play a much less important role. In these tumors, loss of genetic material in the form of deletions and loss of heterozygosity (LOH), resulting in the inactivation of tumor suppressor genes, is more common. In fact, epidemiological, cytogenetic, and molecular analysis of solid tumors led to the discovery of the retinoblastoma gene, *RB*, a cancer susceptibility gene that is also a tumor suppressor now know to be mutated in cancers (12). Today, several tumor suppressor genes have been characterized and are known to play crucial roles in tumorigenesis through loss of function mutations in both solid and hematopoietic malignancies. *P53*, a transcription factor and regulator of apoptosis and response to DNA damage, is commonly inactivated by deletions or by point mutations that result in the production of an inactive protein (13). The more recently discovered *FHIT* tumor suppressor gene, on the other hand, is located in a region of chromosomal fragility at 3p14.2 and is inactivated in most tumors and in premalignant lesions by deletions that result in the absence of protein (for review see Ref. 14). In fact, experimental evidence accumulated during the last three decades has shown that cancer is a multistep genetic disease in which, in most cases, the genetic changes occur as sporadic events during the lifetime of the individual, although in rare cases, one such change can be inherited. Examples of inherited changes that can predispose an individual to cancer include mutations in the *RB*, *APC*, *MSH2*, *MSH3*, and *P16* genes, which predispose to retinoblastoma, colon cancer, and melanoma, respectively.

The specificity and sensitivity of molecular techniques have brought important advances to tumor diagnosis and prognosis, especially for leukemias and lymphomas. In mantle cell lymphoma, for example, the detection of oncogene rearrangements such as *BCL1/CYCLIN D1* rearrangements is used in diagnosis and in follow-up of the disease (for review see Refs. 15 and 16). Furthermore, functional studies of oncogenes, tumor suppressor genes, and tumor susceptibility genes have shown that these are directly involved in the control of one or more of three fundamental cell processes: the rate of cell renewal, the rate of cell death, and the control of genomic stability (for review see Ref. 17). These studies, as well as recent technological advances in targeted cancer therapy, have brought about the first of what will undoubtedly be a growing list of drugs directly targeting the activity of oncogenes and tumor suppressor genes. The widely known trastuzumab (Herceptin; Genentech, San Francisco, CA) approved for treatment of breast cancer

is a monoclonal antibody against the epidermal growth factor-2 (Her2) receptor, the gene for which is amplified in 30% of cases of breast cancer (18). Clearly, in CLL as well, a better understanding of its genetic origen, through the identification and functional characterization of genes altered by the most common chromosomal abnormalities in CLL, will provide important clues to its clinical behavior and new targets for effective therapy.

II. B AND T CELL CHRONIC LYMPHOCYTIC LEUKEMIA

Chronic lymphocytic leukemia is the most common form of adult leukemia in the Western hemisphere. Both B and T-CLL are largely incurable malignancies of mature lymphocytes (Fig. 1). T-CLL/T-PLL, which represents a minority (about 5%) of CLL, is a neoplasm of medullary or postthymic lymphocytes, in most cases CD4+/CD8- T helper cells (19,20). In contrast to B-CLL patients, T-CLL/T-PLL patients often have an aggressive, rapidly progressing disease (19). T-CLL/T-PLL is a relatively common disease among patients with ataxia telangiectasia (AT) an autosomal recessive disorder characterized by, among other symptoms, predisposition to malignancy (21,22). Great progress has been made in the last 6 years in understanding of the molecular origin of T-CLL/T-PLL. In particular, 14q32.1 rearrangements associated with T-PLL/T-CLL have been shown to result in activation of the *TCL-1* and *TCL1b* genes (23,24), and mutations in the *ATM* gene have been shown to occur in cases of sporadic T-PLL/T-CLL, indicating that both genes play crucial roles in lymphoid leukemogenesis.

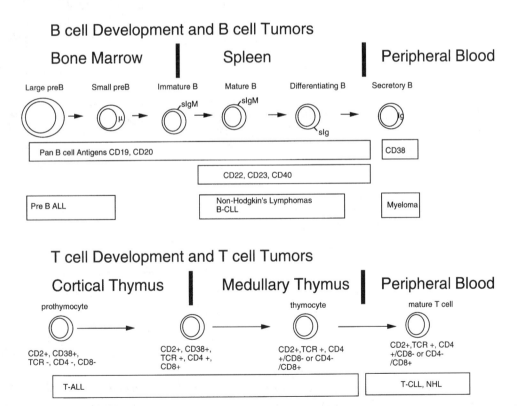

Figure 1   Summary of B and T cell development and corresponding tumors.

In contrast to T-CLL/T-PLL, the molecular origin of B-CLL remains largely unknown. Indeed, B-CLL, which constitutes more than 95% of CLL, remains a challenge for physicians and scientists alike. In individuals older than 70 years of age, B-CLL has an incidence of 10/100,000 making it 10 times more common in the older population than in people younger than 50 (20). CLL is clinically heterogeneous, and although some patients follow an indolent course and survive for 12 years or more, others progress rapidly and succumb to the disease (25,26). B-CLL cells express weak surface immunoglobulins (most often IgM) and pan B-cell antigens such as CD19, CD20. They also coexpress CD5, a T-cell antigen present on the surface of activated lymphocytes (20,25) and on mantle cell lymphoma cells. In contrast to mantle cell lymphomas, B-CLL cells express high levels of CD23. Approximately 40% of patients are initially seen with lymphocytosis of mature-looking lymphocytes (RAI stage 0). These patients show the longest median survival time. In contrast, patients who are first seen with anemia or thrombocytopenia have a median survival time of only 1 to 2 years (RAI stage III/IV). Three to 5% of cases undergo histological transformation into Richter s syndrome or aggressive large B-cell lymphoma, with rapidly growing nodal masses. Several prognostic factors have been well defined, including clinical staging (Rai I-IV [27,28] and Binet A-C [29]), lymphocyte doubling time ($<$12 months worse), extent of marrow involvement (more extensive worse), serum β_{-2} microglobulin level (elevated worse), and serum CD23 level (elevated worse) (20,26–29).

Despite remarkable progress achieved in recent years, treatment options for B-CLL are relatively limited. It is now accepted that indolent disease should not be treated unless there is evidence of progression (30,31). Furthermore, fludarabine, a purine analogue, has been shown to yield a higher or longer response rate (although not higher overall survival) than previously available drugs (30,31). It is a proven, effective treatment that can achieve nearly 30% complete remission (CR) and is recommended as first-line therapy for patients with active disease (31).

One of the reasons for the lack of response of B-CLL to most chemotherapeutic agents may lie in its most salient biological characteristic: B-CLL is a disease of deregulated programmed cell death or apoptosis (32). In fact, B-CLL cells accumulate not because they divide at an accelerated rate but because they survive for an abnormally long time. However, the genetic mechanisms underlying this phenomenon remain largely unknown.

III. CHROMOSOMAL ABNORMALITIES IN T-CHRONIC LYMPHOCYTIC LEUKEMIA

A. Role of the *TCL1* gene in T-Chronic Lymphocytic Leukemia

Most T-CLL/T-PLL carry translocations or inversions of chromosome 14 that juxtapose the 14q32.1 region to the TCR-a/d locus at 14q11. As is the case for other translocations involving antigen receptor genes, these rearrangements place a cellular proto-oncogene under the control of a tissue-specific active enhancer. Using a positional cloning approach, the *TCL1* gene was identified and shown to be overexpressed in T-cell tumors carrying translocations or inversions at 14q32.1 (23,33) (Fig. 2). *TCL1* expression is lymphoid specific and restricted to particular stages of B and T-cell differentiation. Thus, *TCL1* is expressed in CD4$-$/CD8$-$ T-cells but not in single or double positive cells. It is also expressed in pre-B cells and in surface IgM expressing B cells. It is thought that expression

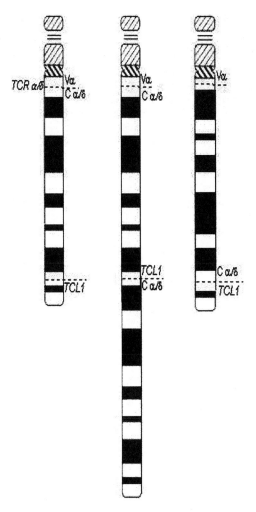

Figure 2 *TCL1* gene rearrangements in T cell leukemias. Left, normal chromosome 14 with the *TCRα/δ* locus located at 14q11 and the *TCL1* locus at 14q32.1. Center: in the t(14;14)(q11;q32) translocation one chromosome 14 brakes at q11 and the other at q32, placing the *TCL1* locus centromeric to the *TCR* Cα/δ locus. Right, the inversion of chromosome 14, inv(14)(q11;q32) splits the *TCR* α/δ locus. The Cα/δ region is thus juxtaposed to the *TCL1* locus with the *TCL1* gene telomeric to the *TCR* α/δ Cα/δ locus.

outside these windows is associated with *TCL1*-mediated leukemogenesis (23). Indeed, transgenic mice overexpressing *TCL1* develop T-cell malignancies with a high incidence late in life, demonstrating that *TCL1* activation can be an initiating event in chronic T cell leukemia (34). A second gene, *TCL1*b, similar to *TCL1* and located within 16 kb of *TCL1* at 14q32.1, was recently isolated and shown to be activated by the same rearrangements (24). The two genes share expression patterns, and the proteins are similar to each other, as well as to a third member of the family, Mtcp1, which is activated in rare cases of T-cell leukemia with a t(X;14)(q28;q11) translocation (24,35 and Fig. 3). Further analysis of the human and murine loci revealed the presence of two additional

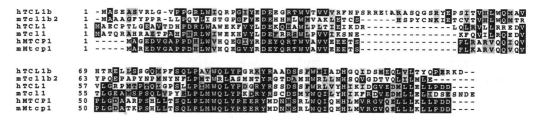

Figure 3 Sequence comparison of the human and murine Tcl1, Tcl1b, and Mtcp1 proteins. Identities are shown by black boxes and similarities are indicated by shaded boxes.

human genes, *TNG1* and *TNG2*, for *TCL1* neighboring gene 1 and 2, which show no homology to known proteins and are also activated by the translocation and duplication of the murine *TCL1b* gene, with five tightly clustered genes conserving similarities within both exons and introns (Fig. 4 and 36). Different experiments have shed some light on the possible function of the Tcl1 protein. Cell fractionation experiments showed that Tcl1 protein is found in both the nucleus and the cytoplasm, and its crystal structure suggests that the protein is involved in the transport of small molecules (37,38). More recently, Tcl1 was shown to physically interact with the Akt kinase (39). *AKT* is a cellular proto-oncogene and its viral homologue causes T-cell lymphoma in mice. *AKT* gene ampli-

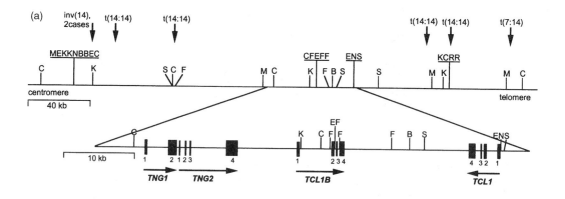

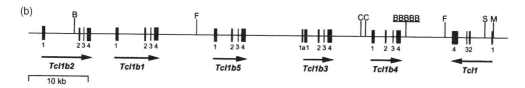

Figure 4 Genomic organization of the human and mouse *TCL1* loci. (a), Human *TCL1* locus. Vertical arrows indicate the positions of cloned 14q32.1 breakpoints occurring in human leukemias. Restriction sites are indicated for *Bss*HII (B), *Cla*I (C), *Eag*I (E), *Sfi*I (S), *Ksp*I (K), *Mlu*I (M), *Not*I (N), and *Sal*I (S). Solid boxes represent exons of the four genes and arrows indicate the direction of transcription. (b), Murine *Tcl1* locus. Restriction sites, exons, and direction of transcription are indicated as in (a).

fication has been observed in breast and ovarian tumors [reviewed in (40)]. Furthermore, underscoring Akt's critical role in tumorigenesis, the protein is involved in the control of gene expression, including the expression of *MYC* and *BCL2*, inhibition of apoptosis, and cell cycle control [for review see (40)]. *Tcl1* was shown to interact with Akt, and this interaction was shown in turn to result in enhanced Akt kinase activity (39). In addition, it was observed that *Tcl1* likely mediates the translocation of Akt to the nucleus (39), where Akt can phosphorylate a variety of nuclear targets (40). It is therefore likely that the interaction between *Tcl1* and Akt1 plays an important role in *TCL1*-mediated leukemogenesis.

B. Role of the *ATM* gene in T-Chronic Lymphocytic Leukemia

Ataxia-Telangiectasia is an autosomal recessive disorder characterized by, among other symptoms, predisposition to malignancy (21,22). As mentioned earlier, although T-CLL/ T-PLL represents a minority of CLL, it is a relatively common disease among AT patients (41). The AT gene, *ATM* (mutated in AT), was mapped to 11q22–23 and identified by positional cloning (42,43). The *ATM* protein shows homology to the catalytic domain of PI-3 kinase and to proteins involved in the control of cell cycle progression, telomere length, and response to DNA damage (for review see Ref. 44). In homozygous *ATM* mutants, T-CLL develops into a T-cell clone carrying a *TCL1*, or rarely *MTCP1*, rearrangement and additional genetic changes (23,33,35). Similarly, in sporadic T-CLL, where *TCL1* translocations are common, loss of heterozygosity (LOH) at 11q22–23 with mutation of the remaining *ATM* allele has been described (45–48). These findings indicate that both *ATM* and *TCL1* play crucial roles in the initiation and progression of T-cell leukemia. It is not clear whether inactivation of the *ATM* gene, which is involved in regulating genomic stability [for review see (49)], actually predisposes the patient to the development of chromosomal rearrangements that in turn lead to leukemia. It has been shown that normal *Atm* protein phosphorylates P53 in response to DNA damage (50), and recent reports suggest that *Atm*'s role in maintaining genomic stability is crucial for its tumorigenic potential. The Nijmegen breakage syndrome (NBS) is an inherited disease characterized by extreme radiation sensitivity, chromosomal instability, and cancer (49). Phosphorylation of the Nbs protein by *Atm* was found to be necessary for the response of cells to gamma-irradiation, demonstrating a crucial role for both proteins in a pathway that controls DNA damage and therefore the accumulation of genetic abnormalities (51,52). *Atm*(−/−) mice develop thymic lymphomas carrying rearrangements in the *Tcr* loci (53). As mentioned earlier, these rearrangements are likely to occur during the physiological process of antigen receptor rearrangement catalyzed in part by the recombinase-activating gene *(Rag)-2*. Mice lacking both the recombinase-activating gene *(Rag)-2* gene and the *ATM* gene develop thymic lymphomas (like the *Atm*(−/−) mice), but the tumors appear later, take longer to evolve, and have chromosomal rearrangements that do not involve the *Tcr* (54). This suggests that in fact *ATM*'s contribution to leukemogenesis in AT patients is related to the increased frequency with which these patients have rearrangements develop.

IV. CHROMOSOMAL ABNORMALITIES IN B-CHRONIC LYMPHOCYTIC LEUKEMIA

Translocations such as t(11;14)(q13;q32) and t(14;18)(q32;21) involving the immunoglobulin locus on chromosome 14 are characteristic of B-cell neoplasms, such as mantle cell lymphoma and follicular lymphoma, respectively. These translocations, which were shown to result in overexpression of cellular proto-oncogenes that either promote cell division (*BCL1/CYCLIN D1* at 11q13) or inhibit cell death (*BCL2* at 18q21) (55–58), are rare in B-CLL. In fact, a minority of B-CLL have been reported to carry rearrangements at 14q32, but most cases are now thought to represent mantle cell lymphoma (59), and although *BCL2* is overexpressed in more than 85% of B-CLLs, *BCL2* gene rearrangements in B-CLL are infrequent events (32,59).

For many years cytogenetic analysis of B-CLL was limited because of the scarcity of dividing cells among B-CLL lymphocytes. A more accurate profile of common chromosomal abnormalities in B-CLL has emerged through the use of fluorescence in situ hybridization (FISH)–based interphase analysis, comparative genomic hybridization (CGH), and microsatellite screening. The two most common chromosomal abnormalities in B-CLL are likely to involve tumor suppressor genes rather than oncogenes. First, is deletion of chromosome 13 at band q14, which occurs in more than 50% of cases. Second, is deletion of chromosome 11q22–23, which occurs in 19% of cases. Trisomy of chromosome 12, which was previously thought to be the most common abnormality, was shown by interphase cytogenetics to occur only in 15% of cases (59,60). Other changes include deletion of 6q (9%) and deletion of 17p13 (10%).

A. 13q14 Deletions

Chromosomal abnormalities involving the long arm of chromosome 13 were initially reported in isolated cases of B-CLL more than 15 years ago. Today we know that homozygous or hemizygous loss at 13q14 occur in more than half of B-CLL, in approximately 50% of mantle cell lymphomas, and in 16% to 40% of multiple myeloma (59–64), suggesting that a tumor suppressor gene at 13q14 is involved in the pathogenesis of these clinically and pathologically diverse group of tumors. As mentioned earlier, the occurrence of high-grade lymphoma during the course of B-CLL (Richter s syndrome) has been reported in about 3% to 5% of cases. Cytogenetic and molecular studies suggest that in many cases the two diseases derive from the same malignant clone (65). It is generally thought that deletions at 13q14 result in inactivation of a tumor suppressor gene following the Knudson hypothesis (i.e., through loss of one allele and mutation of the remaining allele). Inactivation of the retinoblastoma gene (*RB1*) located at 13q14 exemplifies this hypothesis, and *RB1* mutations have been described in many human tumors (66). Therefore, the *RB1* gene was initially thought to be inactivated by 13q14 deletions in B-CLL. Two crucial lines of evidence indicate that a putative tumor suppressor gene different from *RB* is targeted in B-CLL. First, several groups found that most homozygous deletions in B-CLL do not include the *RB* gene and are in fact telomeric to it (67,68). Second, sequence analysis of the remaining *RB* allele in B-CLL cases with loss of heterozygosity (LOH) at 13q14 showed that they retained a wild-type copy of the *RB* gene (69).

The same gene at 13q14 is thought to be targeted by deletions in B-CLL, mantle cell lymphoma, myeloid malignancies, and multiple myeloma. However, although 13q14 loss is clearly associated with poor prognosis in multiple myeloma, in mantle cell lymphoma this abnormality has no obvious prognostic significance (62–64). In B-CLL, 13q14 deletion has no overall impact on survival, but it is associated with more aggressive clinical behavior among patients seen with early stage disease (low β_2-microglobulin or Rai stage 0–11) (70).

Since the first reports of the involvement of a 13q14 putative tumor suppressor gene in B-CLL were published, the locus has been the focus of extensive analysis. The location of the candidate gene has been refined, and three candidates have been cloned and characterized. The first reports indicated homozygous deletion of the *D13S25* locus, a polymorphic marker telomeric to the *RB* gene, and placed the B-CLL suppressor between *RB* and the *D13S31* locus (Fig. 5 and 67,69). Further studies showed a more centromeric location for the gene with homozygous deletions delimited by the *D13S273* and *D13S25* markers (71–74). Loss of heterozygosity studies and yeast artificial cloning of the region were used to further characterize the locus and to define the minimal region of loss. BAC, PAC, and cosmid contigs of the region have been developed (72–80), and two core regions of loss have emerged from a series of studies aimed at identifying the critical gene (Fig. 6). Core regions were defined from the overlap of minimal regions outlined in several studies in which new and known markers were used to define the boundaries of homozygous and

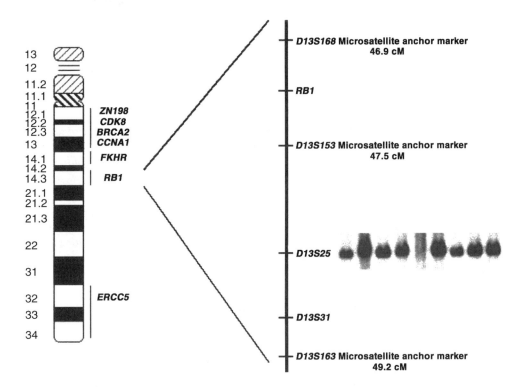

Figure 5 Chromosome 13 ideogram with detail of the chromosomal region deleted in B-CLL, Vertical lines next to the chromosome ideogram indicate the position of genes on the chromosome. *ZN198*, Zinc Finger protein 198; *CDK8*, cyclin-dependent kinase 8; *BRCA2*, breast cancer 2, early onset; *CCNA1*, cyclin A1; *FKHR* forkhead (Drosophila)-homolog1; *RB1*, retinoblastoma 1; *ERCC5*, excision repair cross-complementing rodent repair deficiency, complementation group 5 (xeroderma pigentosum complementation group G). In the locus detail markers are shown from centromere (top) to telomere (bottom). CM, centi Morgan. The inset shows a Southern blot of B-CLL cases in which the B-CLL DNA was hybridized with the *D13S25*-probe. One of the leukemias shows no hybridization signal, indicating the presence of a homozygous deletion of the locus in that case.

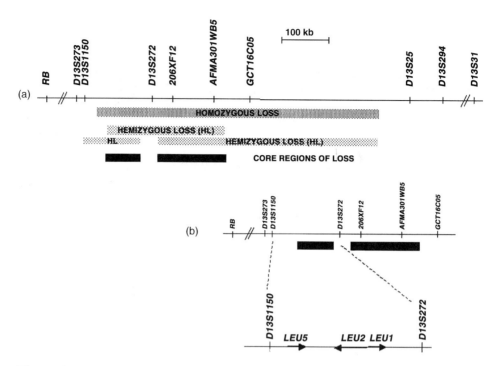

Figure 6 Chromosome 13q14 B-CLL tumor suppressor locus. (a), Map of the region of loss in B-CLL. The extent and position of regions of homozygous and hemizygous loss is shown as are the positions of the core regions of loss. (b), Detail of the region containing the *LEU1, LEU2*, and *LEU5* genes. The arrows indicate the direction of transcription.

hemizygous loss in B-CLL (Fig. 6). The most centromeric of the core regions, in the vicinity of D13S272, contains two candidate genes, *LEU1* and *LEU2* (Fig. 6 and Ref. 81.) The more telomeric region spans less than 300 kb at 13q14 telomeric to *AFMA206XF12*. Three genes have now been identified between *D13S273* and D13S25. *LEU1* and *LEU2* (81) represent two transcriptional units located within a homozygous deletion in CLL. The genes are transcribed in opposite orientation and are separated by only 200 bp. *LEU1* is transcribed into a 1.1 kb mRNA, whereas *LEU2* shows two alternative transcripts of 1.8 and 1.4 kb. The *LEU1* message is detectable in most tissues but not in peripheral blood lymphocytes, whereas *LEU2* shows more specific expression, including expression in lymphoid tissues such as thymus, bone marrow, fetal liver, and peripheral blood lymphocytes. The function of the *Leu1* and *Leu2* proteins, if indeed any protein is made from these transcripts, is not known. Mutational analysis of both genes and of the region between them did not reveal any mutations in B-CLL cases, indicating that they are unlikely to be critical genes in B-cell leukemogenesis. A third gene, *LEU5*, centromeric to the core regions of loss and to the centromeric boundary of homozygous deletions in B-CLL (Fig. 6 and Ref. 78), is homologous to zinc-finger proteins involved in cancer but again shows no alterations in B-CLL. The pattern of allelic loss at 13q14 in B-CLL, with interrupted deletions (74–77) and more than one core region of loss, may be due to genetic heterogeneity within the tumors or to the characteristics of the tumor suppressor gene itself. Homozygous deletions described in B-CLL are relatively large and extend for more than 500 kb from the vicinity of *D13S272* to *D13S25* (Fig. 5). A large gene with relatively few exons separated by large introns could produce a pattern of loss similar to that observed in B-CLL. Further characterization of the region of loss in other malignancies, as well as the availability of the DNA sequence of the region involved will undoubtedly aid in the identification of the critical gene. In fact, the putative B-CLL tumor suppressor is likely to play a crucial role in B-CLL pathogenesis and in the pathogenesis of mantle cell lymphoma and multiple myeloma (MM). Indeed, in MM, 13q14 loss is a marker of poor prognosis and has been found to be associated with the transition from monoclonal gammopathy of undetermined significance (MGUS) to MM. The identification and characterization of the 13q14 tumor suppressor will provide invaluable tools toward the development of novel diagnostic and targeted therapeutic approaches to these diseases.

B.   Deletions of Chromosome 11q22–23

In B-CLL deletions at 11q22–23 that occur in 13% to 20% of cases represent the second most common genetic abnormality and are associated with advanced clinical stage (extensive lymphadenopathy), younger age, and rapid disease progression (59,82–86). In particular, in patients who are less than 55 years old, 11q loss was shown to be associated with reduced survival. Like 13q14 allelic loss, 11q loss is thought to result in inactivation of a tumor suppressor gene. The *ATM* gene, at 11q22–23, is located within the minimal region of loss described in B-CLL (83–85). Several lines of evidence suggested that 11q deletions in B-CLL result in *ATM* gene inactivation. First, the increased incidence of both T and B-cell leukemia in AT patients (22,41) indicates an important role for *ATM* in leukemogenesis. Second, the previously described inactivation of *ATM* in cases of sporadic T-cell leukemias (45–48) showed that *ATM* is not only a cancer predisposition gene but that it can also play a role in the initiation or progression of de novo cancers occurring in a presumably normal genetic background. Third, the finding that absence of Atm protein correlates with poor outcome in B-CLL (86) strongly suggested that the proper function of the Atm protein is directly relevant to B-CLL pathogenesis. To determine whether the *ATM* gene is altered in B-CLL several groups performed single strand conformational polymorphism (SSCP) and direct sequencing analysis of *ATM* exons in sporadic B-CLL cases with LOH at 11q (87,88). These studies have shown that B-CLL cases with LOH at 11q carry mutations in the remaining allele of the *ATM* gene, indicating that *ATM* is involved in B-CLL progression (87,88). Mutations, scattered throughout the protein, and resulting in aberrant mRNA splicing, premature termination of translation, or altered amino acid sequence have been identified (Table 1). Furthermore, both acquired (somatic) and germline *ATM* mutations were identified in B-CLL (87,89 and Table 1). In fact, in a few cases, the mutations were also found in normal cells of the patient, suggesting that the individuals were heterozygous carriers of an *ATM* mutation (87,88). The heterozygous carrier frequency observed in B-CLL was higher than the 1% estimate for the general population, suggesting that *ATM* heterozygotes may be predisposed to B-CLL. However, cancer (including B-CLL) predisposition, is a complex genetic trait with numerous environmental influences, and large studies will be needed to answer this question. Underscoring this complexity is the fact that although 11q is commonly lost in breast cancer, *ATM* is not commonly inactivated in these tumors nor are *ATM* heterozygotes predisposed to breast cancer (90,91). Further population-based studies should shed light on this issue by clarifying the association, if any, of particular *ATM* alleles with particular phenotypes, as well as determining the frequency of mutant alleles in the general population (92). It is not clear how *ATM* contributes to B or T-cell CLL. However, the fact that 80% of tumors

Table 1 ATM Mutations in B-CLL

First allele		Second allele		
Nucleotide	Codon	Nucleotide	Codon	Germline
Deleted		995A→G	332Y→C	WT
1055T_C	3521→T	1048G→A	350A→T	WT
Not deleted		1058delGT	353 frameshift	Carrier
3161C_G	1054P→R	3994ins190	1332 frameshift	Carrier
Not deleted		3910del7	1304 frameshift	WT
Deleted		5071A→C	1691S→R	Carrier
Not deleted		5558A→T	1853D→V	ND
Deleted		5858C→G	1953T→R	ND
Not deleted		6820G→A	2274A→K	ND
Not deleted		7258G→C	2420A→P	ND
Deleted		7271T→G	2424V→G	Carrier
ND		7865C→T	2623R→Stop	ND
Not deleted		8084G→C	2695G→A	WT
Deleted		8412delA	2804 frameshift	ND
Deleted		9023G→A	3008R→H	WT
Deleted		9054A→C	3018L→N	WT
Deleted		9139C→T	3047R→Stop	WT

WT, wild type; ND, not done.
Source: Refs. 87–89.

in AT patients are of lymphoid origin and the finding of *ATM* mutations in non-AT-associated (sporadic) leukemias, clearly indicates that *ATM* inactivation not only interferes with normal lymphoid function and differentiation but also represents an important step in the pathogenesis of these tumors.

Recent experiments have provided clues to the biochemical pathways mediating Atm's function (reviewed in 92,93 and outlined in Fig. 7). Cells respond to genotoxic stress by activating cell cycle checkpoints and DNA repair pathways with the general aim of preventing cells with damaged DNA from proliferating. Atm, whose kinase activity is increased several fold in response to ionizing radiation (IR), has been shown to bind and phosphorylate several proteins involved in these pathways such as p53, c-Abl, Brca1, Nbs1, and the Chk2 kinase (51,52,94–99). Atm was shown to bind p53 and to phosphorylate the protein at serine 15 (Ser 15) (50,94,95), a modification of the p53 protein which occurs in response to DNA damage (reviewed in Ref. 100). Phosphorylation of p53 at Ser 15 stabilizes p53 by inhibiting the interaction of p53 with Mdm2, which in turn results in degradation of the p53 protein. Ser 15 phosphorylation also results in enhanced activity of p53 through sequence-specific DNA binding, thus increasing transcription of p53 target genes such as p21 and 14-3-3, both of which can cause cell cycle arrest (100). Atm was also shown to be critical for the activation of c-Abl after exposure to IR. Atm binds c-Abl, phosphorylates the protein at Ser 465, and is required for the c-abl mediated activation of the Rad51/Rad52 repair complex (96,97). In response to IR, Atm also phosphorylates Brca1, which is involved in DNA repair through its interaction with Rad51. In addition, the activity of another DNA repair complex, Rad50/Mre11/Nbs1, depends on Atm through its phosphorylation of Nbs1 (51,52). Atm exerts control over progression through the G2/S checkpoint by phosphorylating Chk2 soon after exposure to IR (99).

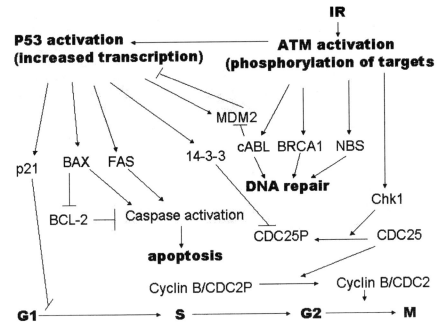

Figure 7   Outline of the *P53* and *ATM* pathways.

The Chk1 and Chk2 kinases phosphorylate and inactivate the Cdc25 phosphatase. Phosphorylated Cdc25 binds 14-3-3 and is thus prevented from dephosphorylating the CYCLIN B/CDC2 complex causing the cell to remain blocked in G2 phase (101). Thus, through its kinase activity, Atm exerts control over a wide variety of proteins directly involved in both cell cycle and DNA damage control. As is clear from the phenotype of AT patients, the function of Atm is not limited to the interactions outlined here and is likely to be involved in other critical cellular processes such as differentiation and senescence.

The pattern of Atm inactivation in B-CLL and in T-cell tumors, loss of one allele and mutation of the remaining allele, is indicative of a classical tumor suppressor inactivation mechanism. It is likely that allelic loss at 11q in B-CLL uncovers the Atm-associated mutator phenotype, which then initiates or accelerates leukemic progression through the accumulation of genetic abnormalities. This possibility becomes especially relevant in light of the known association of 11q loss and of *P53* mutation with adverse outcome and poor prognosis in B-CLL (82–84,86,102). Further studies will be necessary to clarify the biological and clinical significance of *ATM* inactivation and 11q loss in B-CLL.

C.   Trisomy of Chromosome 12

Trisomy 12 occurs in up to 20% of B-CLL and is associated with aggressive disease and atypical morphology (59,103,104), suggesting that one or more genes on chromosome 12 are involved in B-CLL progression. The molecular mechanism by which trisomy 12 contributes to leukemogenesis in B-CLL is still unknown. Microsatellite analysis with chromosome 12 markers has revealed that leukemias carrying three copies of the chromosome retained both alleles of the tested loci, indicating that trisomy results from duplication of one chromosome rather than from loss of one chromosome and triplication of the other (105). Previous studies have also shown partial trisomies, translocations, and amplifications of the 12q12 to 12q22 region of chromosome 12 (59,106). In fact, both dosage effects and rearrangements in candidate genes within this region have been demonstrated in isolated cases. The *MDM2* gene is one such candidate and is located at 12q14–15. The Mdm2 protein binds the *N*-terminus of p53 and inhibits its function by promoting p53 degradation by the proteasome (107). *MDM2* is overexpressed in more than 30% of B-CLL (108,109), although no rearrangements were reported in *MDM2* at the DNA level (110). Chromosome 12 contains a large number of genes directly or indirectly involved

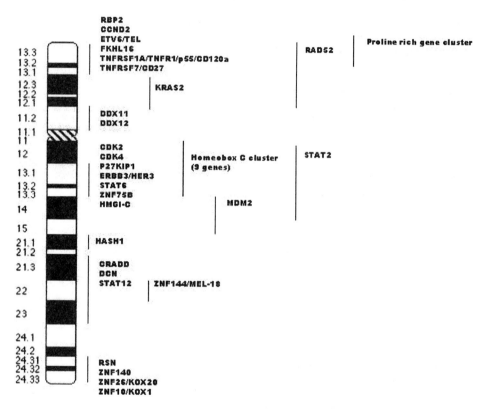

Figure 8 Ideogram of chromosome 12. Vertical lines indicate the position of genes on the chromosome. *RBP2*, *RB* binding protein 2; *CCND2*, cyclin D2; *ETV6/TEL, TEL* oncogenes; *FKHL*, forkhead (Drosophila)-like 16; *TNFRSF1A* and 7; tumor necrosis factor receptor; *KRAS2*, v-Ki-*ras2* Kirsten rat sarcoma 2 viral oncogenes homolog; *DDX11* and 12, DEAD/H box polypeptides 11 and 12; *RAD52*, RAD52 (*S. cerevisiae*) homolog; *CDK2* and 4, cyclin-dependent kinases 2 and 4; *p27KIP1*, cyclin-dependent kinase inhibitor 1 B; *ERBB3/HER3*, v-eRB-b2 avian erythroblastic leukemia viral oncogenes homolog 3; *HMGI-C*, high molecular group protein C; *MDM2*, mouse double minute 2, human homolog of; *STAT2*, 6, and 12, signal transducer and activator of transcription 2, 6, and 12; *HASH1*, achaete-scute complex (*Drosophila*) homolog-like 1; *CRADD*, CASP2 and PRIPK1 domain containing adaptor with death domain; *DCN*, decorin; *RSN*, Reed-Steinberg cell–expressed intermediate filament associated protein; *ZNF140*, 144, 26, 75B, and 10, Zinc finger proteins 140, 144, 26, 75B, and 10.

in cancer (Fig. 8). Among those, the genes for cyclin-dependent kinase 2 and 4, Cdk2 and Cdk4, located at 12q13, within the region amplified in human sarcomas, were also analyzed by Southern blotting, and no abnormalities were detected (110). However, in a case of aggressive B-CLL, *MDM2* amplification was detected with fluorescence in situ hybridization (FISH) (111), suggesting that overexpression and/or amplification of *MDM2* may play a role in B-CLL progression. Increased levels of Mdm2 may contribute to progression in B-CLL by inhibiting p53, which will result in impaired control of DNA damage, cell cycle progression, and cell death. *MDM2* expression is positively regulated by p53, and it has been reported that leukemias that overexpress *MDM2* can carry *P53* mutations (109), suggesting that *P53* mutations may be directly or indirectly responsible for aberrant regulation of *MDM2* expression in some cases. Alternatively, Mdm2 overexpression, such as might occur in cases with *MDM2* gene amplification, combined with p53 inactivation through mutation might be synergistic and enhance the cell's resistance to apoptotic signals.

As shown on Figure 8, the *HMGI-C* gene, a member of the high mobility group (HMG) family, is located at 12q13 and is a candidate for involvement in trisomy 12. *HMGI-C* is involved in the development of benign tumors of mesenchymal origin (for review see Refs 112 and 113). The protein binds DNA and is an architectural factor indirectly involved in transcription (114). Its expression, which does not occur in differentiated adult tissues, is directly associated with cellular transformation (115,116) and has been observed in breast carcinomas and in leukemias (117). A translocation involving chromosome 12 at band q13 in a case of Richter's syndrome, was recently reported to result in rearrangement of the *HMGI-C* gene (118), suggesting that indeed *HMGI-C* rearrangements may play a role in B-CLL pathogenesis.

In acute myelogenous leukemia (AML) trisomy of chromosome 11 was shown to result in self-fusion of the *ALL1* gene at 11q23 and in the formation of a dominant-negative form of *ALL1* (119). A similar mechanism could be involved in B-CLL, resulting in activation of an oncogene or inactivation of a tumor suppressor gene through rearrangement. Further studies of candidate genes at both the DNA and RNA level in a large number of tumors will undoubtedly clarify the role of trisomy 12 in B-cell leukemogenesis.

D. *P53* and *BCL2*

Deletions in the short arm of chromosome 17 occur in up to 17% of B-CLL and are accompanied by mutation of the *P53* tumor suppressor gene located at 17p13 (49,102,120). *P53* gene alterations have been shown to have important implications for the clinical behavior of B-CLL and have been associated with poor survival and drug resistance (102,120).

As outlined before and in Figure 7, the *P53* tumor suppressor gene plays a crucial role in control of the cell's response to DNA damage, cell cycle progression, and cell death (for review see Refs. 92,93, and 100). On exposure of the cell to DNA damaging agents, the protein is stabilized and activated through posttranslational modifications that increase its half-life and enhance its sequence-specific, DNA-binding transcriptional activity (92,93,100). Activated p53 can induce cell cycle arrest and apoptosis. As mentioned previously, p53 induces expression of p21 and the 13-4-3 protein, both of which are involved in cell cycle control (110). p53 also induces the expression of several proapoptotic molecules such as the Killer/Dr5 and Fas/Apo1/Cd95 receptor, as well as the *Bax* protein

(100). Clearly, therefore, mutations in the *P53* gene might alter the leukemic cells' sensitivity to apoptotic signals, including those induced by drugs such as fludarabine, and contribute to disease progression in these tumors. The induction of *BAX* expression by p53 becomes particularly relevant in the context of *BCL2* overexpression which, as mentioned earlier, occurs in more than 80% of B-CLL (121). *Bax* is a proapoptotic member of the *BCL2* gene family. Bax can form heterodimers with Bcl2, and this is known to result in inhibition of the antiapoptotic activity of Bcl2 (reviewed in Ref. 122). These observations suggest that the resistance to chemotherapy observed in tumors with *P53* mutations may be related to loss of regulation of the Bcl2/Bax apoptotic pathway (32). The known activation of p53 by Atm described earlier suggests that the p53 DNA damage/apoptosis pathway plays an important role in B-CLL progression.

As mentioned previously, although *BCL2* gene rearrangements are rare in B-CLL, more than 80% of these leukemias express high levels of *BCL-2* (121). The *BCL2* gene was first isolated through its involvement in the t(14;18) chromosomal translocation characteristic of follicular lymphoma, which places the gene under the control of the immunoglobulin gene transcriptional enhancer (122). Functional studies of Bcl2 have shown that it is a potent inhibitor of programmed cell death or apoptosis (123). Furthermore, it has been shown that proapoptotic signals such as exposure to DNA-damaging agents or chemotherapeutic drugs converge on a pathway regulated by *Bcl2* and *Bcl2* family members and that overexpression of *Bcl2* can protect the cell against any of these signals. Of direct clinical import and of particular significance for B-CLL is the finding that Bcl2 can inhibit the apoptotic effect of every known anticancer drug (32,122). A possible mechanism for the inactivation of Bcl2 has been proposed to occur through Bcl2 phosphorylation induced by antimicrotubule drugs (124). However, Bcl2 phosphorylation was not observed in nondividing cells such as B-CLL cells. A small organic molecule that binds *Bcl2* was recently reported to induce apoptosis in a myeloid leukemia cell line overexpressing *Bcl2* and in a mouse embryonic fibroblast cell line, suggesting a possible means of intervention in B-CLL (125).

E. Other Chromosomal Abnormalities

The t(14;19)(q32.3;q31.1) is a rare but recurrent chromosomal abnormality in B-CLL and other lymphoid tumors. The translocation was shown to result in transcriptional activation of the *BCL3* gene on chromosome 19 through juxtaposition with the immunoglobulin heavy-chain enhancer sequence (126). The Bcl3 protein is a member of the I KappaB family, and it can regulate the immune response and cellular proliferation by modulating the activity of several transcription factors (127,128). Mice overexpressing the Bcl3 protein do not develop tumors but have splenomegaly and accumulation of mature lymphocytes in the lymph nodes, bone marrow, and peritoneal cavity (127). The t(14;19) translocation is rarely the only cytogenetic abnormality in the tumors, and in more than 50% of cases it occurs in conjunction with trisomy 12. Furthermore, a significant fraction of patients with the t(14;19) are younger and, like trisomy 12, the translocation is associated with poor prognosis and aggressive disease (129). Taken together, these observations suggest that BCL3 rearrangement is not an initiating event in B-CLL pathogenesis, but that it may be involved in progression of B-cell leukemia.

Other recurrent chromosomal abnormalities have been reported to occur in less than 10% of B-CLL cases, including deletion of 6q, deletion of 7q, monosomy 21, and 4q abnormalities (59,130–132). The genes targeted by these abnormalities have not been identified, and it is not known what role they might play in B-CLL.

V. CONCLUSION

CLL still represents a major biological and clinical challenge. The *BCL2*, *ATM*, and *P53* genes are known to play important roles in the progression of this malignancy, but the genes targeted by the most common cytogenetic abnormalities in B-CLL remain to be identified. The identification of these genes will provide invaluable tools to improve our understanding of this disease. Therefore, future studies should aim at the identification of novel therapeutic targets through the explanation of its genetic and molecular origin.

REFERENCES

1. PC Nowell, DA Hungerford. A minute chromosome in human granulocytic leukemia. Science 132:1497, 1960.
2. R Dalla Favera, M Bregni, J Erikson, D Patterson, RC Gallo, and CM Croce. Assignment of the human c-MYC oncogene to the region of chromosome 8 which is translocated in Burkitt lymphoma cells. Proc Natl Acad Sci USA 79:7824–7827, 1982.
3. B Amati, H Land. MYC-Max-Mad: A transcription factor network controlling cell cycle progression, differentiation, and death. Curr opin Genet Devel 4:102–108, 1994.
4. L Showe, CM Croce. The role of chromosomal translocations in B- and T-cell neoplasia. Ann Rev Immunol 5:253–277, 1987.
5. FG Haluska, Y Tsujimoto, CM Croce. Mechanisms of chromosome translocation in B- and T-cell neoplasia. Trends Genet 3:11–15, 1987.
6. IT Magrath. Concepts and controversies in lymphoid neoplasia. In: Magrath I, ed. The non-Hodgkin s Lymphomas. London, Arnold and New York: Oxford University Press, 1997, pp 3–46.
7. E Shtivelman, B Lifshitz, RP Gale, E Canaani. Fused transcript for abl and bcr genes in chronic melogenous leukemia. Nature 315:550–554, 1985.
8. JB Konopka, SM Watanabe, ON Witte. An alteration of the human c-abl protein in K562 leukemia cells unmasks associated tyrosine kinase activity. Cell 37:1035–1042, 1984.
9. AM Pendergast, LA Quilliam, ID Cripe, CH Bassing, Z Dai, N Lin, A Batzer, KM Rabun, CJ Der, J Schlessinger, ML Gishizky. BCR-ABL induced oncogenesis is mediated by direct interaction with the SH2 domain of the GRB-2 adaptor protein. Cell 75:175–185, 1993.
10. J Nourse, JD Mellentin, N Galili, J Wikison, E Stanbridge, SD Smith, and ML Cleary. Chromosomal translocation t(1;19) results in synthesis of a homeobox fusion mRNA that codes for a potential chimeric transcription factor. Cell 60:535–546, 1990.
11. MP Kamps, C Murre, X Sun, D Baltimore. A new homeobox gene contributes the DNA binding domain of the t(1;19) translocation protein in pre-B ALL. Cell 60:547–555, 1990.
12. SH Friend, R Benards, S Rogelj, R Weinberg, JM Rapaport, DM Albert, TP Dryja. A human DNA segment with properties of the gene that predisposes to retinoblastoma and osteosarcoma. Nature 323:643–646, 1986.
13. MS Greenblatt, WP Bennett, M Hollstein, CC Harris. Mutations in the P53 tumor suppressor gene: clues to cancer etiology and molecular pathogenesis. Cancer Res, 54:4855–4878, 1994.
14. K Huebner, PN Garrison, LD Barnes, CM Croce. The role of the FHIT/FRA3B locus in cancer. Annu Rev Genet 32:7–31, 1998.
15. G Sozzi, MA Testi, CM Croce. Advances in cancer cytogenetics. J Cell Biochem 32–33 (suppl), 173–182, 1999.

16. M Raffeld. The role of molecular analysis in lymphoma diagnostics. In: Magrath I, ed. The non-Hodgkin s Lymphomas. London, Arnold and New York: Oxford University Press, 1997, pp 109–131.

17. D Hanahan, RA Weinberg. The hallmarks of cancer. Cell 100:57–70, 2000.

18. AN Houghton, DA Scheinberg. Monoclonal antibody therapies-a 'constant' threat to cancer. Nat Med 4:373–374, 2000.

19. E Jaffe, Histopathology and immunology. In: Magrath I, ed. The non-Hodgkin s Lymphomas. London, Arnold and New York: Oxford University Press, 1997, pp 79–108.

20. AS Freeman, LM Nadler. Malignancies of lymphoid cells. In: AS Fauci, E Braunwald, KJ Isselbacher, JD Wilson, JB Martin, DL Kasper, SL Hauser, DL Longo. Harrisson's Principles of Internal Medicine. 14th ed. New York: McGraw-Hill 1998, pp 695–712.

21. RP Sedgwick, E Broder. In: PJ Vinken, GW Bruyn, HL Klawans, eds. Handbook of Clinical Neurology. Amsterdam: Elsevier, 1991, p 347.

22. BD Spector, AH Filipovich, GS Perry. Epidemiology of cancer in ataxia telangiectasia. In: BA Bridges, DG Harnden, eds. Ataxia Telangiectasia, A Cellular and Molecular Link Between Cancer Neuropathology and Immune Deficiency. Chichster: J Wiley, 1982, p 53.

23. L Virgilio, MG Narducci, M Isobe, LG Billips, MD Cooper, CM Croce, G Russo. Identification of the TCL1 gene involved in T cell malignancies. Proc Natl Acad Sci USA 91:12530–12534, 1994.

24. Y Pekarsky, C Hallas, M Isobe, G Russo, CM Croce. Abnormalities at 14q32.1 in T cell malignancies involve two oncogenes. Proc Natl Acad Sci USA 96:2949–2951, 1999.

25. Rai K, Patel D. Chronic lymphocytic leukemia. In: R Hoffman, E Benz, S Shattil, B Furie, H Cohen, L Silberstein, eds. Hematology: Basic Principles and Practice. 2nd ed. New York: Churchill Livingstone, 1995, pp 1308–1322.

26. JA Zwiebel, BD Cheson. Chronic lymphocytic leukemia: Staging and prognostic factors. Semin Oncol 25:42–59, 1998.

27. KR Rai, A Sawitsky, EP Cronkite, AD Chanana, RN Levy, BS Pasternack. Clinical Staging of chronic lymphocytic leukemia. Blood 46:219–234, 1975.

28. KR Rai. A critical analysis of staging in CLL: 1987 UCLA Symposia on Molecular and Cellular Biology. New Series 59:253, 1987.

29. JL Binet, M Lepoprier, G Dighiero, D Charron, P D'Athis, G Vaugier, HM Beral, JC Natali, M Raphael, B Nizet, JY Follezou. A clinical staging system for chronic lymphocytic leukemia: prognostic significance. Cancer 40:855–864, 1977.

30. MJ Keating, S O'Brien, S Lerner, C Koller, M Beran, LE Robertson, EJ Freireich, E Estey, H Kantarjian. Long term follow-up of patients with CLL receiving fludarabine regimens as initial therapy. Blood 92:1165–1171, 1998.

31. BD Cheson. Therapy for previously untreated chronic lymphocytic leukemia: A reevaluation. Semin Hematol 35(suppl 3):14–21, 1998.

32. JC Reed. Molecular biology of chronic lymphocytic leukemia: Implications for therapy. Semin Hematol 35(suppl 3):3–13, 1998.

33. MG Narducci, L Virgilio, M Isobe, A Stoppacciaro, R Elli, M Fiorilli, M Carbonari, A Antonelli, L Chessa, CM Croce, G Russo. TCL1 oncogene activation in preleukemic T-cells from a case of ataxia-telangiectasia. Blood 86:2358–2364, 1995.

34. L Virgilio, C Lazzeri, R Bichi, K Nibu. MG Narducci, G Russo, JL Rothstein, CM Croce. Deregulated expression of TCL1 causes T cell leukemia in mice. Proc Natl Acad Sci USA 95:3885–3889, 1988.

35. MH Stern, J Soulier, M Rosenzwajg, K Nakahara, N Canki-Klein, A Aurians, F Sigans, IR Kirsch. MTCP1: A novel gene on the human chromosome Xq28 translocated to the T-cell receptor alpha/delta locus in mature T-cell proliferations. Oncogene 8:2475–2483, 1993.

36. C Hallas, Y Pekarsky, T Itoyama, J Varnum, R Bichi, J Rothstein, CM Croce. Genomic analysis of human and mouse TCL1 loci reveals a complex of tightly clustered genes. Proc Natl Acad Sci USA 96:14418–14423, 1999.

37. TB Fu, L Virgilio, MG Narducci, A Facchiano, G Russo, CM Croce. Characterization and localization of the TCL1 oncogene product. Cancer Res 54:6297–6301, 1995.

38. Z-Q. Fu, GC DuBoi, SP Song, L Kulikovskaya, L Virgilio, JL Rothstein, CM Croce, IT Weber, RW Harrison. Crystal structure of MTCP-1: implications for the role of TCL1 and MTCP-1 in T cell malignancies. Proc Natl Acad Sci USA 95:3413–3418, 1998.

39. Y Pekarsky, A Koval, C Hallas, R Bichi, M Tresini, S Malstrom, G Russo, P Tsichlis, CM Croce. TCL1 enhances Akt kinase activity and mediates its nuclear translocation. Proc Natl Acad Sci USA 97:3028–3033, 2000.

40. TO Chan, SE Rittenhouse, P Tsichlis. AKT/PKB and other D3 phosphoinositide-regulated kinases: kinase activation by phosphoinositide-dependent phosphorylation. Annu Rev Biochem 68:965–1014, 1999.

41. AMR Taylor, JA Metcalfe, J Thick, YF Mak. Leukemia and lymphoma in ataxia telangiectasia. Blood 87:423–438, 1996.

42. K Savitsky, A Bar-Shira, S Gilad, G Rotman, Y Ziv, L Vanagaite, DA Tagle, S Smith, T Uziel, S Sfez, et al. A single ataxia telangiectasia gene with a product similar to PI-3 kinase. Science 268:1749–1753, 1995.

43. K Savitsky, S Sfez, DA Tagle, Y Ziv, A Sartiel, FS Collins, Y Shiloh, G Rotman. The complete sequence of the coding region of the ATM gene reveals similarity to cell cycle regulators in different species. Hum Mol Genet 4:2025–2032, 1995.

44. VA Zakian. ATM-related genes: What do they tell us about functions of the human gene? Cell 82:685–687, 1995.

45. I Vorechovsky, L Luo, MJ Dyer, D Catovsky, PL Amlot, JC Yaxley, L Foroni, L Hammarstrom, AD Webster, MA Yuille. Clustering of missense mutations in the ataxia-telangiectasia gene in a sporadic T-cell leukemia. Nat Genet 17:96–99, 1997.

46. S Stilgenbauer, C Schaffner, A Litterst, P Liebisch, S Gilad, A Bar-Shira, MR James, P Lichter, H Dohner. Biallelic mutations in the ATM gene in T-prolymphocytic leukemia. Nat Med 3:1155–1559, 1997.

47. MR Yuille, LJ Coignet, SM Abraham, F Yaqub, L Luo, E Matutes, V Brito-Babapulle, I Vorechovsky, MJ Dyer, D Catovsky. ATM is usually rearranged in T-cell prolymphocytic leukemia. Oncogene 16:789–796, 1998.

48. D Stoppa-Lyonnet, J Soulier, A Lauge, H Dastot, R Garand, F Sigaux, MH Stern. Inactivation of the ATM gene in T-cell prolymphocytic leukemia. Blood 91:3920–3926, 1998.

49. Y Shiloh. Ataxia-telangiectasia and the Nijmegen breakage syndrome: related disorders but genes apart. Annu Rev Genet, 31:635–662, 1997.

50. KK Khanna, KE Keating, S Kozlov, S Scott, M Gatei, K Hobson, Y Taya, B Gabrielli, D Chan, SP Lees-Miller, MF Lavin. ATM associates with and phosphorylates P53: mapping the region of interaction. Nat Genet 20:398–400, 1998.

51. X Wu, V Ranganathan, DS Weisman, WF Heine, DN Ciccone, TB O'Neill, KE Crick, KA Pierce, WS Lane, G Rathbun, DM Livingston, DT Weaver. ATM phosphorylation of Nijmegen breakage syndrome protein is required in a DNA damage response. Nature 405:477–482, 2000.

52. DS Lim, ST Kim, B Xu, RS Maser, J Lin, JH Petrini, MB Kastan. *ATM* phosphorylates p95/nbs1 in an S-phase checkpoint pathway. Nature 404:613–617, 2000.

53. C Barlow, S Hirotsune, R Paylor, M Liyanage, M Eckhaus, F Collins, Y Shiloh, JN Crawley, T Ried, D Tagle. A Wynshaw-Boris. ATM-deficient mice: a paradigm of ataxia telangiectasia. Cell 86:159–171, 1996.

54. LK Petiniot, Z Weaver, C Barlow, R Shen, M Eckhaus, SM Steinberg, T Ried, A Wynshaw-Boris, RJ Hodes. Recombinase-activating gene (RAG) 2-mediated V(D)J recombination is not essential for tumorigenesis in ATM-deficient mice. Proc Natl Acad Sci USA 97:6664–6669, 2000.

55. Y Tsujimoto, J Yunis, L Onorato-Showe, PC Nowell, CM Croce. Molecular cloning of the

chromosomal breakpoint of B cell lymphomas and leukemias with the t(11;14) chromosome translocation. Science 224:1403–1406, 1984.

56. Y Tsujimoto, E Jaffe, J Cossman, CM Croce. Clustering of breakpoints on chromosome 11 in human B-cell neoplasms with the t(11;14) chromosome translocation. Nature 315:340–343, 1985.

57. Y Tsujimoto, LR Finger, J Yunis, PC Nowell, CM Croce. Cloning of the chromosome breakpoint of neoplastic B-cells with the t(14;18) chromosome translocation. Science 226: 1097–1099, 1984.

58. Y Tsujimoto, J Cossman, E Jaffe, CM Croce. Involvement of the BCL-2 gene in human follicular lymphoma. Science 228:1440–1443, 1985.

59. H Dohner, S Stilgenbauer, K Dohner, M Bentz, P Lichter, Chromosome aberrations in B-cell chronic lymphocytic leukemia: reassessment based on molecular cytogenetic analysis. J Mol Med 77:266–281, 1999.

60. R Bigoni, A Cuneo, MG Roberti, A Bardi, GM Rigolin, N Piva, G Scapoli, R Spanedda, M Negrini, F Bullrich, ML Veronese, CM Croce, G Castoldi. Chromosome aberrations in atypical chronic lymphocytic leukemia: a cytogenetic and interphase cytogenetic study. Leukemia 11:1933–1940, 1997.

61. S Stilgenbauer, J Nickolenko, J Wilhelm, S Wolf, S Weitz, K Dohner, T Boehm, H Dohner, P Lichter. Expressed sequences as candidates for a novel tumor suppressor gene at band 13q14 in B-cell chronic lymphocytic leukemia and mantle cell lymphoma. Oncogene 16: 1891–1897, 1998.

62. A Cuneo, R Bigoni, GM Rigolin, MG Roberti, A Bardi, N Piva, R Milani, F Bullrich, ML Veronese, C Croce, F Birg, H Dohner, A Hagemeijer, G Castoldi. Cytogenetic profile of follicle mantle lineage: correlation with clinicobiologic features. Bood 93:1372–1380, 1999.

63. N Zojer, R Konigsberg, J Ackermann, E Fritz, S Dallinger, E Kromer, H Kaufmann, L Riedl, H Gisslinger, S Schreiber, R Heinz, H Huber, J Drach. Deletion of 13q remains an independent adverse prognostic variable in multiple myeloma despite its frequent detection by interphase fluorescence in situ hybridization. Blood 95:1925–1930, 2000.

64. R Desikan, B Barlogie, J Sawyer, D Ayers, G Tricot, A Badros, M Zangari, NC Munshi, E Anaissie, D Spoon, D Siegel, S Jagannath, D Vesole, J Epstein, J Shaughnessy, A Fassas, S Lim, P Roberson, J Crowley. Results of high-dose therapy for 1000 patients with multiple myeloma: durable complete remissions and superior survival in the absence of chromosome 13 abnormalities. Blood 95:4008–4010, 2000.

65. FJ Giles, SM O'Brien, MJ Keating. Chronic lymphocytic leukemia in (Richter's) transformation. Semin Oncol 25:117–125, 1998.

66. RA Weinberg. The retinoblastoma gene and gene product. Cancer Surv 12:43–47, 1992.

67. AG Brown, FM Ross, EM Dunne, M Steel, and EM Weir-Thompson. Evidence for a new tumor suppressor locus (DBM) in human B-cell neoplasia telomeric to the retinoblastoma gene. Nat Genet 3:67–72, 1993.

68. LA Hawthorn, R Chapman, D Oscier, J Cowell. The consistent 13q14 translocation breakpoint seen in chronic B-cell leukaemia (BCLL) involves deletion of the D13S25 locus which lies dital to the retinoblastoma predisposition gene. Oncogene 8:1415–1419, 1993.

69. Y Liu, L Szekely, D Grander, S Soderhall, G Juliusson, G Gahrton, S Linder, and S Einhorn. Chronic lymphocytic leukemia cells with deletions at 13q14 commonly have one intact RB1 gene: evidence for a role of an adjacent locus. Proc Natl Acad Sci USA 90:8697–8701, 1993.

70. P Starostik, S O'Brien, C-Y Chung, M Haidar, T Manshouri, H Kantarjian, E Freireich, M Keating, M Albitar. The prognostic significance of 13q14 deletions in chronic lymphocytic leukemia. Leukoc Res 23:795–801, 1999.

71. RM Chapman, MM Corcoran, A Gardiner, LA Hawthorn, JK Cowell, DG Oscier. Frequent homozygous deletions of the D13S25 locus in chromosome region 13q14 defines the location

of a gene critical in leukemogenesis in chronic B-cell lymphocytic leukemia. Oncogene 9: 1289–1293, 1994.

72. Y Liu, M Hermanson, D Grander, M Merup, X Wu, M Heyman, O Rasool, G Juliusson, G Gahrton, R Detlofsson, N Nikiforova, C Buys, S Soderhall, N Yankovsky, E Zabarovsky, S Einhorn. 13q deletions in lymphoid malignancies. Blood 86:1911–1915, 1995.

73. S Stilgenbauer, E Leupolt, S Ohl, G Weiss, M Schroder, K Fischer, M Bentz, P Lichter, H Dohner. Heterogeneity of deletions involving *RB*-1 and the D13S25 locus in B-cell chronic lymphocytic leukemia revealed by fluorescence in situ hybridization. Cancer Res 55:3475–3477, 1995.

74. F Bullrich, ML Veronese, S Kitada, J Jurlander, MA Caligiuri, JC Reed, CM Croce. Minimal region of loss at 13q14 in B-cell chronic lymphocytic leukemia. Blood 88:3109–3115, 1996.

75. S Kalachikov, A Migliazza, E Cayanis, NS Fracchiolla, MF Bonaldo, L Lawton, P Jelenc, X Ye, X Qu, M Chien, R Hauptschein, G Gaidano, U Vitolo, G Saglio, L Resegotti, V Brodjansky, N Yankovsky, P Zhang, MB Soares, J Russo, IS Edelman, A Efstratiadis, R Dalla-Favera, SG Fischer. Cloning and gene mapping of the chromosome 13q14 region deleted in chronic lymphocytic leukemia. Genomics 42:369–377, 1997.

76. I Bouyge-Moreau, G Rondeau, H Avet-Loiseau, MT Andre, S Bezieau, M Cherel, S Saleun, E Cadoret, T Shaikh, MM De Angelis, S Arcot, M Batzer, JP Moisan, MC Devilder. Construction of a 780-kb PAC, BAC, and cosmid contig encompassing the minimal critical deletion involved in B cell chronic lymphocytic leukemia at 13q14.3. Genomics 46:183–190, 1997.

77. S Stilgenbauer, J Nickolenko, J Wilhelm, S Wolf, S Weitz, K Dohner, T Boehm, H Dohner, P Lichter. Expressed sequences as candidates for a novel tumor suppressor gene at band 13q14 in B-cell chronic lymphocytic leukemia and mantle cell lymphoma. Oncogene 16: 1891–1897, 1998.

78. B Kapanadze, V Kashuba, A Baranova, O Rasool, W van Everdink, Y Liu, A Syomov, M Corcoran, A Poltaraus, V Brodyansky, N Syomova, A Kazakov A, R Ibbotson, A van den Berg, R Gizatullin, L Fedorova, G Sulimova, A Zelenin, L Deaven, H Lehrach, D Grander, C Buys, D Oscier, ER Zabarovsky, S Einhorn, N Yankovsky. A cosmid and cDNA fine physical map of a human chromosome 13q14 region frequently lost in B-cell chronic lymphocytic leukemia and identification of a new putative tumor suppressor gene, LEU5, FEBS Lett 426:266–270, 1998.

79. S Bezieau, MC Devilder, G Rondeau, E Cadoret, JP Moisan, I Moreau, Assignment of 48 ESTs to chromosome 13 band q14.3 and expression pattern for ESTs located in the core region deleted in B-CLL. Genomics 52:369–373, 1998.

80. MM Corcoran, O Rasool, Y Liu, A Iyengar, D Grander, RE Ibbotson, M Merup, X Wu, V Brodyansky, AC Gardiner, G Juliusson, RM Chapman, G Ivanova, M Tiller, G Gahrton, N Yankovsky, E Zabarovsky, DG Oscier, S Einhorn. Detailed molecular delineation of 13q14.3 loss in B-cell chronic lymphocytic leukemia. Blood 91:1382–1390, 1998.

81. Y Liu, M Corcoran, O Rasool, G Ivanova, R Ibbotson, D Grander, A Iyengar, A Baranova, V Kashuba, M Merup, X Wu, A Gardiner, R Mullenbach, A Poltaraus, AL Hultstrom, G Juliusson, R Chapman, M Tiller, F Cotter, G Gahrton, N Yankovsky, E Zabarovsky, S Einhorn, D Oscier. Cloning of two candidate tumor suppressor genes within a 10 kb region on chromosome 13q14, frequently deleted in chronic lymphocytic leukemia. Oncogene 15: 2463–2473, 1997.

82. C Fegan, H Robinson, P Thompson, S Wolf, S Weitz, K Dohner, T Boehm, H Dohner, P Lichter. Karyotypic evolution in CLL: identification of a new sub-group of patients with deletions of 11q and advanced progressive disease. Leukemia 9:2003–2008, 1995.

83. H Dohner, S Stilgenbauer, MR James, A Benner, T Weilguni, M Bentz, K Fischer, W Hunstein, P Lichter. 11q deletions identify a new subset of B-cell chronic lymphocytic leukemia characterized by extensive nodal involvement and inferior prognosis. Blood 89:2516–2522, 1997.

84. JR Neilson, R Auer, D White, N Bienz, JJ Waters, JA Whittaker, DW Milligan, CD Fegan. Deletions at 11q identify a subset of patients with typical CLL who show consistent disease progression and reduced survival. Leukemia 11:1929–1932, 1997.

85. S Stilgenbauer, P Liebisch, MR James, M Schroder, B Schlegelberger, K Fischer, M Bentz, P Lichter, H Dohner. Molecular cytogenetic delination of a novel critical genomic region in chromosome bands 11q22.3–23.1 in lymphoprolypherative disorders. Proc Natl Acad Sci USA 15:11837–11847, 1996.

86. P Starostik, T Manshouri, S O'Brien, E Freireich, H Kantarjian, M Haidar, S Lerner, M Keating, M Albitar. Deficiency of the ATM protein expression defines an aggressive subgroup of B-cell chronic lymphocytic leukemia. Cancer Res 58:4552–4557, 1998.

87. F Bullrich, D Rasio, S Kitada, P Starostik, T Kipps, M Keating, M Albitar, JC Reed, CM Croce. ATM mutations in B-cell chronic lymphocytic leukemia. Cancer Res 59:24–27, 1999.

88. T Stankovic, P Weber, G Stewart, T Bedenham, J Murray, PJ Byrd, PA Moss, AM Taylor. Inactivation of ataxia telangiectasia mutated gene in B-cell chronic lymphocytic leukaemia. Lancet 353:26–29, 1999.

89. C Schaffner, S Stilgenbauer, GA Rappold, H Dohner, P Lichter. Somatic ATM mutations indicate a pathogenic role of ATM in B-cell chronic lymphocytic leukemia. Blood 94:748–753, 1999.

90. I Vorechovsky, D Rasio, L Luo, C Monaco, L Hammarstrom, AD Webster, J Zaloudik, G Barbanti-Brodani, M James, G Russo, et al. The ATM gene and susceptibility to breast cancer: analysis of 38 breast tumors reveals no evidence for mutation. Cancer Res 56:2726–2732, 1996.

91. MG FitzGerald, JM Bean, SR Hegde, H Unsal, DJ MacDonald, DP Harkin, DM Finkelstein, KJ Isselbacher, DA Haber. Heterozygous ATM mutations do not contribute to early onset of breast cancer. Nat Genet 15:307–310, 1997.

92. G Rotman, Y Shiloh. ATM: A mediator of multiple responses to genotoxic stress. Oncogene 18:6135–6144, 1999.

93. KK Khanna. Cancer risk and the ATM gene: a continuing debate. J Natl Cancer Inst 92: 795–800, 2000.

94. S Banin, L Moyal, S Shieh, Y Taya, CW Anderson, L Chessa, NI Smorodinsky, C Prives, Y Reiss, Y Shiloh, Y Ziv. Enhanced phosphorylation of P53 by ATM in response to DNA damage. Science 281:1674–1677, 1998.

95. CE Canman, DS Lim, KA Cimprich, Y Taya, K Tamai, K Sakaguchi, E Appella, MB Kastan, JD Siliciano. Activation of the ATM kinase by ionizing radiation and phosphorylation of P53. Science 281:1677–1679, 1998.

96. T Shafman, KK Khanna, P Kedar, K Spring, S Kozlov, T Yen, K Hobson, M Gatei, N Zhang, D Watters, M Egerton, Y Shiloh, S Kharbanda, D Kufe, MF Lavin. Interaction between ATM protein and c-Abl in response to DNA damage. Nature 387:520–523, 1997.

97. R Baskaran, LD Wood, LL Whitaker, CE Canman, SE Morgan, Y Xu, C Barlow, D Baltimore, A Wynshaw-Boris, MB Kastan, JY Wang. Ataxia telangiectasia mutant protein activates c-Abl tyrosine kinase in response to ionizing radiation. Nature 387:516–519, 1997.

98. D Cortez, Y Wang, J Qin, SJ Elledge. Requirement of ATM-dependent phosphorylation of brca1 in the DNA damage response to double-strand breaks. Science 286:1162–1166, 1999.

99. S Matsuoka, M Huang, SJ Elledge. Linkage of ATM to cell cycle regulation by the Chk2 protein kinase. Science 282:1893–1897, 1998.

100. RV Sionov, Y Haupt. The cellular response to P53: the decision between life and death. Oncogene 18:6145–6157, 1999.

101. Y Sanchez, C Wong, RS Thoma, R Richman, Z Wu, H Piwnica-Worms, SJ Elledge. Conservation of the Chk1 checkpoint pathway in mammals: linkage of DNA damage to Cdk regulation through Cdc25. Science 277:1497–1501, 1997.

102. S el Rouby, A Thomas, D Costin, CR Rosenberg, M Potmesil, R Silber, EW Newcomb. P53

gene mutation in B-cell chronic lymphocyticleukemia is associated with drug resistance and is independent of MDR1/MDR3 gene expression. Blood 82:3452–3459, 1993.

103. G Juliusson, DG Oscier, M Fitchett, FM Ross, G Stockdill, MJ Mackie, AC Parker, GL Castoldi, A Guneo, S Knuutila, et al. Prognostic subgroups in B-cell chronic lymphocyticleukemia defined by specific chromosomalabnormalities. N Engl J Med 323:720–724, 1990.

104. JA Garcia-Marco, CM Price, D Catovsky. Interphase cytogenetics in chronic lymphocytic leukemia. Cancer Genet Cytogenet 94:52–58, 1997.

105. S Einhorn, K Burvall, G Juliusson, G Gahrton, T Meeker. Molecular analysis of chromosome 12 in chronic lymphocytic leukemia. Leukemia 3:871–874, 1989.

106. G Gahrton, KH Robert, K Friberg, G Juliusson, P Biberfeld, L Zech. Cytogenetic mapping of the duplicated segment of chromosome 12 in lymphoproliferative disorders. Nature 297: 513–514, 1982.

107. MH Kubbutat, SN Jones, KH Vousden. Regulation of P53 stability by Mdm2. Nature 387: 299–303, 1997.

108. C Bueso-Ramos, Y Yang, E deLeon, P McCown, SA Stass, M Albitar. The human MDM-2 Oncogene is overexpressed in leukemias. Blood 82:2617–2623, 1993.

109. T Watanabe, T Hotta, A Ichikawa, T Kinoshita, H Nagai, T Uchida, T Murate, H Saito. The MDM2 oncogene overexpression in chronic lymphocytic leukemia and low-grade lymphoma of B-cell origin. Blood 84:3158–3165, 1994.

110. F Bullrich, TK MacLachlan, N Sang, T Druck, ML Veronese, SL Allen, N Chiorazzi, A Koff, K Heubner, CM Croce, A Giordano. Chromosomal mapping of members of the cdc2 family of protein kinases, cdk3, cdk6, PISSLRE, and PITALRE, and a cdk inhibitor, p27Kip1, to regions involved in human cancer. Cancer Res. 55:1199–1205, 1995.

111. M Merup, G Juliusson, X Wu, M Jansson, B Stellan, O Rasool, E Roijer, G Stenman, G Gahrton, S Einhorn. Amplification of multiple regions of chromosome 12, including 12q13–15, in chronic lymphocytic leukaemia. Eur J Haematol 58:174–180, 1997.

112. CS Cooper. Translocations in solid tumors Curr Opin Genet Dev 6:71–75, 1996.

113. G Goodwin. The high mobility group protein, HMGI-C. Int J Biochem Cell Biol 30:761–766, 1998.

114. A Wolffe. Architectural factors. Science 264:1100–1101, 1994.

115. MT Berlingieri, G Manfioletti, M Santoro, A Bandiera, R Visconti, V Giancotti, A Fusco. Inhibition of HMGI-C protein synthesis suppresses retrovirally induced neoplastic transformation of rat thyroid cells. Mol Cell Biol 15:1545–1553, 1995.

116. P Rogalla, K Drechsler, G Frey, Y Hennig, B Helmke, U Bonk, J Bullerdiek. HMGI-C expression patterns in human tissues. Implications for the genesis of frequent mesenchymal tumors. Am J Pathol 149:775–779, 1996.

117. B Rommel, P Rogalla, A Jox, CV Kalle, B Kazmierczak, J Wolf, J Bullerdiek. HMGI-C, a member of the high mobility group family of proteins, is expressed in hematopoietic stem cells and in leukemic cells. Leuk. Lymphoma 26:603–607, 1997.

118. B Santulli, B Kazmierczak, R Napolitano, I Caliendo, G Chiappetta, V Rippe, J Bullerdiek, A Fusco. A 12q13 translocation involving the HMGI-C gene in Richter transformation of a chronic lymphocytic leukemia. Cancer Genet Cytogenet 119:70–73, 2000.

119. SA Schichman, E Canaani, CM Croce. Self-fusion of the ALL1 gene. A new genetic mechanism for acute leukemia. JAMA 273:571–576, 1995.

120. R Silber, B Degar, D Costin, EW Newcomb, M Mani, CR Rosenberg, L Morse, JC Drygas, ZN Canellakis, M Potmesil. Chemosensitivity of lymphocytes from patients with B-cell chronic lymphocytic leukemia to chlorambucil, fludarabine, and camptothecin analogs. Blood 84:3440–3446, 1994.

121. M Hanada, D Delia, A Aiello, E Stadtmauer, JC Reed. BCL2 gene hypomethylation and high-level expression in B-cell chronic lymphocytic leukemia. Blood 82:1820–1828, 1993.

122. JC Reed. BCL-2 family proteins: regulators of apoptosis and chemoresistance in hematologic malignancies. Semin Hematol 34(4 suppl 5):9, 1997.

123. Y Tsujimoto, J Cossman, E Jaffe, CM Croce. Involvement of the BCL-2 gene in human follicular lymphoma. Science 228:1440–1443, 1985.

124. S Haldar, A Basu, CM Croce. Bcl2 is the guardian of microtubule integrity. Cancer Res 57: 229–233, 1997.

125. JL Wang, D Liu, ZJ Zhang, S Shan, X Han, SM Srinivasula, CM Croce, ES Alnemri, Z Huang. Structure-based discovery of an organic compound that binds BCL-2 protein and induces apoptosis of tumor cells. Proc Natl Acad Sci USA 97:7124–7129, 2000.

126. TW McKeithan, H Ohno, MO Diaz. Identification of a transcriptional unit adjacent to the breakpoint in the 14;19 translocation of chronic lymphocytic leukemia. Genes Chrom Cancer 3:247–255, 1990.

127. ST Ong, ML Hackbarth, LC Degenstein, DA Baunoch, J Anastasi, TW McKeithan. Lymphadenopathy, splenomegaly, and altered immunoglobulins production in BCL3 transgenic mice. Oncogene 16:2333–2343, 1998.

128. SY Na, JE Choi, HJ Kim, BH Jhun, YC Lee, JW Lee. BCL3, an IkappaB protein, stimulates activating protein-1 transactivation and cellular proliferation. J Biol Chem 274:28491–28496, 1999.

129. L Michaux, J Dierlamm, I Wlodarska, V Bours, H Van den Berghe, A Hegemeijer. t(14;19)/BCL3 rearrangements in lymphoproliferative disorders: a review of 23 cases. Cancer Genet Cytogenet 94:36–43, 1997.

130. S Stilgenbauer, L Bullinger, A Benner, K Wildenberger, M Bentz, K Dohner, AD Ho, P Lichter, H Dohner. Incidence and clinical significance of 6q deletions in B cell chronic lymphocytic leukemia. Leukemia 13:1331–1334, 1999.

131. JM Hernandez, C Mecucci, L Michaux, A Criel, M Stul, P Meeus, I Wlodarska, A Van Orshoven, JJ Cassiman, C De Wolf-Peeters, H Van den Berghe. del(7q) in chronic B-cell lymphoid malignancies. Cancer Genet Cytogenet 93:147–151, 1997.

132. A Cuneo, MG Roberti, R Bigoni, C Minotto, A Bardi, R Milani, A Tieghi, D Campioni, F Cavazzini, C De Angeli, M Negrini, G Castoldi. Four novel non-random chromosome rearrangements in B-cell chronic lymphocytic leukaemia: 6p24–25 and 12p12–13 translocations, 4q21 anomalies and monosomy 21. Br J Haematol 108:559–564, 2000.

3

Chronic Lymphocytic Leukemia
Epidemiological, Familial, and Genetic Aspects

MARIA T. SGAMBATI, MARTHA S. LINET, and SUSAN S. DEVESA

National Cancer Institute, National Institutes of Health, Bethesda, Maryland

I. INTRODUCTION

Chronic lymphocytic leukemia (CLL) is a rare neoplasm that comprises a substantial proportion of all leukemia in middle-aged persons and is the most common type among elderly persons in western populations. The major causes are not known nor is there detailed understanding about how the elusive origin(s) may relate to clinical expression, basic biological mechanisms, or pathogenesis. Nevertheless, a growing body of data exists on demographic patterns, international variation, and etiology as described in earlier reviews (1–9). Also, with the advent of rapid developments in molecular biology, information is increasing on the molecular aspects of CLL. This chapter will emphasize more recent epidemiology work, particularly for familial and genetic aspects of CLL.

Until the last 2 or 3 decades, descriptive and analytical epidemiological investigations frequently considered the leukemias as a single entity or as two major designated categories (i.e., lymphoid and myeloid) plus a heterogeneous grouping of "other and unknown." This grouping made it difficult to analyze the literature where these categories have been used. The Eighth Revision of the International Classification of Diseases (ICD) coding scheme was the first to incorporate the designations of "acute" and "chronic" for the subtypes of lymphoid and myeloid leukemia (3). In both the Eighth and Ninth (10) revisions, the three-digit ICD code 204 designates lymphoid leukemia, whereas a fourth digit is required to differentiate "chronic" (204.1) and "acute" (204.0). An extension of the ICD coding scheme for neoplasms was developed in the mid-1970s and designated as the International Classification of Diseases for Oncology (ICD-O) (11). The ICD-O included codes for morphology and anatomical site in registering incident neoplasms.

The First Edition of the International Classification of Diseases for Oncology (11) added a code for prolymphocytic leukemia (PL) to the CLL categories, whereas the second edition of ICD-O (12) added codes for adult T-cell leukemia/lymphoma and Burkitt's cell leukemia. Population-based cancer registries are increasingly reporting adult T-cell leukemia as a separate entity, but prolymphocytic leukemia is poorly ascertained and rarely reported as a separate entity by most population-based registries. Despite these advances, some recent incidence compilations and many occupational and environmental epidemiological studies do not present results using a fourth digit. Instead, these reports restrict reporting to three-digit codes (lymphocytic leukemia) or even cruder categories (such as leukemia not otherwise specified or acute versus chronic leukemia).

Recent reports show further subclassification of CLL may be appropriate (13). In 1989, the French–American–British (FAB) expert hematology group suggested guidelines for further dividing CLL into typical and atypical CLL (14). Atypical CLL includes CLL, mixed cell type, which has populations of large lymphocytes and CLL/PL, which has a mix of typical CLL cells and prolymphocytes. Molecular data now provide further support for these subcategorizations. In addition, these subtypes are characterized by clinical and prognostic differences (15). Increasingly, clinical reports categorize subtypes of CLL according to cell surface immunophenotypes and immunoglobulin expression, cytogenetic abnormalities (clonal or nonclonal aberrations, karyotype, band patterns in the major breakpoint region), molecular markers, or stage at presentation. Ideally, classifications should incorporate morphological, immunophenotypic, karyotypic, molecular, prognostic, and other features. Because standardized application of such classification approaches in all medical institutions is unlikely in the near future, it will not be possible to evaluate CLL demographic patterns to ascertain the distribution of CLL subtypes with regard to these aspects according to age, gender, racial/ethnic, or geographical differences, nor will it be possible to assess whether there is change in the distribution of CLL subtypes over time.

II. DEMOGRAPHIC PATTERNS

A. Overview

Despite availability of appropriate classification schemes to designate CLL and other subtypes according to major cell type category, newly diagnosed or incident leukemia cases reported to cancer registries and those first identified from death certificates sometimes lack complete information about subtype. For these reasons, population-based mortality data for chronic lymphocytic leukemia are generally difficult to interpret, and population-based incidence data for a given registry must be critically evaluated in light of the proportion of the total leukemia cases that are incompletely designated or unspecified according to subtype. The latter problem also complicates efforts to compare incidence rates for chronic lymphocytic leukemia among cancer registries (5–7). International data are available for various geographical regions reporting to the International Agency for Research on Cancer for the period 1988–92 (16). We selected registries to include that had larger numbers of cases, smaller proportions of unspecified or incompletely specified leukemia cases, and good-quality census data to enable accurate determination of rates. U.S. incidence patterns are summarized in the following, using data from 1973–96 from the nine population-based cancer registries (including five states and four cities comprising about

10% of the U.S. population) of the National Cancer Institute's Surveillance, Epidemiology and End Results (SEER) Program (17).

B. International Incidence Patterns

1. Age-Adjusted Incidence Patterns

Among the four major commonly designated cell types for leukemia, variation in incidence rates was greatest for CLL (6). There was a 26-fold difference between the highest (Canada) and lowest (Japan, Osaka) age-adjusted (world standard) CLL rates for men, and a 38-fold difference between the highest (U.S., Los Angeles non-Hispanic white) and lowest (Japan, Osaka) rates for women (16). The male/female ratio ranged from 1.4 in Zurich, Switzerland, to 3.2 in Shanghai, China. High incidence rates occurred among Caucasian, non-Hispanic populations in North America (rates among men ranged from 3.35–3.69 per 100,000 per year; rates among women ranged from 1.61–1.92 per 100,000 per year), Europe (men, 2.20–3.36; women, 0.90–1.52), and Oceania (men, 2.81–2.96; women, 1.41–1.53). Low rates were seen in east, southeastern, and southern Asia among both genders (men, 0.14–0.58; women, 0.05–0.30) (Fig. 1) (16). Population-based incidence data from Asian populations, compiled in several volumes of Cancer Incidence in Five Continents by the International Agency for Research on Cancer, have demonstrated lower incidence rates for each age group than age-specific rates among other populations, but the difference between Asian and other populations is greatest at older ages. Hospital-based series from Asian populations have only infrequently been described in English-language articles, but CLL comprised only 4.6% of all leukemia among 4174 patients hospitalized at the Peking Union Medical College in Beijing, China (18). B-cell CLL incidence rates were also substantially lower among Asians than among Caucasians on the basis of reports from Japan (19). et al., 1993), China (18,20) and India (21).

C. U.S. Incidence Rates

1. Age-Adjusted Variation Among Racial/Ethnic Groups

As shown in Figure 1, highest rates within the United States in men occurred among blacks in Los Angeles, followed by whites in the SEER and Los Angeles registries, then blacks in the SEER registries, and finally Hispanics in the Los Angeles registry. For women, highest rates were among non-Hispanic whites in Los Angeles, then whites and blacks in SEER, followed by blacks in Los Angeles, and finally lowest rates in Hispanic whites in Los Angeles. Data from an earlier analysis using SEER data provide more information about other ethnic groups in that highest rates for lymphoid leukemia (not further evaluated according to acute or chronic subtypes) were seen among Caucasians, followed by African-Americans, then Hispanics and Chinese-Americans, with lowest and similar rates among Filipinos, Hawaiians, and Japanese-Americans of both sexes (data not shown) (5).

2. Age-Specific Patterns

Chronic lymphocytic leukemia is extremely rare among persons less than age 30 but increases steeply beginning in the fourth decade (Fig. 2). Rates continue to rise exponentially with increasing age and at a steeper rate of increase than other leukemia subtypes until age 70, when the rate of the increase begins to slow somewhat, particularly for black men and for women of both major racial groups. CLL is the predominant leukemia type among

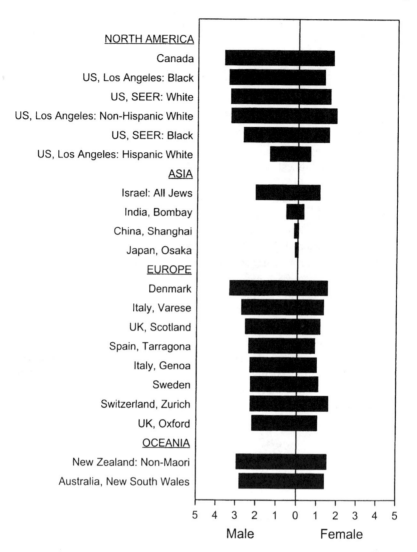

Figure 1 International incidence rates for chronic lymphocytic leukemia per 100,000 (age-adjusted, World Standard) by continent and sex, 1988–1992. (*Source*: Parkin DM, et al. Cancer Incidence in Five Continents, vol. 7. Lyon, France: IARC Scientific Publication Number 143, 1997.)

the elderly, comprising 39% of all leukemia among persons aged 65 or older (17). Incidence rates were higher among men than women at all ages (Fig. 2). For men aged 40–70, rates were similar among Caucasians and African-Americans. Among elderly men, rates were higher in Caucasians than in African-Americans. Rates for Caucasian women were slightly higher than rates for African-American women at virtually all ages. Overall, the median age at diagnosis was older for U.S. whites (66.5) than African-Americans (63.8), because of the differences in population age distribution. Age at diagnosis has risen over time in the United States with the median for all races combined rising from 65.7 years old in 1975–85 to 66.6 years old in 1986–94 (unpublished SEER Program data), largely because of the aging of the population. This pattern has also been observed

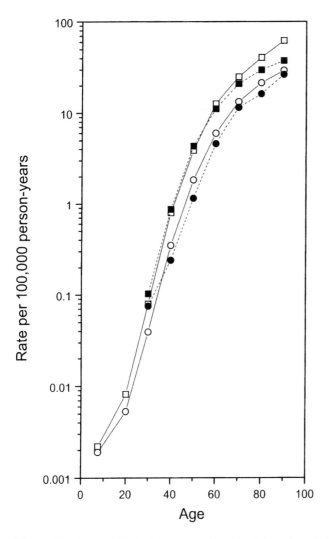

Figure 2   Age-specific incidence rates for chronic lymphocytic leukemia in the nine SEER areas by race and sex, 1973–1996. □, white male; ■, black male; ○, white female; ●, black female. (*Source*: Ries LAG, et al. SEER Cancer Statistics Review, 1973–1996. Bethesda, MD: National Cancer Institute. NIH Pub. No. 99-2789, 1999, pp 262–283.)

in other populations (22), among whom a rising proportion of patients has been diagnosed at an older age.

3.   Age-Adjusted Incidence Trends

Between 1973–76 and 1993–96, age-adjusted (1970 U.S. standard) incidence rates for CLL declined somewhat in all four race-sex groups, although the trends were not linear (Fig. 3). Among Caucasian and African-American men, incidence was fairly stable between 1973–76 and 1989–92, after which incidence rates declined 20%. The decrease began earlier among females of both races. The male predominance in CLL in Western countries was more pronounced earlier in the century (reported male/female ratios ranged

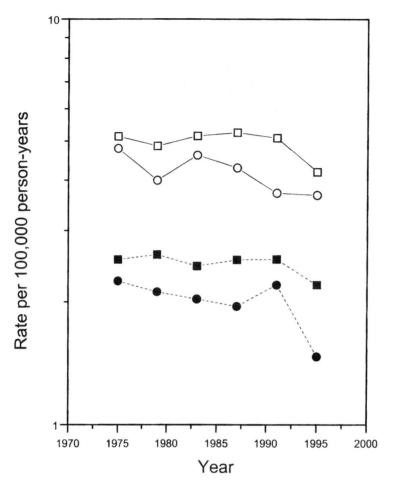

Figure 3   Age-adjusted (1970 U.S. standard) incidence trends for chronic lymphocytic leukemia in the nine SEER areas by race and sex, 1973–76 through 1993–96. □, white male; ■, black male; ○, white female; ●, black female. (*Source*: Ries LAG, et al. SEER Cancer Statistics Review, 1973–1996. Bethesda, MD: National Cancer Institute. NIH Pub. No. 99-2789, 1999, pp 262–283.)

from 2.5 to 3.0) than those reported in more recent studies (male/female ratios ranged from 1.6 to 1.9) (7).

4.   U.S. Population-Based Survival Patterns

For patients with CLL in all age groups, all races, and both sexes combined, the overall 5-year relative survival increased only slightly over the 22 years monitored by the SEER Program registries, from a baseline of 68.2% in 1974–76 to 70.5 in 1989–95 (Table 1). Five-year relative survival rates were similar in Caucasian men and women but were notably lower among African-Americans, although survival was somewhat better in female than in male African-Americans. Those less than age 65 at diagnosis had a higher 5-year relative survival than persons older than age 65 at diagnosis. Interestingly, data from the population-based SEER program are somewhat more positive than data from hospital-based series. In a series of more than 105,000 patients hospitalized for leukemia in a broad spectrum of U.S. hospitals during 1985–95, patients diagnosed with CLL com-

Table 1   Five-Year Relative Survival Rates for Chronic Lymphocytic Leukemia In the U.S. SEER Program by Time Period, Race, Sex, and Age

Period	Age, race, sex	Relative survival CLL
1974–76	All ages, all races, both sexes	68.2
1989–95	All ages, all races, both sexes	70.5[a]
	Caucasian males	72.5
	Caucasian females	71.8
	African-American males	43.6
	African-American females	53.7
	Age < 65 years old	78.8
	Age 65 and older	65.9

[a] $P < 0.05$ for 1989–95 versus 1974–76.
Source: Ries LAG, Rosary CL, Hankey BF, Miller BA, Clegg LX, Edwards, BK, eds. SEER Cancer Statistics Review, 1973–1996, National Cancer Institute. NIH Pub. No. 99–2789. Bethesda, MD, 1999, pp 262–283.

prised 22.6% of the total (23). The average age of the patients in this large series was 69.6 years old at diagnosis of CLL, and overall 5-year relative survival was 48.2% and 10-year relative survival was 22.5%. Five-year relative survival progressively declined with increasing age, from 69.5% for those less than age 40 at diagnosis to 41.7% for those 80 years of age or older at diagnosis. The lower proportion that CLL comprises of total leukemia within the hospital-based (23) compared with the population-based (17) series (22.6% versus 39%, respectively) and the lower overall 5-year relative survival (48.2% during 1985–95 versus 70.5% during 1989–95, respectively), reflects the notable fraction of CLL cases that are not hospitalized for treatment because of mild or absent symptoms (24).

III. OCCUPATIONAL EXPOSURES

A. Overview

For more than 200 years, occupational exposures have been linked with an excess occurrence of cancer. Until the middle of the twentieth century, clinical observations were the primary source of information about cancers associated with occupational exposure. Historically, a specific cancer was clinically linked with a particular carcinogenic exposure when carcinogen exposure levels were high, strong statistical associations between carcinogenic exposure and cancer outcome were observed, cancer was diagnosed in workers still exposed to the putative carcinogen, and sufficient numbers of workers were affected (25).

In the second half of the twentieth century, formal epidemiological assessment was implemented using proportional mortality analysis, and then retrospective cohort studies (following up cohorts of workers retrospectively and comparing cancer risks among exposed versus unexposed groups), and case-control investigations (comparing history of occupational exposures in cancer cases versus controls). Routine surveillance to estimate the occurrence of occupationally induced cancer was initially implemented approximately 45 years ago in England and Wales. More recently, the International Agency for Research on Cancer (IARC) categorized chemical and other agents or industrial processes according to five levels. Group 1 agents were characterized by sufficient evidence of carcinogenicity in humans. Group 2A included agents for which there was *probable* evidence of carcinogenicity in humans, and Group 2B included those with *possible* evidence of carcinogenicity in humans. Group 3 agents were those with insufficient evidence of carcinogenicity. For Group 4 agents, evidence suggested lack of carcinogenicity (26,27).

Occupational cohort studies may provide methodological advantages for evaluating potential etiological associations between CLL (or other cancers) and specific exposures. Advantages include the potential availability of long-term employment records, monitoring data for exposures and serious disease outcomes, and easier identification of potential carcinogens and processes than occurs in the residential environmental setting. Occupational exposures are often higher than those occurring in the residential setting. Nevertheless, failure to consider known nonoccupational carcinogenic exposures (such as cigarette smoking, alcohol consumption, dietary components, or infectious agents) may affect the accuracy of risk estimates for occupational exposures and associated cancers.

B. Physical Agents

1. Ionizing Radiation

Little or no evidence exists that exposure to ionizing radiation is linked with risk of CLL (28–30).

2. Nonionizing Radiation

In a comprehensive assessment of the epidemiological literature on health effects from exposure to power-line frequency electric and magnetic fields (EMF), an expert review committee concluded that there was limited evidence of a relationship between this exposure and risk of CLL. This conclusion was based on three incidence studies that incorporated measurement data (31) and 38 studies relying on job title only (32). In one of the two Swedish measurement studies, Floderus et al. (33) observed a dose-response relationship and a 3.7-fold increased risk for the 22 men whose occupational exposures to EMF were in the 90th or higher percentile of exposure among 250 male CLL cases compared with 1121 population controls. Feychting et al. (34) observed increased risks for CLL among approximately 400,000 persons residing within 300 m of a transmission line in Sweden. Risk was 1.7-fold increased among the 28 CLL cases with estimated EMF workplace exposures of 0.2 microtesla or higher and 2.1-fold increased for 2 of these 28 CLL cases with residential EMF exposures of 0.2 microtesla or greater. Theriault et al. (35) studied 223,292 Canadian and French male utility workers and found CLL risks to be nonsignificantly 1.5-fold increased among the 24 cases whose estimated occupational EMF exposures were 3.1 microtesla-years or greater and nonsignificantly 1.7-fold elevated among the six cases in the 90th exposure percentile or greater. In a meta-analysis of 38 studies of leukemia, the overall risk estimate was 1.6-fold and significantly increased for CLL (and approximately the same level of estimated risk for acute myeloid leukemia [AML]) among studies primarily relying on job title information to define exposure (32).

C. Chemical Agents and Industries with Chemical Exposures

1. Benzene

Although evidence was considered sufficient to designate benzene as a Group 1 carcinogen for acute myeloid leukemia, little evidence has implicated an association with CLL (36–38).

2. Petroleum Industry Workers

In a leukemia type-specific meta-analysis, no excess risk was found for CLL among 208,000 petroleum workers (39). A few studies have described excesses of lymphocytic leukemia or CLL (40,41) or other lymphopoietic malignancies (including non-Hodgkin's lymphoma, multiple myeloma, and possibly leukemia, cell types not specified) (40). However, Marsh et al. (42) other studies of petroleum distribution (43–46), petroleum manufacturing (47), oil and gas production (47,48) or petrochemical production (49) workers have shown no excesses.

3. Gasoline Service Station Workers

Service station workers in Nordic countries had no excess of CLL or other type of leukemia (50).

4. Rubber Workers

Benzene was used extensively in the rubber industry in earlier years, but other chemicals (some contaminated with small amounts of benzene) have been used as replacements in recent times. Excess risks of lymphocytic leukemia were observed in large cohorts of rubber manufacturing workers in the United Kingdom (51,52) and the United States (53,54). More detailed investigations linked solvent exposures of rubber industry workers with increased risk of lymphocytic leukemia (55). The specific solvents implicated included benzene, carbon disulfide, carbon tetrachloride, xylene, and others (56–58), although the notably elevated risks were based on small numbers of lymphocytic leukemia cases in the rubber manufacturing industry. More recent studies in rubber workers in the United Kingdom showed no leukemia excess (59), but a small excess was reported in a detailed review of 12 cohort studies by an IARC committee (60).

5. Styrene and Butadiene

Elevated leukemia and lymphoma risks were reported among some generally small cohorts of workers in plants producing, polymerizing, and/or processing styrene monomers and butadiene (55,61–63). Monomeric styrene and butadiene were implicated in some studies (64), whereas benzene or other solvents were more clearly linked in other investigations (65). No leukemia excesses were observed in large cohorts of workers employed in styrene-butadiene polymer manufacturing and reinforced plastics and composites (styrene-exposed) manufacturing plants (66–68). A notable excess of leukemia among workers exposed to butadiene, but not styrene, in a nested case-control study may indicate a causal association, or possibly a chance of confounding (69). In a retrospective cohort study of 40,683 workers in the reinforced plastics industry from Denmark, Finland, Italy, Norway, Sweden, and the United Kingdom, information on exposure to styrene was reconstructed through job histories, environmental and biological monitoring data, and production records of the plants. There were no excesses of all cancers or of neoplasms of the lymphatic and hematopoietic tissues overall, nor did risk increase with increasing length of exposure. However, mortality from leukemia and lymphoma rose with time since first exposure to a twofold excess 20 years after first exposure (70). Small excess risks of lymphohematopoietic cancers were found in some studies of 1,3-butadiene production facilities (71) particularly among long-time workers. Workers employed in the 1960's in companies producing reinforced plastics in Denmark had elevated risks (72).

6. Ethylene Oxide and Related Chemicals

Ethylene oxide was designated as a probable human carcinogen on the basis of elevated risks for lymphatic leukemia and lymphoma observed in three small Swedish cohorts (73–76) and animal carcinogenicity data (77). Subsequently, excesses of lymphoid leukemia and lymphoma and a significant dose-response effect for these neoplasms were observed among U.S. workers in this industry (78). Non-Hodgkin's lymphoma (but not leukemia) was significantly elevated among U.S. workers from 14 plants producing sterilized medical supplies (79), and elevated leukemia risks were linked with production of ethylene or propylene chlorhydrin, rather than ethylene oxide, at two U.S. facilities (80,81). No excesses were seen in German (82), British (83), or other U.S. plants (84,85), however, leading to an assessment that available data do not provide convincing or consistent evidence of leukemogenicity (86). It is possible that CLL may be linked with ethylene oxide exposure in view of the excess risks seen for non-Hodgkin's lymphoma (NHL) and lymphoid leukemias in those studies evaluating these endpoints. However, investigations focusing on total leukemia mortality could fail to identify excess risks of CLL even if the increases are real because death certificates are often lacking specification of cell type of leukemia.

7. Chemists and Workers in Medical Research

Small excesses of lymphopoietic malignancies (often including a combination of CLL, NHL, and sometimes other neoplasms such as Hodgkin disease or multiple myeloma) have been reported among chemists (87) and workers in biomedical research (88), science technicians (89), clinical laboratory technicians (working in analytical chemistry, pathology, cytology, genetics, and other laboratories) (90), and workers in other types of laboratories (91), but specific chemicals or infectious agents that might be responsible have not been identified. Although excess risks of lymphopoietic tumors have been linked with a high probability of exposure to chemicals, other possibilities could not be ruled out. In most of these studies, risks for CLL have not been separately evaluated from risks for total leukemia.

D. Farmers and Other Agricultural Workers

Many, but not all, studies have shown associations between all types of leukemia and farming (7,92,93). A substantial proportion of the studies have evaluated mortality for all leukemia types combined, although investigations examining risks according to leukemia cell type have implicated farming or farm-related exposures in risk of CLL (94–96). Specific agricultural exposures linked with elevated risk of CLL include DDT (97), animal breeding (98), and working in flour mills (99). Blair and Zahm (93) have postulated that agricultural exposures might affect the immune system. Other agricultural exposures that may be leukemogenic include various agrochemicals (including crop and animal insecticides, herbicides, and fertilizers), infectious agents, or other exposures associated with various forms of livestock, fertilizers, and certain crops. Forage growing and organophosphate insecticides have been associated with elevated risk of hairy cell leukemia (100).

E. Other Occupational Exposures

In a few studies, CLL has also been linked with working in underground coal mining (101), carpet manufacturing (102,103), sawmills or industries using lumber products (27,104), and employment as a barber or hairdresser (105,106) or as a vehicle mechanic (107). Limited data also support associations between CLL and exposure to asbestos (108,109), brick mortar (110), and wood products (97,111).

IV. ENVIRONMENTAL AND LIFESTYLE EXPOSURES

A. Environmental Exposures

There are few studies assessing risks of environmental exposures. Comprehensive assessments have concluded that nonoccupational, environmental exposures to ionizing radiation and nonionizing radiation are not associated with increased risk of CLL (28–31). Although CLL was modestly increased in some studies of farmers and agricultural workers, there is no consistent evidence linking residential pesticide exposures to increased risk of CLL.

1. Cigarette Smoking

Although cigarette smoking has been established as an important risk factor for lung cancer for several decades, it was not until 1986 that smoking was initially linked with increased risk of leukemia (112). An increasing number of cohort and case-control studies reveal increased risks of AML associated with cigarette smoking (7), whereas only three cohort investigations demonstrated elevated risks of lymphocytic leukemia (113–115). One case-control study also demonstrated an increased risk of CLL (116) associated with cigarette smoking. Recent large cohort studies have demonstrated no evidence of an association between cigarette smoking and CLL (117,118).

B. Lifestyle Factors

1. Hair Dyes

CLL, AML, total leukemia, and myelodysplastic syndrome (MDS) have been linked with employment in cosmetology in some investigations (7,119). Risk of CLL was not elevated among men or women using hair dyes in a population-based case-control study in Nebraska (120), nor in large cohorts of women (121) or men and women (56,57,122,123).

2. Diet and Other Lifestyle Factors

There has been little effort to evaluate other potential risk factors for CLL, such as diet or physical activity. In the absence of compelling clinical reports or other evidence linking such factors with CLL, it is unlikely that hypothesis-testing studies will evaluate these factors in the near future.

V. PRIOR MEDICAL HISTORY

The role of prior medical illnesses in the subsequent development of CLL has been investigated in epidemiological studies. Biological hypotheses suggest that infections, allergies, and autoimmune disorders may be associated with long-lasting effects on the immune system, particularly on the B-cell lymphocytes. Autoimmune diseases (lupus erythematosus, multiple sclerosis) may also predispose to CLL given that there is chronic immune dysregulation either arising from or leading to perturbations of lymphocytes.

In a large U.S. case-control study, no association was found between vaccinations or allergy desensitization shots and CLL (124). A small risk of CLL was linked with a history of three infections: syphilis, tuberculosis, and urinary tract infections. The investigators suggested that the association with syphilis might be due to the former use of arsenic in treatment regimens. They also found a small increased risk of CLL associated with history of appendectomy or tonsillectomy. A case-control study of leukemia in Shanghai, China (125) also showed an association with appendectomy; however, because CLL is rare in Asia, the case number was very small. This study also reported associations of

CLL with rheumatoid arthritis, hyperthyroidism, asthma, eczema, chronic infections other than tuberculosis, and use of salicylates. A positive association with prior use of diagnostic x-rays was also reported. In contrast, a case-control study in Yorkshire, England (126), found no association with appendectomy but did find an increased risk of CLL linked with history of migraine, scarlet fever, chronic ear infection, bronchitis, hypertension, and myocardial infarction and a recent history of herpes zoster and a history of malignancy. A large case-control study (127) found no association between various infections and autoimmune disorders and subsequent risk of CLL. However, the investigators reported a small protective effect for allergy-related disorders and surgical ablation of lymphoid tissue. Another case-control study on individuals from California found a decreased risk for CLL in patients with a history of rheumatoid arthritis (RR = 0.3) (128). The investigators also looked at risk of CLL and previous history of tuberculosis, bronchitis, hay fever, eczema, rheumatic fever, and musculoskeletal disease and found no associations.

Overall, results from studies assessing prior medical conditions or treatments and risk of CLL have shown no clear, consistent relationships. In the absence of consistent findings or intriguing clues, it is unclear that this approach is likely to be productive.

VI. FAMILIAL CLL

A family history of CLL or other lymphoproliferative disorders is one of the strongest risk factors for development of CLL. For more than 40 years, familial clustering of CLL, whether with other cases of CLL or other lymphoproliferative disorders, has been reported. In 1947, Videbaek published his seminal work on familial leukemia (129). Videbaek observed that the percentage of lymphoid leukemia was almost double that of myelogenous leukemia in the familial cases. Nearly 30 years later, Gunz published his study of more than 900 individuals in Australia with leukemia (130) and reported findings consistent with Videbaek in that first-degree relatives with leukemia were more frequent in families of cases with CLL than in those with CML. There have subsequently been numerous reports of familial aggregations of CLL (131–137).

Case-control studies show increased risks of leukemia and lymphoproliferative disorders among relatives of cases with CLL (138–140). The etiological factors responsible for these aggregations, whether genetic, shared environmental factors or a combination of both, remain to be explained. Data on possible candidate genes for CLL is reviewed in the following section. One interesting phenomenon observed in CLL is anticipation. Anticipation refers to the worsening severity or earlier age of onset in successive generations (141). Three separate groups of investigators have now reported observing anticipation in familial CLL. Horwitz et al. (141) first described this finding in CLL and AML families, showing a significant difference between the mean age at onset of leukemia in the parental generation and mean age at onset in affected individuals in the offspring generation (66 years versus 51 years). Yuille and colleagues confirmed this finding in 1998 (142), reporting a mean difference in average age of onset between generations of 22.1 years. Goldin et al. (143) observed a similar decrease in average age of onset of CLL between generations (66.7 years versus 50.7). To rule out a bias from changes in clinical screening practices, conservative assumptions about age of onset and information on extrapolated stage at diagnosis were included in the analyses. With this approach, the investigators did not find evidence for temporal changes in clinical screening practices as an explanation for anticipation. Although changes in clinical screening patterns may affect age at diagnosis, this does not appear to be the sole explanation for the observation of anticipation.

Anticipation has been reported in familial occurrence of numerous serious chronic diseases (144). One of the more quoted examples is Huntington disease, in which expansion of trinucleotide repeats (sequences of repeated amino acids) is shown to occur in younger and younger persons in subsequent generations (145). Whether similar genetic alterations may play a role in the anticipation in CLL remains to be determined.

VII. GENETICS OF CLL

Family studies are often the method whereby candidate disease genes are identified. A rapidly expanding body of literature documents genetic changes found in CLL. To date, no specific ''CLL gene'' has been identified, and the molecular pathogenesis of this disease remains largely unknown. Numerous reports on molecular abnormalities in CLL are helping to better delineate prognosis, including survival and response to treatment. This information may aid in therapeutic decision making. In addition to the relationship of specific genetic abnormalities to prognosis, it is also possible that an unknown fraction of genetic abnormalities associated with CLL may also be of etiological importance. This section will review the existing literature on genetic abnormalities associated with CLL from the epidemiological perspective. This information is summarized in Table 2. The reader is also referred to Chapters 2 and 16, which address molecular biology and chromosomal abnormalities of CLL.

A. Chromosome 6

Philip and colleagues evaluated chromosome 6 abnormalities in newly diagnosed cases of CLL using banding techniques (146). The investigators demonstrated alterations in 6% (11 of 193) cases: five cases showed 6p rearrangements, and six cases showed 6q rearrangements. This study also reported that cases with 6q aberrations were diagnosed at a significantly later stage at diagnosis compared with cases without 6q aberrations but this did not translate into a difference in survival. More recent studies point to three areas on the long arm of chromosome 6 that may be the regions of interest in CLL: 6q11-21, 6q21-23, and 6q25-27. Among 285 B-CLL cases evaluated using interphase fluorescent in situ hybridization (FISH), 7% (21 of 285) had 6q21 deletions and 3% (6 of 205) had 6q27 deletions (147). The six cases with 6q27 deletions also had 6q21 deletions. Clinical evaluation showed that patients with 6q deletions had higher white blood cell counts and greater lymphadenopathy compared with patients without 6q deletions, although overall survival did not differ. In a small study from Israel, Amiel et al. (148) found 6q27 deletions in 3 of 14 CLL patients. It is unclear what candidate gene exists at locus 6q21, although recently the TLX gene (a member of the steroid nuclear receptor family and potential tumor suppressor gene) was localized to this region (149).

B. Chromosome 11

Several gene regions on chromosome 11 are of interest as susceptibility loci for CLL. The *ATM* (mutated in ataxia-telangiectasia) gene located at region 11q22-q23 has been investigated as a putative CLL gene. Ataxia-telangiectasia is a rare, autosomal recessive disease characterized by phenotypic pleiotropy, which includes cerebellar degeneration

Table 2 Summary of Genetic Studies of CLL

Authors/year	Study population	Chromosomal abnormality	Method	Cases evaluated	Positive cases n (%)
(Philip et al., 1991)	Denmark	Chromosome 6	G-banding	193	11 (6)
(Gaidano et al., 1994)	Italy	6q27	Southern blot	100	4 (4)
(Amiel et al., 1999)	Israel	6q27 (deletion)	FISH	14	3 (21)
(Stilgenbauer et al., 1996)	Germany	6q21	FISH	285	21 (7)
		6q27		208	6 (3)
(Sola et al., 1999)	France	11q13 [t(11;14)] (Bcl 1/PRAD1 gene)	Rt-PCR and Western blot	111	4 (3)
(Gaidano et al., 1994)	Italy	11q13 [t(11;14)]	Southern blot	100	0
(Cuneo et al., 1997)	Italy	11q13 [t(11;14)]	G-banding and FISH	57	14 (25)
(Stankovic et al., 1999)	United Kingdom	11q22-23 (ATM)	Rt-PCR and Western blot	32	6 (18) (8/20 cases had decreased ATM protein)
(Dohner et al., 1997)	Germany	11q22-23	FISH	214	43 (20)
(Dohner et al., 1993)	Germany	12 (trisomy)	FISH	42	6 (14)
(Que et al., 1993)	United Kingdom	12 (trisomy)	FISH	183	21 (11)
(Cuneo et al., 1994)	Italy	12 (trisomy)	FISH	42	6 (14)
(Criel et al., 1994)	Belgium	12 (trisomy)	G-banding and FISH	111	16 (14)

Reference	Country	Locus	Method	N	Positive (%)
(Avet-Loiseau et al., 1996)	France	12 (trisomy)	FISH	100	16 (16)
(Woessner et al., 1996)	Spain	12 (trisomy)	FISH and G-banding	61	7 (12)
(Gahn et al., 1997)	Germany	12 (trisomy)	FISH	75	15 (20)
(Criel et al., 1997)	Belgium	12 (trisomy)	G-banding	296	32 (11)
(Geisler et al., 1997)	Denmark	12 (trisomy)	G-banding	480	40 (8)
(Acar and Connor, 1998)	Turkey	12 (trisomy)	FISH	26	4 (15)
(Nair et al., 1998)	India	12 (trisomy)	FISH	60	37 (62)
(Liso et al., 1999)	Italy	12 (trisomy)	FISH	23	6 (26)
(Garcia-Marco, 1996)	United Kingdom	13q12	FISH and G-banding	35	28 (80)
(Liu et al., 1992)	Sweden	13q14 (RB1 gene)	Q-banding and Southern blot	27	3 (11)
(Kroft et al., 1997)	United States	13q14	FISH and G-banding	78	23 (30)
(Gahn et al., 1997)	Germany	13q14 (RB1 gene)	FISH	30	6 (20)
(Stilgenbauer et al., 1998)	Germany	13q14	FISH	322	75 (23) RB1 / 121 (38) D13S25
(Hogan et al., 1999)	United States	13q14	FISH	54	26 (48)
(Avet-Loiseau et al., 1996)	France	13q14	FISH	100	31 (31)
(Geisler et al., 1997)	Denmark	Chromosome 17 (17p and 17q)	G-banding	480	8 (2)
(Dohner et al., 1997)	Germany	17p53	FISH	214	21 (10)
(Gaidano et al., 1994)	Italy	17q13 (p53 gene)	SSCP and direct sequencing	100	10 (10)

with progressive ataxia, oculocutaneous telangiectasias, immunodeficiency, sensitivity to ionizing radiation, and a notable predisposition to malignancy (150–152). There is 100-fold increased risk of cancer in patients with AT, and approximately 10% to 15% of patients who are ATM homozygotes develop a lymphoproliferative malignancy (153). Dohner demonstrated 11q22–23 deletions in 20% of cases with CLL (154).

Estimates of 11q deletions in sporadic B-CLL range from 20% to 32% (154,207). Studies of loss of heterozygosity (LOH) in ATM loci have shown 14% to be affected at various markers (155). LOH studies have shown that CLL cases with ATM mutations appear to have more aggressive disease and poorer survival (154). ATM protein expression appears to be markedly decreased in individuals with ATM deletions, and these individuals have shorter survival times than patients with normal ATM protein levels (155). This study showed that survival was significantly shorter in patients less than 55 years of age who also had decreased levels of ATM protein expression. A linkage study of ATM in 24 CLL families did not find evidence for an association (156).

Another site of interest on chromosome 11 is 11q13, the site of the PRAD/cyclin D1. The translocation t(11;14) (also known as BCL1 translocation), which brings the cyclin D1 gene under the control of the IgH gene located at 14q32, is now recognized as a hallmark molecular change in mantle cell lymphoma (157). A few studies have demonstrated this translocation in CLL cases (158,159) and it may be associated with atypical CLL (158) or with cases of poorly characterized B-cell chronic lymphoproliferative disorders (157).

C. Chromosome 12

Trisomy 12 is the most common chromosomal aberration seen in B-CLL with various reports citing 8% to 62% of cases affected (160–166, 208–210). FISH appears to be a more sensitive method for detecting chromosome 12 abnormalities compared with traditional banding techniques (161,162). Trisomy 12 has been associated with poorer survival (160) and with atypical lymphocyte morphology (167–170). It is not yet clear what region of chromosome 12 may be linked with B-CLL, but reports implicate band 12q13 as the site of the potential gene(s) (171,172). Although CLL is thought to be an abnormality of mature B-cells, one study has shown trisomy 12 detectable in CD34+/CD38+ hematological progenitor cells in a subset of CLL patients (165).

D. Chromosome 13

Abnormalities in chromosome 13 are the second most common abnormalities occurring in CLL, occurring in 11% to 48% of cases studied (see Table 2). Initial studies of chromosome 13 abnormalities in CLL seemed to point to the retinoblastoma gene (RBI)—a tumor suppressor gene located at 13q14 (163,173). However, further investigations suggest that alternate loci in the 13q14 regions including D13S25 (174–177), a region in close proximity to the RB1 gene, may in fact be the site of a novel tumor suppressor gene(s) involved in CLL. Another locus, D13S272 in the region of 13q14 and located very close to the *Leu* 1 and *Leu* 2 (leukemia-associated gene 1 and 2), has also been suggested as the site of tumor suppressor gene(s) involved in CLL (178,179); however, another investigation was not able to confirm this finding (180). Although most studies of chromosomal abnormalities in CLL examine peripheral blood lymphocytes and bone marrow lymphocytes, Gahn et al. studied 13q14 deletions in CD34+ selected progenitor cells (165). His group found that 20% of cases carry a 13q14 deletion in these stem cells, suggesting that pluripotent stem cells may undergo clonal transformation in CLL.

Some studies have shown 13q14 abnormalities to be associated with typical lymphocyte morphology in CLL (181), whereas others have not shown any clinical correlation with 13q14 changes (163). Starostik et al. found no difference in survival between patients with and without LOH at 13q14 (182). However, in patients with low β_2-microglobulin levels, individuals with LOH at 13q14 had significantly shorter survival than individuals without LOH, but these results were based on small numbers. When analyzed by stage, early-stage patients (Rai 0-II) with 13q14 LOH had a significantly shorter survival. Hogan showed that individuals with monosomy in the 13q14 region (RB1, D13S319, or D13S25 loci) had a longer treatment-free survival than individuals with diploidy at these loci, although the difference was not statistically significant (183). The other region of interest on chromosome 13 is the BRCA1 gene, encompassing 13q12; however, data on the role of this region have been mixed (184,185).

E. Chromosome 17

The p53 tumor suppressor gene, located at 17p13.1 is the most common genetic abnormality in cancer, and mutations of p53 have been associated with the Li-Fraumeni syndrome (186). However, p53 abnormalities appear to be infrequent findings in sporadic CLL (187). Approximately 10% of CLL cases are reported to have p53 abnormalities (154,188), and Gaidano et al. showed that these were due to mutations in the p53 gene rather than inactivation of p53 by amplification of the MDM2 gene. Mutations in p53 may be a more frequent finding in atypical subtypes of CLL such as CLL-PL (CLL-prolymphocytic subtype) (189), and it is possible that p53 plays a role in transformation of CLL to intermediate or high-grade non-Hodgkins lymphoma (190).

F. Immunoglobulin Gene Rearrangements and CLL

Until recently, B-CLL was thought to arise from naïve B-lymphocytes as demonstrated by germline configurations of V_H immunoglobulin gene sequences. New observations show that V_H genes may be either mutated or unmutated and that this finding may represent a novel prognostic indicator. Hamlin (191) evaluated 84 patients with CLL and found that 45% of cases had unmutated V_H genes and 55% had mutated V_H genes. Clinical correlation showed a significant correlation with mutation status: among stage A patients, individuals with mutated V_H genes had a median survival of 293 months compared with individuals with unmutated V_H genes who had a median survival of 95 months. Two groups have looked at V_H gene use in familial CLL. One group evaluated 12 families (Italian and French) and found that gene use was nonrandom and differed from frequencies reported among nonrelated patients (192). In contrast, another group evaluated 11 families (United States) and found a pattern of V_H gene use similar to sporadic CLL cases (193). These findings suggest that B-CLL is indeed a heterogeneous disease, not only at the clinical level but at the molecular level as well, and that CLL may arise from either memory B-cells or naïve B-cells.

G. Telomeres, Telomerase, and CLL

Telomeres are present on the end of eukaryotic chromosomes and function to prevent chromosome instability and DNA degradation. Telomeres are repeated amino acid sequences that are synthesized by the enzyme telomerase. Shortened telomeres and increased telomerase activity may play a role in human tumors. Several studies have looked at the relationship of telomere length and telomerase activity in CLL. Bechter et al. (194) showed that shorter telomere length was associated with a significantly shorter survival, and higher telomerase activity was observed in patients with more advanced disease. Trentin et al. (195) found higher telomerase activity in CLL versus normal lymphocytes, and higher activity was more often found in individuals with progressive rather than stable disease.

Although no single gene has been identified as a susceptibility gene for CLL, it is clear from mounting data that several chromosomal regions repeatedly show abnormalities. It is possible that one of the genes described earlier is in fact the "CLL gene," whereas the others play a role in the carcinogenesis pathway for CLL development. Another possibility is that CLL may be more heterogeneous than previously recognized and that multiple genetic paths can lead to the same phenotypic outcome—the development of CLL. Therefore, it is important in future genetic studies to continue to make clinicopathological correlations in an effort to better understand the genetic events that lead to CLL. In addition, because epidemiological studies of CLL seek to identify exposures that are etiologically associated with CLL, it will undoubtedly be useful to evaluate whether specific exposures are etiologically linked with distinct genetic abnormalities that characterize CLL, particularly those that are found to play an important role in the pathogenesis of this malignancy.

VIII. SECOND MALIGNANCIES SUBSEQUENT TO CLL

Because CLL is a cancer of the immune system, and immune dysfunction has been posited to play a role in carcinogenesis, second cancers may play an important role in the natural history of CLL. Second cancers may be particularly important in those patients with indolent CLL or early-stage disease, whose survival might otherwise be similar to those without CLL. Also of interest is whether therapy for CLL may play a role in development of second cancers.

Numerous case reports of second malignancies after CLL and more than 15 studies of populations of CLL patients with second malignancies have been published in the literature. Seven studies will be the focus of review here (Table 3). In addition, several studies have evaluated either specific types of cancer after CLL (e.g., lung, renal) or second malignancies after a specified treatment (fludarabine). These studies will also be mentioned in the text portion only of this section. Studies of second malignancies after CLL vary in numbers of primary CLL patients and method. Some authors chose to exclude cases that were diagnosed simultaneously with CLL and another malignancy or within 3 to 6 months of the diagnosis of CLL. Even if CLL is diagnosed simultaneously or shortly before a second malignancy, CLL could have existed for several years before diagnosis. Although the origins of CLL and a second malignancy may differ, a common etiological agent could contribute to both. Several studies had treatment data available and analyzed the contribution of this factor to development of second tumors.

Of the seven studies listed in Table 3, three are population based and four are hospital based. The studies are based on populations from Canada (196,197), the United States (198–200), and Europe (201,202). Numbers of CLL cases varied from 102 to 9456, and the range of second cancers diagnosed in each study was 13 to 840. The rates for second cancers ranged from 6.2% to 15.7%. In addition, in studies with small numbers of second tumors, the cancer subtype analyses may be based on a few cases only. The person-year

Table 3   Summary of Studies of Second Malignancies in CLL

Authors/year	Number of cases of CLL/study population	Type of registry	Total number of second malignancies	Relative risk (RR) of second malignancy (observed-expected ratio)
(Stavraky et al., 1970)	$n = 258$ (825 person-years)/Canada	Hospital	13	1.29 (for all sites) 1.89 (skin only)[a]
(Manusow and Weinerman, 1975)	$n = 102$ (395 person-years)/Canada	Hospital	16	3.18 (all sites) 8.14 (skin only)[a]
(Greene et al., 1978)	$n = 4869$ (16,584 person years)/United States	Population	234	1.1 (all sites) 6.7 (melanoma) 5.3 (connective tissue) 1.5 (lung)
(Davis et al., 1987)	$n = 419$ (1399 person years)/United States	Population	57	2.3 (non-lymphoid) 22.5 (soft tissue)[b] 4.2 (lung) 3.3 (colon) 2.7 (other sites) 5.6 (lymphoid)
(Travis et al., 1992)	$n = 9456$ (39,943 person-years)/United States	Population	840	1.28 (all sites, excluding NHL) 7.69 (Hodgkins disease) 3.97 (eye) 2.79 (melanoma) 1.98 (brain and central nervous system) 1.90 (lung) 1.20 (prostate) 1.51 (other ill-defined or unknown sites)
(Bertoldero et al., 1994)	$n = 212$/Italy	Hospital	19	1.4 (all sites) 16.7 (tongue)[c] 10 (thyroid)[c] 10 (gallbladder)[c] 3.5 (lung)
(Lauvin et al., 1996)	$n = 248$/France	Hospital	22 (non-lymphoma)	Risks not calculated (see text)

[a] Subtypes of skin cancer not given.
[b] Based on 2 cases.
[c] Based on 1 case.

follow-up ranged from 395 person-years to 39,943 person-years and was not given in two studies. With regard to gender, most of the studies showed risk of a second cancer not to be significantly different for men and women. Six of the seven studies calculated risk ratios on the basis of observed versus expected number of cancer cases. The two earliest studies give risks for skin cancer only, but the subtypes of skin cancer are not given, so comparison to later studies that tend to separate melanoma from nonmelanoma skin cancer is difficult. Most studies included second hematopoietic malignancies in the analyses; however, because cases of non-Hodgkins lymphoma and possibly other B-cell neoplasms may represent a clonal evolution of the underlying B-CLL, it may be more appropriate to exclude these types of cancers. Recent evidence shows that Hodkgin's disease (HD) arises from the B-cell lymphocyte (203). It is possible that HD after CLL represents a disease transformation or clonal selection similar to Richter syndrome.

All of the studies in Table 3 showed consistent increases in second malignancies of all sites, with risks ranging from 1.1 to 3.18. Davis et al analyzed lymphoid malignancies separately from nonlymphoid malignancies and found an increased risk of 5.6 for NHL, HD, and multiple myeloma (199). Travis et al. also found an increased risk for HD of 7.69 based on 13 cases (200). The risk of lung cancer as a second primary tumor was elevated in four of the studies, with risks ranging from 1.5 to 4.2 (198–201). Soft tissue sarcomas and connective tissue tumors were noted to be elevated in two studies with risk of 5.3 (198) and 22.5 (199); however, the second study is based on only two observed cases. Two studies showed elevated risks for skin cancer of 1.89 and 8.14; however, subtypes (basal cell, squamous cell, melanoma) were not given (196,197). Two studies showed elevated risks of 2.79 and 6.7 for melanoma (198,200), and Travis et al. also found an elevated risk of 3.97 for ocular melanoma (based on four cases) (200). Chemotherapy and radiation may have contributed to the increased risk of melanoma, lung cancer, and HD (198,200).

In a cohort of young (≤ 55 years old) CLL patients in Italy observed over a 10-year period, Mauro and colleagues found a second cancer rate of 4% compared with 14% among an older (> 55 years old) CLL cohort (204). The investigators also noted a similar rate of second malignancies between both treated (9.5%) and untreated (11%), although a higher rate of Richter's transformation (5.9% versus 1.2%) was seen among younger cases. Nucleoside analogues, primarily fludarabine, are now an important part of CLL treatment. Two large studies have reported follow-up of patients who have received either fludarabine or other nucleoside analogues for CLL. Among 174 patients treated with fludarabine as initial therapy between 1986 and 1993, six individuals (3%) died of second malignancies: liver cancer ($n = 1$), lung cancer ($n = 2$), ovarian cancer ($n = 1$), colon cancer ($n = 1$), and head and neck cancer ($n = 1$) (205). In the same study, one patient had HD develop, and nine patients had a Richter's transformation develop. In another study, Cheson et al. reviewed data on 724 patients who had received fludarabine for relapsed and refractory CLL (206). Among the 595 individuals for whom information on second malignancies was available, 83 (14%) second malignancies were reported. However, when NHL (18 cases), nonmelanotic skin cancer (3 cases), cancers diagnosed before or within 2 months of starting fludarabine (36 cases), or with a missing diagnosis date (3 cases) were excluded, this number fell to 23. With these exclusions, an excess risk of second cancers (1.65) was still seen. Of these 23 second cancers, the highest number of second tumors included lung ($n = 6$), gastrointestinal ($n = 5$), and bladder ($n = 2$). No cases of melanoma were reported, and 1 case each of sarcoma and CNS cancer was observed.

The risk of second malignancies appears consistently increased among individuals with CLL. There may be a higher rate of melanoma, sarcoma and other connective tissue cancers, lung, and colon cancer, although these increases have not been as consistently observed, and small numbers of cases make risk ratios somewhat unstable. Although treatment may play a role in this increased risk, it does not solely explain the rate of second malignancies, which are also seen among untreated patients. In addition, fludarabine does not appear to pose any greater risk than older treatments such as chlorambucil. It is likely that a combination of immune dysregulation, which is intrinsically part of CLL, underlying genetic alterations, and environmental and lifestyle exposures (such as benzene and cigarette smoking), may contribute to the development of second cancers.

IX. SUMMARY

In summary, research has led to an improved understanding of the natural history and biology of CLL. Within the past 20 years, the heterogeneity of the disease has become clear based on clinical observation. Advances in molecular biology are leading to insights into the genetic changes that accompany CLL. Despite all the progress, much remains to be understood about this disease. Although there are certain suspect etiological exposures such as certain prior medical conditions, the associated risks have not been overwhelmingly large or consistent. New techniques to evaluate small and complex chromosomal changes seem to pinpoint several possible candidate gene regions for CLL. In the coming years, future research should focus on better understanding the clinical heterogeneity of CLL and attempting to explain the specific molecular markers that may be important in defining etiologically distinct subtypes of the disease. Rather than there being a single pathway to the development of CLL, it is more likely that there are multiple potential leukemogenic pathways with various environmental and genetic factors interacting. Future epidemiological studies of environmental and other risk factors should attempt to include biospecimen collection as part of the study in an effort to identify "at-risk" phenotypes—that is, certain individuals who may be more susceptible to carcinogenic effects of certain agents.

REFERENCES

1. RA Cartwright, SM Bernard. Epidemiology. In: JA Whittaker, B Delemotte, eds. Leukaemia. Oxford: Blackwell Scientific Publications, 1985, pp 3–23.
2. MS Linet. The Leukemias: Epidemiologic Aspects. (6). New York: Oxford University Press. Monographs in epidemiology and biostatistics, 1985.
3. MS Linet, WA Blattner. The epidemiology of chronic lymphocytic leukemia. In: AS Polliack, D Catovsky, eds. Chronic lymphocytic leukemia. Chur, Switzerland: Harwood Academic Press, 1988, pp 11–32.
4. MS Linet, SS Devesa. Descriptive epidemiology of the leukemias. In: ES Henderson, TA Lister, eds. Leukemia. Philadelphia: W.B. Saunders Co., 1990, pp 207–224.
5. SC Finch, MS Linet. Chronic leukaemias. Baillieres Clin Haematol 5:27–56, 1992.
6. FD Groves, MS Linet, SS Devesa. Patterns of occurrence of the leukaemias. Eur J Cancer 31A:941–949, 1995.
7. MS Linet, RA Cartwright. The leukemias. In: D Schottenfeld, JF Fraumeni Jr., eds. Cancer Epidemiology and Prevention. New York: Oxford University Press, 1996, pp 841–892.
8. FD Groves, MS Linet, SS Devesa. Epidemiology of leukemia: Overview and patterns of occurrence. In: E Henderson, TA Lister, eds. Leukemia. Philadelphia: WB Saunders, 1996, pp 145–159.
9. GE Marti, FD Groves, MS Linet. Descriptive epidemiology of chronic lymphocytic leukemia. In: GE Marti, R Vogt, V Zenger, eds. Proceedings of the USPHS Workshop on Laboratory and Epidemiologic Approaches to Determining the Role of Environmental Exposures as Risk

Factors for B-Cell Chronic Lymphocytic Leukemia and Other B-cell Lymphoproliferative Disorders. Atlanta, Georgia: DHHS, PHS CDC, FDA, ATSDR, 1997, pp 165–172.

10. World Health Organization. International Classification of Disease. 9th ed. Geneva: World Health Organization, 1977.

11. World Health Organization. International Classification of Diseases for Oncology, Geneva, Switzerland: World Health Organization, 1976.

12. CL Percy, V Van Holten, C Muir. World Health Organization. International Classification of Diseases for Oncology. Second Edition. Geneva, Switzerland: World Health Organization, 1990.

13. A Criel, L Michaux, C De Wolf-Peeters. The concept of typical and atypical chronic lymphocytic leukaemia. Leuk Lymphoma 33:33–45, 1999.

14. JM Bennett, D Catovsky, MT Daniel, et al. Proposals for the classification of chronic (mature) B and T lymphoid leukaemias. French-American-British (FAB) Cooperative Group. J Clin Pathol 42:567–584, 1989.

15. A Criel, G Verhoef, R Vlietinck, et al. Further characterization of morphologically defined typical and atypical CLL: a clinical, immunophenotypic, cytogenetic and prognostic study on 390 cases. Br J Haematol 97:383–391, 1997.

16. DM Parkin, SL Whelan, J Ferlay, L Raymond, J Young. Cancer Incidence in Five Continents. Vol. 7. IARC Scientific Publication Number 143. Lyon, France, 1997.

17. LAG Ries, CL Kosary, BF Hankey, BA Miller, LX Clegg, BK Edwards. SEER Cancer Statistics Review, 1973–1996. NIH Pub. No. 99-2789. Bethesda, MD: National Cancer Institute, 1999, pp 262–283.

18. DR Boggs, SC Chen, ZN Zhang, A Zhang. Chronic lymphocytic leukemia in China. Am J Hematol 25:349–354, 1987.

19. H Asou, M Takechi, K Tanaka, et al. Japanese B cell chronic lymphocytic leukaemia: a cytogenetic and molecular biological study. Br J Haematol 85:492–497, 1993.

20. PM Chen, SH Lin, SF Fan, et al. Genotypic characterization and multivariate survival analysis of chronic lymphocytic leukemia in Taiwan. Acta Haematol 97:196–204, 1997.

21. TS Kumaravel, D Chendil, M Arif, et al. Cytogenetic and molecular genetic studies on Indian patients with chronic lymphocytic leukemia. Int J Hematol 64:31–37, 1996.

22. C Rozman, F Bosch, E Montserrat. Chronic lymphocytic leukemia: a changing natural history? Leukemia 11:775–778, 1997.

23. LF Diehl, LH Karnell, HR Menck. The American College of Surgeons Commission on Cancer and the American Cancer Society. The National Cancer Data Base report on age, gender, treatment, and outcomes of patients with chronic lymphocytic leukemia. Cancer 86:2684–2692, 1999.

24. M Keating. Chronic lymphocytic leukemia. In: ES Henderson, TA Lister, MF Greaves, eds. Leukemia. Philadelphia: W.B. Saunders Co., 1996, pp 554–586.

25. RR Monson. Occupational Epidemiology. Boca Raton, Fl: CRC Press, 1990.

26. L Tomatis, C Agthe, H Bartsch, et al. Evaluation of the carcinogenicity of chemicals: a review of the Monograph Program of the International Agency for Research on Cancer (1971 to 1977). Cancer Res 38:877–885, 1978.

27. IARC. Chemicals, groups of chemicals, complex mixtures, physical and biological agents and exposure circumstances to be evaluated in future IARC monographs. Report of an ad-hoc working group. IARC Intern. Rep. No. 931005. Lyon, France, 1993.

28. JD Boice Jr, CE Land, DL Preston. Ionizing radiation. In: D Schottenfeld, JF Fraumeni, Jr. eds. Cancer Epidemiology and Prevention, New York: Oxford University Press, 1996, pp 319–354.

29. JD Boice Jr, JH Lubin. Occupational and environmental radiation and cancer. Cancer Causes Control 8:309–322, 1997.

30. E Ron. Ionizing radiation and cancer risk: evidence from epidemiology. Radiat Res 150: S30–S41, 1998.

31. CJ Portier, MS Wolfe. Assessment of Health Effects from Exposure to Power-Line Frequency Electric and Magnetic Fields. Working Group Report. NIH Pub. No. 98-3981, 108–116.

United States, National Institute of Environmental Health Sciences. U.S. National Institutes of Health. USDHHS, 1998.

32. LI Kheifets, AA Afifi, PA Buffler, ZW Zhang, CC Matkin. Occupational electric and magnetic field exposure and leukemia. A meta-analysis. J Occup Environ Med 39:1074–1091, 1997.

33. B Floderus, T Persson, C Stenlund, A Wennberg, A Ost, B Knave. Occupational exposure to electromagnetic fields in relation to leukemia and brain tumors: a case-control study in Sweden. Cancer Causes Control 4:465–476, 1993.

34. M Feychting, U Forssen, B Floderus. Occupational and residential magnetic field exposure and leukemia and central nervous system tumors. Epidemiology 8:384–389, 1997.

35. G Theriault, M Goldberg, AB Miller, et al. Cancer risks associated with occupational exposure to magnetic fields among electric utility workers in Ontario and Quebec, Canada, and France: 1970–1989. Am J Epidemiol, 139:550–572, 1994.

36. RA Rinsky, AB Smith, R Hornung, et al. Benzene and leukemia. An epidemiologic risk assessment. N Engl J Med 316:1044–1050, 1987.

37. DF Utterback, RA Rinsky. Benzene exposure assessment in rubber hydrochloride workers: a critical evaluation of previous estimates. Am J Ind Med 27:661–676, 1995.

38. RB Hayes, SN Yin, M Dosemeci, et al. Benzene and the dose-related incidence of hematologic neoplasms in China. Chinese Academy of Preventive Medicine—National Cancer Institute Benzene Study Group. J Natl Cancer Inst 89:1065–1071, 1997.

39. GK Raabe, O Wong. Leukemia mortality by cell type in petroleum workers with potential exposure to benzene. Environ Health Perspect, 104(Suppl 6):1381–92:1381–1392, 1996.

40. PA Bertazzi, AC Pesatori, C Zocchetti, R Latocca. Mortality study of cancer risk among oil refinery workers. Int Arch Occup Environ Health 61:261–270, 1989.

41. C Wongsrichanalai, E Delzell, P Cole. Mortality from leukemia and other diseases among workers at a petroleum refinery. J Occup Med 31:106–111, 1989.

42. GM Marsh, PE Enterline, D McCraw. Mortality patterns among petroleum refinery and chemical plant workers. Am J Ind Med 19:29–42, 1991.

43. O Wong, F Harris, TJ Smith. Health effects of gasoline exposure. II. Mortality patterns of distribution workers in the United States. Environ Health Perspect 101(suppl 6):63–76, 1993.

44. L Rushton. A 39-year follow-up of the U.K. oil refinery and distribution center studies: results for kidney cancer and leukemia. Environ Health Perspect 101(suppl 6):77–84, 1993.

45. AR Schnatter, TW Armstrong, MJ Nicolich, et al. Lymphohaematopoietic malignancies and quantitative estimates of exposure to benzene in Canadian petroleum distribution workers. Occup Environ Med 53:773–781, 1996.

46. O Wong, L Trent, F Harris. Nested case-control study of leukaemia, multiple myeloma, and kidney cancer in a cohort of petroleum workers exposed to gasoline. Occup Environ Med 56:217–221, 1999.

47. Y Honda, E Delzell, P Cole. An updated study of mortality among workers at a petroleum manufacturing plant. J Occup Environ Med 37:194–200, 1995.

48. N Sathiakumar, E Delzell, P Cole, I Brill, J Frisch, G Spivey. A case-control study of leukemia among petroleum workers. J Occup Environ Med 37:1269–1277, 1995.

49. BJ Divine, CM Hartman, JK Wendt. Update of the Texaco mortality study 1947–93: Part II. Analyses of specific causes of death for white men employed in refining, research, and petrochemicals. Occup Environ Med 56:174–180, 1999.

50. E Lynge, A Andersen, R Nilsson, et al. Risk of cancer and exposure to gasoline vapors. Am J Epidemiol 145:449–458, 1997.

51. AJ Fox, PF Collier. A survey of occupational cancer in the rubber and cablemaking industries: analysis of deaths occurring in 1972–74. Br J Ind Med 33:249–264, 1976.

52. HG Parkes, CA Veys, JA Waterhouse, A Peters. Cancer mortality in the British rubber industry. Br J Ind Med 39:209–220, 1982.

53. TF Mancuso. Epidemiological investigation of occupational cancers in the rubber industry. In: C Levinson, ed. The New Multinational Health Hazards. Geneva: ICF, 1975, pp 80–136.

54. E Delzell, RR Monson. Mortality among rubber workers. III. Cause-specific mortality, 1940–1978. J Occup Med 23:677–684, 1981.

55. AJ McMichael, R Spirtas, JF Gamble, PM Tousey. Mortality among rupper workers: Relationship to specific jobs. J Occup Med 18:178–185, 1976.

56. EWJ Arp, PH Wolf, H Checkoway. Lymphocytic leukemia and exposures to benzene and other solvents in the rubber industry. J Occup Med 25:598–602, 1983.

57. TC Wilcosky, H Checkoway, EG Marshall, HA Tyroler. Cancer mortality and solvent exposures in the rubber industry. Am Ind Hyg Assoc J 45:809–811, 1984.

58. H Checkoway, T Wilcosky, P Wolf, H Tyroler. An evaluation of the associations of leukemia and rubber industry solvent exposures. Am J Ind Med 5:239–249, 1984.

59. T Sorahan, HG Parkes, CA Veys, JA Waterhouse, JK Straughan, A Nutt. Mortality in the British rubber industry 1946–85. Br J Ind Med 46:1–10, 1989.

60. M Kogevinas, M Sala, P Boffetta, N Kazerouni, H Kromhout, S Hoar-Zahm. Cancer risk in the rubber industry: a review of the recent epidemiological evidence. Occup Environ Med 55:1–12, 1998.

61. RR Monson, KK Nakano. Mortality among rubber workers. I. White male union employees in Akro, Ohio. Am J Epdemiol, 103:284–296, 1976.

62. JT Hodgson, RD Jones. Mortality of styrene production, polymerization and processing workers at a site in northwest England. Scand J Work Environ Health 11:347–352, 1985.

63. TD Downs, MM Crane, KW Kim. Mortality among workers at a butadiene facility. Am J Ind Med 12:311–329, 1987.

64. MG Ott, RC Kolesar, HC Scharnweber, EJ Schneider, JR Venable. A mortality survey of employees engaged in the development or manufacture of styrene-based products. J Occup Med 22:445–460, 1980.

65. RR Monson, LJ Fine. Cancer mortality and morbidity among rubber workers. J Natl Cancer Inst 61:1047–1053, 1978.

66. O Wong. A cohort mortality study and a case-control study of workers potentially exposed to styrene in the reinforced plastics and composites industry. Br J Ind Med 47:753–762, 1990.

67. GM Matanoski, C Santos-Burgoa, L Schwartz. Mortality of a cohort of workers in the styrene-butadiene polymer manufacturing industry (1943–1982). Environ Health Perspect, 86:107–17:107–117, 1990.

68. P Cole, E Delzell, J Acquavella. Exposure to butadiene and lymphatic and hematopoietic cancer. Epidemiology, 4:96–103, 1993.

69. C Santos-Burgoa, GM Matanoski, S Zeger, L Schwartz. Lymphohematopoietic cancer in styrene-butadiene polymerization workers. Am J Epidemiol 136:843–854, 1992.

70. M Kogevinas, G Ferro, R Saracci, et al. Cancer mortality in an international cohort of workers exposed to styrene. IARC Sci Publ 127:289–300, 1993.

71. BJ Divine, JK Wendt, CM Hartman. Cancer mortality among workers at a butadiene production facility. IARC Sci Publ 127:345–362, 1993.

72. HA Kolstad, E Lynge, J Olsen, N Breum. Incidence of lymphohematopoietic malignancies among styrene-exposed workers of the reinforced plastics industry. Scand J Work Environ Health 20:272–278, 1994.

73. C Hogstedt, O Rohlen, BS Berndtsson, O Axelson, I Ehrenberg. A cohort study of mortality and cancer incidence in ethylene oxide production workers. Br J Ind Med 36:276–280, 1979.

74. C Hogstedt, N Malmqvist, B Wadman. Leukemia in workers exposed to ethylene oxide. JAMA 241:1132–1133, 1979.

75. C Hogstedt, L Aringer, A Gustavsson. Ethylene oxide and cancer-review of the literature and follow-up of two studies. Arbete Halsa 1:1984.

76. C Hogstedt, L Aringer, A Gustavsson. Epidemiologic support for ethylene oxide as a cancer-causing agent. JAMA 255:1575–1578, 1986.

77. WM Snellings, CS Weil, RR Maronpot. A two-year inhalation study of the carcinogenic potential of ethylene oxide in Fischer 344 rats. Toxicol Appl Pharmacol 75:105–117, 1984.

78. L Stayner, K Steenland, A Greife, et al. Exposure-response analysis of cancer mortality in a cohort of workers exposed to ethylene oxide. Am J Epidemiol 138:787–798, 1993.
79. K Steenland, L Stayner, A Greife, et al. Mortality among workers exposed to ethylene oxide. N Engl J Med 324:1402–1407, 1991.
80. HL Greenberg, MG Ott, RE Shore. Men assigned to ethylene oxide production or other ethylene oxide related chemical manufacturing: a mortality study. Br J Ind Med 47:221–230, 1990.
81. LO Benson, MJ Teta. Mortality due to pancreatic and lymphopoietic cancers in chlorohydrin production workers. Br J Ind Med 50:710–716, 1993.
82. A Theiss, R Frentzel-Beyme, R Link. Mortality study on employees exposed to alkylene oxides (ethylene oxide/propylene oxide) and their derivatives. 249–259. 1981. Geneva, International Labor Office. Prevention of Occupational Cancer—International Symposium. Occupational and Health Series. No. 46.
83. MJ Gardner, D Coggon, B Pannett, EC Harris. Workers exposed to ethylene oxide: a follow up study. Br J Ind Med 46:860–865, 1989.
84. RW Morgan, KW Claxton, BJ Divine, SD Kaplan, VB Harris. Mortality among ethylene oxide workers. J Occup Med 23:767–770, 1981.
85. MJ Teta, LO Benson, JN Vitale. Mortality study of ethylene oxide workers in chemical manufacturing: a 10 year update. Br J Ind Med 50:704–709, 1993.
86. RE Shore, MJ Gardner, B Pannett. Ethylene oxide: an assessment of the epidemiological evidence on carcinogenicity. Br J Ind Med 50:971–997, 1993.
87. WJ Hunter, BA Henman, DM Bartlett, G Le, I. Mortality of professional chemists in England and Wales, 1965–1989. Am J Ind Med 23:615–627, 1993.
88. S Cordier, ML Mousel, C Le Goaster, et al. Cancer risk among workers in biomedical research. Scand J Work Environ Health 21:450–459, 1995.
89. C Burnett, C Robinson, J Walker. Cancer mortality in health and science technicians. Am J Ind Med 36:155–158, 1999.
90. P Gustavsson, C Reuterwall, J Sadigh, M Soderholm. Mortality and cancer incidence among laboratory technicians in medical research and routine laboratories (Sweden). Cancer Causes Control 10:59–64, 1999.
91. M Dosemeci, M Alavanja, R Vetter, B Eaton, A Blair. Mortality among laboratory workers employed at the U.S. Department of Agriculture. Epidemiology, 3:258–262, 1992.
92. A Blair, SH Zahm, NE Pearce, EF Heineman, JF Fraumeni, Jr. Clues to cancer etiology from studies of farmers. Scand J Work Environ Health 18:209–215, 1992.
93. A Blair, SH Zahm. Agricultural exposures and cancer. Environ Health Perspect, 103(suppl 8):205–8:205–208, 1995.
94. A Blair, DW White. Leukemia cell types and agricultural practices in Nebraska. Arch Environ Health 40:211–214, 1985.
95. LM Brown, A Blair, R Gibson, et al. Pesticide exposures and other agricultural risk factors for leukemia among men in Iowa and Minnesota. Cancer Res 50:6585–6591, 1990.
96. C Kelleher, J Newell, C MacDonagh-White, et al. Incidence and occupational pattern of leukaemias, lymphomas, and testicular tumours in western Ireland over an 11 year period. J Epidemiol Community Health 52:651–656, 1998.
97. U Flodin, M Fredriksson, B Persson, O Axelson. Chronic lymphatic leukaemia and engine exhausts, fresh wood, and DDT: a case-referent study. Br J Ind Med 45:33–38, 1988.
98. D Amadori, O Nanni, F Falcini, et al. Chronic lymphocytic leukaemias and non-Hodgkin's lymphomas by histological type in farming-animal breeding workers: a population case-control study based on job titles. Occup Environ Med 52:374–379, 1995.
99. MC Alavanja, A Blair, MN Masters. Cancer mortality in the U.S. flour industry. J Natl Cancer Inst 82:840–848, 1990.
100. J Clavel, D Hemon, L Mandereau, B Delemotte, F Severin, G Flandrin. Farming, pesticide use and hairy-cell leukemia. Scand J Work Environ Health 22:285–293, 1996.

101. PA Gilman, RG Ames, MA McCawley. Leukemia risk among U.S. white male coal miners. A case-control study. J Occup Med 27:669–671, 1985.

102. RA Cartwright, JG Miller, DA Scarisbrick. Leukaemia in a carpet factory: an epidemiological investigation. J Soc Occup Med 37:42–43, 1987.

103. TR O'Brien, P Decoufle. Cancer mortality among northern Georgia carpet and textile workers. Am J Ind Med 14:15–24, 1988.

104. J Burkhardt. Leukemia in hospitals with occupational exposure to the sawmill industry. West J Med 137:155–159, 1982.

105. JJ Spinelli, RP Gallagher, PR Band, WJ Threlfall. Multiple myeloma, leukemia, and cancer of the ovary in cosmetologists and hairdressers. Am J Ind Med 6:97–102, 1984.

106. MJ Teta, J Walrath, JW Meigs, JT Flannery. Cancer incidence among cosmetologists. J Natl Cancer Inst 72:1051–1057, 1984.

107. KL Hunting, H Longbottom, SS Kalavar, F Stern, E Schwartz, LS Welch. Haematopoietic cancer mortality among vehicle mechanics. Occup Environ Med 52:673–678, 1995.

108. E Kagan, RJ Jacobson, KY Yeung, DJ Haidak, GH Nachnani. Asbestos-associated neoplasms of B cell lineage. Am J Med 67:325–330, 1979.

109. DA Schwartz, TL Vaughan, NJ Heyer, et al. B cell neoplasms and occupational asbestos exposure. Am J Ind Med 14:661–671, 1988.

110. L Markovic-Denic, S Jankovic, J Marinkovic, Z Radovanovic. Brick mortar exposure and chronic lymphocytic leukemia. Neoplasma 42:79–81, 1995.

111. E Lynge. A follow-up study of cancer incidence among workers in manufacture of phenoxy herbicides in Denmark. Br J Cancer 52:259–270, 1985.

112. H Austin, P Cole. Cigarette smoking and leukemia. J Chron Dis 39:417–421, 1986.

113. L Garfinkel, P Boffetta. Association between smoking and leukemia in two American Cancer Society prospective studies. Cancer 65:2356–2360, 1990.

114. LJ Kinlen, E Rogot. Leukaemia and smoking habits among United States veterans. BMJ, 297:657–659, 1988.

115. MS Linet, JK McLaughlin, AW Hsing, et al. Cigarette smoking and leukemia: results from the Lutheran Brotherhood Cohort Study. Cancer Causes Control 2:413–417, 1991.

116. LM Brown, GD Everett, R Gibson, LF Burmeister, LM Schuman, A Blair. Smoking and risk of non-Hodgkin's lymphoma and multiple myeloma. Cancer Causes Control. 3:49–55, 1992.

117. GD Friedman. Cigarette smoking, leukemia, and multiple myeloma. Ann Epidemiol 3:425–428, 1993.

118. J Adami, O Nyren, R Bergstrom, et al. Smoking and the risk of leukemia, lymphoma, and multiple myeloma (Sweden). Cancer Causes Control, 9:49–56, 1998.

119. L Miligi, CA Seniori, P Crosignani, et al. Occupational, environmental, and life-style factors associated with the risk of hematolymphopoietic malignancies in women. Am J Ind Med 36:60–69, 1999.

120. SH Zahm, DD Weisenburger, PA Babbitt, RC Saal, JB Vaught, A Blair. Use of hair coloring products and the risk of lymphoma, multiple myeloma, and chronic lymphocytic leukemia. Am J Public Health 82:990–997, 1992.

121. F Grodstein, CH Hennekens, GA Colditz, DJ Hunter, MJ Stampfer. A prospective study of permanent hair dye use and hematopoietic cancer. J Natl Cancer Inst 86:1466–1470, 1994.

122. MJ Thun, SF Altekruse, MM Namboodiri, EE Calle, DG Myers, CWJ Heath. Hair dye use and risk of fatal cancers in U.S. women. J Natl Cancer Inst 86:210–215, 1994.

123. SF Altekruse, SJ Henley, MJ Thun. Deaths from hematopoietic and other cancers in relation to permanent hair dye use in a large prospective study (United States). Cancer Causes Control 10:617–625, 1999.

124. KA Rosenblatt, TD Koepsell, JR Daling, et al. Antigenic stimulation and the occurrence of chronic lymphocytic leukemia. Am J Epidemiol 134:22–28, 1991.

125. W Zheng, XO Shu, RP Pan, YT Gao, JF Fraumeni, Jr. Prior medical conditions and the risk of adult leukemia in Shanghai, People's Republic of China. Cancer Causes Control 4:361–368, 1993.

126. RA Cartwright, SM Bernard, CC Bird, et al. Chronic lymphocytic leukaemia: case control epidemiological study in Yorkshire. Br J Cancer 56:79–82, 1987.

127. M Linet, LD McCaffrey, RL Humphrey, et al. Chronic lymphocytic leukemia and acquired disorders affecting the immune system: a case-control study. J Natl Cancer Inst 77:371–378, 1986.

128. MM Doody, AG Glass, GD Friedman, LM Pottern, JDJ Boice, JF Fraumeni, Jr. Leukemia, lymphoma, and multiple myeloma following selected medical conditions. Cancer Causes Control 3:449–456, 1992.

129. A Videbaek. Familial leukemia. A preliminary report. Acta Medica Scand 127:26–52, 1947.

130. FW Gunz, JP Gunz, AM Veale, CJ Chapman, IB Houston. Familial leukaemia: a study of 909 families. Scand J Haematol 15:117–131, 1975.

131. EB Reilly, SI Rapaport, NW Karr, H Mills, RA Cartwright. Familial chronic lymphatic leukemia. Arch Inter Med 90:87–89, 1952.

132. FW Gunz, W Dameshek. Chronic lymphocytic leukemia in a family, including twin brothers and a son. JAMA 164:1323–1325, 1957.

133. JF Fraumeni Jr, CL Vogel, VT DeVita. Familial chronic lymphocytic leukemia. Ann Intern Med 71:279–284, 1969.

134. M Schweitzer, CJ Melief, JE Ploem. Chronic lymphocytic leukaemia in 5 siblings. Scand J Haematol 11:97–105, 1973.

135. WA Blattner, W Strober, AV Muchmore, RM Blaese, S Broder, JF Jr. Fraumeni. Familial chronic lymphocytic leukemia. Immunologic and cellular characterization. Ann Intern Med 84:554–557, 1976.

136. F Brok-Simoni, G Rechavi, N Katzir, I Ben-Bassat. Chronic lymphocytic leukaemia in twin sisters: monozygous but not identical. Lancet 1:329–330, 1987.

137. F Fernhout, RB Dinkelaar, A Hagemeijer, K Groeneveld, E van Kammen, JJ van Dongen. Four aged siblings with B cell chronic lymphocytic leukemia. Leukemia 11:2060–2065, 1997.

138. MS Linet, ML Van Natta, R Brookmeyer, et al. Familial cancer history and chronic lymphocytic leukemia. A case-control study. Am J Epidemiol 130:655–664, 1989.

139. J Cuttner. Increased incidence of hematologic malignancies in first-degree relatives of patients with chronic lymphocytic leukemia. Cancer Invest 10:103–109, 1992.

140. Z Radovanovic, L Markovic-Denic, S Jankovic. Cancer mortality of family members of patients with chronic lymphocytic leukemia. Eur J Epidemiol 10:211–213, 1994.

141. M Horwitz, EL Goode, GP Jarvik. Anticipation in familial leukemia. Am J Hum Genet 59:990–998, 1996.

142. MR Yuille, RS Houlston, D Catovsky. Anticipation in familial chronic lymphocytic leukaemia. Leukemia 12:1696–1698, 1998.

143. LR Goldin, M Sgambati, GE Marti, L Fontaine, N Ishibe. Anticipation in familial chronic lymphocytic leukemia. Am J Hum Genet 65:265–269, 1999.

144. MG McInnis. Anticipation: an old idea in new genes. Am J Hum Genet 59:973–979, 1996.

145. NG Ranen, OC Stine, MH Abbott, et al. Anticipation and instability of IT-15 (CAG)n repeats in parent-offspring pairs with Huntington disease. Am J Hum Genet 57:593–602, 1995.

146. P Philip, C Geisler, MM Hansen, et al. Aberrations of chromosome 6 in 193 newly diagnosed untreated cases of chronic lymphocytic leukemia. Cancer Genet Cytogenet 53:35–43, 1991.

147. S Stilgenbauer, L Bullinger, A Benner, et al. Incidence and clinical significance of 6q deletions in B cell chronic lymphocytic leukemia. Leukemia 13:1331–1334, 1999.

148. A Amiel, I Mulchanov, A Elis, et al. Deletion of 6q27 in chronic lymphocytic leukemia and multiple myeloma detected by fluorescence in situ hybridization. Cancer Genet Cytogenet 112:53–56, 1999.

149. A Jackson, P Panayiotidis, L Foroni. The human homologue of the *Drosophila* tailless gene (TLX): characterization and mapping to a region of common deletion in human lymphoid leukemia on chromosome 6q21. Genomics 50:34–43, 1998.

150. K Savitsky, A Bar-Shira, S Gilad, et al. A single ataxia telangiectasia gene with a product similar to PI-3 kinase. Science 268:1749–1753, 1995.

151. I Vorechovsky, L Luo, A Lindblom, et al. ATM mutations in cancer families. Cancer Res 56:4130–4133, 1996.

152. KD Brown, A Chakravarti. Multiple ATM-dependent pathways: an explanation for pleiotropy. Am J Hum Genet 64:46–50, 1999.

153. AM Taylor, JA Metcalfe, J Thick, YF Mak. Leukemia and lymphoma in ataxia telangiectasia. Blood 87:423–438, 1996.

154. H Dohner, S Stilgenbauer, MR James, et al. 11q deletions identify a new subset of B-cell chronic lymphocytic leukemia characterized by extensive nodal involvement and inferior prognosis. Blood 89:2516–2522, 1997.

155. P Starostik, T Manshouri, S O'Brien, et al. Deficiency of the ATM protein expression defines an aggressive subgroup of B-cell chronic lymphocytic leukemia. Cancer Res 58:4552–4557, 1998.

156. S Bevan, D Catovsky, A Marossy, et al. Linkage analysis for ATM in familial B cell chronic lymphocytic leukaemia. Leukemia 13:1497–1500, 1999.

157. V Levy, V Ugo, A Delmer, et al. Cyclin D1 overexpression allows identification of an aggressive subset of leukemic lymphoproliferative disorder. Leukemia 13:1343–1351, 1999.

158. A Cuneo, R Bigoni, M Negrini, et al. Cytogenetic and interphase cytogenetic characterization of atypical chronic lymphocytic leukemia carrying BCL1 translocation. Cancer Res 57:1144–1150, 1997.

159. B Sola, V Salaun, JJ Ballet, X Troussard. Transcriptional and post-transcriptional mechanisms induce cyclin-D1 over-expression in B-chronic lymphoproliferative disorders. Int J Cancer 83:230–234, 1999.

160. G Juliusson, DG Oscier, M Fitchett, et al. Prognostic subgroups in B-cell chronic lymphocytic leukemia defined by specific chromosomal abnormalities. N Engl J Med 323:720–724, 1990.

161. H Dohner, S Pohl, M Bulgay-Morschel, S Stilgenbauer, M Bentz, P Lichter. Trisomy 12 in chronic lymphoid leukemias—a metaphase and interphase cytogenetic analysis. Leukemia 7:516–520, 1993.

162. A Cuneo, R Bigoni, M Balboni, et al. Trisomy 12 in chronic lymphocytic leukemia and hairy cell leukemia: a cytogenetic and interphase cytogenetic study. Leuk Lymphoma 15:167–172, 1994.

163. H Avet-Loiseau, MC Devilder, R Garand, et al. 13q14 deletions are not primary events in B-cell chronic lymphocytic leukemia: a study of 100 patients using fluorescence in situ hybridization. Clin Cancer Res 2:1673–1677, 1996.

164. R Bigoni, A Cuneo, MG Roberti, et al. Chromosome aberrations in atypical chronic lymphocytic leukemia: a cytogenetic and interphase cytogenetic study. Leukemia 11:1933–1940, 1997.

165. B Gahn, C Schafer, J Neef, et al. Detection of trisomy 12 and Rb-deletion in CD34+ cells of patients with B-cell chronic lymphocytic leukemia. Blood 89:4275–4281, 1997.

166. H Acar, MJ Connor. Detection of trisomy 12 and centromeric alterations in CLL by interphase- and metaphase-FISH. Cancer Genet Cytogenet 100:148–151, 1998.

167. TH Que, JG Marco, J Ellis, et al. Trisomy 12 in chronic lymphocytic leukemia detected by fluorescence in situ hybridization: analysis by stage, immunophenotype, and morphology. Blood 82:571–575, 1993.

168. A Criel, I Wlodarska, P Meeus, et al. Trisomy 12 is uncommon in typical chronic lymphocytic leukaemias. Br J Haematol 87:523–528, 1994.

169. S Woessner, F Sole, A Perez-Losada, L Florensa, RM Vila. Trisomy 12 is a rare cytogenetic finding in typical chronic lymphocytic leukemia. Leuk Res 20:369–374, 1996.

170. DG Oscier, E Matutes, A Copplestone, et al. Atypical lymphocyte morphology: an adverse prognostic factor for disease progression in stage A CLL independent of trisomy 12. Br J Haematol, 98:934–939, 1997.

171. M Merup, G Juliusson, X Wu, et al. Amplification of multiple regions of chromosome 12, including 12q13-15, in chronic lymphocytic leukaemia. Eur J Haematol 58:174–180, 1997.

172. AD Stock, TR Dennis. A translocation breakpoint at chromosome band 12q13 associated with B-cell chronic lymphocytic leukemia. Cancer Genet Cytogenet 111:166–168, 1999.

173. Y Liu, D Grander, S Soderhall, G Juliusson, G Gahrton, S Einhorn. Retinoblastoma gene deletions in B-cell chronic lymphocytic leukemia. Genes Chromosomes Cancer 4:250–256, 1992.

174. AG Brown, FM Ross, EM Dunne, CM Steel, EM Weir-Thompson. Evidence for a new tumor suppressor locus (DBM) in human B-cell neoplasia telomeric to the retinoblastoma gene. Nat Genet 3:67–72, 1993.

175. LA Hawthorn, R Chapman, D Oscier, JK Cowell. The consistent 13q14 translocation breakpoint seen in chronic B-cell leukaemia (BCLL) involves deletion of the D13S25 locus which lies distal to the retinoblastoma predisposition gene. Oncogene 8:1415–1419, 1993.

176. Y Liu, L Szekely, D Grander, et al. Chronic lymphocytic leukemia cells with allelic deletions at 13q14 commonly have one intact RBI gene: evidence for a role of an adjacent locus. Proc Natl Acad Sci USA 90:8697–8701, 1993.

177. S Stilgenbauer, J Nickolenko, J Wilhelm, et al. Expressed sequences as candidates for a novel tumor suppressor gene at band 13q14 in B-cell chronic lymphocytic leukemia and mantle cell lymphoma. Oncogene 16:1891–1897, 1998.

178. Y Liu, M Corcoran, O Rasool, et al. Cloning of two candidate tumor suppressor genes within a 10 kb region on chromosome 13q14, frequently deleted in chronic lymphocytic leukemia. Oncogene 15:2463–2473, 1997.

179. MM Corcoran, O Rasool, Y Liu, et al. Detailed molecular delineation of 13q14.3 loss in B-cell chronic lymphocytic leukemia. Blood 91:1382–1390, 1998.

180. G Rondeau, I Moreau, S Bezieau, E Cadoret, JP Moisan, MC Devilder. Exclusion of Leu1 and Leu2 genes as tumor suppressor genes in 13q14.3-deleted B-CLL. Leukemia 13:1630–1632, 1999.

181. SH Kroft, WG Finn, NE Kay, LC Peterson. Isolated 13q14 abnormalities and normal karyotypes are associated with typical lymphocyte morphology in B-cell chronic lymphocytic leukemia. Am J Clin Pathol 107:275–282, 1997.

182. P Starostik, S O'Brien, CY Chung, et al. The prognostic significance of 13q14 deletions in chronic lymphocytic leukemia. Leuk Res 23:795–801, 1999.

183. WJ Hogan, A Tefferi, TJ Borell, R Jenkins, CY Li, TE Witzig. Prognostic relevance of monosomy at the 13q14 locus detected by fluorescence in situ hybridization in B-cell chronic lymphocytic leukemia. Cancer Genet Cytogenet 110:77–81, 1999.

184. JA Garcia-Marco. Frequent somatic deletion of the 13q12.3 locus encompassing BRCA2 in chronic lymphocytic leukemia. Blood 88:1568–1575, 1996.

185. P Panayiotidis, K Ganeshaguru, C Rowntree, SA Jabbar, VA Hoffbrand, L Foroni. Lack of clonal BCRA2 gene deletion on chromosome 13 in chronic lymphocytic leukaemia [see comments]. Br J Haematol 97:844–847, 1997.

186. T Frebourg, N Barbier, YX Yan, et al. Germ-line p53 mutations in 15 families with Li-Fraumeni syndrome. Am J Hum Genet 56:608–615, 1995.

187. G Juliusson, D Oscier, G Gahrton. Cytogenetic findings and survival in B-cell chronic lymphocytic leukemia. Second IWCLL Compilation of Data on 622 Patients. Leukemia and Lymphoma Supplement:21–25, 1991.

188. G Gaidano, EW Newcomb, JZ Gong, et al. Analysis of alterations of oncogenes and tumor suppressor genes in chronic lymphocytic leukemia. Am J Pathol 144:1312–1319, 1994.

189. D Lens, MJ Dyer, JM Garcia-Marco, et al. p53 abnormalities in CLL are associated with excess of prolymphocytes and poor prognosis. Br J Haematol 99:848–857, 1997.

190. A Cuneo, C de Angeli, MG Roberti, et al. Richter's syndrome in a case of atypical chronic lymphocytic leukaemia with the t(11;14)(q13;q32): role for a p53 exon 7 gene mutation. Br J Haematol 92:375–381, 1996.

191. TJ Hamblin, Z Davis, A Gardiner, DG Oscier, FK Stevenson. Unmutated Ig V(H) genes are associated with a more aggressive form of chronic lymphocytic leukemia [see comments]. Blood 94:1848–1854, 1999.

192. O Pritsch, X Troussard, C Magnac, et al. VH gene usage by family members affected with chronic lymphocytic leukaemia. Br J Haematol 107:616–624, 1999.

193. A Sakai, GE Marti, S Pittaluga, JW Touchman, F Fend, M Raffeld. Analysis of expressed immunoglobulin heavy chain genes in familial B-CLL. Blood 95(4):1413–1419, 2000.

194. OE Bechter, W Eisterer, G Pall, W Hilbe, T Kuhr, J Thaler. Telomere length and telomerase activity predict survival in patients with B cell chronic lymphocytic leukemia. Cancer Res 58:4918–4922, 1998.

195. D Manusow, BH Weinerman. Subsequent neoplasia in chronic lymphocytic leukemia. JAMA 232:267–269, 1975.

196. KM Stavraky, TA Watson, DF White, EM Miles. Chronic lymphocytic leukemia and subsequent cancer in the same patient. Cancer 26:410–414, 1970.

197. missing refs.

198. MH Greene, RN Hoover, JF Fraumeni, Jr. Subsequent cancer in patients with chronic lymphocytic leukemia—a possible immunologic mechanism. J Natl Cancer Inst 61:337–340, 1978.

199. JW Davis, NS Weiss, BK Armstrong. Second cancers in patients with chronic lymphocytic leukemia. J Natl Cancer Inst 78:91–94, 1987.

200. LB Travis, RE Curtis, BF Hankey, JF Fraumeni, Jr. Second cancers in patients with chronic lymphocytic leukemia. J Natl Cancer Inst 84:1422–1427, 1992.

201. G Bertoldero, G Scribano, L Podda, R Berti, G Amadori. Occurrence of second neoplasms in chronic lymphocytic leukemia. Experience at Padua Hospital between 1979 and 1991. Ann Hematol 69:195–198, 1994.

202. R Lauvin, Y Le Breton-Kashi, P Jego, B Grosbois, R Leblay. Primary malignant tumors (lymphoma excluded) in patients with chronic lymphocytic leukemia. A series of 22 cases from a retrospective study of 248 patients. Ann Med Interne (Paris) 147:389–392, 1996.

203. H Kanzler, R Kuppers, S Helmes, et al. Hodgkin and Reed-Sternberg-like cells in B-cell chronic lymphocytic leukemia represent the outgrowth of single germinal-center B-cell-derived clones: potential precursors of Hodgkin and Reed-Sternberg cells in Hodgkin's disease. Blood 95(3):1023–31; 95:1023–1031, 2000.

204. FR Mauro, R Foa, D Giannarelli, et al. Clinical characteristics and outcome of young chronic lymphocytic leukemia patients: a single institution study of 204 cases. Blood 94:448–454, 1999.

205. MJ Keating, S O'Brien, S Lerner, et al. Long-term follow-up of patients with chronic lymphocytic leukemia (CLL) receiving fludarabine regimens as initial therapy. Blood 92:1165–1171, 1998.

206. BD Cheson, DA Vena, J Barrett, B Freidlin. Second malignancies as a consequence of nucleoside analog therapy for chronic lymphoid leukemias. J Clin Oncol 17:2454–2460, 1999.

207. ML Larramendy, SM Siitonen, Y Zhu, M Hurme, L Vilpo, JA Vilpo, S Knuutila. Optimized mitogen stimulation induces proliferation of neoplastic cells in chronic lymphocytic leukemia: significance for cytogenetic analysis. The Tampere Chronic Lymphocytic Leukemia Group. Cytogenetic Cell Genet 82:215–221, 1998.

208. CH Geisler, P Philip, BE Christensen, et al. In B-cell chronic lymphocytic leukaemia chromosome 17 abnormalities and not trisomy 12 are the single most important cytogenetic abnormalities for the prognosis: a cytogenetic and immunophenotypic study of 480 unselected newly diagnosed patients. Leuk Res 21:1011–1023, 1997.

209. CN Nair, A Chougule, S Dhond. et al. Trisomy 12 in chronic lymphocytic leukemia—geographical variation. Leuk Res 22:313–317, 1998.

210. V Liso, S Capalbo, A Lapietra, V Pavone, A Guarini, G Specchia. Evaluation of trisomy 12 by fluorescence in situ hybridization in peripheral blood, bone marrow and lymph nodes of patients with B cell chronic lymphocytic leukemia. Haematologica 84:212–217, 1999.

4

The Origin and Nature of the Chronic Lymphocytic Leukemia Lymphocyte

PAOLO GHIA and FEDERICO CALIGARIS-CAPPIO

University of Torino, Torino, Italy

I. INTRODUCTION

B-cell chronic lymphocytic leukemia (B-CLL) is characterized by the relentless accumulation of small, resting, long-lived B cells, that typically coexpress on the surface faint levels of immunoglobulins (Ig) and the CD5 molecule. CD5 is also present on the membrane of mantle zone lymphoma (MZL) cells, but differs from CLL cells in any other respect.

CD5 (Ly-1 in the mouse) is a 67-kDa surface glycoprotein originally reported to identify a T helper subset (1) but subsequently defined as a pan-T cell marker. As for the B cell lineage, the CD5 molecule had initially been believed to be a tumor marker for B cells, because murine B cell lymphomas (2) and human CLL (3) were found to express this molecule. Subsequently, CD5 was demonstrated to be present also on some normal B cells both in humans (4) and mice (5,6). These findings led to identification of a B cell subset, the CD5$^+$ B cell subset, which would have created more debate in immunology than few other issues (7). Also, because this subset is disproportionally highly represented in B-CLL, it has become the prototype of "normal counterpart" in the quest for normal equivalent cells of lymphoid malignancies. It is the purpose of this chapter to critically review the origin and nature of B-CLL malignant cells in light of the role and significance of normal CD5$^+$ B cells.

II. B CELL SUBSETS: THE DEVELOPMENT AND REPERTOIRE OF CD5$^+$ B CELLS (B-1 CELLS)

The investigation of the expression and the significance of CD5 (Ly-1) allowed the identification of discrete B cell subsets both in mouse and man. The finding that the T cell

Table 1 B Cell Subsets in the Mouse: Differences in Surface Marker Expression

Marker	B-1a	B-1b	Conventional B cells
Ly-1/CD5	+	−	−
Mac1/CD11b	+	+	−
FcεR/CD23	−	−	+
IgM	+++	+++	+
IgD	± to ++	± to ++	+++

marker CD5 was expressed by a small proportion of normal B cells led to a new nomenclature of B cells based on the concept that they may comprise at least two main populations/lineages that were termed B-1 and B-2 cells. The former encompasses the CD5$^+$ population, the latter represents the "conventional" CD5$^-$ B lymphocytes (8).

A. In the Mouse

In normal mice, B-1 cells can be distinguished from conventional B cells on the basis of the phenotype, the anatomical location, and the functional properties (9).

1. Surface Phenotype (Table 1)

B-1 cells express bright IgM, dull-to-moderate levels of IgD, Mac1 (CD11b) but not the FcεR (CD23). In contrast, conventional B cells (B-2 cells) are dull for IgM and bright for IgD, negative for Mac1 and positive for FcεR.

2. Anatomical Localization (Table 2)

Conventional B cells develop late during ontogeny and are generated throughout life from newly produced unrearranged progenitors that differentiate in the bone marrow (BM). In adults, they predominate in the spleen and lymph nodes. In contrast, B-1 cells arise early in ontogeny and originate from the fetal omentum. They are a small fraction of the splenic B cells; are virtually absent in adult BM, lymph nodes, and peripheral blood; and predominate in the peritoneal and pleural cavities. They maintain their number in adult animals by self-replenishment (10,11) (i.e., by division of fully mature B-1 cells). In the absence of a continuous supply from the BM, the size of the B-1 population is kept constant by

Table 2 B Cell Subsets in the Mouse: Progenitor Distribution During Different Stages of Development

Stage	B-1a	B1-b	Conventional B cells
Fetal	Omentum, liver	Omentum, liver	Liver
Postnatal	Spleen Peritoneal cavity	Bone marrow	Bone marrow
Adult	Peritoneal, pleural cavities	Peritoneal, pleural cavities	Bone marrow

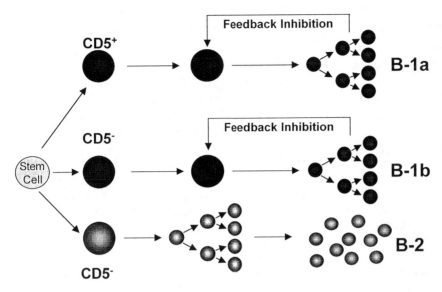

Figure 1   Development and feedback regulation of B cell lineages. Reconstitution studies showed that B-1a, B-1b, and conventional B cells are distinct lineages. Feedback inhibition regulates the de novo production of both B-1a and B-1b cells.

the self-renewal capacity of B-1 cells. Also, starting during the first weeks of life, B-1 cells exert a feedback regulation that limits the de novo production from progenitors, thereby preventing the entry of newly arisen B-1 cells into the peripheral pool (12,13) (Fig. 1).

3. "Sister" Populations: B-1a and B-1b Cells

On the basis of CD5 expression, B-1 cells can be further subdivided into two independent "sister" populations, B-1a and B-1b. B-1a cells are CD5$^+$ and constitute most of B-1 cells in normal animals. B-1b cells have the same phenotypic and functional characteristics of B-1a cells but do not express detectable levels of CD5 (14).

The two "sister" populations also differ, because they derive from different progenitors and have a different ability to persist into adulthood (15). Both B-1 cell populations arise early in ontogeny. B-1a progenitors are abundant in fetal omentum and liver but diminish with age and are very rare (or nonfunctional) in adult BM. In contrast, B-1b progenitors are active in fetal tissues, steadily persist into adulthood, and are present in adult BM. Nevertheless, the supply of B-1b cells from the BM also appears to be restricted by negative feedback mechanisms that prevent the entrance of newly generated cells into the adult peripheral pool of B-1 cells.

The lineage distinction between different B cell populations mainly relies on reconstitution experiments. Adult BM readily reconstitutes conventional B cells and B-1b cells but only poorly CD5$^+$B cells. On the other hand, 13-day fetal omentum reconstitutes B-1a and B-1b cells but not conventional B cells, whereas fetal liver (13 and 14 day) is capable of reconstituting all three lineages. It is of interest that the distinction between the conventional B and B-1 (B-1a and B-1b) lineages is also reflected by the genetically controlled variation in their frequencies in different mouse strains (14).

4. Antibody Repertoire and Functional Properties

B-1 cells have been postulated to play a major role in the production of IgM antibodies (Ab). Actually they can produce all Ig isotypes and make major contributions to serum IgM, IgG3, and IgA. Furthermore, they are responsible for a large percentage of the IgA-producing plasma cells in the gut. They are able to respond well to some multivalent antigens that are T-independent (TI) but do, however, also produce T-dependent (TD) responses. Thus, although B-1 cells are selective with respect to antigen (Ag), they are capable of making both TI and TD responses (9).

Two features of Abs produced by B-1 cells are noteworthy (16). First, B-1 cells produce Ig of low affinity and broad specificity for microorganism coat antigens (Ags) such as polysaccharides, lipids, and proteins of bacterial components. Second, they preferentially produce Abs against auto-Ags, particularly polyreactive natural autoAbs. Analyses of the epitopes recognized by these autoAbs suggest that they tend to cross-react with bacterial Ag and vice versa. It is noteworthy to underline that the V region genes expressed by B-1–produced Abs carry little or no somatic mutations. This phenomenon is likely the result of their limited ability to form germinal centers, as indicated also by the limited capacity to undergo isotype-switching (17–19).

Because of their ability to produce multireactive antibodies, B-1 cells are considered carriers of ''natural immunity.'' Three distinct functions have been attributed to B-1 cells, which are not mutually exclusive (16). First, they may provide natural protection against infection by microorganisms by means of the production of broad-specificity Abs. Second, they may favor the clearance of denatured self-Ags by means of the production of polyreactive autoaAbs. Third, they are possibly involved in the induction of autoimmune diseases by means of the production of pathogenic autoAb. The involvement of B-1 cells in the occurrence of autoimmune diseases remains controversial. Some evidence suggests a scenario in which B-1 cells can be activated by environmental factors such as enteric bacteria to produce autoAbs that subsequently can cause autoimmune manifestations. This appears to be true in transgenic mice carrying Ig genes derived from a hybridoma producing an anti-red blood cell (RBC) (20).

In summary, B-1 cells differ from conventional B cells because they produce a more restricted set of low-affinity, broad-specificity germline Abs that react with ubiquitous microorganisms, whereas conventional B cells produce a larger, more diversified set of Abs capable of specific high-affinity interactions.

5. Effect of Age on CD5$^+$ B Cells

Virtually all mice over the age of 15 months have clonal populations of B-1 cells detectable within the pools of splenic and peritoneal lymphocytes (21). The B-1 repertoire, which is fixed early in development, becomes progressively restricted as animals age, because new entrants in the B-1 pool are prevented by the feedback mechanism. Clonal populations expand to occupy a progressively greater proportion of the B cell pool. This may be related to the fact that in the elderly the Ab response to Ags that stimulate CD5$^+$B cells is well preserved in contrast to that stimulating conventional B cells (22). It is intriguing to hypothesize that the B cell clonal populations present in old mice may be the precursors of the murine CLL-like disorders that are characterized by clonal expansion of CD5$^+$ B cells and frequently occur in elder mice (23). Surprisingly, despite the high numbers of CD5$^+$ B cells and the high levels of serum autoAbs, autoimmune disorders are less common in older than in younger animals.

B. In Man

In man, as in mice, CD5$^+$ B cells predominate in the fetus and neonate (24). They represent most B cells in the fetal circulation and decrease to 60% to 80% in the umbilical cord blood. They are also the first B cells that appear in the fetal liver and in the developing lymph nodes. They become 5% to 30% of the circulating B cells in the adult peripheral blood, 10% in the adult spleen, and less than 30% in lymph nodes, where they are mainly located within the follicular mantle zone (FMZ) (25). Actually, most virgin B cells (IgM$^+$, IgD$^+$, CD38$^-$) express CD5. As in mice, most B cells in the peritoneal cavity are CD5$^+$ (19% to 76% of the B cells) (26), and CD5$^+$ B cells are virtually absent in human adult BM. Human B-1 cells, as in the mouse, very rarely show a small number of mutated Ig sequences and are thus thought to be primarily involved in immune responses to TI antigens and not to participate in germinal center (GC) reactions (27,28).

As in mice, human B-1 cells have been claimed to be mainly involved in the production of polyreactive low-affinity Abs. Interestingly enough, there is evidence indicating that CD5$^-$ B cells are also involved in the production of these Abs. Therefore, the hypothesis of a prevalent role of CD5$^+$ B cells in autoimmune diseases remains speculative (29).

C. CD5: Sign of a Separate Lineage or Activation Marker?

Although experimental evidence indicates that, especially in the mouse, CD5$^+$ B cells may constitute a separate lineage, no conclusions can be definitely drawn in humans, and the possibility that CD5 might just be an activation marker cannot be ruled out (30).

The role of CD5 as a molecular watershed is confused by several observations. First, CD5 has a different significance in different species, (e.g., all rabbit B cells are CD5$^+$) (31). Next, as mentioned earlier, the strongest evidence of the existence of a separate lineage comes from reconstitution experiments in mice, in which different cell populations appear to develop from different progenitors at different stages of ontogeny. The situation is quite different in humans in whom, besides the ontogenetic data previously described, it has become clear that after BM transplantation using neonatal and adult BM cells, both B cell subsets are readily reconstituted. Furthermore, even murine conventional B cells can be induced to express high levels of surface CD5 after sIg cross-linking, in clear contrast to lipopolysaccharide (LPS), which is not capable of inducing this phenotype (32). Anti-IgM Ab, together with IL-6, is capable of inducing not only the expression of CD5 but also an overall phenotype typical of CD5$^+$ peritoneal B cells (33). Human CD5$^-$ B cells can be induced to express the CD5 phenotype after stimulation with the polyclonal B cell stimulator *Staphylococcus aureus* Cowan strain I (SAC) (34). Finally, the expression of CD5 can be down-modulated by exposing CD5$^+$ B cells to exogenous cytokines (e.g., IL-1 or IL-2) (35) and by stimulating them with Epstein-Barr virus (EBV) (36).

If CD5 were merely an activation marker, one could envision that most, if not all, B cells might potentially express CD5, provided they are placed in the proper environment and/or exposed to the right activation/differentiation conditions. Still, the possibility remains that two kinds of CD5$^+$B cells may coexist. A distinct CD5$^+$ lineage, originating early in ontogeny and corresponding functionally to the classical B-1 subset (''constitutive phenotype''), might be present together with a CD5$^+$ subset, generated by the activation of some members of the conventional B cell population (''induced'' phenotype) (30).

III. GENERAL FEATURES OF CHRONIC LYMPHOCYTIC LEUKEMIA B CELLS

Chronic lymphocytic leukemia cells are characterized by distinct phenotype, typical unresposiveness to exogenous stimuli, absence of measurable proliferation, and defective apoptosis. Despite a unique and monotonously uniform immunophenotype, no consistent molecular or cytogenetic abnormalities have been so far identified. The absence of a single abnormality in CLL raises the possibility that multiple distinct defects might converge on certain critical signaling points and feed into a common pathway that would result into extended survival, protection from apoptosis, and inappropriate accumulation of neoplastic cells. However, experimental evidence has been recently gathered, indicating that the term "CLL," we still use to define a single nosological entity more likely covers a wide spectrum of different forms of disease. It is therefore reasonable to foresee that in the near future a molecular "splitting" will clear up the phenotypic "lumping."

A. Surface Phenotype

All the membrane Ags typical of mature B cells, such as CD19, CD20, CD21, CD24, and CD40, are expressed by the malignant cells, but it is the contemporaneous presence of CD5, CD23, and faint to undetectable sIg that represents the characteristic trait of the disease (37). This triad helps to distinguish CLL from most B cell malignancies and especially from the leukemic variants of non-Hodgkin lymphomas. Although most CLL cases express either IgM alone or both IgM and IgD on their cell surface, heavy chain class switching has been reported, with a definite, albeit small, subset expressing IgG or IgA. Finally, there are few CLL in which the mechanism of allelic exclusion appears to have failed. In these cases, κ and λ light chains are coexpressed in association with a single H chain, suggesting that the onset of malignancy occurred at an early stage, when the activity of recombinase genes was still present (38).

The CLL immunophenotype suggests a relationship with the normal CD5$^+$ B cells present in B mantles of secondary lymphoid follicles, so that it has become customary to consider them as the likely normal cellular counterparts of B-CLL. It is certainly true that several characteristics of normal B-1 cells are shared by malignant CLL cells (reviewed in Ref. (39)), including the low expression of CD20 (40), the ability to form rosettes with mouse erythrocytes (41), and the expression of myelomonocytic antigens (42). However, as extensively discussed elsewhere (43), the differences between normal and malignant CD5$^+$ B cells are likewise significant. It should be remembered that normal CD5$^+$ B cells do not have the low to undetectable levels of sIg that are so typical of malignant B-CLL and that their phenotypic features are synchronous with the cell cycle phases, whereas B-CLL cells show an asynchronism between the phenotype that is activated and the position within the cell cycle that is fully resting. Also, the unusual adhesive properties and the peculiar cytoskeleton organization of malignant B-CLL cells are shared only by cells of the monocyte-macrophage lineage (44). Finally, it is extremely difficult to transform B-CLL cells with EBV, even if they express a functional EBV receptor (45), whereas this difficulty is remarkably absent in normal CD5$^+$ B.

B. Functional Characteristics

1. Functional Hyporesponsiveness

The low levels of sIg that are so typical of B-CLL are seen only in normal B lymphocytes that have been anergized by interaction with self-Ags. This feature is mirrored by a typical

Ag receptor nonresponsiveness, which again closely resembles both functionally and bio-chemically the behavior of tolerant autoreactive B cells. In truth, the response of B-CLL cells to the activation of the B cell receptor (BCR) is heterogeneous (see following) but rarely results in proliferation.

The BCR complex is composed of the membrane form of the Ig molecule and the noncovalently associated Ig α/β (CD79a/CD79b) heterodimer. The extracelluar domain of CD79b is lacking in most B-CLL patients (46). Recently, it has been claimed that the diminished display of BCR on the membrane of B-CLL cells is due to the occurrence of somatic mutations predicted to affect CD79b expression (47). However, other groups have failed to identify causal mutations both in random and familial cases of CLL and detected only polymorphic changes or silent mutations that can not lead to a truncated CD79b protein (48,49). An alternative explanation is offered by the detection of a CD79b trun-cated form that arises by alternative splicing of CD79b gene and lacks exon 3 that encodes the extracellular Ig-like domain. This alternatively spliced variant was found in all B-CLL cases analyzed, thereby suggesting a role for the alternative splicing of CD79b gene in causing the reduced expression of BCR on the surface of B-CLL cells (49). It is of interest that the spliced variant levels are higher in activated normal B cells compared with resting B cells and that in vivo activated germinal center B cells are essentially CD79b negative. This raises the interesting possibility that B cells physiologically use alternative splicing of CD79b to down-regulate BCR expression on activation and suggests that the lack of CD79b in B-CLL reflects the state of activation of the B cell that underwent the malignant transformation. The possibility that CLL cells are living in a "frustrated" state of activa-tion is also witnessed by the fact that they may synthesize and secrete a wide variety of cytokines (50). Still, none of them is individually and consistently able to force the G0 block of B-CLL cells. Some cytokines have been suggested to act as autocrine growth factors or to exert an inhibitory activity on surrounding cells. However, their role in the natural history of the disease is still unclear, and the fact remains that more than 99% of circulating malignant CLL cells are in the G0/early G1 phase of the cell cycle and that virtually no mitogenic signal active on normal B cells can stimulate CLL cells to prolif-erate.

2. Functional Heterogeneity

The overall general picture previously described that depicts CLL cells as bland, frustrated cells is disturbed by the existence of a heterogeneity among individual cases in terms of cell morphology, karyotypic abnormalities, and functional characteristics. Functional differences have been observed in several independent studies of laboratory manipulation of malignant CLL cells and may mirror the clinical heterogeneity, with some patients surviving for prolonged periods without therapy and others that pursue an aggressive course that demands intensive treatment.

Although leukemic cells from most patients are prone to apoptotic death within a short period of time in culture, some survive for up to 3 weeks (51). Some cytokines have been shown to prevent in vitro apoptosis or even induce proliferation of individual B-CLL cases, with a marked heterogeneity of response from case to case. For example, a subset of samples was found to be proliferating, albeit weakly, in response to IL-2, whereas another did not. In addition, considering as parameters the cell response to anti-Ig antibod-ies and the expression of CD38, B-CLL were divided into two groups. The CD38-positive subset has been invariably found to enter apoptosis when stimulated through IgM (52) and to increase both survival and differentiation when stimulated by IgD (53). In contrast the CD38-negative subset appears to be completely resistant to these stimuli. Another element of discrimination may be represented by the expression of A-myb gene, which encodes a transcription factor that is related both functionally and structurally to the *v-myb* oncogene. Two groups of patients have been identified that were either positive (25% of the cases) or negative (75% of the cases) for the expression of the gene (54).

Furthermore, elevated serum thymidine kinase levels appear to identify a subgroup at high risk of disease progression in early, nonsmouldering CLL (55).

More recent evidence of CLL heterogeneity comes from investigations of Ig genes in both IgM-expressing and non-IgM-expressing B-CLL cases. The analyses of the structure of clonal Ig in CLL is likely to become the real turnaround in this central issue, because it can help differentiate entities that have a distinct clinical outcome.

3. The Antibody Repertoire

Several independent studies have established that the use of IgH chain variable region (V_H) genes among B-CLL cells is not random (56). Overall, the Abs expressed in CLL are not representative of the Abs expressed in the fetal repertoire or in B-cells of normal adults. Analyses of the V_H gene families used in CLL point to a statistically significant difference in comparison with both fetal and adult normal CD5$^+$ B cells. However, when the single V_H genes are analyzed, it becomes evident that few genes account for more than half the cases and that the most are similarly overused in the normal CD5$^+$ B cell repertoire. The exception is the overrepresentation of the V_H 1–69 gene. This gene has been consistently shown to be the most widely used V_H gene in CLL, accounting for more than two thirds of all V_H1 genes used and being present in about 20% of all patients (57). This gene is frequently represented in normal CD5$^+$ B cells and encodes for Ig with rheumatoid factor (RF) activity (56), possibly indicating a triggering role for B-cell superAgs. In fact, a high proportion of CLL B cells display natural autoAb activity and frequently behave as RF (58) as it would be expected from their putative origin from normal CD5$^+$ B cells. Despite the fact that autoimmune-associated phenomena are frequently observed in CLL, it is intriguing that in most cases the pathogenetic autoAbs are not secreted by the malignant clone. All these observations indicate that CLL B cells express a distinctive and selected Ig repertoire, which seemingly is not derived from a "normal, nonneoplastic" repertoire of pathogenic autoAbs.

The nonrandom use of V_H genes helps to define that the CLL cell derives from a mature B cell compartment but does not allow one to conclude whether these receptor restrictions come from developmental forces or are driven by Ag encounters. As in the course of TD immune reactions, somatic mutations are introduced into rearranged V genes in B cells, the study of V gene sequences allows discrimination at the B cell stage of differentiation. It has been always assumed that B-CLL cells would accumulate little, if any, somatic mutations, thus resembling normal CD5$^+$ B cells. On these bases, B-CLL cells were considered to be mature, but naive, Ag-inexperienced lymphocytes. However, starting from the observation of Schroeder and Dighiero (38), several groups have accumulated data on the presence of somatic mutations in CLL. It is now clear that about 50% of IgM$^+$ B-CLL and about 75% of the non-IgM$^+$ B-CLL exhibit high levels of somatic mutations and that replacement mutations accumulate in the complementary determining regions (CDR) (59). These data indicate that a proportion of malignant clones have been triggered in a TD fashion, (i.e., they have undergone a germinal center experience and are probably memory cells) (Fig. 2). This is in clear contrast with the fact that the normal CD5$^+$ B cell population is characterized by unmutated V genes (27,28). To explain these discrepancies it may be recalled that normal CD5$^+$ B cells usually do not participate in TD immune reactions. However, if in rare cases CD5$^+$ B cells are drawn into the GCs,

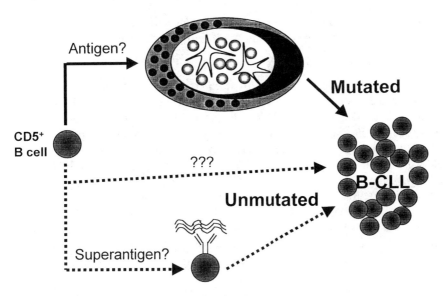

Figure 2 Sequence analyses of the V_H genes expressed in B-CLL cells show that at least two subsets exist. The malignant cells that carry somatic mutations seem to have undergone antigen selection, likely in germinal center reactions. The unmutated subset could either arise from a T-independent stimulation through the BCR (e.g., superantigens) or from an insofar unknown stimulus (CD5?).

the vigorous proliferative expansion and the processes of somatic hypermutations and/or class switching typical of GC might put the long-lived $CD5^+$ B cells at an increased risk for malignant transformation.

The presence of somatic mutations has been correlated with other features of CLL, and especially with the clinical course and the response to therapy (60). It has been shown (61) that the cases with trisomy 12, which are usually associated with advanced disease and a less favorable prognosis, show a minimal level of mutations. In contrast, cases with 13q14 abnormality, that have a better prognosis, show significant levels of somatic diversification. Very similar data, obtained quite independently by two groups, have shown that the survival of mutated patients is strikingly better than the survival of unmutated patients (60,62). One study (62) has also provided evidence that patients experiencing a worse clinical outcome not only lack somatic mutations but also express high surface levels of CD38 on the leukemic cells.

In summary, the presence and the characteristics of the somatic mutations suggest that a subset of CLL is derived from memory B cells that have passed through the GC stage of Ag selection and B-cell differentiation. Therefore, CLL may arise from either pregerminal center naive B cells or germinal center exposed B cells. However, both the data from V_H gene sequences and the BCR properties discussed before suggest that in most CLL the malignant cells are activated. It remains to be established through which pathway they have been activated, whether the classical TD pathway that implies a GC experience and the development of somatic mutations or a TI pathway, triggered either by autoAgs or by conventional TI Ags, that would be nonmutational (Fig. 2). Taken together these data bring in a number of intriguing and yet unanswered questions. It may actually be asked whether Ag stimulation may be a promoting factor in the evolution of certain CLL clones. Should B-CLL cells have an in vivo reactivity with a specific Ag, it may be asked which consequence might this reactivity have for the cell and the patient and also whether Ag selection is continuing to occur during the course of the disease.

4. The Role of CD5

The CD5 molecule can associate with the BCR complex after sIgM ligation and serves as a substrate for BCR-induced tyrosine kinase activity, raising the possibility that CD5 has a functional role in sIgM-induced signals (63). In fact, CD5 negatively regulates directly or indirectly sIgM signaling. When CD5 associates with sIgM on B-1 cells, it prevents sIgM-mediated proliferative signals. The negative regulatory function of CD5 appears to affect only sIgM signaling, because LPS- and CD40-mediated signaling that bypass sIgM dependent signal transduction remain unaltered in CD5-deficient B-1 cells.

BCR-mediated proliferation signals, but not those inducing apoptosis, are impaired in B-1 cells. In fact, ligation of sIgM and of CD5 on resting tonsillar B cells results in apoptosis (64). Thus, the presence of CD5 somehow redirects B-1 cells from a proliferative to an apoptotic pathway in response to sIgM ligation. If the interaction of CD5 with sIgM is prevented, a significant proliferative response can be restored after sIgM-mediated activation.

Because the normal B-1 cell repertoire is primarily directed against microbial and self-Ag, the regulation of the BCR signaling by CD5 may have evolved as a mechanism to check the uncontrolled expansion of B-1 cells. The CD5-mediated negative regulation can be overcome, however, with strong growth signals provided by mitogenic moieties of microbial antigens (e.g., LPS) or by T cell help (e.g., CD40L).

In contrast with this negative regulatory effect, it has been suggested that CD5 may also contribute to survival and expansion of B cells through its interaction with V_H framework regions of surface Ig (65). It has been shown that CD5 is an endogenous ligand selective for B-cell surface Ig framework region sequences (65). The Ig-CD5 interaction maps on both molecules to domains different from the ones recognized in a classic Ag-Ab reaction. These interactions of V_H framework regions with CD5 as a ligand may be necessary to maintain, select, or expand B-1 cells (66). CD5 interaction with sIg, as well as endogenous Ags or (in mucosal sites) exogenous (microbial) superAgs, can provide B cells with continual stimulation and might prevent their elimination from the immune system (65). This mechanism has clear implications for the pathogenesis of CLL. It might contribute to autostimulatory growth of transformed B cells with a particular V_H, perhaps skewing the normal V_H repertoire and contributing to the lifelong production of malignant lymphocytes. The same mechanism can also be at work for CD72, the first CD5 ligand identified that is expressed on all B lymphocytes, including CLL malignant cells (67).

In conclusion, because of the expression of CD5, the $CD5^+$ population appears to be more susceptible to apoptosis than the $CD5^-$ population but also more prone to autostimulatory growth signals. It is, therefore, striking that $CD5^+$ B cells have such a propensity to give rise to a malignancy that is characterized by defective apoptosis and lack of proliferation.

C. Defective Apoptosis: Typical Feature of Chronic Lymphocytic Leukemia

1. Apoptosis Cascade

B-chronic lymphocytic leukemia has emerged as the prototype of malignancies characterized by a defective apoptosis that leads to a progressive and relentless accumulation of monoclonal B cells in the BM, lymphoid tissues, and peripheral blood. Apoptosis is a physiological process pivotal in the regulation of tissue homeostasis that is characterized by distinctive biochemical and morphological changes. It is marked by a sequence of events that involves an initiation or triggering step, a cascade of intracellular signaling steps, and a final execution phase, which is irreversible and represents a point of no return for the cell. Among the apoptosis-inducing signals, binding of the Fas ligand to the Fas receptor (CD95), members of the tumor necrosis factor (TNF) and TNF receptor family, respectively, is considered one of the most potent (68). Leukemic cells from B-CLL patients do not exhibit significantly increased apoptosis after CD95 ligation (69). This is likely because malignant B-CLL cells are either negative or only weakly positive for Fas expression. After activation with SAC + IL-2, α- or γ-IFN or through CD40 ligation (70), the neoplastic cells upregulate the expression of Fas, but unexpectedly remain generally resistant to anti-Fas mAb-induced apoptosis (70,71). This resistance is not due to mutated FAS protein (71). One can then speculate that such a resistance would allow tumor cells to escape, in vivo, from Fas/FasL-mediated regulatory control of $CD4^+$ lymphocytes and from antitumor cytotoxicity of $CD8^+$ cells. In agreement with this hypothesis, the CD95-deficient (*lpr*) mice have lethal B-cell lymphoma develop only when they are deficient in T cells (72).

Beside the role of intrinsic defects, one alternative and attractive hypothesis can be offered to explain the mechanism of resistance to CD95 apoptosis in malignant B cells. When a normal B cell is stimulated through BCR by a cognate Ag, it becomes resistant to Fas-mediated apoptosis (73–75). Because a high proportion of CLL cases appear to be Ag-experienced, this possibility does not seem so bizarre for neoplastic B lymphocytes also (Fig. 3).

Several proteins involved in regulating the intracellular cascade leading to apoptosis have been cloned. The bcl-2 family of proteins is among the key regulators of programmed cell death. Bcl-2 has been originally cloned from the t(14;18) translocation (76), present in most of follicular lymphomas, and turned out to be a major suppressor of apoptosis. All the other members of the family positively and negatively contribute to cell death (77). Some of them are death suppressors (bcl-x_L, mcl-1), some others are death inducers (bax, bcl-x_s, bak), some others are just regulators (bad). A delicate balance of homodimers and heterodimers of these proteins modulates the proapoptotic signal, either permitting or inhibiting the amplifying cascade after the cytochrome C release from the mitochondria, as well as the final execution phase. This results in the proteolytic activation of the caspases, proteins that belong to a family of cysteine proteinases and are considered to be the key executioners of programmed cell death, able to dismantle and package the cell by cleaving key cellular components.

A constitutive and altered expression of some of the genes involved in such a cascade could explain the diminished cell death. Analyses of the bcl-2 family members did not show conclusive data. It is clear that most B-CLL cells express high levels of bcl-2 proteins in the absence of any detectable t(14;18) translocation (78). This is perhaps due to a complete demethylation of both copies of the gene, leading to up-regulation of its expression. However, there is no agreement on the role of bcl-2 levels and modulation during the onset of spontaneous apoptosis in vitro, and during the in vivo responses to chemotherapy. Discrepancies can also be found on the role of bcl-2 in Fas resistance. Some workers suggested that, when present, CD95-induced apoptosis is independent of bcl-2 expression (70,79), whereas others indicated the opposite (80).

In addition, CLL cells commonly also contain bax and bak proteins and not appreciable levels of bcl-x_L and bad. It is also interesting to note that two thirds of the patients with CLL express the antiapoptotic protein called mcl-1 (81). Perhaps the overall bcl-2/

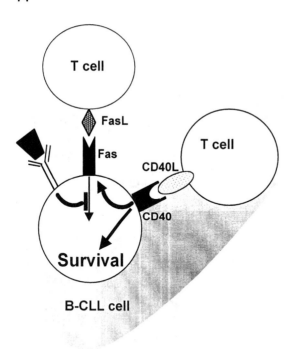

Figure 3 A possible scenario of molecules involved in B-CLL cell survival. Stimulation through CD40 of the malignant cells could induce the expression of Fas (CD95), whose death signal would be inhibited by a contemporaneous signal delivered through the BCR (by an antigen? a superantigen?). The overall result would be a survival signal for the CLL cell.

bax ratio may determine chemosensitivity of B-CLL cells, or the presence of higher levels of mcl-1 may explain the failure to achieve a complete remission, but no definitive conclusions can be drawn so far. What is clear is that CLL cells retain the capacity to activate caspases spontaneously, as well as in response to chemotherapy (e.g., exposure to dexamethasone and fludarabine) (69). Further studies are needed to determine the precise role of each gene and to dissect the specific defects that can prevent the timely activation of apoptosis.

2.   Survival Signals

B-CLL cells express the CD40 molecule on the membrane. CD40 is a transmembrane glycoprotein that belongs to the TNF receptor superfamily. Its natural ligand (CD40L) is a member of the TNF family that is expressed on activated T cells (82). CLL can respond to both the soluble form of the ligand (CD40L/CD154) and to anti-CD40 mAbs. Contrasting results obtained in the past on the effect of CD40 ligation on CLL cells are explained by the fact that the sensitivity of the malignant cells depends on the intensity of the signal. Only strong cross-linking of the receptor gives rise to a response, enhancing CLL viability in vivo and rescuing CLL cells from spontaneous apoptosis. Moreover, the CD40-stimulation is able to counteract the therapeutic effect of apoptogenetic drugs in vivo (83), namely of fludarabine. High levels of CD40L were present in the plasma of CLL patients examined (84), perhaps explaining the fact that the capacity of patients' autologous plasma to rescue CLL cells from spontaneous apoptosis could be reversed by anti-CD40L antibodies. The experimental evidences of a possible role for CD40L$^+$ nontumoral cells in CLL appear to be justified by the presence of CD4$^+$ helper T cells in involved BM and lymph nodes (85).

In addition, the presence of functional CD40 on the surface of leukemic B-CLL cells can support a further mechanism that protects the neoplastic clone from a cytolytic immune response. The CD40 molecules on the surface of malignant B cells are capable of inducing down-modulation and endocytosis of CD40L expressed on activated T cells (86). This seems in contrast with the previous scenario where CD40 ligation can induce cell survival of malignant cells. A situation of acquired CD40L deficiency would occur when the proportion of CD4$^+$ T cells relative to that of leukemic cells declines below a critical level. In CLL patients such proportions are generally noted in the later stages of disease, when probably the CD40-mediated survival is no longer critical for the maintenance of the disease.

The question remains whether the CD40-mediated antiapoptotic pathway is part of the pathogenetic mechanism of the disease and can contribute to the prolonged life span and accumulation of the leukemic cells.

IV. CONCLUSIONS

A multitude of experimental data have insofar failed to precisely reveal the origin of CLL cells. Irrespective of the caveats concerning the role and significance of CD5 and despite the sometimes harsh dispute over the possibility that CD5$^+$ B cells may or may not represent a separate B-cell lineage, it still remains reasonable to consider CD5$^+$ B cells as the normal counterpart of B-CLL. Anergy, activation, anti-self-reactivity, and defective apoptosis are the key features of the malignant cell. However, it is worth mentioning that, in contrast to many other neoplasias, the precise dissection of the nature of the malignant cell in B-CLL, although fundamental, is insufficient to understand the pathogenesis of the disease. Several findings indicate that besides an extensive search of intrinsic defects of the neoplastic cell, a likewise scrupulous investigation of the role of the microenvironment in which the malignant cells seed is necessary to more properly define the pathogenesis of CLL. Bystander, nontumoral cells, the numerous extrinsic factors they produce, and the interactions they entail play a fundamental, although insufficient, role in the onset and progression of B-CLL (87).

ACKNOWLEDGMENTS

This work was supported by Associazione Italiana per la Ricerca sul Cancro (A.I.R.C.)-Milano and by MURST (Ministero per l'Università e la Ricerca Scientifica e Tecnologica).

REFERENCES

1. H Cantor, EA Boyse. Functional subclasses of T lymphocytes bearing different Ly antigens. II. Cooperation between subclasses of Ly+ cells in the generation of killer activity. J Exp Med 141:1390–1399, 1975.
2. LL Lanier, NL Warner, JA Ledbetter, LA Herzenberg. Expression of Lyt-1 antigen on certain murine B cell lymphomas. J Exp Med 153:998–1003, 1981.
3. L Boumsell, A Bernard, V Lepage, L Degos, J Lemerle, J Dausset. Some chronic lymphocytic

leukemia cells bearing surface immunoglobulins share determinants with T cells. Eur J Immunol 8:900–904, 1978.

4. F Caligaris-Cappio, M Gobbi, M Bofill, G Janossy. Infrequent normal B lymphocytes express features of B-chronic lymphocytic leukemia. J Exp Med 155:623–628, 1982.

5. K Hayakawa, RR Hardy, DR Parks, LA Herzenberg. The ''Ly-1 B'' cell subpopulation in normal, immunodefective, and autoimmune mice. J Exp Med 157:202–218, 1983.

6. V Manohar, E Brown, WM Leiserson, TM Chused. Expression of Lyt-1 by a subset of B lymphocytes. J Immunol 129:532–538, 1982.

7. AB Kantor. The development and repertoire of B-1 cells (CD5 B cells). Immunol Today 12: 389–391, 1991.

8. AB Kantor. A new nomenclature for B cells. Immunol Today 12:388, 1991.

9. AB Kantor, LA Herzenberg. Origin of murine B cell lineages. Annu Rev Immunol 11:501–538, 1993.

10. K Hayakawa, RR Hardy, AM Stall, LA Herzenberg. Immunoglobulin-bearing B cells reconstitute and maintain the murine Ly-1 B cell lineage. Eur J Immunol 16:1313–1316, 1986.

11. K Hayakawa, RR Hardy, LA Herzenberg. Progenitors for Ly-1 B cells are distinct from progenitors for other B cells. J Exp Med 161:1554–1568, 1985.

12. PA Lalor, LA Herzenberg, S Adams, AM Stall. Feedback regulation of murine Ly-1 B cell development. Eur J Immunol 19:507–513, 1989.

13. PA Lalor, AM Stall, S Adams, LA Herzenberg. Permanent alteration of the murine Ly-1 B repertoire due to selective depletion of Ly-1 B cells in neonatal animals. Eur J Immunol 19: 501–506, 1989.

14. AM Stall, S Adams, LA Herzenberg, AB Kantor. Characteristics and development of the murine B-1b (Ly-1 B sister) cell population. Ann N Y Acad Sci 651:33–43, 1992.

15. AB Kantor, AM Stall, S Adams, LA Herzenberg. Differential development of progenitor activity for three B-cell lineages. Proc Natl Acad Sci U S A 89:3320–3324, 1992.

16. M Murakami, T Honjo. Involvement of B-1 cells in mucosal immunity and autoimmunity. Immunol Today 16:534–539, 1995.

17. DM Tarlinton, M McLean, GJ Nossal. B1 and B2 cells differ in their potential to switch immunoglobulin isotype. Eur J Immunol 25:3388–3393, 1995.

18. I Forster, H Gu, K Rajewsky. Germline antibody V regions as determinants of clonal persistence and malignant growth in the B cell compartment. Embo J 7:3693–3703, 1988.

19. J Braun, L King. Unique V gene usage by B-Ly1 cell lines, and a discordance between isotype switch commitment and variable region hypermutation [published erratum appears in J Mol Cell Immunol 4:239, 1989]. J Mol Cell Immunol 4:121–127, 1989.

20. M Murakami, K Nakajima, K Yamazaki, T Muraguchi, T Serikawa, T Honjo. Effects of breeding environments on generation and activation of autoreactive B-1 cells in anti-red blood cell autoantibody transgenic mice. J Exp Med 185:791–794, 1997.

21. D Tarlinton, AM Stall, LA Herzenberg. Repetitive usage of immunoglobulin VH and D gene segments in CD5+ Ly-1 B clones of (NZB × NZW)F1 mice. Embo J 7:3705–3710, 1988.

22. M Weksler, R Schwab, D Ai-hao. Aging and the immune system. In: RR Rich, ed. Clinical Immunology: Principles and Practice. St. Louis: Mosby–Year Book, Inc., 1996, pp 789–795.

23. AM Stall, MC Farinas, DM Tarlinton, PA Lalor, LA Herzenberg, S Strober. Ly-1 B-cell clones similar to human chronic lymphocytic leukemias routinely develop in older normal mice and young autoimmune (New Zealand Black-related) animals. Proc Natl Acad Sci U S A 85:7312–7316, 1988.

24. M Bofill, G Janossy, M Janossa, GD Burford, GJ Seymour, P Wernet, E Kelemen. Human B cell development. II. Subpopulations in the human fetus. J Immunol 134:1531–1538, 1985.

25. M Gobbi, F Caligaris-Cappio, G Janossy. Normal equivalent cells of B cell malignancies: analysis with monoclonal antibodies. Br J Haematol 54:393–403, 1983.

26. S Nisitani, M Murakami, T Akamizu, T Okino, K Ohmori, T Mori, M Imamura, T Honjo.

Preferential localization of human CD5+ B cells in the peritoneal cavity. Scand J Immunol 46:541–545, 1997.

27. HP Brezinschek, SJ Foster, RI Brezinschek, T Dorner, R Domiati-Saad, PE Lipsky. Analysis of the human VH gene repertoire. Differential effects of selection and somatic hypermutation on human peripheral CD5(+)/IgM+ and CD5(−)/IgM+ B cells. J Clin Invest 99:2488–2501, 1997.

28. M Fischer, U Klein, R Kuppers. Molecular single-cell analysis reveals that CD5-positive peripheral blood B cells in healthy humans are characterized by rearranged Vkappa genes lacking somatic mutation. J Clin Invest 100:1667–1676, 1997.

29. G Dighiero. Natural autoantibodies, tolerance, and autoimmunity. Ann N Y Acad Sci 815: 182–192, 1997.

30. P Youinou, C Jamin, PM Lydyard. CD5 expression in human B-cell populations. Immunol Today 20:312–316, 1999.

31. C Raman, KL Knight. CD5+ B cells predominate in peripheral tissues of rabbit. J Immunol 149:3858–3864, 1992.

32. YZ Cong, E Rabin, HH Wortis. Treatment of murine CD5-B cells with anti-Ig, but not LPS, induces surface CD5: two B-cell activation pathways. Int Immunol 3:467–476, 1991.

33. HH Wortis, M Teutsch, M Higer, J Zheng, DC Parker. B-cell activation by crosslinking of surface IgM or ligation of CD40 involves alternative signal pathways and results in different B-cell phenotypes. Proc Natl Acad Sci U S A 92:3348–3352, 1995.

34. K Morikawa, F Oseko, S Morikawa. Induction of CD5 antigen on human CD5-B cells by stimulation with *Staphylococcus aureus* Cowan strain I. Int Immunol 5:809–816, 1993.

35. F Caligaris-Cappio, M Riva, L Tesio, M Schena, G Gaidano, L Bergui. Human normal CD5+ B lymphocytes can be induced to differentiate to CD5-B lymphocytes with germinal center cell features. Blood 73:1259–1263, 1989.

36. M Nakamura, SE Burastero, AL Notkins, P Casali. Human monoclonal rheumatoid factor-like antibodies from CD5 (Leu-1)+B cells are polyreactive. J Immunol 140:4180–4186, 1988.

37. F Caligaris-Cappio, TJ Hamblin. B-cell chronic lymphocytic leukemia: A bird of a different feather. J Clin Oncol 17:399–408, 1999.

38. HW Schroeder Jr., G Dighiero. The pathogenesis of chronic lymphocytic leukemia: analysis of the antibody repertoire. Immunol Today 15:288–294, 1994.

39. F Caligaris-Cappio. B-chronic lymphocytic leukemia: a malignancy of anti-self B cells. Blood 87:2615–2620, 1996.

40. JH Antin, SG Emerson, P Martin, N Gadol, KA Ault. Leu-1+ (CD5+) B cells. A major lymphoid subpopulation in human fetal spleen: phenotypic and functional studies. J Immunol 136:505–510, 1986.

41. G Stathopoulos, EV Elliott. Formation of mouse or sheep red-blood-cell rosettes by lymphocytes from normal and leukaemic individuals. Lancet 1:600–601, 1974.

42. F Morabito, EF Prasthofer, NE Dunlap, CE Grossi, AB Tilden. Expression of myelomonocytic antigens on chronic lymphocytic leukemia B cells correlates with their ability to produce interleukin 1. Blood 70:1750–1757, 1987.

43. F Caligaris-Cappio, D Gottardi, A Alfarano, A Stacchini, MG Gregoretti, P Ghia, MT Bertero, A Novarino, L Bergui. The nature of the B lymphocyte in B-chronic lymphocytic leukemia. Blood Cells 19:601–613, 1993.

44. F Caligaris-Cappio, L Bergui, L Tesio, G Corbascio, F Tousco, PC Marchisio. Cytoskeleton organization is aberrantly rearranged in the cells of B chronic lymphocytic leukemia and hairy cell leukemia. Blood 67:233–239, 1986.

45. AB Rickinson, S Finerty, MA Epstein. Interaction of Epstein-Barr virus with leukaemic B cells in vitro. I. Abortive infection and rare cell line establishment from chronic lymphocytic leukaemic cells. Clin Exp Immunol 50:347–354, 1982.

46. AP Zomas, E Matutes, R Morilla, K Owusu-Ankomah, BK Seon, D Catovsky. Expression of

the immunoglobulin-associated protein B29 in B cell disorders with the monoclonal antibody SN8 (CD79b). Leukemia 10:1966–1970, 1996.

47. AA Thompson, JA Talley, HN Do, HL Kagan, L Kunkel, J Berenson, MD Cooper, A Saxon, R Wall. Aberrations of the B-cell receptor B29 (CD79b) gene in chronic lymphocytic leukemia. Blood 90:1387–1394, 1997.

48. B Payelle-Brogard, C Magnac, FR Mauro, F Mandelli, G Dighiero. Analysis of the B-cell receptor B29 (CD79b) gene in familial chronic lymphocytic leukemia. Blood 94:3516–3522, 1999.

49. A Alfarano, S Indraccolo, P Circosta, S Minuzzo, A Vallario, R Zamarchi, A Fregonese, F Calderazzo, A Faldella, M Aragno, C Camaschella, A Amadori, F Caligaris-Cappio. An alternatively spliced form of CD79b gene may account for altered B-cell receptor expression in B-chronic lymphocytic leukemia. Blood 93:2327–2335, 1999.

50. V Pistoia. Production of cytokines by human B cells in health and disease. Immunol Today 18:343–350, 1997.

51. P Panayiotidis, K Ganeshaguru, SA Jabbar, AV Hoffbrand. Interleukin-4 inhibits apoptotic cell death and loss of the bcl-2 protein in B-chronic lymphocytic leukaemia cells in vitro. Br J Haematol 85:439–445, 1993.

52. S Zupo, L Isnardi, M Megna, R Massara, F Malavasi, M Dono, E Cosulich, M Ferrarini M. CD38 expression distinguishes two groups of B-cell chronic lymphocytic leukemias with different responses to anti-IgM antibodies and propensity to apoptosis. Blood 88:1365–1374, 1996.

53. S Zupo, R Massara, M Dono, E Rossi, F Malavasi, ME Cosulich, M Ferrarini. Apoptosis or plasma cell differentiation of CD38-positive B-chronic lymphocytic leukemia cells induced by cross-linking of surface IgM or IgD. Blood 95:1199–1206, 2000.

54. J Golay, M Luppi, S Songia, C Palvarini, L Lombardi, A Aiello, D Delia, K Lam, DH Crawford, A Biondi, T Barbui, A Rambaldi, M Introna. Expression of A-myb, but not c-myb and B-myb, is restricted to Burkitt's lymphoma, sIg+ B-acute lymphoblastic leukemia, and a subset of chronic lymphocytic leukemias. Blood 87:1900–1911, 1996.

55. M Hallek, I Langenmayer, C Nerl, W Knauf, H Dietzfelbinger, D Adorf, M Ostwald, R Busch, I Kuhn-Hallek, E Thiel, B Emmerich. Elevated serum thymidine kinase levels identify a subgroup at high risk of disease progression in early, nonsmoldering chronic lymphocytic leukemia. Blood 93:1732–1737, 1999.

56. TJ Kipps. Signal transduction pathways and mechanisms of apoptosis in CLL B-lymphocytes: their role in CLL pathogenesis. Hematol Cell Ther 39(suppl 1):S17–27, 1997.

57. TJ Kipps, E Tomhave, LF Pratt, S Duffy, PP Chen, DA Carson. Developmentally restricted immunoglobulin heavy chain variable region gene expressed at high frequency in chronic lymphocytic leukemia. Proc Natl Acad Sci U S A 86:5913–5917, 1989.

58. TJ Kipps, DA Carson. Autoantibodies in chronic lymphocytic leukemia and related systemic autoimmune diseases. Blood 81:2475–2487, 1993.

59. F Fais, F Ghiotto, S Hashimoto, B Sellars, A Valetto, SL Allen, P Schulman, VP Vinciguerra, K Rai, LZ Rassenti, TJ Kipps, G Dighiero, H Schroeder, M Ferrarini, N Chiorazzi. Chronic lymphocytic leukemia B cells express restricted sets of mutated and unmutated antigen receptors. J Clin Invest 102:1515–1525, 1998.

60. TJ Hamblin, Z Davis, A Gardiner, DG Oscier, FK Stevenson. Unmutated Ig V(H) genes are associated with a more aggressive form of chronic lymphocytic leukemia. Blood 94:1848–1854, 1999.

61. DG Oscier, A Thompsett, D Zhu, FK Stevenson. Differential rates of somatic hypermutation in V(H) genes among subsets of chronic lymphocytic leukemia defined by chromosomal abnormalities. Blood 89:4153–4160, 1997.

62. RN Damle, T Wasil, F Fais, F Ghiotto, A Valetto, SL Allen, A Buchbinder, D Budman, K Dittmar, J Kolitz, SM Lichtman, P Schulman, VP Vinciguerra, KR Rai, M Ferrarini, N Chio-

razzi. Ig V gene mutation status and CD38 expression as novel prognostic indicators in chronic lymphocytic leukemia. Blood 94:1840–1847, 1999.

63. G Bikah, J Carey, JR Ciallella, A Tarakhovsky, S Bondada. CD5-mediated negative regulation of antigen receptor-induced growth signals in B-1 B cells. Science 274:1906–1909, 1996.

64. JO Pers, C Jamin, R Le Corre, PM Lydyard, P Youinou. Ligation of CD5 on resting B cells, but not on resting T cells, results in apoptosis. Eur J Immunol 28:4170–4176, 1998.

65. R Pospisil, RG Mage. CD5 and other superantigens as "ticklers" of the B-cell receptor. Immunol Today 19:106–108, 1998.

66. R Pospisil, G Silverman, GE Marti, A Aruffo, MA Bowen, RG Mage. CD5 is a potential selecting ligand for B-cell surface immunoglobulin: a possible role in maintenance and selective expansion of normal and malignant B cells. Leuk Lymphoma 36:353–365, 2000.

67. H Van de Velde, I von Hoegen, W Luo, JR Parnes, K Thielemans. The B-cell surface protein CD72/Lyb-2 is the ligand for CD5. Nature 351:662–665, 1991.

68. PH Krammer. CD95(APO-1/Fas)-mediated apoptosis: live and let die. Adv Immunol 71:163–210, 1999.

69. LM Osorio, M Aguilar-Santelises. Apoptosis in B-chronic lymphocytic leukaemia [in process citation]. Med Oncol 15:234–240, 1998.

70. D Wang, GJ Freeman, H Levine, J Ritz, MJ Robertson. Role of the CD40 and CD95 (APO-1/Fas) antigens in the apoptosis of human B-cell malignancies. Br J Haematol 97:409–417, 1997.

71. P Panayiotidis, K Ganeshaguru, L Foroni, AV Hoffbrand. Expression and function of the FAS antigen in B chronic lymphocytic leukemia and hairy cell leukemia. Leukemia 9:1227–1232, 1995.

72. SL Peng, ME Robert, AC Hayday, J Craft. A tumor-suppressor function for Fas (CD95) revealed in T cell-deficient mice. J Exp Med 184:1149–1154, 1996.

73. C Lagresle, P Mondiere, C Bella, PH Krammer, T Defrance. Concurrent engagement of CD40 and the antigen receptor protects naive and memory human B cells from APO-1/Fas-mediated apoptosis. J Exp Med 183:1377–1388, 1996.

74. JC Rathmell, SE Townsend, JC Xu, RA Flavell, CC Goodnow. Expansion or elimination of B cells in vivo: dual roles for CD40- and Fas (CD95)-ligands modulated by the B cell antigen receptor. Cell 87:319–329, 1996.

75. TL Rothstein, JK Wang, DJ Panka, LC Foote, Z Wang, B Stanger, H Cui, ST Ju, A Marshak-Rothstein. Protection against Fas-dependent Th1-mediated apoptosis by antigen receptor engagement in B cells. Nature 374:163–165, 1995.

76. Y Tsujimoto, J Cossman, E Jaffe, CM Croce. Involvement of the bcl-2 gene in human follicular lymphoma. Science 228:1440–1443, 1985.

77. DT Chao, SJ Korsmeyer. BCL-2 family: regulators of cell death. Annu Rev Immunol 16:395–419, 1998.

78. M Schena, LG Larsson, D Gottardi, G Gaidano, M Carlsson, K Nilsson, F Caligaris-Cappio. Growth- and differentiation-associated expression of bcl-2 in B-chronic lymphocytic leukemia cells. Blood 79:2981–2989, 1992.

79. T Mainou-Fowler, VA Craig, AJ Copplestone, MD Hamon, AG Prentice. Effect of anti-APO1 on spontaneous apoptosis of B cells in chronic lymphocytic leukaemia: the role of bcl-2 and interleukin 4. Leuk Lymphoma 19:301–308, 1995.

80. MY Mapara, R Bargou, C Zugck, H Dohner, F Ustaoglu, RR Jonker, PH Krammer, B Dorken. APO-1 mediated apoptosis or proliferation in human chronic B lymphocytic leukemia: correlation with bcl-2 oncogene expression. Eur J Immunol 23:702–708, 1993.

81. S Kitada, J Andersen, S Akar, JM Zapata, S Takayama, S Krajewski, HG Wang, X Zhang, F Bullrich, CM Croce, K Rai, J Hines, JC Reed. Expression of apoptosis-regulating proteins in chronic lymphocytic leukemia: correlations with in vitro and in vivo chemoresponses. Blood 91:3379–3389, 1998.

82. IS Grewal, RA Flavell. CD40 and CD154 in cell-mediated immunity. Annu Rev Immunol 16:111–135, 1998.
83. MF Romano, A Lamberti, P Tassone, F Alfinito, S Costantini, F Chiurazzi, T Defrance, P Bonelli, F Tuccillo, MC Turco, S Venuta. Triggering of CD40 antigen inhibits fludarabine-induced apoptosis in B chronic lymphocytic leukemia cells [published erratum appears in Blood 15;93:214, 1999]. Blood 92:990–995, 1998.
84. A Younes, V Snell, U Consoli, K Clodi, S Zhao, JL Palmer, EK Thomas, RJ Armitage, M Andreeff. Elevated levels of biologically active soluble CD40 ligand in the serum of patients with chronic lymphocytic leukaemia. Br J Haematol 100:135–141, 1998.
85. G Pizzolo, M Chilosi, A Ambrosetti, G Semenzato, L Fiore-Donati, G Perona. Immunohistologic study of bone marrow involvement in B-chronic lymphocytic leukemia. Blood 62:1289–1296, 1983.
86. M Cantwell, T Hua, J Pappas, TJ Kipps. Acquired CD40-ligand deficiency in chronic lymphocytic leukemia. Nat Med 3:984–989, 1997.
87. P Ghia, F Caligaris-Cappio. The indispensable role of microenvironment in the natural history of low grade B cell neoplasms. Adv Cancer Res 79:157–174, 2000.

5

Immunoglobulin Variable Region Gene Characteristics and Surface Membrane Phenotype Define B-CLL Subgroups with Distinct Clinical Courses

NICHOLAS CHIORAZZI

North Shore–Long Island Jewish Research Institute, North Shore University Hospital, and New York University School of Medicine, Manhasset, New York

MANLIO FERRARINI

Istituto Nazionale per la Ricerca sul Cancro, and Università di Genova, Genova, Italy

I. INTRODUCTION

B cell chronic lymphocytic leukemia (B-CLL) cases are clinically heterogeneous, because some patients survive for prolonged periods without requiring definitive therapy, whereas others die rapidly despite aggressive treatment (1,2). However at the cellular level, the disease has been considered homogeneous, resulting from the accumulation of a leukemic clone derived from a normal CD5$^+$ B lymphocyte (3). In addition, these B lymphocytes have been termed "incompetent" (4).

Recent data, however, suggest that B-CLL cases are also heterogeneous *at the cellular level* and can be divided into at least two subgroups on the basis of the molecular and phenotypic features of the monoclonal leukemic B cells. Furthermore, these data suggest that the leukemic B-CLL cells derive from immunocompetent and probably antigenically experienced B lymphocytes. These two distinctions, (i.e., that the leukemic cells of different patients are *not* homogeneous and that they do *not* derive from immature incompetent B lymphocytes) appear to be significant. Most importantly, the distinctions provide clinicians with tools to subdivide patients with B-CLL into groups that follow different clinical courses. Moreover, they will likely provide the basic and clinical investigator with clues to decipher differences in disease pathogenesis.

In this chapter, we will review the information that led to the definition of these B-CLL subgroups. These subgroups are defined by the characteristics of the immunoglobulin (Ig) variable region (V) genes expressed by the clone of B-CLL cells (i.e., the presence or absence of V gene mutations) and also by surface membrane phenotype of the B-CLL cells (i.e., the percentage of the B-CLL clone that expresses CD38). In addition, we will review the current knowledge on the differences in clinical course and outcome that patients in these subgroups experience. We believe that the subcategorization of patients with B-CLL using these laboratory parameters will aid clinicians in designing new therapeutic protocols, in choosing which patients to treat, and perhaps in deciding on which modalities to use.

II. THE EXPRESSION OF Ig GENES AND THE DEVELOPMENT AND MATURATION OF NORMAL B LYMPHOCYTES

A. Rearrangement of V Genes to Encode an Antibody Molecule

The genes encoding the heavy (H) and light (L) chain components of an antibody molecule are located in distinct clusters on different chromosomes. In man, the genes for the H chain lie on chromosome 14 and for the L chain on chromosomes 2 (κ chains) and 22 (λ chains). These clusters contain multiple genes for the variable (V) portions of the Ig molecules located at the 5' end of each locus and genes for the constant (C) portions of Ig molecules at the 3' end of these loci. Between these two regions, the D and J_H gene segments for the H chain and the J_L segments for the L chains reside.

The somatic DNA rearrangements that lead to the formation of gene segments encoding a complete Ig molecule within an individual B cell proceed in a defined order, beginning with the H chain locus (5,6). The initial rearrangement involves the recombination of a D segment with a J_H segment, with deletion of the intervening DNA (Fig. 1). This recombination event results in a DNA fragment that will encode the third complementarity determining region (CDR) and the fourth framework region (FR) of the V region of the H chain. Subsequently, any one of a series of 44 functional V_H gene segments is rearranged to this DJ_H segment to yield the 5' portion of the V region of the Ig molecule (FR1, CDR1, FR2, CDR2, and FR3). Additional diversity in the CDR3 region can develop by either the addition or deletion of nucleotides at the D-J_H or at the V_H-DJ_H junctions. These additional nucleotides are inserted by terminal deoxynucleotidyl transferase (7,8) or removed by exonucleases. The process of modifying the nucleotide sequence at the D-J_H and V_H-DJ_H junctions is referred to as coding end processing (9).

Similar processes occur at the L chain loci, although these involve only two gene segments (V_L and J_L). In general, V genes of the κ locus are rearranged first. If these attempts on both chromosomes fail to yield a functional L chain, rearrangements of the V genes of the λ locus occur.

The gene segments that code for the C_H and C_L peptides do not recombine at the DNA level with the rearranged $V_H DJ_H$ or $V_L J_L$ segments. Rather, processing of the primary

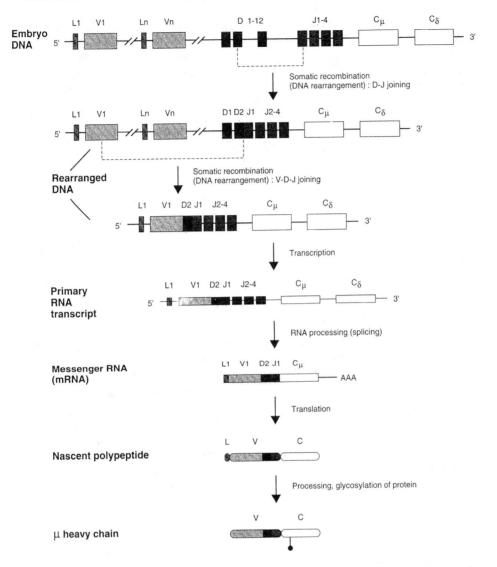

Figure 1 Sequence of gene rearrangement, transcription, and synthesis of the Ig μ H chain. In this example, the V region of the μ chain is encoded by the exons V1, D2, and J1. V genes are indicated as V1 to Vn; C_H genes 3′ of Cδ are not shown. (Adapted with permission from AK Abbas, AH Lichtman, JS Pober, eds, *Cellular and Molecular Immunology*, 3rd ed. Philadelphia: W.B. Saunders Company, 1991, 78.)

RNA nuclear transcripts derived from these segments leads to the fully endowed, functional mRNA transcript that can be translated into a μ H chain and either a κ or λ L chain.

B. Maturation of B Lymphocytes

B lymphocytes develop in the bone marrow from specific precursor cells in a sequential manner also. Stem cells give rise to pro-B cells that in turn lead to pre-B cells, and then to immature B cells, and finally to mature B cells (10). Although the earliest cells in this sequence do not express Ig genes, the expression of these genes and the synthesis of Ig gene products subsequently occurs in a well-defined and fairly rigidly adhered to order. These events are essential for the development of mature B cells. Figure 2 illustrates these stages of B cell development and the Ig genes that are rearranged, transcribed, and translated into Ig molecules at these various stages.

Mature B lymphocytes exit the bone marrow, begin to circulate, and localize eventually at different sites of the peripheral lymphoid organs (11). Virgin IgM$^+$/IgD$^+$ B cells localize primarily in the mantle zone of lymphoid follicles. Although several factors are likely to influence their subsequent fate, the mode of antigenic stimulation and the specificity of the BCR play a fundamental role.

When BCR encounter an antigen with adequate and appropriate affinity, a signal is transduced to the inside of the B lymphocyte, indicating that it should proliferate and/or differentiate into a plasma cell (12). Antigens differ in the ways in which they stimulate B cells, in particular in their need to and capacity to elicit T cell help for the B cells (13). Therefore, they are classified as T cell–independent or T cell–dependent antigens. T cell–independent antigens usually are multimeric molecules that display repeating antigenic epitopes in long linear arrays. These arrays can effectively cross-link multiple BCR molecules and thereby induce B cell activation. T cell–independent antigens cannot be processed well into fragments that can be presented to T cells in association with major histocompatibility (MHC) molecules. The antibody responses induced by T cell–independent antigens are usually different than those induced by T cell–dependent antigens. They are primarily of the IgM isotype, and the affinity of these antibodies does not change appreciably over time. B lymphocytes that express the CD5 antigen classically are thought to respond to T cell–independent antigens (14,15).

When T cell–dependent antigens bind to and stimulate B cells, they are internalized, digested, and displayed as fragments on the B cell surface in association with MHC molecules (16). These antigen-MHC fragments are recognized by specific T cells, allowing them to provide costimulatory signals to the B cell in the forms of contact-mediated and soluble cytokine-mediated help. The signals needed to promote these processes result from a dynamic interplay between the B cell and the T cell (17,18). This interplay involves pairs of cell interaction molecules (e.g., CD40 with CD40 ligand, B7.1 and B7.2 with CD28) and cytokines that are up- and down-regulated in a coordinated manner based on each preceding cellular communication. As a consequence of these T-dependent antigen-initiated interactions, these B cells may switch the isotype they produce, migrate to germinal centers, and undergo a number of changes in the Ig V_H and V_L genes aimed at increasing the affinity of the antibody produced (10). Memory B cells that characteristically express only surface IgM or IgG, exit the germinal centers and enter in part into the B lymphocyte circulating pool or seed into the marginal zone or marginal zone equivalent areas (13,19).

Figure 2   A summary of the development of human B cells. The stages in B cell development, their location, the state of the Ig genes, the expression of cell surface molecules, and the expression of essential intracellular proteins are shown. CD38 is also expressed on mature activated B cells, especially those stimulated by antigen. (Adapted with permission from CA Janeway, Jr., P Travers, eds, Immunobiology. The Immune System in Health and Disease. 2nd ed. New York: Garland Publishing Inc, 1996, 5:27.)

B cells		Heavy-chain genes	Light-chain genes	Intra-cellular proteins	Surface marker proteins
Stem cell		Germline	Germline		CD34 CD45
Early pro-B cell		D–J rearranged	Germline	RAG-1 RAG-2 TdT λ5, VpreB	CD34, CD45 MHC class II CD10, CD19 CD38
Late pro-B cell		V–DJ rearranged	Germline	TdT λ5, VpreB	CD45R MHC class II (Dμ) CD10, CD19 CD38, CD20 CD40
Large Pre-B cell	pre-B receptor	VDJ rearranged	Germline	RAG-1 RAG-2 μ λ5, VpreB	CD45R MHC class II preB-R CD19, CD38 CD20, CD40
Small Pre-B cell	μ	VDJ rearranged	V–J rearrangement	μ	CD45R MHC class II CD19, CD38 CD20, CD40
Immature B cell	IgM	VDJ rearranged. μ heavy chain produced in membrane form	VJ rearranged		CD45R MHC class II IgM CD19, CD20 CD40
Mature naive B cell	IgD IgM	VDJ rearranged. μ chain produced in membrane form. Alternative splicing yields μ + δ mRNA	VJ rearranged		CD45R MHC class II IgM, IgD CD19, CD20 CD21, CD40
Lympho-blast	IgM	VDJ rearranged. Alternative splicing yields secreted μ chains	VJ rearranged	Ig	CD45R MHC class II CD19, CD20 CD21, CD40
Memory B cell	IgG	Isotype switch to Cγ, Cα, or Cε. Somatic hypermutation	VJ rearranged. Somatic hypermutation		CD45R MHC class II IgG, IgA CD19, CD20 CD21, CD40
Plasma cell	IgG	Isotype switch and alternative splicing yields secreted γ, α, or ε chains	VJ rearranged	Ig	Plasma cell antigen-1 CD38

ANTIGEN INDEPENDENT

ANTIGEN DEPENDENT

TERMINAL DIFFERENTIATION

BONE MARROW

PERIPHERY

The scheme of mature B cell circulation and development outlined earlier is still incomplete, because new data continuously add to its complexity. For example, it is now known that marginal zone B cells are comprised also of virgin B cells and of B cells capable of T cell–independent responses (20–22). Likewise, memory cells may be found within the IgM$^+$/IgD$^+$ B cell pool (23–25).

C. Events That Contribute to the Shaping of the Antigen-Binding Repertoire

The expression of the Ig H and L chain genes are not merely markers but serve critical functions in the development of B cells. Indeed, those B cells that do not perform these Ig rearrangement, transcription, and translation events successfully are lost from the developing repertoire. This is made clear by the facts that spontaneous or induced alterations in these genes or in their expression have profound influences on B cell development (10). By the time a surface BCR is present—either at the pre-B cell with a BCR that includes a surrogate L chain or at the immature B cell with a BCR that includes a classical L chain—signals through the receptor have profound effects on the developing B lymphocyte.

The degree to which a BCR can interact with autologous structures (autoantigens) affects the B lymphocyte's subsequent development. Although autoreactivity may be tolerated (and possibly preferred) at the pre-B cell stage, it is clear that such reactivity is selected against in immature and mature B cells. B cells with BCR of sufficient affinity for immobilized, cell-bound antigens are either deleted from the repertoire by apoptosis (26) or are induced to undergo secondary V gene rearrangements (receptor editing) that might salvage the cell by creating a new nonautoreactive BCR (27–29). B cells expressing BCR with affinity for soluble autoantigens are handled somewhat differently. These cells are rendered unresponsive to the antigen but may exit the bone marrow as anergic B cells that express reduced numbers of surface BCR molecules (30,31). These B cells have several phenotypic and functional characteristics similar to B-CLL cells.

The mature functional (as well as anergic) B cells that exit the bone marrow do not express BCR comprised of all possible V gene segments in all possible combinations. In other words, the repertoire of emerging mature B cells is not completely random. This is a reflection of both the positive and negative (against autoreactivity) selection events (32), as well as apparent, and not well understood, genetic preferences for the recombination of certain gene segments (33–40). This concept is important for understanding the BCR repertoires expressed by B lymphocytes involved in diseases such as B-CLL.

A series of events crucial for shaping the antibody repertoire can occur in the periphery in the germinal centers of lymphoid follicles (10,41). Here, the B cells that respond to an antigen, with the help of T cells and other accessory cells such as follicular dendritic cells, undergo changes in the V_H/V_L genes that consist primarily in the accumulation of point mutations. Thus, accumulation of these mutations marks a cell that has passed or has not traversed a germinal center. This information may be very important for B-CLL cells, because B-CLL cases can be segregated into two groups on the basis of the presence or absence of Ig V gene mutations (vide infra). Although CD5$^+$ B cells frequently respond to T cell–independent antigen, it is likely that at least one subset of B-CLL originated from cells that had responded to antigen in a T cell–dependent fashion and had passed through germinal centers (42).

The Ig V gene nucleotide mutational changes occurring in the germinal center are random, and it is therefore likely that some mutations will result in B cells with receptors that either lose affinity for the selecting antigen or develop receptors for autoantigen (41,43). This requires that the immune system have mechanisms to either modify the BCR of these B cells or to eliminate them. Two important mechanisms of receptor modification include receptor editing of the L chain (27–29) and receptor revision of the H chain (43–46). Apoptosis is the mechanism responsible for clonal deletion.

III. IMMUNOGLOBULIN V GENES IN B-CLL

Over the years, there has been considerable interest in the Ig V genes expressed by the leukemic B cells of B-CLL patients and in the structure of the BCR encoded by these V genes. This interest comes from the belief that antigen binding to the BCR, and subsequent stimulation of the B cell, might be involved in the pathogenesis of this disease.

Understanding the V genes and the structure of the BCR expressed by the leukemic B cells can provide information about the immunocompetency, differentiation stage, and subset designation of B-CLL cells and the B lymphocytes from which they derive. For instance, if antigen binding to the BCR is involved in the evolution from a normal B cell to a leukemic cell, it would be most unlikely for this to have occurred in an ''incompetent'' precursor B cell that could not transduce and respond to signals delivered through its BCR. In addition, this B lymphocyte by definition would not be ''naïve.'' Furthermore, antigen-binding might lead indirectly to the transformation of distinct subsets of B cells at discrete stages of maturation. This could occur in several ways. First, because some B cell lineages (e.g., CD5$^+$ B cells in mice; (47,48) appear to express restricted sets of BCR because of apparent biased V gene use, then certain antigens and antigenic determinants might support the leukemic evolutionary process. In addition, because antigen-binding leads to cellular differentiation, engagement of the BCR might allow the B lymphocyte to progress through certain stages of maturation that may be more likely to favor malignant transformation (e.g., the germinal center reaction).

Finally, if B-CLL is a disease of B lymphocytes that react with specific antigens or restricted sets of antigens, studies of the structure of the BCR and the genes that encode it may infer information about the nature and identity of the antigen(s). Although several B cell lymphoproliferative disorders appear to be associated with viral infection (e.g., Burkitt's lymphoma, primary effusion lymphomas, Castleman's disease, and possibly multiple myeloma; 49–53), there has been only one example suggesting that an infectious agent may be involved in B-CLL. These were studies indicating that B-CLL patients from the Caribbean were infected with HTLV-1 (54–56) and that the antigen receptors of some of these B-CLL cells reacted with antigens derived from HTLV-1 (57). This observation suggests that a virus or its expressed foreign proteins could be selected by the BCR and either directly transform the B cell or serve as chronic antigenic stimuli to select out and expand those B cells that would eventually develop a transforming event. In this respect, B-CLL would differ from these other lymphoproliferative disorders in which latent viral infection per se induces cell proliferation and promotes both the clonal expansion and the accumulation of additional genetic changes. In these instances, the clonal stimulation and expansion do not involve the BCR.

Antigen binding and stimulation could be relevant, therefore, before and/or after the ultimate leukemogenic event. Chronic stimulation, by either foreign antigens or au-

Table 1 V Gene Findings Suggestive of Antigen Reactivity, Drive, and Selection

Biased use of individual V_H and/or V_L gene families
Biased use of individual V_H and/or V_L genes
Selective pairing of individual V_H and V_L genes
Accumulation of more replacement mutations than predicted by statistical algorithms in the CDR
   and/or accumulation of less replacement mutations than predicted in the FR
Presence of relatively unique CDR3 motifs in the rearranged $V_H DJ_H$ or $V_L J_L$ genes

toantigens, could lead to the preleukemic expansion of discrete B cell clones, and within these stimulated and dividing clones, critical molecular defects might arise that could combine to lead to the leukemia. Furthermore, ongoing antigen binding to the BCR of the leukemic clone might also alter its in vivo behavior by modifying its growth rate, impeding spontaneous or induced apoptosis, or by other ill-defined mechanisms.

In summary, studies of the V genes expressed by B-CLL cells and the structure of the BCR they encode may provide information about the immunobiology of the B-CLL cell and clues to the evolution to the leukemic state. In particular, such analyses can address the following questions:

Are B-CLL cases diverse or restricted in their Ig V gene characteristics?
Do B-CLL cells derive from immunologically competent or immunologically incompetent B cells?
Is there a potential role of antigen reactivity and drive in the disease?
What are the maturation stage(s) and subset designation(s) of the B cell clone(s) transformed in the disease?

The information derived from Ig V gene analyses that support a role for the potential role of antigen reactivity and drive in a lymphoid disease is listed in Table 1. The data relevant to each of these points in B-CLL are summarized in the following sections.

IV. Ig V GENE CHARACTERISTICS OF B-CLL CELLS

A. Gene Use

The first reports that B-CLL cells use a restricted set of V genes were published by Kipps et al. (58–60). This principle has now been confirmed by several groups for V_H gene use.

Normal $CD5^+$ B lymphocytes use genes of the various V_H families in the following order: $V_H3 > V_H1 = V_H4 > V_H5 > V_H2 > V_H7$ (40). When the data from all of the studies of V_H gene use in B-CLL that are currently available (42,61–71) are pooled, the statistical analyses indicate that V_H gene family use is not comparable to the normal B cell repertoire (Fig. 3). In B-CLL, V_H1 family genes are expressed more frequently, and V_H3 family genes are expressed less frequently than in normal $CD5^+$ B lymphocytes (42). In addition, there is a significant overrepresentation of two individual genes among B-CLL cases—the V_H 1–69 gene and the V_H 4-34 gene (Fig. 4). This overrepresentation of V_H 1-69 in B-CLL is apparently restricted to distinct alleles (72).

Because the total number of B-CLL cases in these V_H gene analyses is ~300, it seems likely that this distribution of V_H genes is representative of the disease. However, several caveats need to be considered regarding the comparison of gene use in the B-CLL versus normal B cell repertoires. The first is the recently appreciated fact that the normal

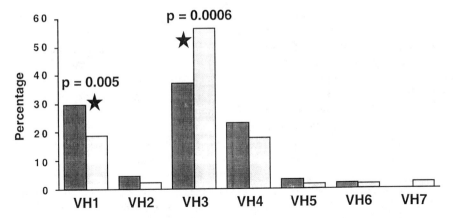

Figure 3 Comparison of V_H gene family use between the available IgM$^+$ B-CLL cases and normal blood B cells. The IgM$^+$ B-CLL cases represent a pool of those reported in the literature (42,61–71). Normal IgM$^+$ CD5$^+$ blood B cell sequences were derived from analyses of single cells from two controls (40). Statistical comparisons were performed using Fisher's exact test. (Adapted with permission from Ref. 42.)

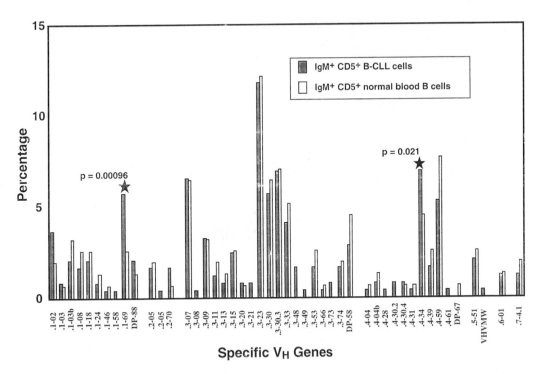

Figure 4 Comparison of V_H gene use between the available IgM$^+$ B-CLL cases and normal blood B cells. The IgM$^+$ B-CLL cases and the normal IgM$^+$ CD5$^+$ blood B cell sequences are as described in the legend to Figure 3 (42,61–71). Normal IgM$^+$ CD5$^+$ blood B cell sequences were derived from analyses of single cells from two controls (40). Statistical comparisons were performed using Fisher's exact test. (Adapted with permission from Ref. 42.)

B cell repertoire is developmentally skewed on the basis of gene rearrangements that are selected by various mechanisms either in the bone marrow or in the periphery (27–29,33–40,43–46). Second, it is unclear whether these V gene biases are maintained throughout adulthood or whether they change with age, either in all individuals or in selected individuals on the basis of their antigenic exposures. Indeed, age-related V_H gene bias is seen in inbred strains of mice (73,74). Furthermore, oligoclonal B cell expansions containing restricted V_H genes are common in aging mice (75), and as certain strains of mice age, they develop monoclonal gammopathies and B-CLL–like leukemias and lymphomas (76–78). Finally, the V gene sequences of $CD5^+$ B cells that are available as controls derive from only a limited number of normal individuals that are of ages considerably younger than most B-CLL patients (40), and therefore potential differences in V_H expression among normals (e.g., Ref. 79) must be considered. Despite these potentially confounding issues, however, at this point it seems reasonable to accept a bias in V_H gene use in B-CLL.

B. Pairing of Specific V_H and V_L Genes

There are not extensive data on this issue in B-CLL. It has been suggested that IgM-expressing cases are more likely to express V_L genes of the VκIIIb family, although these data are derived from limited numbers of cases (80,81), and this issue probably requires further study. The most convincing data on selective pairing of Ig V_H and V_L genes in B-CLL cells are derived from cases that express surface membrane IgG (82). In a cohort of 21 patients, 5 were found to express V genes that code for remarkably similar BCR (83). In all five cases, the rearranged $V_H DJ_H$ segments consisted of a V_H4-39 gene linked to a D6-13 segment in turn linked to a J_H5 segment. The rearranged $V_L J_L$ genes of each of these B-CLL cells were comprised of the same Vκ1 gene (O12); the J_L segment in all but one of these patients was Jκ1. Therefore, at least in this isotype-switched subset of B-CLL cases, pairing of specific V_H, D, and J_H segments and specific V_L and J_L genes can occur.

C. Occurrence of Somatic Mutations in the Ig V Genes Expressed by B-CLL Cells

Initial studies of B-CLL cells suggested that the V genes of these cells (or the B cells from which they derive) undergo little, if any, somatic mutation (58–60,84–87). These findings were consistent with murine data, suggesting that the $CD5^+/Ly1^+/B1$ B cell lineage is characterized by a restricted V gene repertoire that rarely accumulates mutations (88). However, the concept of a lack of somatic mutation in B-CLL cells has now been modified. Interest in this issue was stimulated by a statistical review of available B-CLL sequences by Schroeder and Dighiero that suggested that B-CLL might represent the clonal expansion of both unmutated and mutated $CD5^+$ B cells (61). Analyses of IgG^+ B-CLL cases (89,90) and cases defined by chromosomal abnormalities (119) supported this view.

However, the pivotal study that documented this point was that of Fais et al. (42), which clearly demonstrated that ~50% of randomly chosen IgM^+ B-CLL cases and ~75% of IgG^+ and IgA^+ cases exhibited significant numbers of V_H gene mutations ($\geq$2% differences from most similar germline genes). These cases all exhibited the clinical and laboratory characteristics typical of B-CLL patients. In addition, each case expressed only one V_H or V_L gene (i.e., did not lack allelic exclusion, a feature that has been shown to occur in 5%–10% of B-CLL cases (91)).

The degree of V gene mutation that occurred in these B-CLL cells was considerable, because >30% of the IgM$^+$ B-CLL cells and >65% of the isotype-switched B-CLL cells exhibited >5% differences from their germline gene counterparts (42). Furthermore, there was a 10-fold greater percentage of B-CLL cells expressing mutations in the >5% range compared with normal CD5$^+$ B lymphocytes (3.5% versus 31.8%); this frequency even exceeded that reported for CD5$^-$ B cells (~17.6% versus 31.8%; Fig. 5). On the basis of these data, Fais et al. concluded that B-CLL cases are heterogeneous at the level of the leukemic cell and therefore can be segregated into two subgroups on the basis of the presence or absence of significant numbers of V$_H$ gene mutations (42). Hamblin et al. subsequently reported data in another large cohort of well-characterized B-CLL patients confirming this observation (71).

One of the reasons for the discrepancy between the initial studies of mutations in B-CLL cells and those reported recently may relate to the observation that V$_H$ gene mutations in B-CLL are distributed nonstochastically and appear to relate to the V$_H$ family gene expressed in the B-CLL cell (42). A V$_H$ family-related hierarchy in the likelihood that a B-CLL cell will express V$_H$ gene mutations appears to exist (V$_H$3 > V$_H$4 > V$_H$1). Therefore, patient cohorts that are small and that are inadvertently skewed in V$_H$ gene

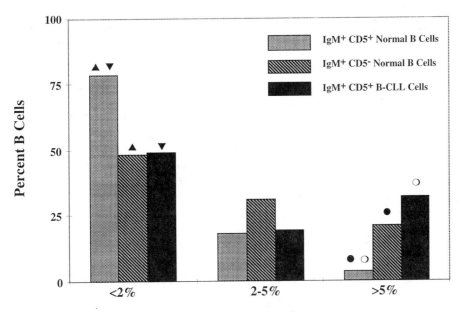

Percent Difference from Progenitor Germline Gene

Figure 5 Comparison of extent of V$_H$ gene mutation between normal peripheral blood IgM$^+$ CD5$^+$ and IgM$^+$ CD5$^-$ B cells, and IgM$^+$ CD5$^+$ B-CLL cells. The IgM$^+$ CD5$^+$ blood B cells (n = 144) and the IgM$^+$ CD5$^-$ B cells (n = 206) are from Ref. 40; the IgM$^+$ CD5$^+$ B-CLL cells (n = 63) are from the study of Fais et al. (42). Statistically significant differences (Fisher's exact test) were found in the <2% group between the CD5$^+$ and the CD5$^-$ normal B cells (regular triangle) and between the CD5$^+$ normal cells and the B-CLL cells (inverted triangle) with a P value for both of <0.00005. Similarly, within the >5% group, statistically significant differences were found between the same two comparisons (closed and open circles, respectively) with a p value for both of <0.000001. (Adapted with permission from Ref. 42.)

family expression might demonstrate different levels of somatic mutation. It is still unclear why B-CLL cells display these differences in mutation. This may reflect differences in the types of antigens that have driven the individual B cells before their leukemic transformation and/or differences in the maturation stages at which they were transformed into leukemic cells (42,71,92).

D. Accumulation of More Than Predicted Replacement (R) Mutations in the CDR and Less in the FR

B cells with receptors that have been selected by antigen often display a higher than predicted frequency of replacement (R) mutations in the CDR and/or a lower percentage of R mutations in the FR (24,93,94). These comparisons need to take into account the inherent susceptibility to develop amino acid replacements in the different regions of the V_H gene (95). Using algorithms that incorporate these considerations, ~20% of B-CLL cells demonstrate selection for R mutations in their CDR and ~60% demonstrate a selection against R mutations in the FR (42).

Therefore, the cases with more R mutations in CDR may derive from B lymphocytes that were selected for clonal expansion on the basis of their reactivity with specific antigens. The cases with less R mutations in FR may derive from B lymphocytes that were selected for the expression of an intact BCR, which is consistent with the notion that mature B cells must receive trophic signals through the BCR to maintain viability (96).

E. Presence of Relatively Unique CDR3 Motifs

The CDR3 of both the H and L chains are the most variable parts of the BCR (5,97), and these regions are most likely to make intimate contact with antigen (98). CDR3 structure is a function of the specific gene segments that are rearranged and recombined, as well as the extent of coding end processing that occurs during these recombination events. Therefore, CDR3 structure can be analyzed at several levels, including gene segment use, nucleotide or amino acid composition, length, and charge.

The use of D gene families in B-CLL appears comparable to other antibodies in the databases (99). In one study, D3 genes were found most frequently, followed by D6 and D2 family genes (42), which is consistent with the normal repertoire (99). The most frequently used D3 segment was D3-3 (previously known as DXP4), that was found in a considerably greater proportion than in the normal repertoire. Johnson et al. (72) found that this specific D segment was used most often among B-CLL cells expressing the V_H 1-69 gene, a finding that was corroborated in one large random study (42) but not in another (71). In general, D segments in B-CLL cells are expressed in their hydrophilic reading frames (42), which is typical of the normal adult B cell repertoire (99,100).

J_H family use among B-CLL cells as a group does not appear to differ significantly from the normal CD5$^+$ B cell repertoire (42). However, J_H use differs among B-CLL cells that express different V_H family genes (42,72). Thus, ~90% of the B-CLL cases that use V_H 3-07 genes are associated with a J_H4 gene segment, whereas only <20% of the 1-69 genes used this segment (42). In contrast, 50% to 70% of the B-CLL cases that use 1-69 genes use a J_H6 segment (42,72), whereas few of the B-CLL cases that use 3-07 genes use a J_H6 segment (42).

HCDR3 length also apparently varies according to the V_H family incorporated into the rearranged gene of the B-CLL cells ($V_H4 > V_H1 > V_H3$; Ref. 42). These differences are even more obvious when comparing the most frequently used genes in the three major families. For instance, in the study by Fais et al. (42), the average HCDR3 length of all the 3-07 genes was 12.90 aa. In contrast, the average HCDR3 length among all of the 4-34$^+$B-CLL cells was 17.0 aa. The 4-34$^+$ B-CLL cells could be segregated into two groups: those with HCDR3 lengths longer than the average (19.92) that usually contained a J_H6 or J_H5 segment and those shorter than the average (12.33) that usually contained a J_H4 segment. The HCDR3 lengths among the 1-69$^+$ B-CLL cells was 17.85 (42). In the study of Johnson et al. (72), the HCDR3 lengths of 1-69–expressing B-CLL cells were even longer (19.0 aa).

The HCDR3 of IgM$^+$ B-CLL cases frequently contain relatively long stretches of tyrosines (Y) at their 3′ ends coded for by a J_H6 segment (42,72). Furthermore, when the acidic and basic amino acids and HCDR3 charges as defined by an estimated pI were determined, most of the IgM$^+$ B-CLL HCDR3 segments were much more acidic than usual. Those IgM$^+$ B-CLL cells expressing V_H1 genes had the lowest estimated pI, whereas those B-CLL cells expressing V_H3 genes had an average estimated pI of 4.61. The V_H4-expressing B-CLL cells displayed intermediate values (42).

Thus, there appear to be three HCDR3 categories in B-CLL cells on the basis of length, amino acid composition, and charge, and each of these appears to vary according to the V_H gene family expressed in the B-CLL cell (42).

V. SUMMARY OF Ig V GENE ANALYSES IN B-CLL

Collectively, these data suggest that:

B-CLL cases are restricted in regard to their Ig V gene characteristics. They segregate into two groups on the basis of the presence or absence of significant numbers ($\geq 2\%$) of somatic mutations. The "unmutated group" ($<2\%$ differences from germline gene) is more likely to express V_H1 family genes, in particular the V_H 1-69 gene, with a HCDR3 that is longer than average, is composed of a J_H6 segment possibly linked to a D3-3 (DXP-4) segment, contains several tyrosine residues, and is more acidic in charge. In contrast, the "mutated group" ($\geq 2\%$ differences from germline gene) is more likely to express V_H3 family genes, in particular the V_H 3-07 or 3-21 genes, with a HCDR3 that is shorter than average, is composed of a J_H4 segment, and is much less acidic in charge. An intermediate group composed of V_H4 family genes that have characteristics of either the unmutated or mutated group also exist. Thus, the BCR of these two subgroups is significantly different structurally. Figure 6 illustrates three prototypic BCR structures.

At least half of the B-CLL cases (those with Ig V gene mutations) derive from immunologically competent B cells. Because the current state of our knowledge suggests that somatic mutations are induced in B lymphocytes that have been triggered by T-dependent antigens and have probably migrated to germinal centers, the B-CLL precursors must have been competent and representative of the subset of cells from which they derive.

There is probably a potential role of antigen reactivity and drive in the disease. These data remain circumstantial. However, the data that favor this are (1) the apparent biases in V_H gene use (V_H1-69 and V_H4-34) globally in B-CLL and the probable biases in J_H and possibly in D segment use in the unmutated versus mutated subgroups of B-CLL, (2) the preservation of BCR structure indicated by

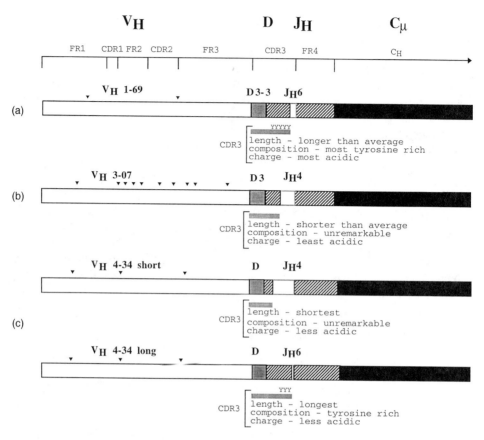

Figure 6 Prototypic variable regions of surface membrane IgM receptors in B-CLL. Schematic representations of the proposed V_H 1-69 (a), V_H 3-07 (b), and V_H 4-34 (c) prototypic V regions. Inverted triangles represent possible mutations. (Adapted with permission from Ref. 42.)

the lack of R replacements in the FR of most of the mutated B-CLL cases and the enhancement of R replacements in the CDR of some mutated cases, and (3) the unique HCDR3 motifs that distinguish the unmutated and mutated B-CLL cases from each other and from normal CD5[+] B cells. Whether these antigenic selections occurred as a result of the normal aging process remains to be determined.

At least the subgroup of B-CLL cases that contain Ig V gene mutations must have derived from mature antigenically experienced (not naïve) B cells that had probably reached the postgerminal center stage of maturation. This conclusion is based on the current state of our knowledge of mature B lymphocyte maturation. The following data support this conclusion.

VI. MATURATION AND ACTIVATION STAGES OF B-CLL CELLS

Initial studies of B-CLL cells suggested that they were naïve, antigen-inexperienced B lymphocytes. This was based on their surface membrane phenotype (IgM[+]/IgD[+]) and on the apparent lack of Ig V gene mutations. However, on the basis of the documentation of somatic mutations in approximately half of the cases (42), at least these cases most likely derive from previously stimulated/postgerminal center B cells. It still remains unclear whether unmutated B-CLL cells are naïve B cells or are B cells that have been antigen-stimulated cells but have not accumulated mutations. If the latter is true, the lack of mutation in some of these cells may reflect stimulation by antigens that cannot turn on the mutation machinery and/or the germinal center reaction (e.g., T-independent antigens) or may reflect a selection for unmutated V genes. As mentioned earlier, based on D and J_H gene use and HCDR3 motifs (42,72), antigen selection may have occurred in these unmutated B-CLL cells. However, these studies are only suggestive, and again the possibility that these "selections" reflect normal B cell development or the aging process must be considered.

Although B-CLL cells appear to be resting B cells, published data suggest that in vivo activation, albeit abortive, may have occurred. It has been reported that in both B-CLL and normal $CD5^+$ B cells cyclin D2 levels are selectively elevated without elevations of the other cyclins that follow in cell cycle progression (101). In addition, nuclear factor ATp (NF-ATp) can be increased in B-CLL cells (102). Both of these findings suggest that B-CLL cells or their precursors were triggered and attempted to enter the cell cycle. Finally, a recent study demonstrated the expression of CD40 ligand on the surface of B-CLL cells, again suggesting cellular activation (103). Thus, the molecular studies of V_H gene mutation reviewed earlier and these cellular studies suggest that in vivo activation of B-CLL cells or their precursors may have occurred.

The antigen specificity of the BCR of the B-CLL cell may again be relevant in this regard. Studies from our laboratory (104) and those of others (105,106) have shown that IgM^+ B-CLL cells synthesize polyreactive and autoreactive mAb. These findings are compatible with their $CD5^+$ B cell lineage (15) and may relate to the activated phenotype seen in B-CLL. Interestingly, autoantibody production increases with age in mice (107) and man (108), and $CD5^+$ B cell numbers increase in mice during the aging process (14). Thus, it is possible that the autoreactivity that is characteristic of $CD5^+$ B cells may be involved in the clonal expansions seen in aging mice and men and in B-CLL cells or their precursors.

To more accurately define the stage of maturation at which B-CLL cells are arrested, Damle et al. studied the surface membrane expression of IgD and CD38 on $CD5^+/CD19^+$ B cells in a series of well-characterized cases (92). Analyses of CD38 and IgD expression were chosen because they distinguish B cells at various stages of differentiation (39,109). These studies indicated that CD38 expression was heterogeneous among B-CLL cases. In some cases, few (<30%), if any, members of the B-CLL clone expressed CD38, whereas in other cases the percentages were much higher and approached 100%. Thus, the B-CLL cases could again be subdivided into two categories, although in this instance the subgrouping was based on the percentage of the B-CLL clonal members that expressed 30% or more $CD38^+$ cells (92). (For convenience, the B-CLL subgroup with <30% $CD38^+$ B-CLL cells will be referred to as $CD38^-$, and the group with ≥30% $CD38^+$ B-CLL cells will be referred to as $CD38^+$.)

To identify even more accurately the activation and maturation states of B-CLL cases, both as a whole and based on CD38 expression and subcategorization, our laboratories recently studied the surface membrane expression of a large battery of markers on $CD5^+/CD19^+$ B-CLL cells using a three-color immunofluorescence approach (110,111). CD5+/CD19+ B cells from age-matched healthy donors were analyzed as controls. Specifically, the expression of IgM, IgD, CD22, CD23, CD24, CD25, CD27, CD30, CD38, CD39, CD40, CD40 ligand (CD154), CD44, CD45RA, CD62L (L-selectin), CD69, CD71, CD72, CD77, CD79b, CD80, CD86, CD95, HLA-DR, Syndecan-1 (CD138), FcγR, and FcγRIIb was studied.

Compared with normal CD5$^+$/CD19$^+$ B cells, significantly higher percentages of B-CLL cases (not subgrouped on the basis of CD38 expression) expressed CD23, CD25, CD27, CD39, CD69, and CD71 (110,111). In contrast, significantly lower percentages of B-CLL cells expressed CD22, CD38, CD40, CD40L, CD62L, CD72, CD77, CD79b, CD80, CD95, and FcγRIIb. When the density of antigen expression was measured, B-CLL cells exhibited a significantly higher density of CD27 but significantly lower density of IgM, IgD, CD22, CD38, and FcγRIIb than normal CD5$^+$ cells.

When the B-CLL cases were segregated on the basis of the percentages of CD38$^+$ cells and then analyzed for these same markers, significantly more B-CLL cells from the CD38$^+$ cases expressed CD69 and CD40, whereas significantly more B-CLL cells from the CD38$^-$ cases expressed CD71, CD62L, and CD39. Although the percentages of HLA-DR$^+$ B-CLL did not differ between the two groups, the surface density of HLA-DR was significantly higher on B-CLL cells from the CD38$^+$ cases. Interestingly, the percentage of B-CLL cells expressing CD69 correlated inversely to the percentage of cells expressing CD71; higher percentages of CD69$^+$ cells and lower percentages of CD71$^+$ cells were found in the CD38$^+$ group, and vice versa in the CD38$^-$ group (110,111).

Therefore, B-CLL cases can also be subdivided into two subgroups on the basis of surface membrane phenotype (i.e., expression of CD38). Furthermore, the CD38$^+$ group has an extended phenotype of greater expression of CD40 and CD69; in contrast, the CD38$^-$ group is characterized by greater expression of CD39, CD62L, and CD71. Because CD69 expression is a marker of cells in an earlier state of activation and precedes CD71 expression (112,113), it seems likely that the CD38$^+$ cases represent B cells that were frozen at a more proximal time in relation to antigen exposure. However, because both the CD38$^+$ and the CD38$^-$ subgroups express certain activation markers in excess of each other and of normal CD5$^+$ B cells, it also seems likely that all cases of B-CLL derive from immunologically competent, antigen-activated B cells. Nevertheless, we cannot exclude completely the possibility that the transformation process has dysregulated the expression of the genes for these markers and led to these distinct surface membrane phenotypes. If this is the case, the striking differences in phenotype may indicate differences in the transformation process or the ability of B cells at different stages of differentiation to be affected by the same process.

Finally, besides differing in their expression of surface markers, CD38$^+$ and CD38$^-$ B CLL cells differ in certain functional features, in particular their abilities to be triggered through the BCR. For example, cross-linking of surface Ig in vitro activates the signal transducing cascade in CD38$^+$ B-CLL cells as documented by both Ca^{++} mobilization and tyrosine protein phosphorylation (114). Surprisingly, the results of this signal transduction differ on the basis of which Ig isotype is cross-linked. Activation by means of surface IgM causes apoptosis, whereas activation by means of surface IgD induces prolonged in vitro survival and plasma cell differentiation (115). In contrast, cross-linking of surface Ig in CD38$^-$ B-CLL cells does not result in the delivery of activation signals; the cells appear to be unable to respond and may be anergic. These findings may have relevance for the understanding the different effects caused by the encounter with a potential antigen in CD38$^+$ and CD38$^-$ B-CLL cells.

VII. SUMMARY OF MATURATION AND ACTIVATION STAGES OF B-CLL CELLS

Collectively, these data suggest that:

B-CLL cases can also be subdivided into two subgroups on the basis of surface membrane phenotype (i.e., the expression of CD38).

The B-CLL cells in the CD38$^+$ subgroup usually express more CD69, whereas the B-CLL cells in the CD38$^-$ group usually express more CD71. Therefore, these two subgroups of B-CLL cells have significant differences in surface membrane phenotype.

The CD38$^+$ cases probably represent B cells that were frozen at a more proximal time in relation to antigen exposure than the CD38$^-$ cases. This is based on the findings that CD69 expression is a marker of cells in an earlier state of activation and precedes CD71 expression.

There are functional differences between CD38$^+$ and CD38$^-$ B-CLL cells. This is based on the differences in the ability to transduce signals through the BCR. This may lead to differences in the in vivo biology of these two subgroups of B-CLL cases if signals through the BCR continue to affect the function of the leukemic B cell.

All cases of B-CLL *derive from* immunologically competent, antigen-activated B cells. This is based on the findings that both the CD38$^+$ and the CD38$^-$ subgroups express markers characteristic of cellular activation, although the subgroups differ in the precise activation markers that they express in excess of each other and of normal CD5$^+$ B cells.

VIII. COMPARISON OF THE B-CLL SUBGROUPS DEFINED BY Ig V GENE CHARACTERISTICS AND SURFACE MEMBRANE PHENOTYPE

Because both the molecular (i.e., V gene mutation status) and cellular (i.e., CD38 expression) parameters suggest that B-CLL cases segregate into two subgroups of approximately equal numbers, we determined whether these two sets of subgroups were overlapping (92,116). As in other analyses, care was taken to only include B-CLL cases that exhibited characteristic clinical and laboratory features and to exclude those cases that expressed more than one V_H or V_L gene (i.e., lacked allelic exclusion; Ref 91). The B-CLL cases were classified as "unmutated" if they differed by <2% from the most similar germline gene in *both* the expressed V_H and V_L genes and "mutated" if they displayed ≥2% differences in *either* the expressed V_H or V_L gene.

The following statistical analyses represent our most recent data (116), and they agree favorably with our initial report (92). The unmutated and mutated groups differ significantly in the percentages of CD38$^+$ B-CLL cells (means, 63.9% versus 7.3%, respectively; P = 0.00001). When the percentages of CD38-expressing cells are plotted individually (Fig. 7), the cases segregate into two distinct sets, with 30% CD38$^+$ cells serving as the cutoff. There is a clear inverse relationship between CD38 expression and V gene mutation status. The kappa coefficient calculated for association between these two subgroups of CD38$^+$ B-CLL cases versus the unmutated and mutated groups is -0.81, indicating a strong inverse relationship.

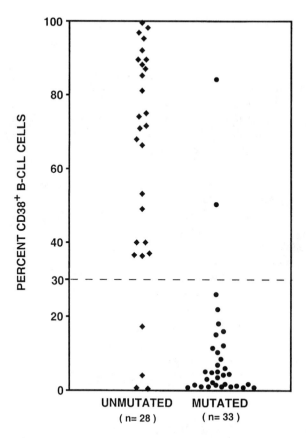

Figure 7 Percentage of CD38$^+$/CD5$^+$/CD19$^+$ cells among mutated and unmutated B-CLL cases. The percentage of CD38-expressing B-CLL cells among 61 patients whose Ig V$_H$ and V$_L$ gene sequences were determined. Unmutated cases (◆) display <2.0% differences from the most similar germline gene; mutated samples (●) display ≥2% differences. PBMC were analyzed for surface expression of CD19/CD5/CD38 by triple color immunofluorescence using anti-CD19-APC, anti-CD5-FITC, and anti-CD38-PE. Isotype-matched negative controls were used in all assays to determine positive from negative results. (Adapted with permission from Ref. 116.)

The specificity of high percentages of CD38$^+$B cells (≥30%) indicating the presence of <2% mutations is 94%, with a sensitivity of 86%. The positive predictive value of ≥30% CD38$^+$ B cells indicating the "unmutated" genotype is 94.6%. Conversely, the specificity of low percentages of CD38$^+$ B cells (<30%) indicating the presence of ≥2% mutations is 94%, with a sensitivity of 86%. The negative predictive value of <30% CD38$^+$ B cells indicating the "mutated" genotype is 84.6%. These CD38 criteria indicate V gene mutation status with 90% accuracy (116).

Despite our relatively strong inverse correlation between V gene mutation status and CD38 expression, Hamblin et al. recently reported that they were unable to reproduce these data using a different immunofluorescence approach in a somewhat smaller subgroup of patients for whom only V$_H$ sequence data were available (117). In addition, they pointed out that the CD38$^+$ subgroup did not show an overexpression of V$_H$1 family genes, in particular V$_H$ 1-69 genes, as previously reported in B-CLL (42,61,63,71,72) as being characteristic of the Ig V gene unmutated group. Therefore, at this juncture, it is important to view these two markers (V gene mutation status and CD38 expression) as independent variables that usually, but do not necessarily, overlap. The frequency with which the two sets of markers overlap will require more extensive studies of more comparable patient populations (i.e., cases for which both V_H and V_L gene sequences are known and for which allelic exclusion is verified) using similar technical approaches (e.g., three-color immunoflourescence of $CD5^+/CD19^+/CD38^+$ cells).

IX. CLINICAL COURSES OF B-CLL SUBGROUPS

A. Clinical Courses of Subgroups Based on Ig V Gene Mutation Status

In 1999, Damle et al. and Hamblin et al. reported, in back-to-back articles, that Ig V gene mutation status correlated inversely with disease course and survival (72,92). Because collectively these two studies reported results on 147 patients, it seems likely that these data are reliable.

Specifically, both groups found those patients with B-CLL cells that expressed V genes with <2% mutations ("unmutated") experienced a more aggressive clinical course and shorter survival than the patients with ≥2% V gene mutations ("mutated"; Fig. 8a). The median survival of the patients in the unmutated group in the study by Damle et al. was 9 years, whereas median survival for the mutated group was not reached for the duration of follow-up (92). Furthermore, the median survival of the unmutated cases in the Rai intermediate risk group (Fig. 9a) that are the most heterogeneous in treatment requirements and survival and whose outcome is the most difficult to predict (1,2) was 9 years compared with 17 years for the mutated cases (92). In the study by Hamblin et al. (71) median survival for the unmutated group was 117 months (9.7 years) and for the mutated group 293 months (24.4 years). In addition, the median survival for Binet stage A patients with unmutated V_H genes was 95 months (7.9 years) compared with 293 months (24.4 years) for patients in the mutated group (71). Furthermore, the patients in the unmutated group progressed more often and more rapidly to more advanced clinical Binet stages. Similar data were subsequently published by Maloun et al. (118).

Finally, Damle et al. showed that the treatment histories of the patients with unmutated and mutated V genes were different, because >75% of the patients in the mutated group required no or minimal treatment, whereas only ~20% of the unmutated cases required no or minimal therapy (92). Furthermore, even though ~95% of the patients in the unmutated group received fludarabine, only two achieved a durable clinical response (92).

It is interesting that the B-CLL cells of the unmutated subgroup reported by Hamblin and coworkers (71,119) were more likely to express trisomy 12 than the mutated group, and those B-CLL cells of the mutated subgroup were more likely to express 13q14 abnormalities. These data may relate to the shorter survival of the unmutated group.

B. Clinical Courses of Subgroups on the Basis of CD38 Expression

In addition to reporting the preceding data on the prognostic value of Ig V gene mutation status, Damle et al. reported on the value of CD38 expression in this regard (92). These investigators found significant differences in chemotherapy requirements and survival as a function of the percentages of $CD38^+$ leukemic cells. Thus, ~70% of the cases with

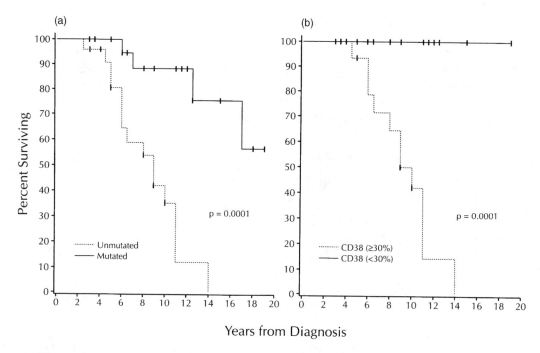

Figure 8 Survival based on V gene mutation status and CD38 expression. (a) Kaplan-Meier plot comparing survival based on the absence ("unmutated": · · · ·) or presence ("mutated":—) of significant numbers (≥2%) of V gene mutations in 47 B-CLL cases (unmutated: 24 cases; mutated: 23). Median survival of unmutated group: 9 years; median survival of mutated group not reached ($P = 0.0001$; log-rank test). (b) Kaplan-Meier plot comparing survival based on the detection of ≥30% (· · · · ·) or <30% CD38+ B-CLL cells (≥30%, 17 cases; <30%, 19). Median survival of the ≥30% CD38+ group, 10 years; median survival of the <30% CD38+ group, not reached ($P = 0.0001$; log-rank test). (Adapted with permission from Ref. 92.)

<30% CD38+ B-CLL cells required either no or minimal chemotherapy compared with ~23% of the cases with ≥30% CD38+ B-CLL cells; conversely, >75% of the ≥30% CD38+ cases required either continuous chemotherapy or chemotherapy with two or more agents or regimens.

Furthermore, median survival for the patients in the ≥30% CD38+ group was 10 years, compared with undetermined in the <30% CD38+ group, because all patients in this group were alive for the duration of follow-up (Fig. 8b). Highly significant differences in survival also were found among the patients in the Rai intermediate risk group (Fig. 9b), with median survival for the ≥30% CD38+ patients being reached in 10 years, whereas all patients in the <30% CD38+ group remained alive throughout the years of follow-up (92). Hamblin et al. recently reported in a letter (117) that they also found a significant inverse correlation between CD38 expression and survival in B-CLL patients. Therefore, the validity of this prognostic marker is confirmed.

Thus, Ig V gene mutation status and CD38 expression are novel and valuable independent markers of prognosis in B-CLL. Because these markers appear to be stable over time, it is likely that they are identifying inherent differences between the two types of B lymphocytes transformed in this disease that lead to inherent differences in the level

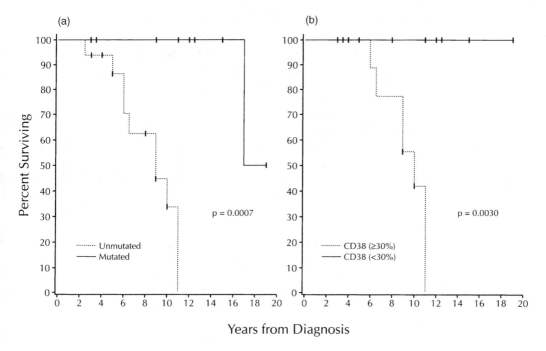

Figure 9   Survival based on V gene mutation status and CD38 expression among B-CLL patients who stratify to the Rai intermediate risk category. (a) Kaplan-Meier plot comparing V gene mutation status with survival among the cases within the Rai intermediate risk category (unmutated, 16 cases; mutated, 9). Median survival of the mutated group; 9 years; median survival of the unmutated group, 17 years (P = 0.0007; log-rank test). (b) Kaplan-Meier plot comparing numbers of CD38+ B-CLL cells with survival among the cases within the Rai intermediate risk category ($\geq$30%, 11 cases; <30%, 9). Median survival of the 30% CD38+ group, 10 years; median survival of the <30% CD38+ group, not reached (P = 0.0030; log-rank test). None of the patients in the <30% CD38+ group died during the follow-up period. (Adapted with permission from Ref. 92.)

of disease aggressivity. As mentioned earlier, these markers more often than not overlap (accuracy ~90%). However, because the two markers do not overlap completely (92, 116,117), further studies of comparable patient sets using comparable technical approaches will be necessary to determine whether the two markers are interchangeable and, more importantly, whether one or another or both approaches has greater usefulness to the clinician in determining clinical course and outcome.

X.   CONCLUDING REMARKS AND SPECULATIONS

The data reviewed in the preceding sections indicate that B-CLL cases can be viewed as heterogeneous at the level of the leukemic cell from at least two viewpoints: Ig V gene characteristics (predominantly V gene mutation status) and surface membrane phenotype (predominantly CD38 expression). These molecular and cellular parameters identify two sets of subgroups that appear to be overlapping but not identical.

Furthermore, these data suggest that B-CLL cells derive from immunocompetent B lymphocytes that have been driven by specific antigens sometime during their preleukemic development and possibly after their transformation into leukemic cells. This notion is based on the facts that these cells express surface membrane molecules and Ig V gene mutations indicative of BCR-mediated triggering and cellular activation and maturation. Indeed, it seems likely that the leukemic transformation of the precursor B lymphocyte corresponds temporally with antigen encounter. For the unmutated and CD38[+] groups, this encounter is probably more recent than for the mutated and CD38[-] groups; this speculation is based on the surface membrane phenotypes mentioned earlier.

The currently available data support the speculation that the differences in cellular phenotype and V gene characteristics reflect differences in the types of antigenic stimuli received by the B-CLL precursor cells (i.e., T-dependent versus T-independent) and the level of maturation that these antigens and ancillary cells have been able to promote. Thus, the two sets of B-CLL cases characterized in this study appear to represent B cells transformed at different stages of B cell differentiation and/or activation.

It seems clear that the mutated and CD38[-] B-CLL cases derive from B cells that have been stimulated by T cell–dependent antigens that induced migration to secondary lymphoid organs in which they underwent a germinal center reaction and developed Ig V gene mutations. Thus, these mutated and CD38[-] B-CLL cases derive from post-GC/ memory cells (39,109), possibly from the small subset of IgM[+]/IgD[+] memory cells found in the blood (24), bone marrow (23), or tonsils (25). Although it is unclear whether these cell subsets express surface membrane CD5, this may not be incongruous, because in man CD5 expression appears to be activation state-dependent (120).

In contrast, the unmutated and CD38[+] B-CLL cases could be derived from either naïve B cells or activated B cells that have not entered a GC and therefore have not had the opportunity to develop Ig V gene mutations. On the basis of analyses of HCDR3 characteristics of unmutated B-CLL cases (42,72,83) and on the surface membrane phenotypes described previously, we favor the hypothesis that the unmutated and the CD38[+] B-CLL cells derive from B lymphocytes that have been activated by antigen. Therefore, the lack of Ig V gene mutations in these cells could indicate either that the B-CLL transforming event occurred after stimulation with a T cell–dependent antigen but before entering a lymphoid follicle or that the transforming event occurred after stimulation with a T cell–independent (auto)antigen, because both T-independent antigens and autoantigens normally cannot elicit T cell help and cannot lead to a GC reaction or V gene mutations. The latter may be a more reasonable possibility, considering that resting CD5[+] human B cells respond well to such stimuli (121) and that CD5[+] B-CLL cells frequently produce autoantibodies (104–106).

We believe that on the basis of their differentiation and activation differences, these two sets of B-CLL cells have inherently different biological properties that lead to different clinical outcomes. For example, if the mutated and CD38[-] B-CLL cells represent memory cells that were activated in the past by T cell–dependent exogenous antigens, they would be expected to be relatively inactive and to remain so, because they would rarely encounter the appropriate foreign antigen. Therefore, as B-CLL cells, they might grow slowly and be more likely to undergo spontaneous apoptosis. Indeed, recent data emphasize the need for B lymphocytes to receive intermittent trophic signals through an intact BCR to promote cell survival (96). Furthermore, because the in vitro data suggest that the CD38[-] B-CLL cells cannot transduce an activating signal through their BCR (114), they would be unable to receive such trophic survival signals.

Conversely, if the unmutated and CD38[+] cases derive from B cells that were chronically stimulated through the BCR by autoantigens, they might be expected to be more active and to remain so because they would be more likely to encounter the appropriate autoantigen. This would be particularly true if the stimulatory signals were delivered by IgD, which often is the dominant isotype expressed by B-CLL cells. Therefore, as B-CLL cells, they might cycle more than memory cells and also be more likely to receive survival signals through the BCR (96) that could abort either spontaneous apoptosis or that induced by chemotherapeutic agents.

Finally, we believe that it is unlikely that CD38 is relevant solely as a marker of cellular differentiation and clinical course. We favor the hypothesis that it also functions as a signaling molecule and therefore may be directly relevant to the differences in disease aggressivity. CD38 is known to play a role as an accessory molecule in BCR-mediated signal transduction (122,123), as well as inducing B cell proliferation directly in some experimental systems (124). Indeed, CD38 can increase or decrease a B lymphocyte's chance for survival (125,126), depending on the state of maturation/activation of the cell. CD38-mediated signaling induces death by apoptosis in immature B cells (127) and rescues from apoptosis in mature B cells (125,126). Further studies will be necessary to determine whether CD38 is providing important signals to the B-CLL cell through its ligand CD31 that is expressed in the bone marrow or other lymphoid and nonlymphoid compartments (128).

ACKNOWLEDGMENTS

Supported in part by US PHS grant AI 10811 from the NIH NIAID and grant CA 81554 from the NIH NCI, and by the Jean Walton Fund for Lymphoma and Myeloma Research, the Joseph Eletto Leukemia Research Fund, and the Sass Foundation for Medical Research.

REFERENCES

1. K Rai, D Patel. Chronic lymphocytic leukemia. In: R Hoffman, E Benz, S Shattil, B Furie, H Cohen, L Silberstein, eds. Hematology: Basic Principles and Practice. New York: Churchill Livingstone, 1995, pp 1308–1321.
2. JA Zwiebel, BD Cheson. Chronic lymphocytic leukemia: staging and prognostic factors. Semin Oncol 25:42–59, 1998.
3. F Caligaris-Cappio, M Gobbi, M Bofill, G Janossy. Infrequent normal B lymphocytes express features of B-chronic lymphocytic leukemia. J Exp Med 155:623–628, 1982.
4. W. Dameshek. Chronic lymphocytic leukemia: an accumulative disease of immunologically incompetent lymphocytes. Blood 29:566, 1967.
5. S Tonegawa. Somatic generation of antibody diversity. Nature 302:575–581, 1983.
6. FW Alt, EM Oltz, F Young, J Gorman, G Taccioli, J Chen. VDJ recombination. Immunol Today 13:306–314, 1992.
7. SV Desiderio, GD Yancopoulos, M Paskind, E Thomas, MA Boss, N Landau, FW Alt, D Baltimore. Insertion of N regions into heavy-chain genes is correlated with expression of terminal deoxytransferase in B cells. Nature 311:752–755, 1984.
8. T Komori, A Okada, V Stewart, FW Alt. Lack of N regions in antigen receptor variable region genes of TdT-deficient lymphocytes [published erratum appears in Science 1993 Dec 24;262(5142):1957]. Science 261:1171–1175, 1993.
9. B Nadel, S Tehranchi, AJ Feeney. Coding end processing is similar throughout ontogeny. J Immunol 154:6430–6436, 1995.
10. K Rajewsky. Clonal selection and learning in the antibody system. Nature 381:751–758, 1996.

11. I MacLennan, E Chan. The dynamic relationship between B-cell populations in adults. Immunol Today 14:29–34, 1993.

12. T Kurosaki. Molecular mechanisms in B cell antigen receptor signaling. Curr Opin Immunol 9:309–318, 1997.

13. YJ Liu, J Zhang, PJ Lane, EY Chan, IC MacLennan. Sites of specific B cell activation in primary and secondary responses to T cell-dependent and T cell-independent antigens. Eur J Immunol 21:2951–2962, 1991.

14. LA Herzenberg, AM Stall, PA Lalor, C Sidman, WA Moore, DR Parks, LA Herzenberg. The Ly-1 B cell lineage. Immunol Rev 93:81–102, 1986.

15. TJ Kipps. The CD5 B cell. Adv Immunol 47:117–185, 1989.

16. A Lanzavecchia. Receptor-mediated antigen uptake and its effect on antigen presentation to class II-restricted T lymphocytes. Annu Rev Immunol 8:773–793, 1990.

17. RJ Noelle, DM Shepherd, HP Fell. Cognate interaction between T helper cells and B cells. VII. Role of contact and lymphokines in the expression of germ-line and mature gamma 1 transcripts. J Immunol 149:1164–1169, 1992.

18. EA Clark, JA Ledbetter. How B and T cells talk to each other. Nature 367:425–428, 1994.

19. YJ Liu, S Oldfield, IC MacLennan. Memory B cells in T cell-dependent antibody responses colonize the splenic marginal zones. Eur J Immunol 18:355–362, 1988.

20. A Tierens, J Delabie, L Michiels, P Vandenberghe, C De Wolf-Peeters. Marginal-zone B cells in the human lymph node and spleen show somatic hypermutations and display clonal expansion. Blood 93:226–234, 1999.

21. J Spencer, ME Perry, DK Dunn-Walters. Human marginal-zone B cells. Immunol Today 19: 421–426, 1998.

22. M Dono, S Zupo, A Augliera, VL Burgio, R Massara, A Melagrana, M Costa, CE Grossi, N Chiorazzi, M Ferrarini. Subepithelial B cells in the human palatine tonsil. II. Functional characterization. Eur J Immunol 26:2043–2049, 1996.

23. E Paramithiotis, MD Cooper. Memory B lymphocytes migrate to bone marrow in humans. Proc Natl Acad Sci U S A 94:208–212, 1997.

24. U Klein, K Rajewsky, R Kuppers. Human immunoglobulin (Ig)M+IgD+ peripheral blood B cells expressing the CD27 cell surface antigen carry somatically mutated variable region genes: CD27 as a general marker for somatically mutated (Memory) B cells. J Exp Med 188:1679–1689, 1998.

25. M Dono, S Zupo, N Leanza, G Melioli, M Fogli, A Melagrana, N Chiorazzi, M Ferrarini. Heterogeneity of tonsillar subepithelial B lymphocytes, the splenic marginal zone equivalents. J Immunol 164:5596–5604, 2000.

26. DA Nemazee, K Burki. Clonal deletion of B lymphocytes in a transgenic mouse bearing anti-MHC class I antibody genes. Nature 337:562–566, 1989.

27. D Gay, T Saunders, S Camper, M Weigert. Receptor editing: an approach by autoreactive B cells to escape tolerance. J Exp Med 177:999–1008, 1993.

28. MZ Radic, J Erikson, S Litwin, M Weigert. B lymphocytes may escape tolerance by revising their antigen receptors. J Exp Med 177:1165–1173, 1993.

29. SL Tiegs, DM Russell, D Nemazee. Receptor editing in self-reactive bone marrow B cells. J Exp Med 177:1009–1020, 1993.

30. SB Hartley, MP Cooke, DA Fulcher, AW Harris, S Cory, A Basten, CC Goodnow. Elimination of self-reactive B lymphocytes proceeds in two stages: arrested development and cell death. Cell 72:325–335, 1993.

31. R Carsetti, G Kohler, MC Lamers. Transitional B cells are the target of negative selection in the B cell compartment. J Exp Med 181:2129–2140, 1995.

32. JI Healy, CC Goodnow. Positive versus negative signaling by lymphocyte antigen receptors. Annu Rev Immunol 16:645–670, 1998.

33. GD Yancopoulos, SV Desiderio, M Paskind, JF Kearney, D Baltimore, FW Alt. Preferential

utilization of the most JH-proximal VH gene segments in pre-B-cell lines. Nature 311:727–733, 1984.

34. RM Perlmutter, JF Kearney SP Chang, LE Hood. Developmentally controlled expression of immunoglobulin VH genes. Science 227:1597–1601, 1985.

35. HW Schroeder, Jr., JL Hillson, RM Perlmutter. Early restriction of the human antibody repertoire. Science 238:791–793, 1987.

36. I Suzuki, L Pfister, A Glas, C Nottenburg, EC Milner. Representation of rearranged VH gene segments in the human adult antibody repertoire. J Immunol 154:3902–3911, 1995.

37. JL Hillson, IR Oppliger, EH Sasso, EC Milner, MH Wener. Emerging human B cell repertoire. Influence of developmental stage and interindividual variation. J Immunol 149:3741–3752, 1992.

38. P Kraj, SP Rao, AM Glas, RR Hardy, EC Milner, LE Silberstein. The human heavy chain Ig V region gene repertoire is biased at all stages of B cell ontogeny, including early pre-B cells. J Immunol 158:5824–5832, 1997.

39. V Pascual, YJ Liu, A Magalski, O de Bouteiller, J Banchereau, JD Capra. Analysis of somatic mutation in five B cell subsets of human tonsil. J Exp Med 180:329–339, 1994.

40. HP Brezinschek, SJ Foster, RI Brezinschek, T Dorner, R Domiati-Saad, PE Lipsky. Analysis of the human VH gene repertoire. Differential effects of selection and somatic hypermutation on human peripheral CD5(+)/IgM+ and CD5(−)/IgM+ B cells. J Clin Invest 99:2488–2501, 1997.

41. G Kelsoe. Life and death in germinal centers (redux). Immunity 4:107–111, 1996.

42. F Fais, F Ghiotto, S Hashimoto, B Sellars, A Valetto, SL Allen, P Schulman, VP Vinciguerra, K Rai, LZ Rassenti, TJ Kipps, G Dighiero, H Schroeder, M Ferrarini, N Chiorazzi. Chronic lymphocytic leukemia B cells express restricted sets of mutated and unmutated antigen receptors. J Clin Invest 102:1515–1525, 1998.

43. D Nemazee, M Weigert. Revising B cell receptors. J Exp Med 191:1813–1817, 2000.

44. C Chen, Z Nagy, EL Prak, M Weigert. Immunoglobulin heavy chain gene replacement: a mechanism of receptor editing. Immunity 3:747–755, 1995.

45. PC Wilson, K Wilson, Y-J Liu, J Banchereau, V Pascual, JD Capra. Receptor revision of immunoglobulin heavy chain variable region genes in normal human B lymphocytes. J Exp Med 191:1881–1894, 2000.

46. K Itoh, E Meffre, E Albesiano, A Farber, D Dines, P Stein, SE Asnis, R Furie, R Jain, N Chiorazzi. Immunoglobulin heavy chain variable region gene replacement as a mechanism for receptor revision in rheumatoid aarthritis synovial tissue B lymphocytes. J Exp Med 192:1151–1164, 2000.

47. PA Lalor, G Morahan. The peritoneal Ly-1 (CD5) B cell repertoire is unique among murine B cell repertoires. Eur J Immunol 20:485–492, 1990.

48. CA Pennell, LW Arnold, G Haughton, SH Clarke. Restricted Ig variable region gene expression among Ly-1+ B cell lymphomas. J Immunol 141:2788–2796, 1988.

49. Y Chang, J Ziegler, H Wabinga, E Katangole-Mbidde, C Boshoff, T Schulz, D Whitby, D Maddalena, HW Jaffe, RA Weiss, PS Moore. Kaposi's sarcoma-associated herpesvirus and Kaposi's sarcoma in Africa. Uganda Kaposi's Sarcoma Study Group. Arch Intern Med 156:202–204, 1996.

50. E Cesarman, Y Chang, PS Moore, JW Said, DM Knowles. Kaposi's sarcoma-associated herpesvirus-like DNA sequences in AIDS-related body-cavity-based lymphomas. N Engl J Med 332:1186–1191, 1995.

51. J Soulier, L Grollet, E Oksenhendler, P Cacoub, D Cazals-Hatem, P Babinet, MF d'Agay, JP Clauvel, M Raphael, L Degos, et al. Kaposi's sarcoma-associated herpesvirus-like DNA sequences in multicentric Castleman's disease. Blood 86:1276–1280, 1995.

52. B Klein, XG Zhang, ZY Lu, R Bataille. Interleukin-6 in human multiple myeloma. Blood 85:863–872, 1995.

53. R Burger, F Neipel, B Fleckenstein, R Savino, G Ciliberto, JR Kalden, M Gramatzki. Human

herpesvirus type 8 interleukin-6 homologue is functionally active on human myeloma cells. Blood 91:1858–1863, 1998.

54. W Blattner, C Saxinger, J Clark, D Mann. Human T-cell leukemia/lymphoma virus-associated lymphoreticular neoplasia in Jamaica. Lancet 2:61–64, 1983.

55. J Clark, B Hahn, D Mann. Molecular and immunologic analysis of an HTLV-positive CLL case from Jamaica. Cancer 56:495–499, 1986.

56. A Peterman, M Jerdan, S Staal, B Bender, H Streicher, J Schupbach, L Resnick. Evidence for HTLV-I associated with mycosis fungoides and B-cell chronic lymphocytic leukemia. Arch Dermatol 122:568–571, 1986.

57. D Mann, P DeSantis, G Mark, A Pfeifer, M Newman, N Gibbs, M Popovic, M Sarngadharan, R Gallo, J CLark. HTLV-I-associated B-cell CLL: indirect role for retrovirus in leukemogenesis. Science 236:1103–1106, 1987.

58. TJ Kipps, E Tomhave, PP Chen, DA Carson. Autoantibody-associated kappa light chain variable region gene expressed in chronic lymphocytic leukemia with little or no somatic mutation. Implications for etiology and immunotherapy. J Exp Med 167:840–852, 1988.

59. LF Pratt, L Rassenti, J Larrick, B Robbins, PM Banks, TJ Kipps. Ig V region gene expression in small lymphocytic lymphoma with little or no somatic hypermutation. J Immunol 143:699–705, 1989.

60. LX Pan, TC Diss, HZ Peng, AJ Norton, PG Isaacson. Nodular lymphocyte predominance Hodgkin's disease: a monoclonal or polyclonal B-cell disorder? Blood 87:2428–2434, 1996.

61. HW Schroeder, Jr., G Dighiero. The pathogenesis of chronic lymphocytic leukemia: analysis of the antibody repertoire. Immunol Today 15:288–294, 1994.

62. A Shen, C Humphries, P Tucker, F Blattner. Human heavy-chain variable region gene family nonrandomly rearranged in familial chronic lymphocytic leukemia. Proc Natl Acad Sci U S A 84:8563–8567, 1987.

63. TJ Kipps, E Tomhave, LF Pratt, S Duffy, PP Chen, DA Carson. Developmentally restricted immunoglobulin heavy chain variable region gene expressed at high frequency in chronic lymphocytic leukemia. Proc Natl Acad Sci U S A 86:5913–5917, 1989.

64. LA Spatz, KK Wong, M Williams, R Desai, J Golier, JE Berman, FW Alt, N Latov. Cloning and sequence analysis of the VH and VL regions of an anti-myelin/DNA antibody from a patient with peripheral neuropathy and chronic lymphocytic leukemia. J Immunol 144:2821–2828, 1990.

65. DF Friedman, EA Cho, J Goldman, CE Carmack, EC Besa, RR Hardy, LE Silberstein. The role of clonal selection in the pathogenesis of an autoreactive human B cell lymphoma. J Exp Med 174:525–537, 1991.

66. A Matolcsy, P Casali, RG Nador, YF Liu, DM Knowles. Molecular characterization of IgA- and/or IgG-switched chronic lymphocytic leukemia B cells. Blood 89:1732–1739, 1997.

67. V Cherepakhin, SM Baird, GW Meisenholder, TJ Kipps. Common clonal origin of chronic lymphocytic leukemia and high-grade lymphoma of Richter's syndrome. Blood 82:3141–3147, 1993.

68. AS, Korganow, T Martin, JC Weber, B Lioure, P Lutz, AM Knapp, JL Pasquali. Molecular analysis of rearranged VH genes during B cell chronic lymphocytic leukemia: intraclonal stability is frequent but not constant. Leuk Lymphoma 14:55–69, 1994.

69. W Ikematsu, H Ikematsu, T Otsuka, S Okamura, S Kashiwagi, Y Niho. Surface phenotype and immunoglobulin heavy chain gene usage in chronic B-cell leukemias. Ann N Y Acad Sci 764:492–495, 1995.

70. L Foroni, A Werner, M Papaioannou, J Yaxley, M Attard, A Hoffbrand. The VH usage in B cell chronic lymphocytic leukemia cells is a random event and it is not disease related (abst). Blood 88:238a, 1996.

71. TJ Hamblin, Z Davis, A Gardiner, DG Oscier, FK Stevenson. Unmutated Ig VH genes are associated with a more aggressive form of chronic lymphocytic leukemia. Blood 94:1848–1854, 1999.

72. TA Johnson, LZ Rassenti, TJ Kipps. Ig VH1 genes expressed in B cell chronic lymphocytic leukemia exhibit distinctive molecular features. J Immunol 158:235–246, 1997.

73. AM Stall, MC Farinas, DM Tarlinton, PA Lalor, LA Herzenberg, S Strober, LA Herzenberg. Ly-1 B-cell clones similar to human chronic lymphocytic leukemias routinely develop in older normal mice and young autoimmune (New Zealand Black-related) animals. Proc Natl Acad Sci U S A 85:7312–7316, 1988.

74. AC Viale, JA Chies, F Huetz, E Malenchere, M Weksler, AA Freitas, A Coutinho. VH-gene family dominance in ageing mice. Scand J Immunol 39:184–188, 1994.

75. J LeMaoult, S Delassus, R Dyall, J Nikolic-Zugic, P Kourilskv, M Weksler. Clonal expansions of B lymphocytes in old mice. J Immunol 158:3868–3874, 1997.

76. J Radl. Age-related monoclonal gammapathies: clinical lessons from the aging C57BL mouse. Immunol Today 11:234–236, 1990.

77. TW van den Akker, R Brondijk, J Radl. Influence of long-term antigenic stimulation started in young C57BL mice on the development of age-related monoclonal gammapathies. Int Arch Allergy Appl Immunol 87:165–170, 1988.

78. C van Arkel, CM Hopstaken, C Zurcher, NA Bos, FG Kroese, HF Savelkoul, R Benner, J Radl. Monoclonal gammopathies in aging mu, kappa-transgenic mice: involvement of the B-1 cell lineage. Eur J Immunol 27:2436–2440, 1997.

79. EH Sasso, T Johnson, TJ Kipps. Expression of the immunoglobulin VH gene 51pl is proportional to its germline gene copy number. J Clin Invest 97:2074–2080, 1996.

80. F Goni, PP Chen, B Pons-Estel, DA Carson, B Frangione. Sequence similarities and cross-idiotypic specificity of L chains among human monoclonal IgM kappa with anti-gamma-globulin activity. J Immunol 135:4073–4079, 1985.

81. S Fong, PP Chen, TA Gilbertson, RI Fox, JH Vaughan, DA Carson. Structural similarities in the kappa light chains of human rheumatoid factor paraproteins and serum immunoglobulins bearing a cross-reactive idiotype. J Immunol 135:1955–1960, 1985.

82. M Wakai, S Hashimoto, M Omata, ZM Sthoeger, SL Allen, SM Lichtman, P Schulman, VP Vinciguerra, B Diamond, M Dono, et al. IgG+, CD5+ human chronic lymphocytic leukemia B cells. Production of IgG antibodies that exhibit diminished autoreactivity and IgG subclass skewing. Autoimmunity 19:39–48, 1994.

83. A Valetto, F Ghiotto, F Fais, S Hashimoto, SL Allen, SM Lichtman, P Schulman, VP Vinciguerra, BT Messmer, DS Thaler, M Ferrarini, N Chiorazzi. A subset of IgG+ B-CLL cells expresses virtually identical antigens receptors that bind similar peptides. Blood 92:431a, 1998.

84. TC Meeker, JC Grimaldi, R O'Rourke, J Loeb, G Juliusson, S Einhorn. Lack of detectable somatic hypermutation in the V region of the Ig H chain gene of a human chronic B lymphocytic leukemia. J Immunol 141:3994–3998, 1988.

85. R Kuppers, A Gause, K Rajewsky. B cells of chronic lymphatic leukemia express V genes in unmutated form. Leuk Res 15:487–496, 1991.

86. DF Friedman, JS Moore, J Erikson, J Manz, J Goldman, PC Nowell, LE Silberstein. Variable region gene analysis of an isotype-switched (IgA) variant of chronic lymphocytic leukemia. Blood 80:2287–2297, 1992.

87. SD Wagner, L Luzzatto. V kappa gene segments rearranged in chronic lymphocytic leukemia are distributed over a large portion of the V kappa locus and do not show somatic mutation. Eur J Immunol 23:391–397, 1993.

88. RR Hardy, K Hayakawa. Developmental origins, specificities and immunoglobulin gene biases of murine Ly-1 B cells. Int Rev Immunol 8:189–207, 1992.

89. S Hashimoto, M Wakai, J Silver, N Chiorazzi. Biased usage of variable and constant-region Ig genes by IgG+, CD5+ human leukemic B cells. Ann N Y Acad Sci 651: 477–479, 1992.

90. S Hashimoto, M Dono, M Wakai, SL Allen, SM Lichtman, P Schulman, VP Vinciguerra, M Ferrarini, J Silver, N Chiorazzi. Somatic diversification and selection of immunoglobulin

heavy and light chain variable region genes in IgG+ CD5+ chronic lymphocytic leukemia B cells. J Exp Med 181:1507–1517, 1995.

91. LZ Rassenti, TJ Kipps. Lack of allelic exclusion in B cell chronic lymphocytic leukemia. J Exp Med 185:1435–1445, 1997.

92. RN Damle, T Wasil, F Fais, F Ghiotto, A Valetto, SL Allen, A Buchbinder, D Budman, K Dittmar, J Kolitz, SM Lichtman, P Schulman, VP Vinciguerra, KR Rai, M Ferrarini, N Chiorazzi. Ig V gene mutation status and CD38 expression as novel prognostic indicators in chronic lymphocytic leukemia. Blood 94:1840–1847, 1999.

93. TH Jukes, JL King. Evolutionary nucleotide replacements in DNA. Nature 281:605–606, 1979.

94. MJ Shlomchik, A Marshak-Rothstein, CB Wolfowicz, TL Rothstein, MG Weigert. The role of clonal selection and somatic mutation in autoimmunity. Nature 328:805–811, 1987.

95. B Chang, P Casali. The CDR1 sequences of a major proportion of human germline Ig VH genes are inherently susceptible to amino acid replacement. Immunol Today 15:367–373, 1994.

96. KP Lam, R Kuhn, K Rajewsky. In vivo ablation of surface immunoglobulin on mature B cells by inducible gene targeting results in rapid cell death. Cell 90:1073–1083, 1997.

97. I Sanz. Multiple mechanisms participate in the generation of diversity of human H chain CDR3 regions. J Immunol 147:1720–1729, 1991.

98. EA Padlan. Anatomy of the antibody molecule. Mol Immunol 31:169–217, 1994.

99. SJ Corbett, IM Tomlinson, ELL Sonnhammer, D Buck, G Winter. Sequence of the human immunoglobulin diversity (D) segment locus: a systematic analysis provides no evidence for the use of DIR segments, inverted D segments, "minor" D segments or D-D recombination. J Mol Biol 270:587–597, 1997.

100. FM Raaphorst, CS Raman, J Tami, M Fischbach, I Sanz. Human Ig heavy chain CDR3 regions in adult bone marrow pre-B cells display an adult phenotype of diversity: evidence for structural selection of DH amino acid sequences. Int Immunol 9:1503–1515, 1997.

101. A Delmer, F Ajchenbaum-Cymbalista, R Tang, S Ramond, AM Faussat, JP Marie, R Zittoun. Overexpression of cyclin D2 in chronic B-cell malignancies. Blood 85:2870–2876, 1995.

102. K Schuh, A Avots, HP Tony, E Serfling, C Kneitz. Nuclear NF-ATp is a hallmark of unstimulated B cells from B-CLL patients. Leuk Lymphoma 23:583–592, 1996.

103. EJ Schattner, J Mascarenhas, I Reyfman, M Koshy, C Woo, SM Friedman, MK Crow. Chronic lymphocytic leukemia B cells can express CD40 ligand and demonstrate T-cell type costimulatory capacity. Blood 91:2689–2697, 1998.

104. ZM Sthoeger, M Wakai, DB Tse, VP Vinciguerra, SL Allen, DR Budman, SM Lichtman, P Schulman, LR Weiselberg, N Chiorazzi. Production of autoantibodies by CD5-expressing B lymphocytes from patients with chronic lymphocytic leukemia. J Exp Med 169:255–268, 1989.

105. BM Broker, A Klajman, P Youinou, J Jouquan, CP Worman, J Murphy, L Mackenzie, R Quartey-Papafio, M Blaschek, P Collins, et al. Chronic lymphocytic leukemic (CLL) cells secrete multispecific autoantibodies. J Autoimmun 1:469–481, 1988.

106. L Borche, A Lim, JL Binet, G Dighiero. Evidence that chronic lymphocytic leukemia B lymphocytes are frequently committed to production of natural autoantibodies. Blood 76:562–569, 1990.

107. K Zhao, R Gueret, M Weksler. Age-associated increases in serum levels of IgM and autoantibodies reflect absolute but not relative changes in antibody repertoire. Aging: Immunol Infect Dis 5:233–238, 1994.

108. K Zhao, Y Wang, R Gueret, A Coutinho, M Weksler. Dysregulation of the humoral immune response in old mice. Internat Immunol 7:929–934, 1995.

109. EA Clark, PJ Lane. Regulation of human B-cell activation and adhesion. Annu Rev Immunol 9:97–127, 1991.

110. RN Damle, F Fais, F Ghiotto, A Valetto, E Albesiano, T Wasil, FM Batliwalla, SL Allen, P Shulman, VP Vinciguerra, KR Rai, M Ferrarini, N Chiorazzi. Chronic lymphocytic leukemia: A proliferation of B cells at two distinct stages of differentiation. In B1 Lymphocytes

in B Cell Neoplasia (M. Potter, F. Melchers, eds.). Curr Top Microbiol Immunol 2000; 252: 285–293.

111. RN Damle, X-J Yan, E Albesiano, F Ghiotto, A Valetto, S Allen, P Shulman, V Vinciguerra, K Raj, M Ferrarini, N Chiorazzi. Differences in expression of surface markers among B-CLL subgroups indicate arrests at distinct stages of B cell maturation. Blood 96:368a, 2000.

112. R Biselli, PM Matricardi, R D'Amelio, A Fattorossi. Multiparametric flow cytometric analysis of the kinetics of surface molecule expression after polyclonal activation of human peripheral blood T lymphocytes. Scand J Immunol 35:439–447, 1992.

113. E Arva, B Andersson. Kinetics of cytokine release and expression of lymphocyte cell-surface activation markers after in vitro stimulation of human peripheral blood mononuclear cells with Streptococcus pneumoniae. Scand J Immunol 49:237–243, 1999.

114. S Zupo, L Isnardi, M Megna, R Massara, F Malavasi, M Dono, E Cosulich, M Ferrarini. CD38 expression distinguishes two groups of B-cell chronic lymphocytic leukemias with different responses to anti-IgM antibodies and propensity to apoptosis. Blood 88:1365–1374, 1996.

115. S Zupo, R Massara, M Dono, E Rossi, F Malavasi, ME Cosulich, M Ferrarini. Apoptosis or plasma cell differentiation of CD38-positive B-chronic lymphocytic leukemia cells induced by cross-linking of surface IgM or IgD. Blood 95:1199–1206, 2000.

116. R Damle, T Wasil, S Allen, P Shulman, K Rai, M Ferrarini, N Chiorazzi. Updated data on V gene mutation status and CD38 expression in B-CLL. Blood 95:2456–2457, 2000.

117. T Hamblin, J Orchard, A Gardiner, D Oscier, Z Davis, F Stevenson. Immunoglobulin V genes and CD38 expression on CLL. Blood 95:2455–2456, 2000.

118. K Maloum, F Davi, H Merle-Beral, O Pritsch, C Magnac, F Vuillier, G Dighiero, X Troussard, F Mauro, J Benichou. Expression of unmutated VH genes is a detrimental prognostic factor in chronic lymphocytic leukemia. Blood 96:377–379, 2000.

119. DG Oscier, A Thompsett, D Zhu, FK Stevenson. Differential rates of somatic hypermutation in V(H) genes among subsets of chronic lymphocytic leukemia defined by chromosomal abnormalities. Blood 89:4153–4160, 1997.

120. S Zupo, M Dono, R Massara, G Taborelli, N Chiorazzi, M Ferrarini. Expression of CD5 and CD38 by human CD5-B cells: requirement for special stimuli. Eur J Immunol 24:1426–1433, 1994.

121. S Zupo, M Dono, L Azzoni, N Chiorazzi, M Ferrarini. Evidence for differential responsiveness of human CD5+ and CD5-B cell subsets to T cell-independent mitogens. Eur J Immunol 21:351–359, 1991.

122. FE Lund, N Yu, KM Kim, M Reth, MC Howard. Signaling through CD38 augments B cell antigen receptor (BCR) responses and is dependent on BCR expression. J Immunol 157: 1455–1467, 1996.

123. L Santos-Argumedo, C Teixeira, G Preece, PA Kirkham, RM Parkhouse. A B lymphocyte surface molecule mediating activation and protection from apoptosis via calcium channels. J Immunol 151:3119–3130, 1993.

124. G Shubinsky, M Schlesinger. The CD38 lymphocyte differentiation marker: new insight into its ectoenzymatic activity and its role as a signal transducer. Immunity 7:315–324, 1997.

125. S Zupo, E Rugari, M Dono, G Taborelli, F Malavasi, M Ferrarini. CD38 signalling by agonistic monoclonal antibody prevents apoptosis of human germinal center B cells. Eur J Immunol 24:1218–1222, 1994.

126. A Funaro, M Morra, L Calosso, MG Zini, CM Ausiello, F Malavasi. Role of the human CD38 molecule in B cell activation and proliferation. Tissue Antigens 49:7–15, 1997.

127. M Kumagai, E Coustan-Smith, DJ Murray, O Silvennoinen, KG Murti, WE Evans F Malavasi, D Campana. Ligation of CD38 suppresses human B lymphopoiesis. J Exp Med 181: 1101–1110, 1995.

128. F Malavasi, A Funaro, M Alessio, LB DeMonte, CM Ausiello, U Dianzani, F Lanza, E Magrini, M Momo, S Roggero. CD38: a multi-lineage cell activation molecule with a split personality. Int J Clin Lab Res 22:73–80, 1992.

6

Apoptosis Dysregulation in Chronic Lymphocytic Leukemia

JOHN C. REED and SHINICHI KITADA

The Burnham Institute, La Jolla, California

I. INTRODUCTION

It is now well established that defects in the normal mechanisms that control programmed cell death (PCD) occur commonly in cancers. Cell numbers in the body are governed not only by cell division, which determines the rate of cell production, but also by cell death, which sets the rate of cell loss. In the course of a typical day, an average adult produces, and in parallel eradicates, $\sim$50 to 70 billion cells, representing approximately 1 million cells per second. Normally, these two processes of cell division and cell death are tightly coupled so that no net increase in cell numbers occurs or so that such increases represent only temporary responses to environmental stimuli. However, alterations in the expression or function of genes that control PCD can upset this delicate balance, contributing to the expansion of neoplastic cells (reviewed in Ref. 1).

Many types of human cancers are characterized by combinations of defects in both the genes that control the cell division cycle and those involved in PCD. However, some types of malignancies are heavily skewed toward either defective division or death. B-CLL represents a quintessential example of a human malignancy that appears to result primarily from defects in cell death regulation as opposed to cell proliferation. At least in the early stages of the disease, most patients have a monoclonal expansion of circulating mature naive B-cells, $\sim$99% of which represent G_0 phase quiescent cells (2–5). It is assumed therefore that the gradual accumulation of these malignant B cells occurs because they enjoy a selective survival advantage relative to their normal B-cell counterparts, which have average half-lives of only 5 to 7 days as opposed to many months for B-cell chronic lymphocytic leukemia (B-CLL) cells (6).

To date, it remains enigmatic what events contribute to the neoplastic expansion of B-CLL cells in vivo. Clearly, the presence of certain nonrandom cytogenetic abnormalities in B-CLLs suggests the involvement of one or more genes that are likely to play a role in cell death regulation. A prime candidate in this regard is the putative tumor suppressor gene on 13q14, which appears to become inactivated in >75% of B-CLLs (7). Defective regulation of cell death through immune cell interactions is also a possible contributor to the outgrowth of noncycling B-CLL cells. In this regard, numerous lymphokines and cytokines (both secreted and cell surface) have been reported to deliver either antiapoptotic or proapoptotic signals to B lymphocytes. Thus, the immune networks that participate in the production of these factors and that may be aberrantly controlled in B-CLL represent another potential point of dysregulation. Let us then consider what constitutes the core components of the apoptosis machinery and examine what we know about the status of these components in B-CLL.

A. The Core Cell Death Machinery

Clues to the dysregulation of PCD in B-CLL seem likely to be found by studying the core cell death machinery. The molecules that participate in the fundamental steps of PCD have been defined in large part through genetic studies of PCD in simple organisms such as the free-living nematode *Caenorhabiditis elegans* (8). Three essential genes have thus been identified, termed CED-3, CED-4, and CED-9, which control the commitment step that decides the ultimate life/death fate of individual cells. Homologues of each of these cell death genes have been identified in humans and other mammalian species, often occurring in families comprised of multiple members. These proteins are well conserved throughout metazoan evolution, suggesting that they define the core elements of the cell death pathway.

1. CED-3/Caspases

CED-3 is a cysteine proteinase with specificity for asparatic acid residues in the P_1 position of its substrates. In *C. elegans*, all programmed cell deaths that occur during the development of this simple animal depend on the presence of an intact CED-3 gene (9). In mammalian species, at least 14 CED-3 homologs have been identified, termed caspases-1 through -14 (10). These proteases exist as inactive zymogens in all animal cells but can be activated by proteolytic cleavage of their proforms at conserved asparatic acid residues, thus generating the subunits of the enzymatically active proteases that consist of heterotetramers comprised of two large and two small subunits. Because caspases both cleave substrates at Asp residues and are themselves activated by cleavage at Asp residues, the potential for proteolytic cascades exists and indeed has been documented in some scenarios (reviewed in Ref. 11). The concept of upstream initiator and downstream effector caspases that operate within a proteolytic cascade thus has emerged (10,11). Relevant to their mechanisms of activation, all the upstream initiator caspases contain large prodomains, and many of these prodomains have been shown to bind other proteins involved in triggering the cascade. The downstream caspases, which function as the ultimate effectors of apoptosis, uniformly possess small prodomains and are probably activated predominantly, if not exclusively, by proteolytic cleavage by upstream caspases. The irreversible cleavage of specific protein substrates in cells by these downstream effector caspases is what directly or indirectly then accounts for the biochemical and morphological changes that are recognized as apoptosis.

How does the first protease become activated? In most cases, this is probably achieved by the "induced-proximity" method (reviewed in Ref. 12). This model is predicated on the observation that the proforms of most caspases are not entirely devoid of activity, but rather possess at least weak protease activity ($\sim$1% of the fully active enzyme where tested to date). When these proenzymes are brought into close apposition, they can transproteolyse each other, thereby generating the processed autonomously active proteases.

Caspase activation has been documented in B-CLL cells, when successfully induced to undergo apoptosis by chemotherapeutic drugs (13). Although little is known about the expression of various caspases in B-CLLs, the levels of one of the cell death proteases, caspase-3, are variable in B-CLLs, although all peripheral blood B-CLLs tested ($n = 48$) did express this procaspase. Interestingly, expression of caspase-3 is not constitutive in normal B-cells. Rather, caspase-3 expression is dynamically regulated. For example, it has been reported that apoptosis-prone germinal center B-cells contain high levels of procaspase-3, whereas long-live mantle zone B cells contain little of this protein (14). Thus, the relative levels of at least some caspases may fluctuate, depending on the stage of differentiation or activation of B-cells, raising the possibility that it may be possible to modulate caspase expression in B-CLLs with the aim of rendering these cells more sensitive to apoptotic stimuli. Moreover, because examples exist of caspase gene disruption in solid tumors, it is possible (though not proven) that aggressive B-CLLs could suffer from loss of expression of one or more of these cell death proteases.

2. CED-4/Apaf-1

Diverse mechanisms may induce caspase activation in mammalian cells. In *Caenorhabditis elegans*, the only documented mechanism depends on CED-4, another essential gene for PCD in the nematode. CED-4 is an adenosine triphosphate (ATP)–binding protein and putative ATPase that binds to CED-3 (15,16). CED-4 uses the energy of ATP hydrolysis to induce conformational changes in the proform of CED-3 that allow it to cleave itself, thus generating an autonomously active, processed protease.

A mammalian homologue of CED-4 has been identified, termed Apaf-1 (apoptotic protease activating factor-1). The human Apaf-1 protein, however, is structurally more complex than the worm CED-4 (17). For example, in addition to a CED-4–like domain containing a putative ATP-binding P-loop, the Apaf-1 protein possesses an *N*-terminal domain that shares homology to the prodomains of human caspases-2 and -9 and to the prodomain of the worm CED-3 protein. This *N*-terminal domain, called a caspase-associated recruitment domain (CARD domain), has been shown to mediate interactions with the prodomain of caspase-9, thus allowing Apaf-1 to induce autoprocessing of this particular caspase (18).

In addition, however, the CED-4–like domain within Apaf-1 is flanked on its carboxyl-side by 14 tandem copies of a WD domain. This C-terminal region of the protein appears to function as a negative regulatory domain that holds Apaf-1 in a latent, inactive state in cells, preventing it from binding caspase-9. The presence of this negative regulatory domain thus defines a fundamental difference between the human Apaf-1 and worm CED-4 proteins. The human protein requires an activation step to interact with caspases and induce cell death, whereas the worm CED-4 protein has constitutive caspase-binding and death-inducing activity.

The only known mechanism for activating Apaf-1 is cytochrome c, which binds to Apaf-1, apparently relieving the repression applied by the WD domains (18). Cytochrome c is normally sequestered inside mitochondria, between the inner and outer membranes of these organelles. However, it becomes released into the cytosol after exposure of cells to a variety of proapoptotic stimuli, including chemotherapeutic drugs (19–21). Gene ablation studies in mice have documented an essential role for Apaf-1 in the induction of apoptosis by means of the cytochrome c/mitochondrial pathway (22,23). Moreover, fibroblasts derived from Apaf-1 knock-out mice exhibit defects in p53-induced apoptosis and are easily transformed in vitro, suggesting that Apaf-1 functions as a tumor suppressor gene (24). Although little is known about Apaf-1 expression in B-CLLs, recent data indicate that expression of this proapoptotic protein may be variable among CLLs, implying that differences in Apaf-1 levels could potentially equate to differences in apoptosis-sensitivity among B-CLLs (25).

At least one additional Apaf-1–related gene has been described in humans, Nod-1/ CARD-4. This protein also has a CARD domain and nucleotide-binding domain (NB-domain), but contains several leucine-rich repeats (LRRs) instead of WD repeats (26,27). Nod-1/CARD-4 can also associate with procaspase-9 and induce apoptosis, but its overall significance in apoptosis regulation remains poorly defined, and its expression in B-CLL is unexplored to date.

3. CED-9/Bcl-2

In *C. elegans*, a potent death-suppressing protein has been identified, termed CED-9. The CED-9 gene product has been reported to bind to CED-4, preventing it from activating the caspase, CED-3 (16,28–30). CED-9's homologues in human cells constitute the Bcl-2 family of apoptosis-regulatory proteins. At least 20 members of the Bcl-2 family have been identified in mammalian species to date (reviewed in Refs. 1,31). Some Bcl-2 family proteins such as Bcl-2, Bcl-X_L, Bcl-W, Mcl-1, Boo/Diva, and Al/Bfl-1 suppress apoptosis analogous to CED-9. Moreover, at least some of the Bcl-2 family proteins, Boo/Diva and possibly Bcl-X_L, can bind to the CED-4 homologue Apaf-1 (32), suggesting further parallels between the mammalian and nematode cell death machinery. In addition, introduction of the human Bcl-2 protein into CED-9–deficient worms partly restores apoptosis defects in these animals, demonstrating the enormous evolutionary conservation of these core components of the cell death regulatory machinery. However, human Bcl-2 does not bind the CED-4 protein, suggesting an alternative mechanism. In this regard, some Bcl-2 family proteins share structural similarity with pore-forming/ion-channel proteins and may function at least in part by forming channels in the intracellular membranes where they typically reside: namely, the outer mitochondrial membrane, endoplasmic reticulum, and nuclear envelope (reviewed in Ref. 33). Thus, in addition to functions related to protein interactions, some Bcl-2 family proteins possess an intrinsic function as ion-channel/pore-forming proteins, directly controlling the integrity of membranes and governing processes such as release of cytochrome c from mitochondria (34,35).

In *C. elegans*, an antagonist of CED-9 has been identified, EGL-1, which binds to CED-9 and prevents it from forming complexes with CED-4 (36,37). Analogous proteins are also found in humans, including Bcl-X_S, Bad, Hrk, Bim, Bik, Blk, APR/Noxa, and Bcl-G_S (reviewed in Refs. 38,39). These apoptosis-inducing members of the Bcl-2 family function as antagonists of Bcl-2 and its antiapoptotic relatives through mechanisms that involve formation of heterodimers, essentially functioning as transdominant inhibitors of Bcl-2 and its related cytoprotective proteins (reviewed in Ref. 40). All these proteins share a short region of sequence homology (~15–20 amino-acids in length) with the other

Bcl-2 family proteins, called a BH3 domain, but are otherwise quite diverse in sequence and presumably structure. The BH3 domain mediates dimerization among Bcl-2 family proteins and is responsible for the binding of these proapoptotic proteins to cytoprotective members of the Bcl-2 family such as Bcl-2, Bcl-X$_L$, Mcl-1, and others (reviewed in Ref. 41). In *C. elegans*, the production of EGL-1 is controlled at the transcriptional level, dictating whether this CED-9 antagonist is present or absent (42). In humans, expression of some of the "BH3-only" proteins is also controlled at a transcriptional level. For example, APR/Noxa is a p53-inducible gene, which contributes to apoptosis induction by this important tumor suppressor in at least some types of cells (43). However, several of the mammalian BH3-only proteins are constitutively present in cells, and their activity is controlled either through interactions with other proteins or by posttranslational modifications. For example, isoforms of the BH3-only protein Bim are sequestered in association with microtubules by interactions with dynein light chain. Disruption of this interaction allows Bim to translocate to the surface of mitochondria, bind Bcl-2/Bcl-X$_L$ and related antiapoptotic proteins, and trigger cytochrome c release and apoptosis (44). Thus, proteins such as Bim may provide important connections between microtubule-altering drugs and apoptotic responses.

Unlike the simpler nematode, additional classes of Bcl-2 family proteins have been observed in humans that are not found in the worm. The largest of these subfamilies includes the mammalian proapoptotic proteins, Bax, Bak, Bok/Mtd, and Bid. These proteins most likely share structural similarity with pore-forming proteins and directly or indirectly induce cytochrome c release from mitochondria by means of their effects on membrane integrity. Although none of these apoptosis inducers is found in the genome of *C. elegans*, the fly *Drosophila melanogaster* contains at least one protein having striking sequence and functional similarity to mammalian Bok (45). The activity of these killer Bcl-2-family proteins can be controlled either by altering their relative levels, affecting their intracellular location, or inducing conformational changes by means of protein interactions. For example, *bax* is another p53-inducible gene, and thus in some types of cells, p53 triggers increases in Bax protein production associated with induction of apoptosis (46). For example, in normal lymphocytes, DNA damaged induced by x-irradiation induces striking increases in *bax* expression (47). However, in B-CLLs, even when p53 remains wild-type, *bax* is not induced, implying a defect in this p53-response mechanism (48,49). In most nonlymphoid cells, Bax protein is constitutively present, but in a latent state in the cytosol, awaiting poorly defined activating signals to induce its translocation to mitochondria and insertion into mitochondrial membranes (50,51). In contrast, Bak is constitutively associated with membranes but appears to rely on dimerization with the BH3 domain of Bid to trigger conformational changes that allow it to fully insert into membranes and trigger cytochrome c release (reviewed in Ref. 52).

Many examples exist of alterations in the expression of either apoptosis-suppressing or apoptosis-inducing members of the Bcl-2 family in human cancers (reviewed in Refs. 53–55). In B-CLL, it has been reported that high levels of Bcl-2 protein exist in most cases examined (56–60). Moreover, higher levels of Bcl-2 protein or higher ratios of Bcl-2: Bax have been associated with more aggressive behavior of B-CLLs, including progressive disease, refractoriness to chemotherapy, and shorter overall survival (reviewed in Ref. 61). However, not all studies have identified an association between Bcl-2 or Bax expression and outcome in B-CLL, implying that other factors play a role. Another antiapoptotic Bcl-2 family member, Mcl-1, is present at aberrantly high levels in roughly half of B-CLLs. Higher levels of Mcl-1 were associated with a failure to achieve complete remission in patients treated using single-agent regimens with either chlorambucil or fludarabine (48).

4. IAP Family Proteins

IAP family proteins constitute a novel group of apoptosis suppressers that are conserved throughout animal evolution, with homologues identified in *Drosophila*, baculoviruses, mice, humans, and other species (62–69). Interestingly, however, *C. elegans* appears to lack apoptosis-suppressing IAPs, revealing yet another difference in the cell death machinery of worms and men (reviewed in Refs. 70,71). Although the mechanism by which IAP-family proteins suppress cell death remains debated, the only clearly identified activity for these proteins thus far is as inhibitors of caspases. Specifically, several of the human IAP family proteins have been reported to directly bind and potently inhibit particular members of the caspase family of cell death proteases (72–74). Interestingly, not all caspases are targets of IAP suppression. To date, only caspases-3, -7, and -9 have been reported to be bound and inhibited by IAPs. Caspases-1, -6, -8, and -10 are not. The significance of this selective inhibition of caspases by IAPs is that those caspases inhibited operate in the distal portions of the proteolytic cascades that lead to apoptosis, with some such as caspases-3 and -7 functioning as the ultimate effectors of apoptosis that cleave the various proteins responsible for the death of the cell. Caspases-3 and -7 represent a point of convergence of many, if not most, apoptosis cell death pathways. Interesting, the IAP target caspase-9 is the protease that is acted on by Apaf-1, representing the first protease within the mitochondria/cytochrome c pathway for caspase activation (Fig. 1).

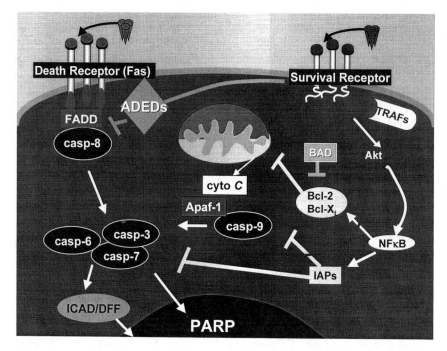

Figure 1   Summary of cell survival and cell death pathways. See text for details.

Although the expression of IAPs in B-CLL has not been examined to date, overexpression of some IAPs occurs in cancers. For example, the IAP-family member Survivin is overexpressed in a large proportion of human cancers (69), providing evidence that alterations in the expression of these proteins can occur in the course of tumorigenesis. Higher levels of Survivin have been associated with adverse prognosis in several types of solid tumors, although Survivin is not generally expressed in low-grade B-cell malignancies (reviewed in Refs. 75,76). Elevated levels of the IAP member XIAP occur in acute myelogenous leukemia (AML) and are associated with poor responses to chemotherapy, shorter remission duration, and perhaps shorter overall survival (77).

B. Signal Transduction and Apoptosis Regulation

The core machinery of the cell death pathway communicates with the external and internal world of the cells by interfacing with multiple signal transduction pathways. Some of those that may be particularly germane to B-CLL are discussed here.

1.   TNF-Family Death Receptors

Although many mechanisms for caspase activation probably exist, one of the most striking is exemplified by the tumor necrosis factor (TNF) family of cytokine receptors (reviewed in Ref. 78). Several TNF family receptors are known to transduce signals that result in apoptosis, including TNF-R1 (CD120a), Fas (CD95), DR3 (Wsl-1; Tramp); DR4 (Trail-R1); DR5 (Trail-R2); and DR6. These death receptors contain a conserved cytosolic domain known as a death domain (DD) that is responsible for recruiting adapter proteins such as Fadd/Mort-1 to the receptor complex after binding of ligand. The Fadd/Mort-1 protein contains both a DD domain and an additional protein-interaction domain called a death effector domain (DED). The DED of Fadd/Mort-1 binds certain caspases that contain homologous DEDs within their prodomains, caspases-8 and -10. The oligomerization of caspases within the death receptor complex results in transprocessing of the zymogens by the induced proximity method (reviewed in Refs. 11,12). Processing of caspase-8 removes the DED-containing prodomain, thus releasing the activated protease into the cytosol, where it can cleave and activate other downstream procaspases such as caspase-3.

Fas plays a critical role in regulating homeostasis of lymphoid cell populations in vivo. Cytolytic T cells and natural killer (NK) cells heavily rely on surface expression of Fas-ligand (FasL) to trigger apoptosis in target cells (reviewed in Refs. 79–81). Mice with defects in this receptor or its ligand develop a lymphoproliferative syndrome accompanied by autoimmune problems caused primarily by excessive immunoglobulin production (82,83). Hereditary mutations in Fas have also been described in humans, again causing a lymphoproliferative and autoimmune disorder (84). In both humans and mice, mutations are found in the DD, preventing proper signaling by this receptor. During activation, most lymphocytes are induced to express Fas, thus rendering them potentially vulnerable to Fas-mediated apoptosis. Cells that receive appropriate signals by way of antigen-receptors and costimulatory molecules express proteins that make them resistant to Fas, allowing them to survive and clonally expand. Thus, when antigen becomes limiting at the end of an immune response, Fas expression on activated lymphocytes ensures apoptotic elimination of excess lymphocytes and a return of lymphocyte counts to normal.

B-CLLs have been reported to be profoundly resistant to Fas (CD95)-induced apoptosis (85–89), suggesting the possibility of defects in the apoptotic signaling pathway used by Fas and other TNF-family death receptors. In this regard, several DED-containing inhibitors of death receptor signaling have been described. One of these is Flip, also known as Flame, I-Flice, CASH, Rick, and Usurpin (reviewed in Ref. 90). The Flip protein is a homologue of caspases-8 and -10, which contains DED domains but lacks proteolytic activity. In most circumstances, Flip competes with caspases for binding to Fadd/Mort-1, thus functioning as a transdominant inhibitor of these caspases involved in TNF-family cytokine signaling. Flip production is dynamically regulated in B-CLLs, with CD40-delivering signals that up-regulate the levels of this antiapoptotic protein (87). Other DED-containing antiapoptotic proteins that include BAR and Bap31, which are both membrane-anchored proteins found predominantly in association with mitochondrial and endoplasmic reticulum membranes, respectively (91,92). The expression of these other antiapoptotic DED-containing proteins (ADEDs) in B-CLL has not been explored. Regardless of the mechanism, defects in the Fas-signaling pathway of B-CLLs may have at least two important implications. First, roadblocks to Fas-induced apoptosis make it more difficult for immune effector cells to trigger apoptosis of B-CLL cells, particularly because CTLs rely so heavily on Fas for killing target cells. Second, in some types of leukemia cells, it appears that genotoxic stress injury induces expression of Fas-ligand, Fas, or other members of the TNF family of death receptors (93), thus resulting in activation of the DED containing cell death protease, caspase-8, and apoptosis. Consequently, defects in the Fas-pathway may contribute to chemoresistance in some circumstances. How relevant TNF-family death receptors are for chemoresponses by B-CLL cells in particularly, and cancers in general, remains controversial (94–96).

2. NF-κB

The transcription factor NF-κB plays important roles in apoptosis. In its classic form, NF-κB consists of a p50 and p65 heterodimer, where the p50 subunit contains the DNA-binding domain, which binds specific target sequences in the genome and the p65 (RelA) subunit carries the transactivation domain for recruiting transcriptional coactivators (reviewed in Refs. 97–100). However, several p50 and p65 homologous proteins exist, constituting the broader NF-κB (Rel) family. NF-κB activity is regulated at many levels, but the most impressive is by its sequestration in the cytosol by the IκB-family proteins. When bound to IκB, NF-κB cannot enter the nucleus and thus is unable to regulate gene expression. Many receptor signal transduction pathways can trigger NF-κB activation by inducing degradation of IκB proteins. Kinase-induced phosphorylation of IκB on ser32 and ser36 signals for binding of phosphorylated IκB by an F-box protein, β-Trcp, which then recruits IκB to a large multiprotein E3 ubiquitin-ligase complex (the SCF complex), resulting in its polyubiquitination and then subsequent degradation by the 26s proteosome (101–103).

TNF-family cytokine receptors are well known for their ability to induce NF-κB. Many members of the TNFR family interact by way of their cytosolic intracellular domains with TRAF-family proteins. At least six TRAF-family members are known in humans to date. Several TRAF-family proteins bind various protein kinases that are capable of inducing IκB phosphorylation and thereby activating NF-κB. These adapter proteins thus bridge the kinases to various TNF-family receptors, providing the link to a pathway for NF-κB induction. Among the TNF-family receptors known to directly bind TRAFs by means of their cytosolic domains and to induce NF-κB are p75-TNFR2 (CD120b), CD27, CD30, CD40, BCMA, and others (reviewed in Ref. 104). Additional TNF-family receptors-can indirectly bind TRAFs, by means of adapter proteins, thus recruiting TRAFs to the receptor complexes, including TNFR1, DR3, and DR6 (reviewed in Ref. 105).

Little is known about TRAF-family gene expression in B-CLLs thus far. However, TRAF1 levels are reportedly elevated compared with normal peripheral blood B cells in about half of previously untreated B-CLLs and in >80% of posttreatment refractory CLLs (106). Interestingly, overexpression of TRAF1 in lymphoid cells in transgenic mice results in resistance to activation-induced apoptosis but is not associated with lymphocytosis (107). In contrast, mice expressing a mutant (dominant-negative) of TRAF2 develop a striking lymphoproliferative disorder (108).

Elevated levels of NF-kB activity have been consistently detected in B-CLLs, and stimulation through TNF-family receptors such as CD40 results in further NF-kB activity (109). The reason for the higher baseline levels of NF-kB in B-CLLs is unknown. One possible explanation is that B-CLLs may aberrantly express ligands for certain TNF-family receptors on their surface, thus resulting in autocrine stimulation. For example, roughly 15% to 30% of B-CLLs express CD40-ligand (CD40L) on their surface, whereas normal B-cells do not express this ligand (109–111). Note that CD40L, similar to many members of the TNF-family, is displayed on the cell surface as as type-II receptor rather than directly secreted. All B cells, including B-CLLs, express the receptor CD40. Thus, the expression of ligand and receptor on the same cell may result in autocrine stimulation of NF-kB. Elevated levels of soluble CD40L have also been detected in the sera of B-CLL patients, and plasma from these patients can rescue B-CLL cells from apoptosis in culture, by means of a mechanisms that is blocked by addition of anti-CD40L antibody (112).

CD27 and its ligand CD70 are also commonly coexpressed on B-CLL cells, whereas normal resting B cells rarely express either CD27 or CD70 (110,113), implying aberrant regulation of the expression of these molecules in B-CLL. In addition, although CD30-ligand CD30L is found on normal B cells, the receptor CD30 is not. In contrast, a subset of B-CLL patients express CD30L and also ectopically express CD30 on their B-CLL cells (110,114), suggesting yet another instance in which a pathological autocrine loop might be established.

How does NF-κB suppress apoptosis? The answer is by inducing transcription of several antiapoptotic genes, including cytoprotective members of the Bcl-2 family (Bcl-X_L, Bfl-1), IAP-family proteins (cIAP2 and possibly cIAP1 and XIAP in some cell-types), and others (115–120).

3. Akt

The protein kinase Akt (also known as PKB) plays an important role in apoptosis suppression. This kinase is activated in response to phospholipid second messengers generated by phosphatidyl inositol 3′ kinase (PI3K) (reviewed in Ref. 121). Many growth factor receptors, neutrophin receptors, and lymphokine receptors stimulate increases in PI3K and Akt activity. Akt has multiple ways of suppressing apoptosis, probably only some of which have been delineated thus far. For example, Akt can phosphorylate the proapoptotic Bcl-2 family protein BAD, thus preventing it from dimerizing with Bcl-2 and Bcl-X_L and thereby abrogating its activity (122–124). Akt can also phosphorylate and inactive forkhead-family transcription factors that are responsible induction of Fas-ligand gene expression and induction of apoptosis (125). Finally, Akt can phosphorylate human caspase-9, inactivating this apical caspase in the cytochrome c/mitochondrial pathway for apoptosis (126). The status of Akt activity in B-CLLs has scarely been explored to date. However, one of the TRAF-family members known to be recruited to CD40 receptor complexes, TRAF6, can induce activation of PI3K and Akt (127). Also, the protein encoded by the TCL1 gene of T-cell CLL/PLL binds Akt and enhances its activity (128,129).

C. Therapeutic Implications

Advances in basic knowledge about the core machinery of apoptosis and the various signal transduction pathway that provide inputs into it are beginning to reveal strategies for overcoming apoptosis resistance in cancers in general. Many of the lessons learned are likely to find applicability to B-CLL as well.

For example, antisense oligonucleotides targeting Bcl-2 have been applied against B-cell malignancies for promoting apoptosis (130,131) and are currently in phase III clinical trials. Strategies for generation of small-molecule inhibitors of the Bcl-2 protein have also been developed on the basis of information about how BH3 peptides antagonize this protein within the context of natural Bcl-2 suppression by proapoptotic Bcl-2 family proteins (132,133). The TNF-family ligand, TRAIL, which binds and induces apoptosis by means of the death receptors DR4 and DR5, is scheduled to soon enter clinical trials for cancer patients. Anti-CD40L antibodies may also soon find their way into clinical trials, thus blocking one of the NF-κB-inducing members of this family, which is particularly important for B-cell survival. Small-molecule inhibitors of the NF-κB-inducing kinases, IKKα and IKKβ, have also been discovered (134), and could find applicability for the treatment of CLL and other cancers. In addition, small-molecule inhibitors of Akt would be expected to bc provide a powerful tool in the arsenal of anticancer agents, particularly given evidence of hyperactivity of Akt in ~80% of human cancers caused by inactivation of the PTEN gene, Akt gene amplification, and other mechanisms documented in tumors. Altogether, these and other examples suggest that knowledge about apoptosis mechanisms in cancers and leukemias will provide rich opportunities for drug discovery and progress in the war on malignancies of all kinds.

II. SUMMARY

Chronic lymphocytic leukemia represents a quintessential example of a human malignancy that is caused primarily by defects in programmed cell death rather than cell cycle regulation. The mature circulating B-lymphocytes that comprise CLL in most patients are largely quiescent G_0 phase cells, which accumulate not because they are dividing more rapidly than normal but because they survive longer than their normal counterparts. This prolonged survival of B-CLL cells is caused by defects in the normal pathways for programmed cell death (apoptosis). Many studies have documented that defects in apoptosis pathways also commonly contribute to chemoresistance, rendering tumor cells less sensitive to the cytotoxic actions of currently available anticancer drugs. Alternations in apoptosis pathways also can render malignant cells impervious to the cytotoxic responses of immune cells. Most likely, therefore, the current incurability of B-CLL can be attributed largely to the underlying defects that prevent these leukemic cells from undergoing programmed cell death. This chapter has discussed some of the major pathways that control apoptosis and summarized current information about some of the ways that these pathways may be abnormal in B-CLL. Therapeutic implications were also discussed.

REFERENCES

1. JC Reed. Bcl-2 and the regulation of programmed cell death. J Cell Biol 124:1–6, 1994.
2. G Dighiero, P Travade, S Chevret, P Fenaux, C Chastang, J-L Binet. B-cell chronic lymphocytic leukemia: present status and future directions. Blood 78:1901–1914, 1991.
3. S O'Brien, A del Giglio, M Keating. Advances in the biology and treatment of B-cell chronic lymphocytic leukemia. Blood 85:307–318, 1995.
4. F Caligaris-Cappio. B-chronic lymphocytic leukemia: a malignancy of anti-self B cells. Blood 87:2615–2620, 1996.
5. T Kipps. Chronic lymphocytic leukemia. Curr Opin Hematol 4:268–276, 1997.
6. ICM MacLennan, D Gray. Antigen-driven selection of virgin and memory B cells. Immunol Rev 91:61–66, 1986.
7. F Bullrich, ML Veronese, S Kitada, et al. Minimal region of loss at 13q14 in B-cell chronic lymphocytic leukemia. Blood 88:3109–3115, 1996.
8. MO Hengartner, HR Horvitz. Programmed cell death in Caenorhabditis elegans. Curr Opin Genet Dev 4:581–586, 1994.
9. J Yuan, S Shaham, S Ledoux, H Ellis, H Horvitz. The C. elegans cell death gene ced-3 encodes a protein similar to mammalian interleukin-1 beta-converting enzyme. Cell 75:641–652, 1993.
10. ES Alnemri, DJ Livingston, DW Nicholson, et al. Human ICE/CED-3 protease nomenclature. Cell 87:171, 1996.
11. GS Salvesen, VM Dixit. Caspases: Intracellular signaling by proteolysis. Cell 1997; 91:443–446.
12. GS Salvesen, VM Dixit. Caspase activation: the induced-proximity model. Proc Natl Acad Sci USA 96:10964–10967, 1999.
13. B Bellosillo, M Dalmau, D Colomer, J Gil. Involvement of CED-3/ICE proteases in the apoptosis of B-chronic lymphocytic leukemia cells. Blood 89:3378–3384, 1997.
14. S Krajewski, RD Gascoyne, JM Zapata, et al. Immunolocalization of the ICE/Ced-3-family protease, CPP32 (Caspase-3), in non-Hodgkin's lymphomas (NHLs), chronic lymphocytic leukemias (CLL), and reactive lymph nodes. Blood 89:3817–3825, 1997.
15. A Chinnaiyan, D Chaudhary, K O'Rourke, E Koonin, V Dixit. Role of CED-4 in the activation of CED-3. Nature 388:728–729, 1997.
16. S Seshagiri, L Miller. *Caenorhabditis elegans* CED-4 stimulates CED-3 processing and CED-3 induced apoptosis. Curr Biol 7:455–460, 1997.
17. H Zou, WJ Henzel, X Liu, A Lutschg, X Wang. Apaf-1, a human protein homologous to C. elegans CED-4, participates in cytochrome c-dependent activation of caspase-3. Cell 90:405–413, 1997.
18. P Li, D Nijhawan, I Budihardjo, et al. Cytochrome c and dATP-dependent formation of Apaf-1/Caspase-9 complex initiates an apoptotic protease cascade. Cell 91:479–489, 1997.
19. X Liu, CN Kim, J Yang, R Jemmerson, X Wang. Induction of apoptotic program in cell-free extracts: requirement for dATP and Cytochrome C. Cell 86:147–157, 1996.
20. J Yang, X Liu, K Bhalla, et al. Prevention of apoptosis by Bcl-2: release of cytochrome c from mitochondria blocked. Science 275:1129–1132, 1997.
21. RM Kluck, E Bossy-Wetzel, DR Green, DD Newmeyer. The release of cytochrome c from mitochondria: a primary site for Bcl-2 regulation of apoptosis. Science 275:1132–1136, 1997.
22. H Yoshida, YY Kong, R Yoshida, et al. Apaf1 is required for mitochondrial pathways of apoptosis and brain development. Cell 94:739–750, 1998.
23. F Cecconi, G Alvarez-Bolado, BI Meyer, KA Roth, P Gruss. Apaf1 (CED-4 homolog) regulates programmed cell death in mammalian development. Cell 94:727–737, 1998.
24. M Soengas, R Alarcon, H Yoshida, et al. Apaf-1 and caspase-9 in p53-dependent apoptosis and tumor inhibition. Science 284:156–159, 1999.

25. L Leoni, Q Chao, H Cottam, et al. Induction of an apoptotic program in cell-free extracts by 2-chloro-2′-deoxyadenosine 5′-triphosphate and cytochrome c. Proc Natl Acad Sci USA 95:9567–9571, 1998.

26. N Inohara, T Koseki, L Del Peso, et al. Nod1, an Apaf-1-like activator of caspase-9 and nuclear factor-kB. J Biol Chem 274:14560–14567, 1999.

27. J Bertin, W-J Nir, C Fischer, et al. Human CARD4 Protein is a Novel CED-4/Apaf-1 cell death family member that activates NF-κB. J Biol Chem 274:12955–12958, 1999.

28. MS Spector, S Desnoyers, DJ Heoppner, MO Hengartner. Interaction between the C. elegans cell-death regulators CED-9 and CED-4. Nature 385:653–656, 1997.

29. AM Chinnaiyan, K O'Rourke, BR Lane, VM Dixit. Interaction of CED-4 with CED-3 and CED-9: a molecular framework for cell death. Science 275:1122–1126, 1997.

30. D Wu, HD Wallen, G Nunez. Interaction and regulation of subcellular localization of CED-4 by CED-9. Science 275:1126–1129, 1997.

31. G Kroemer. The proto-oncogene Bcl-2 and its role in regulating apoptosis. Nat Med 8:614–620, 1997.

32. G Pan, K O'Rourke, VM Dixit. Caspase-9, Bcl-X_L, and apaf-1 form a ternary complex. J Biol Chem 273:5841–5845, 1998.

33. S Schendel, M Montal, JC Reed. Bcl-2 family proteins as ion-channels. Cell Death Differ 5:372–380, 1998.

34. T Rosse, R Olivier, L Monney, et al. Bcl-2 prolongs cell survival after Bax-induced release of cytochrome c[see comments]. Nature 391:496–499, 1998.

35. JM Jürgensmeier, Z Xie, Q Deveraux, L Ellerby, D Bredesen, JC Reed. Bax directly induces release of cytochrome c from isolated mitochondria. Proc Natl Acad Sci USA 5:4997–5002, 1998.

36. B Conradt, H Horvitz. The C. elegans protein EGL-1 is required for programmed cell death and interacts with the Bcl-2-like protein CED-9. Cell 93:519–529, 1998.

37. L del Peso, VM Gonzalez, G Nunez. Caenorhabditis elegans EGL-1 Disrupts the Interaction of CED-9 with CED-4 and Promotes CED-3 Activation. J Biol Chem 273:33495–33500, 1998.

38. J Reed. Bcl-2 family proteins. Oncogene 17:3225–3236, 1998.

39. JC Reed. Mechanisms of apoptosis. Am J Pathol 157:1415–1430, 2000.

40. JC Reed. Double identity for proteins of the Bcl-2 family. Nature 387:773–776, 1997.

41. A Kelekar, CB Thompson. Bcl-2-family proteins—the role of the BH3 domain in apoptosis. Trends Cell Biol 8:324–330, 1998.

42. B Conradt, H Horvitz. The tra-1a sex determination protein of C. elegans regulates sexually dimorphic cell deaths by repressing the egl-1 cell death activator gene. Cell 98:317–327, 1999.

43. A Hirao, YY Kong, S Matsuoka, et al. DNA damage-induced activation of p53 by the checkpoint kinase Chk2. Science 287:1824–1827, 2000.

44. H Puthalakath, D Huang, L O'Reilly, S King, A Strasser. The proapoptotic activity of the Bcl-2 family member bim is regulated by interaction with the dynein motor complex. Mol Cell 3:287–296, 1999.

45. H Zhang, Q Huang, N Ke, et al. Drosophila pro-apoptotic bcl-2/bax homologue reveals evolutionary conservation of cell death mechanisms. J Biol Chem 275:27303–27306, 2000.

46. T Miyashita, JC Reed. Tumor suppressor p53 is a direct transcriptional activator of human Bax gene. Cell 80:293–299, 1995.

47. S Kitada, S Krajewski, T Miyashita, M Krajewska, JC Reed. γ-Radiation induces upregulation of Bax protein and apoptosis in radiosensitive cells in vivo. Oncogene 12:187–192, 1996.

48. S Kitada, J Andersen, S Akar, et al. Expression of apoptosis-regulating proteins in chronic lymphocytic leukemia: Correlations with in vitro and in vivo chemoresponses. Blood 91: 3379–3389, 1998.

49. JB Johnston, P Daeninck, L Verburg, et al. P53, MDM-2, BAX and BCL-2 and drug resistance in chronic lymphocytic leukemia. Leukemia Lymphoma 26:435–449, 1997.

50. KG Wolter, YT Hsu, CL Smith, A Nechushtan, XG Xi, RJ Youle. Movement of bax from the cytosol to mitochondria during apoptosis. J Cell Biol 139:1281–1292, 1997.

51. A Nechushtan, C Smith, Y-T Hsu, R Youle. conformation of the Bax C-terminus regulates subcellular location and cell death. EMBO J 18:2330–2341, 1999.

52. SJ Korsmeyer, MC Wei, M Saito, S Weiler, KJ Oh, PH Schlesinger. Pro-apoptotic cascade activates BID, which oligomerizes BAK or BAX into pores that result in the release of cytochrome c. Cell Death Differ 2000; in press.

53. JC Reed. Bcl-2 and B-cell neoplasia: dysregulation of programmed cell death in cancer. In: JR Bertino, ed. Encyclopedia of Cancer Vol. 1. San Diego: Academic Press, 1997, pp 125–145.

54. JC Reed. Bcl-2 family proteins: Regulators of apoptosis and chemoresistance in hematologic malignancies. Semin Hematol 34:9–19, 1997.

55. JC Reed. Bcl-2 family proteins and the hormonal control of cell life and death in normalcy and neoplasia. In: G Litwack, ed. Vitamins and Hormones. Vol. 53. San Diego: Academic Press, 1997, pp. 99–138.

56. M Schena, L Larsson, D Gottardi, et al. Growth—and differentiation-associated expression of Bcl-2 in B-chronic lymphocytic leukemia cells. Blood 79:2981–2989, 1992.

57. M Hanada, D Delia, A Aiello, E Stadtmauer, J Reed. Bcl-2 gene hypomethylation and high-level expression in B-cell chronic lymphocytic leukemia. Blood 82:1820–1828, 1993.

58. DJ McConkey, J Chandra, S Wright, et al. Apoptosis sensitivity in chronic lymphocytic leukemia is determined by endogenous endonuclease content and relative expression of BCL-2 and BAX. J. Immunol. 156:2624–2630, 1996.

59. C Pepper, T Hoy, D Bentley. Bcl-2/Bax ratios in chronic lymphocytic leukemia and their correlation with in vitro apoptosis and clinical resistance. Br J Oncol 76:935–938, 1998.

60. LE Robertson, W Plunkett, K McConnell, MJ Keating, TJ McDonnell. Bcl-2 expression in chronic lymphocytic leukemia and its correlation with the induction of apoptosis and clinical outcome. Leukemia 10:456–459, 1996.

61. J Reed. Chronic lymphocytic leukemia: a disease of disregulated programmed cell death. Clin Immunol Newslett 17:125–140, 1998.

62. RJ Clem, LK Miller. Control of programmed cell death by the baculovirus genes p35 and IAP. Mol Cell Biol 14:5212–5222, 1994.

63. NE Crook, RJ Clem, LK Miller. An apoptosis-inhibiting baculovirus gene with a zinc finger-like motif. J Virol 67:2168–2174, 1993.

64. BA Hay, DA Wassarman, GM Rubin. Drosophila homologs of baculovirus inhibitor of apoptosis proteins function to block cell death. Cell 83:1253–1262, 1995.

65. N Roy, MS Mahadevan, M McLean, et al. The gene for neuronal apoptosis inhibitory protein is partially deleted in individuals with spinal muscular atrophy. Cell 80:167–178, 1995.

66. M Rothe, M-G Pan, WJ Henzel, TM Ayres, DV Goeddel. The TNFR2-TRAF signaling complex contains two novel proteins related to baculoviral inhibitor of apoptosis proteins. Cell 83:1243–1252, 1995.

67. P Liston, N Roy, K Tamai, et al. Suppression of apoptosis in mammalian cells by NAIP and a related family of IAP genes. Nature 379:349–353, 1996.

68. C Duckett, V Nava, R Gedrich, et al. A conserved family of cellular genes related to the baculovirus iap gene and encoding apoptosis inhibitors. EMBO J 15:2685–2689, 1996.

69. G Ambrosini, C Adida, D Altieri. A novel anti-apoptosis gene, survivin, expressed in cancer and lymphoma. Nat Med 3:917–921, 1997.

70. J Abrams. An emerging blueprint for apoptosis in drosophila. Trends Cell Biol 9:435–440, 1999.

71. JC Reed, JR Bischoff. Bringing chromosomes through cell division—and surviving the experience. Cell 102:545–548, 2000.

72. QL Deveraux, R Takahashi, GS Salvesen, JC Reed. X-linked IAP is a direct inhibitor of cell death proteases. Nature 388:300–304, 1997.

73. N Roy, QL Deveraux, R Takashashi, GS Salvesen, JC Reed. The c-IAP-1 and c-IaP-2 proteins are direct inhibitors of specific caspases. EMBO J, 16:6914–6925, 1997.

74. QL Deveraux, N Roy, HR Stennicke, et al. IAPs block apoptotic events induced by caspase-8 and cytochrome c by direct inhibition of distinct caspases. EMBO J 17:2215–2223, 1998.

75. Q Deveraux, J Reed. IAP family proteins: Suppressors of apoptosis. Genes Dev 13:239–252, 1999.

76. DC Altieri, C Marchisic. Survivin apoptosis: An interloper between cell death and cell proliferation in cancer. Biol Dis 79:1327, 1999.

77. I Tamm, S Kornblau, H Segall, et al. Expression and prognostic significance of iap-family genes in human cancers and myeloid leukemias. Clin Can Res 6:1796–1803, 2000.

78. D Wallach, M Boldin, E Varfolomeev, R Beyaert, P Vandenabeele, W Fiers. Cell death induction by receptors of the TNF family: towards a molecular understanding. FEBS Lett 410:96–106, 1997.

79. DR Green, RP Bissonnette, JM Glynn, Y Shi. Activation-induced apoptosis in lymphoid systems. Semin Hematol 4:379–388, 1992.

80. S Nagata, P Golstein. The Fas death factor. Science 267:1449–1456, 1995.

81. J Wang, MJ Lenardo. Molecules involved in cell death and peripheral tolerance. Curr Opin Immunol 9:818–825, 1997.

82. R Watanabe-Fukunaga, CI Brannan, NG Copeland, NA Jenkins, S Nagata. Lymphoproliferation disorder in mice explained by defects in Fas antigen that mediates apoptosis. Nature 356:314–317, 1992.

83. T Takahashi, M Tanaka, CI Brannan, et al. Generalized lymphoproliferative disease in mice, caused by a point mutation in the Fas ligand. Cell 76:969–976, 1994.

84. GH Fisher, FJ Rosenberg, SE Straus, et al. Dominant interfering fas gene mutations impair apoptosis in a human autoimmune lymphoproliferative syndrome. Cell 81:935–946, 1995.

85. P Garrone, E-M Neidhardt-Berard, E Garcia, et al. B-chronic lymphocytic leukemia cells display reduced susceptibility to Fas-induced apoptosis. Blood 1997:In press.

86. P Panayiotidis, K Ganeshaguru, L Foroni, AV Hoffbrand. Expression and function of the FAS antigen in B chronic lymphocytic leukemia and hairy cell leukemia. Leukemia 9:1227–1232, 1995.

87. S Kitada, J Zapata, M Andreeff, J Reed. Bryostatin and CD40-ligand enhance apoptosis resistance and induce expression of cell survival genes in B-cell chronic lymphocytic leukaemia. Br J Hematol 106:995–1004, 1999.

88. N Laytragoon-Lewin, E Duhony, XF Bai, H Mellstedt. Downregulation of the CD95 receptor and defect CD40-mediated signal transduction in B-chronic lymphocytic leukemia cells. Eur J Haematol 61:266–271, 1998.

89. D Wang, GJ Freeman, H Levine, J Ritz, MJ Robertson. Role of the CD40 and CD95 (APO-1/Fas) antigens in the apoptosis of human B-cell malignancies. Br J Haematol 97:409–417, 1997.

90. D Wallach. Placing death under control. Nature 388:123–126, 1997.

91. FWH Ng, M Nguyen, T Kwan, et al. p28 Bap31, a Bcl-2/Bcl-X$_L$ -and procaspase-8-associated protein in the endoplasmic reticulum. J Cell Biol 39:327–338, 1997.

92. H Zhang, Q Xu, S Krajewski, et al. BAR: An apoptosis regulator at the intersection of caspase and bcl-2 family proteins. Proc Natl Acad Sci USA 97:2597–2602, 2000.

93. C Friesen, I Herr, PH Krammer, K-M Debatin. Involvement of the CD95 (APO-1/Fas) receptor/ligand system in drug induced apoptosis in leukemia cells. Nat Med 2:574–577, 1996.

94. CM Eischen, TJ Kottke, LM Martins, et al. Comparison of apoptosis in wild-type and Fas-resistant cells: chemotherapy-induced apoptosis is not dependent on Fas/Fas ligand interactions. Blood 90:935–943, 1997.

95. A Villunger, A Egle, M Kos, et al. Drug-induced apoptosis is associated with enhanced Fas (Apo-1/CD95) ligand expression but occurs independently of Fas(Apo-1/CD95) signaling in human T-acute lymphatic leukemia cells. Cancer Res 57:3331–3334, 1997.

96. M Kastan. On the TRAIL from p53 to apoptosis? Nat Genet 17:130–131, 1997.

97. M Barkett, TD Gilmore. Control of apoptosis by Rel/NF-kappaB transcription factors. Oncogene 18:6910–6924, 1999.

98. T Maniatis. A ubiquitin ligase complex essential for the NF-κB, Wnt/Wingless, and hedgehog signaling pathways. Genes Dev 13:505–510, 1999.

99. IM Verma, J Stevenson. IkappaB kinase: beginning, not the end. Proc Natl Acad Sci USA 94:11758–11760, 1997.

100. I Stancovski, D Baltimore. NF-KB activation: the IKB kinase revealed? Cell 91:299–302, 1997.

101. SJ Elledge, JT Winston, P Strack, P Beer-Romero, CY Chu. The SCFb-TRCP-ubiquitin liagse complex associates specifically with phosphorylated destruction motifs in IkBa and β-catenin and stimulates IkBa ubiquitination in vitro. Genes Dev 13:270–283, 1999.

102. JT Winston, P Strack, P Beer-Romero, CY Chu, SJ Elledge, JW Harper. The SCF^{B-TRCP}-ubiquitin ligase complex associates specifically with phosphorylated destruction motifs in IκBα and β-catenin and stimulates IκBα ubiquitination in vitro. Genes Dev 13:270–283, 1999.

103. H Suzuki, T Chiba, M Kobayashi, et al. IkBa Ubiquitination is catalyzed by an SCF-like complex containing Skp1, cullin-1, and two F-box/WD40-Repeat Proteins, βTrCP1 and βTrCP2. Biochem Biophys Res Commun 256:127–132, 1999.

104. RH Arch, RW Gedrich, CB Thompson. Tumor necrosis factor receptor-associated factors (TRAFs)—a family of adapter proteins that regulates life and death. Genes Dev 12:2821–2830, 1998.

105. A Ashkenazi, V Dixit. Death receptors: signaling and modulation. Science 281:1305–1308, 1998.

106. JM Zapata, M Krajewska, S Krajewski, et al. TRAF-family protein expression in normal tissues and lymphoid malignancies. J Immunol 2000; In press.

107. DE Speiser, SY Lee, B Wong, et al. A regulatory role for TRAF1 in antigen-induced apoptosis of T cells. J Exp Med 185:1777–1783, 1997.

108. SY Lee, A Reichlin, A Santana, KA Sokol, MC Nussenzweig, Y Choi. TRAF2 is essential for JNK but not NF-kB activation and regulates lymphocyte proliferation and survival. Immunity 7:703–713, 1997.

109. RR Furman, Z Asgary, JO Mascarebhas, H-C Liou, EJ Schattner. Modulation of NF-kB activity and apoptosis in chronic lymphocytic leukemia B cells. J Immunol 164:2200–2206, 2000.

110. L Trentin, R Zambello, R Sancetta, et al. B lymphocytes from patients with chronic lymphoproliferative disorders are equipped with different costimulatory molecules. Can Res 57:4940–4947, 1997.

111. E Schattner, J Mascarenhas, I Reyfman, et al. CLL B cells can express CD40 ligand and demonstrate T-cell type costimulatory capacity. Blood 91:2689–2697, 1998.

112. A Younes, V Snell, U Consoli, et al. Elevated levels of biologically active soluble CD40 ligand in the serum of patients with chronic lymphocytic leukemia. Br J Haematol 100:135–141, 1998.

113. EA Ranheim, MJ Cantwell, TJ Kipps. Expression of CD27 and its ligand, CD70, on chronic lymphocytic leukemia B cells. Blood 85:3556–3565, 1995.

114. A Younes, U Consoli, S Zhao, et al. CD30 ligand is expressed on resting normal and malignant human B lymphocytes. Br J Haematol 93:569–571, 1996.

115. D Stroka, A Badrichani, F Bach, C Ferran. Overexpression of A1, an NF-κB-inducible, anti-apoptotic Bcl gene inhibits endothelial cell activation. Blood 93:3803–3810, 1999.

116. G Cheng, H Lee, H Dadgostar, Q Cheng, J Shu. NF-kB-mediated up-regulation of bcl-x and

bfl-1/al is required for cd40 survival signaling in B lymphocytes. Proc Natl Acad Sci USA 96:9136–9141, 1999.

117. C Stehlik, R de Martin, I Kumabashiri, A Schmid, B Binder, J Lipp. Nuclear factor (NF)-κB-regulated X-chromosome-linked iap gene expression protects endothelial cells from tumor necrosis factor α-induced apoptosis. J Exp Med 188:211–216, 1998.

118. C Stehlik, R de Martin, B Binder, J Lipp. Cytokine induced expression of porcine inhibitor of apoptosis protein (iap) family member is regulated by NF-κB. Biochem Biophys Res Commun 243:827–832, 1998.

119. MX Wu, Z Ao, KVS Prasad, R Wu, SF Schlossman. IEX-1L, an apoptosis inhibitor involved in NF-kB-mediated cell survival. Science 281:998–1001, 1998.

120. H Lee, P Dempsey, T Parks, X Zhu, D Baltimore, G Cheng. Specificities of CD40 signaling: Involvement of TRAF2 in CD40-induced NF-κB activation and intercellular adhesion molecule-1 up-regulation. Proc Natl Acad Sci USA 96:1421–1426, 1999.

121. S Datta, A Brunet, M Greenberg. Cellular survival: A play in three Akts. Genes Dev 13: 2905–2927, 1999.

122. SR Datta, H Dudek, X Tao, et al. Akt phosphorylation of BAD couples survival signals to the cell-intrinsic death machinery. Cell 91:231–241, 1997.

123. L del Peso, M González-García, C Page, R Herrera, G Nunez. Interleukin-3-induced phosphorylation of BAD through the protein kinase Akt. Science 278:687–689, 1997.

124. P Blume-Jensen, R Janknecht, T Hunter. The Kit receptor promotes cell survivial via activation of PI 3-kinase and subsequent Akt-mediated phosphorylation of Bad on Ser136. Curr Biol 8:779–782, 1998.

125. A Brunet, A Bonni, MJ Zigmond, et al. Akt promotes cell survival by phosphorylating and inhibiting a forkhead transcription factor. Cell 96:857–868, 1999.

126. M Cardone, N Roy, H Stennicke, et al. Regulation of cell death protease caspase-9 by phosphorylation. Science 282:1318–1321, 1998.

127. BR Wong, D Besser, N Kim, et al. TRANCE, a TNF family member, activates Akt/PKB through a signaling complex involving TRAF6 and c-Src. Mol Cell 4:1041–1049, 1999.

128. Y Pekarsky, A Koval, C Hallas, et al. Tcl1 enhances akt kinase activity and mediates its nuclear translocation. Proc Natl Acad Sci USA 3028–3033, 2000.

129. J Laine, G Kunstle, T Obata, et al. The protooncogene TCL1 is an akt kinase coactivator. Mol Cell 6:395–407, 2000.

130. JC Reed, C Stein, C Subasinghe, et al. Antisense-mediated inhibition of BCL2 protooncogene expression and leukemic cell growth and survival: comparisons of phosphodiester and phosphorothioate oligodeoxynucleotides. Can Res 50:6565–6570, 1990.

131. A Webb, D Cunningham, F Cotter, et al. BCL-2 antisense therapy in patients with non-Hodgkin lymphoma. Lancet 349:1137–1141, 1997.

132. M Sattler, H Liang, D Nettesheim, et al. Structure of Bcl-xL-Bak peptide complex: recognition between regulators of apoptosis. Science 275:983–986, 1997.

133. J-L Wang, D Liu, Z-J Zhang, et al. Structure-based discovery of an organic compound that binds Bcl-2 protein and induces apoptosis of tumor cells. Proc Natl Acad Sci USA 97:7124–7129, 2000.

134. A Rossi, P Kapahi, G Natoli, et al. Anti-inflammatory cyclopentenone prostaglandins are direct inhibitors of IkappaB kinase. Nature 403:103–108, 2000.

7

Cytokines and Regulatory Molecules in the Pathogenesis and Clinical Course of B-Cell Chronic Lymphocytic Leukemia

ENRICA ORSINI and ROBIN FOA

University "La Sapienza," Rome, Italy

I. INTRODUCTION

B-cell chronic lymphocytic leukemia (B-CLL) is a unique accumulative disorder, characterized by a low proliferative activity and by the progressive accumulation of clonal B lymphocytes blocked in the early phases (G0/G1) of the cell cycle. For a long time it had been postulated that in the pathogenesis of the disease, still largely unknown, as well as in its clinical course, an important role must be played by the dysregulation of intercellular mechanisms that normally control the progression through the cell cycle. Over the years, several altered cytokine networks have been described as capable of influencing the life span of B-CLL cells in vivo, and the neoplastic clone itself is known to produce a number of soluble factors, some of which potentially implicated in autocrine loops. Moreover, defective apoptosis (programmed cell death) and deregulation of some cell cycle regulatory genes have been shown to contribute to the malignant process in B-CLL.

Cell growth processes are governed in eukaryotic cells by complex mechanisms involving positive kinase complexes, as well as negative regulatory elements. Cell-to-cell contacts and signaling through membrane molecules and several soluble cytokines may variably influence this cell cycle machinery. The arrest of B-CLL cells in the early phases of the cell cycle suggests the importance of investigating the intracellular regulatory processes operational within the malignant clone and the residual accessory cell populations, as well as the influence of soluble and membrane extracellular signals.

In addition to contributing in the unraveling of the pathogenesis of the disease and of the mechanisms that govern the accumulation process unique to this disease, a better understanding of the role of these molecules may also help to shed light on the not yet understood marked heterogeneity in the clinical course of B-CLL patients with apparent similar biological properties. This is clinically relevant, because an early identification of parameters that may help to define the progressive or stable nature of individual patients would have important implications for the management of the disease.

In this chapter, we will focus in particular on the possible role that different cytokines and regulatory molecules may play in B-CLL. Although we will necessarily also touch on apoptosis, the latter will be more accurately discussed in an accompanying chapter of this volume.

II. CYTOKINES AND GROWTH FACTORS

In normal B cells, proliferation and differentiation, as well as programmed cell death, are under the control of several cytokines and growth factors. It is thus conceivable that the abnormal growth and accumulation of the malignant cell population in B-CLL might be greatly influenced by deregulated cytokine pathways. Indeed, different lines of evidence suggest that cytokines may participate in autocrine or paracrine loops affecting B-CLL cell growth through the induction or inhibition of cell proliferation, protection from or induction of apoptosis, and up- and down-modulation of apoptosis-related genes. More-over, the fact that B-CLL cells often die rapidly in vitro in contrast with their long life span in vivo suggests that cytokine networks may be providing an instrumental survival advantage in vivo. Over the years, the possible involvement of several cytokines in B-CLL has been investigated and the number of candidate molecules is constantly grow-ing. Figure 1 graphically represents the possible role that different cytokines may have

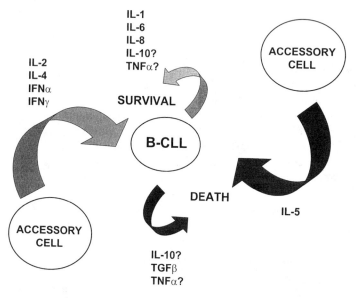

Figure 1   Autocrine and paracrine cytokines that may influence B-CLL cell survival and death.

in B-CLL. More detailed information on release, receptor expression, and potential activities of different cytokines in B-CLL is reported in Table 1. Some of the cytokines that have gained more attention and their possible role in B-CLL will be individually discussed in the following.

A. Interleukin-1

Interleukin-1 (IL-1), initially described as lymphocyte-activating factor (LAF) and endogenous pyrogen, is a nonspecific mediator of inflammation and an immunostimulant. IL-1 activities are mediated by two distinct proteins named IL-1α and IL-1β (1,2). Both molecules are produced by monocytes/macrophages but also by a number of different cell types (3). Two distinct receptors for IL-1 have been cloned, named type I and type II, both capable of binding IL-1α and IL-1β (4). The IL-1 receptors are also widely distributed on a variety of cell types, including fibroblasts and T and B cells. IL-1 induces a multitude of biological activities, such as fever, production of acute-phase reactants, coactivation of lymphocytes, chemotaxis of polymorphonuclear cells, and proliferation of fibroblasts and endothelial cells (5). In the setting of the immune response processes, macrophage-derived IL-1 induces the up-regulation of IL-2 receptors on T cells and also acts as a growth factor for B cells. In the latter, the cytokine may be spontaneously produced in the absence of any apparent stimulus (6) and has been described as one of the factors regulating the progression through the cell cycle into late G1 in B lymphocytes (7).

The ability of B-CLL cells to spontaneously produce IL-1β has been demonstrated many years ago (6,8) and associated with the expression, on malignant B cells, of antigens considered specific for myelomonocytic cells, such as CD14 and CD11b (9). The production of IL-1 by B-CLL lymphocytes has been correlated with the stage of the disease. In fact, although cells from patients with stable disease were found to secrete near normal levels of IL-1β, B cells from patients with progressive B-CLL produced lower amounts of the cytokine (10).

Apart from disease status, other cytokines may also influence IL-1 production by B-CLL cells. Tumor necrosis factor α (TNFα) has been reported capable of inducing in vitro mRNA for IL-1α and IL-1β, and also for IL-6 and TNFα itself. This effect is abrogated by the addition of interferon α (IFNα), so that the blocking of autocrine growth factor loops has been indicated as one way IFNα may mediate its therapeutic effects (11).

Because B-CLL lymphocytes not only constitutively produce IL-1 but also express the IL-1β receptor (12), this cytokine has been investigated as a possible autocrine growth factor. However, although differentiation and activation of B-CLL malignant lymphocytes, characterized by an increment in surface immunoglobulins (Ig) and in CD23 antigen expression, have been described after treatment with IL-1β (13), in many reports this cytokine failed to induce proliferation of B-CLL cells (13,14). Mainou-Fowler et al. (15) reported a proliferative effect of IL-1 in vitro in a proportion of pokeweed mitogen–treated B-CLL cases but also an inhibition of B-CLL cell responses to IL-2.

Given the accumulative nature of B-CLL and the role of defective apoptosis in the pathogenesis of the disease, cytokines may play an important role in the survival of malignant lymphocytes acting on the regulation of programmed cell death. Indeed, IL-1 is capable of protecting B-CLL cells from apoptosis, both spontaneous and induced by hydrocortisone (16), supporting its potential role as an autocrine survival factor in B-CLL.

Table 1 Cytokines in B-CLL

Cytokine	Release	Receptor	Activities
IL-1β	Yes	Yes	Induces differentiation and activation
			Inhibits spontaneous and cortisone-dependent apoptosis
			Potential autocrine survival factor
			Possible immunomodulatory activities
IL-2	?	Yes	Costimulates proliferation
			Modulates expression of IL-2R
			Reduced availability for T and NK cells
IL-4	No	Yes	Inhibits spontaneous and IL-2–dependent proliferation
			Increases CD40-mediated proliferation
			Protects from spontaneous, steroid, IL-5, and Fas signaling-induced apoptosis
			Increased production by T lymphocytes
IL-5	No	Probable	Increases spontaneous apoptosis
			May increase proliferation
IL-6	Yes	Yes	Inhibits TNFα-mediated proliferation
			Protects from spontaneous and steroid-induced apoptosis
			Possible role in B-CLL autoimmune phenomena
IL-8	Yes	Yes	Upmodulates IL-8 mRNA
			Inhibits apoptosis
			Possible autocrine survival factor
IL-10	Yes	Yes	Contrasting data: may induce or prevent apoptosis
			Possible inhibitory effect on host Th-1 and APC compartments
TNFα	Yes	Yes (contrasting data)	Contrasting data: may increase or inhibit proliferation
			May suppress apoptosis
			Up-modulates p55 IL-2 receptor
TGFβ	Yes	Yes	Inhibits DNA synthesis in a proportion of cases
			Incapable of inducing apoptosis in most B-CLL
			Possible role in bone marrow failure and in immunodeficiency
IFNα	?	Yes	Can induce proliferation
			Inhibits apoptosis
IFNγ	On activation	Probable	Costimulates proliferation
			Inhibits apoptosis
G-CSF	On activation	Yes	Decreases spontaneous apoptosis

In summary, in B-CLL IL-1 might potentially act as an autocrine cytokine capable of promoting the survival of the leukemic clone. However, given the immunomodulatory activities of this cytokine, a role in the stimulation of a tumor-specific T-cell response and in the immunological control of the disease, as suggested by the reported reduced levels of IL-1 in patients with progressive disease, cannot be ruled out.

B. Interleukin-2

Interleukin-2 is a natural glycoprotein secreted mainly by CD4+ T cells. Resting lymphocytes do not secrete IL-2, but activation by means of the antigen receptor leads to the induction of both IL-2 and high-affinity IL-2 receptor. Interleukin-2 is critical for the development of immune response, inducing the proliferation and activation of T lymphocytes, as well as the generation of lymphokine-activated killer (LAK) cells capable of lysing different human neoplastic cells. In addition, it may promote the production of other cytokines, such as granulocyte-macrophage colony-stimulating factor (GM-CSF), IFNγ, and TNFα (17).

Chronologically, IL-2 has been the first cytokine thoroughly investigated in B-CLL and the first cytokine for which a potential involvement in the disease has been suggested. This is based on a number of evidences. B-CLL cells frequently show a weak expression of the α chain of the IL-2 receptor (p55) coupled, in some cases, by the intermediate affinity β chain (p75) receptor; the common γ chain (p64) is always expressed (for a review see Ref. 18). IL-2 may have an active role on the leukemic cell population, because it can up-regulate the expression of the p55 antigen of the IL-2 receptor and induce a costimulatory effect on B-CLL cells, particularly after a primary signal (19). In fact, IL-2 increases thymidine incorporation in anti-IgM and in anti-CD40 activated B-CLL cells (20).

In addition to acting directly or indirectly on the leukemic clone, IL-2 might have an important role also in the pathogenesis of the multiple dysfunctions of the accessory T and NK cell compartments described over the years in B-CLL patients. In fact, B-CLL cells may absorb exogenous IL-2 (21). This proves that, in B-CLL, the IL-2 receptor complex is functional. In addition, B-CLL patients show increased serum levels of the soluble IL-2 receptor, with a trend toward higher values in patients with more invasive disease (22). These latter two observations have potential practical implications. Both circumstances—the absorption (''sponge'' effect) by the overwhelming leukemic B cells and the binding of IL-2 by the soluble IL-2 receptor (23)—are likely to contribute to a decreased availability of the IL-2 produced in normal or reduced amounts by the residual T-cell compartment (21,24). The decreased availability of IL-2 to exert in vivo its physiological activities may thus play a contributory role in some of the defects encountered within the nonleukemic accessory cell compartment in B-CLL (25). This is further confirmed by the evidence that exogenous IL-2 may enhance the T-cell colony–forming capacity (25) and cytotoxic function in B-CLL (26).

The studies on IL-2 represent the first demonstration that an impaired cellular cross-talk between leukemic and accessory lymphoid populations is operational in B-CLL and may have an impact on the clinical course of the disease.

C. Interleukin-4

Interleukin-4 is a T-cell–derived lymphokine that costimulates normal B-cell proliferation in the presence of anti-IgM or anti-CD40 antibody (27). Most data suggest that IL-4 promotes the proliferation and differentiation of normal B cells after activation by other mechanisms, with the exception of IL-2–mediated activation, after which IL-4 inhibits proliferation (28,29).

Although neoplastic B-CLL cells do not produce IL-4, this cytokine might have a role in the disease, because CD19+ B-CLL cells have been shown to express the IL-4 receptor on their surface (30,31), and functional effects of IL-4 on malignant B-CLL cell development have been described. The different environmental systems used in vitro may influence the role of IL-4 on B-CLL proliferation, making the real in vivo effect difficult to anticipate. In fact, contradicting data have been reported by different authors. IL-4 has been shown capable of inhibiting both spontaneous and IL-2– or TNFα-induced ^{3}H-thymidine uptake by B-CLL cells (28,32,33). In contrast, a proliferative effect on leukemic B-CLL cells has been documented when B-CLL lymphocytes are activated by the CD40 pathway, but not on B-CLL cells activated by surface Ig (20). The influence of different signaling pathways used for activation, sometimes supporting and sometimes inhibiting the IL-4–induced growth of B-CLL cells, suggests an altered signal transduction rather than an impaired functionality of IL-4 receptors on these cells (20). In fact, defects in the signal transduction pathway secondary to surface IgM cross-linking have been described in B-CLL cells (34,35).

The possibility that IL-4 may play a role on the apoptotic program of B-CLL cells has been recently suggested. In several studies, IL-4 was shown capable of protecting B-CLL cells from apoptotic death, both spontaneous and induced by steroids, IL-5, and Fas signaling. An implication of Bcl-2 has also been reported, because the inhibition of apoptosis in B-CLL cells mediated by IL-4 was found to correlate with increased levels of Bcl-2. This association has, however, not been confirmed by all authors (16,36–38).

The antiapoptotic effect of IL-4 on B-CLL cells might play a particularly important role in the clinical course of the disease in view of the shift to Th2 cytokine production recently reported. It has, in fact, been shown that B-CLL T lymphocytes may express IL-4 (39) and, as discussed later, our group has recently reported the expansion in B-CLL of a T-cell subset capable of expressing and releasing CD30 and IL-4 (40). Thus, in B-CLL nonneoplastic T cells may indirectly contribute, through the production of increased levels of IL-4, to the expansion and accumulation of the neoplastic clone (Fig. 2). The relevance in vivo of the IL-4 protective effect against cytotoxicity and apoptotic death has still to be demonstrated. However, an enhanced susceptibility of B-CLL cells to the antiapoptotic effect of IL-4 in previously treated patients has been reported; this could be a consequence of drug selection and one of the mechanisms of acquired drug resistance (42).

D. Interleukin-6

Interleukin-6 is a multifunctional cytokine, produced by a variety of cell populations. Its biological activities include the stimulation of B- and T-cell growth and differentiation, multilineage hematopoiesis, production of acute-phase proteins by hepatocytes, osteoclast formation, and platelet production (43). IL-6 is primarily a B-cell growth and differentiation factor, known to be essential for normal B-cell development and for normal megakaryocyte maturation. Thus, an abnormal expression of IL-6 may be involved in the pathogenesis of a variety of diseases, among which are B-cell malignancies, such as multiple myeloma.

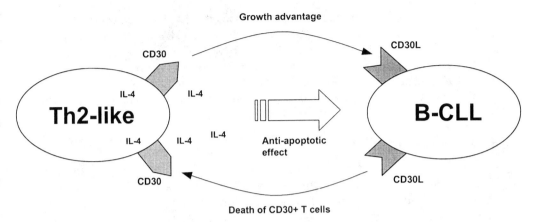

Figure 2 Th2 cells in B-CLL. The CD30-expressing Th2-like population, overrepresented in B-CLL, may mediate a proliferative signal for B-CLL tumor cells through the CD30L and an anti-apoptotic effect through the release of IL-4. In contrast, death of CD30+ T cells can be induced by B-CLL cells through the ligation of the CD30 molecule (modified from Ref. 41).

Interleukin-6 binds first to a low-affinity α subunit, an 80-kDa glycoprotein called IL-6 receptor or gp80. This IL-6/IL-6 receptor complex recruits the signal transducing β subunit, a 130-kDa glycoprotein called gp130, and this association leads to the formation of the high-affinity IL-6 receptor complex and to signal transduction. Gp130 does not bind IL-6 or IL-6 receptor on their own (44,45). Moreover, the IL-6 receptor is often secreted in a soluble form that binds IL-6 and is biologically active as an agonist, making cells expressing gp130, but not the IL-6 receptor, responsive to IL-6 (46,47).

B-CLL lymphocytes express the gp80 chain of the IL-6 receptor in most cases, and serum levels of IL-6 receptor have been reported to be significantly greater in B-CLL patients than in age-matched controls (48). A link with the tumor cell mass has been suggested, because the highest values of soluble IL-6 receptor have been recorded in Binet's stage B patients.

It has been reported that B-CLL lymphocytes may produce a biologically active IL-6 protein (49), but the role of this cytokine in B-CLL might be different from what was observed in other B-cell neoplasms, in which IL-6 has a growth simulation effect. In fact, IL-6 not only does not induce B-CLL cell proliferation but is also capable of decreasing TNFα-induced B-CLL cell growth (50,51). Because TNFα can induce IL-6 expression in B-CLL lymphocytes, IL-6 has been suggested to act in B-CLL as a negative feedback regulator of an autocrine TNFα action. On the other hand, more recent reports include IL-6 between the cytokines capable of protecting B-CLL cells from both spontaneous and steroid-induced apoptosis (15,16,52). The mechanism proposed as responsible for this effect is a delay in the down-regulation of Bcl-2 in vitro (53).

The true in vivo production of IL-6 by B-CLL cells and its biological relevance also remain controversial. Serum levels of IL-6 in B-CLL patients have been reported to be either normal (54) or increased in patients with indolent disease, whereas progressive B-CLL patients seem to lose their ability to produce IL-6 (55). The latter observation has been confirmed also in vitro in a more recent article, in which B-CLL cells from patients with advanced stages of disease were found unable to produce high levels of IL-6 after stimulation with the phorbol ester PMA (56). On the other hand, higher levels of IL-6 in the serum of advanced/progressive B-CLL patients compared with indolent cases have also been detected by other groups (52,57).

Finally, the spontaneous secretion of IL-6 by B-CLL cells in vivo might play a role in the autoimmune phenomena often observed in patients with B-CLL. In fact, higher levels of in vitro IL-6 production have been reported in cells from B-CLL patients with autoimmune hemolytic anemia than from control B-CLL samples (58).

E. Interleukin-8

Interleukin-8/NAP-1 is a member of the proinflammatory supergene family, with an important role in acute inflammation through binding to and activation of the IL-8 receptors on neutrophils and mononuclear cells. In fact, IL-8 displays potent and specific neutrophil activation and chemoattractant properties (59). The chemotactic activity of IL-8 appears to also affect T lymphocytes and basophils (60). Interleukin-8 is produced in response to several inflammatory stimuli, including microbial products and cytokines, such as TNFα and IL-1 (61). The natural cellular sources of IL-8 production have been described to be, among others, monocytes/macrophages, T cells, large granular lymphocytes, but there is no evidence of IL-8 production by normal B cells (62,63).

Unlike their normal counterpart, B-CLL cells express and release constitutively IL-8 (31). Circulating levels of IL-8 are also significantly greater in serum samples from B-CLL patients than from normal donors (31,64). The circulating levels of IL-8 have been found to correlate with the mRNA expression of Bcl-2 by B-CLL cells, suggesting that the effects of IL-8 might be exerted through a Bcl-2–dependent pathway. Moreover, a potential prognostic role has been proposed for this cytokine, because stage A patients with levels of IL-8 greater than the median value are more likely to progress to a more advanced clinical stage than those with levels less than the median value (64).

Although B-CLL cells express the IL-8 receptor, exogenous IL-8 has failed to show any in vitro proliferative activity on leukemic B-CLL cells. However, the addition of IL-8 at doses comparable with the levels of IL-8 released constitutively by B-CLL cells can prolong their survival (65). Again, the antiapoptotic effect of IL-8 is associated with an increased expression of Bcl-2 mRNA. Conversely, endogenous IL-8 neutralization by incubation in the presence of anti-IL-8 antibodies is capable of inducing the in vitro death of B-CLL cells (65). Coupled to the ability of IL-8 to up-modulate IL-8 mRNA in B-CLL cells, these findings support a potential autocrine role of IL-8 in the process of cell accumulation characteristic of this disease.

It is worth recalling that IL-8 is so far the only cytokine for which a biological action on B-CLL cells has been demonstrated at the same dose range released constitutively by the leukemic cells.

F. Interleukin-10

Interleukin-10 was initially identified as cytokine synthesis inhibitory factor (CSIF) for its ability to inhibit the synthesis of IFNγ, TNFα, IL-1, IL-3, and several other cytokines by activated mononuclear cells (66,67). The molecular mechanisms involved in this inhibitory function are different and include transcriptional and posttranscriptional means (68). Interleukin-10 is produced by monocytes/macrophages, B cells, Th1 and Th2 T-cell clones, and some CD8+ cells (69); its effect is probably indirect, through the synthesis of monokines such as IL-1, IL-6, and TNFα (70). In addition, IL-10 may modulate accessory cell functions through the inhibitory effect on dendritic cell maturation and activation (71).

It has been reported that B-CLL lymphocytes express IL-10 mRNA (72), as well as its receptor (73). IL-10 mRNA expression in B-CLL has been found to correlate inversely with progression of disease, because it has been associated with stable disease (72). However, literature data on the in vivo production of IL-10 during the natural history of the disease have been equivocal. Egle et al. (74) reported that the levels of IL-10 were significantly greater in patients with Rai stages III and IV compared with stages 0 to II, and the same results have been recently confirmed by another group (75). In contrast, in a previous report, the median serum IL-10 values were found not to differ between healthy controls and B-CLL patients, although some of the latter may exhibit elevated levels without any clinical relevance (76).

Interleukin-10 may prevent programmed cell death of both normal human germinal center B cells and Epstein-Barr virus blasts (77,78), but contrasting data are reported in the literature on the effects of IL-10 on the survival of neoplastic B-CLL cells. Indeed, this cytokine has been reported to both inhibit and induce apoptosis of B-CLL lymphocytes. In the study by Fluckiger et al. (79) IL-10 was found capable of inhibiting the spontaneous thymidine incorporation in a proportion of B-CLL samples and, in addition, of inducing B-CLL cells to die from apoptosis with a concomitant decrease in Bcl-2 protein levels. Addition of IL-2, IL-4, IFNγ, and anti-CD40 monoclonal antibody prevented this IL-10–mediated apoptosis of B-CLL cells. In contrast, other authors have suggested that IL-10 might act as an autocrine growth factor for B-CLL cells, because in their study B-CLL lymphocytes spontaneously released IL-10 in culture and this cytokine enhanced the survival of B-CLL cells in a dose-dependent fashion by inhibiting the process of apoptotic cell death (80). More recently, in an extensive study on the IL-10 receptor expression by B-CLL cells, Jurlander and colleagues (73) also found that IL-10 could prolong survival of B-CLL cells, with a pattern of STAT protein phosphorylation identical to the pattern of IL-10 receptor activation observed in normal B cells. The authors also reported that the activation pathway leading to IL-10–mediated B-CLL cell survival was similar to that induced through the receptors for IFNα and IFNγ, cytokines known to inhibit apoptosis in B-CLL cells (81,82). The potential heterogeneity of IL-10–induced effects on B-CLL cells is further underlined by a recent article in which IL-10 was found capable of increasing the in vitro apoptotic B-CLL cell numbers in stage 0 patients, but not in stage I and II patients (83). Data from our group indicate that leukemic B-CLL cells express variable levels of intracytoplasmic IL-10 and that exogenous IL-10 can induce an antiapoptotic signal on leukemic B-CLL cells (unpublished).

IL-10 may also play an important role in the clinical course of B-CLL not only by influencing the growth and survival of the neoplastic clone but also through its effects on the residual T-cell compartment. Interleukin-10 is known to inhibit the secretion of type 1 cytokines, thus its production by the neoplastic clone could represent a factor that affects the shift toward a Th-2–type response and the overexpression of type 2 cytokines reported in B-CLL patients (40). Moreover, IL-10 might contribute to T-cell hyporesponsiveness in B-CLL patients through its direct inhibitory effect on the antigen-presenting cell compartment and through the down-modulation of major histocompatibility complex (MHC) class II and B7 expression on peripheral blood dendritic cells (84,85). Although no data are available on the functional status of professional antigen-presenting cells in B-CLL patients, dendritic cell defects have been reported in other malignancies and shown to represent a constitutive part of the general tumor-associated immunodepression. On the basis of these data, further investigation on the role of IL-10 in B-CLL is required.

G. Tumor Necrosis Factor α

Tumor necrosis factor-α is a cytokine produced by macrophages but also by B and T lymphocytes and NK cells. It shares a large number of heterogenous activities with IL-1, including the induction of inflammatory responses, immune modulation, and regulation of tumor cell growth (86). It is also a growth factor for different normal cell populations (e.g., T lymphocytes, B lymphocytes, and fibroblasts). Two transmembrane receptors for TNFα with a different molecular weight, p55 and p75, have been identified. The p75 high-affinity receptor appears to mediate the proliferative effect of TNFα at low concentrations. At high concentrations, TNFα may also bind the low affinity receptor p55, which appears, however, to use a separate signaling pathway from the p75 receptor (87,88).

TNFα belongs to the number of cytokines produced and released by B-CLL cells, and its potential role in the regulation of proliferation of the neoplastic clone has been suggested. Leukemic lymphocytes from patients with B-CLL have been shown to express the TNFα mRNA and to release TNFα spontaneously in vitro (89,90). Moreover, elevated serum levels of TNFα are detectable in patients with B-CLL compared with normal controls, with a progressive increase in relation to the stage of the disease (91,92). In B-CLL patients receiving IFNα therapy, serum levels of TNFα have been found to correlate significantly with changes in lymphocyte count (93). However, it has been suggested that other sources apart from B-CLL lymphocytes, such as cells belonging to the monocyte/ macrophage lineage, may contribute to the increased amounts of serum TNFα (91).

Normal B cells produce TNFα and express TNFα receptors on stimulation; in these cells, TNFα costimulates DNA synthesis. Although some authors could not demonstrate a constitutive expression of the TNFα receptor on B-CLL cells (94), different reports described that freshly isolated neoplastic cells from B-CLL patients were positive for both the p55 and p75 receptor types (95,96). The situation may be more complicated in vivo, because B-CLL patients have elevated serum levels of soluble TNFα receptor, and the latter appears more pronounced in advanced disease. In this situation, because of the competitive effects of the receptor soluble form, the net effect of TNFα on the surface of the neoplastic cells as a growth factor could be less relevant (96).

Supporting the potential role of TNFα as an autocrine growth factor in B-CLL, Cordingley et al. first showed that ^{3}H-thymidine incorporation by B-CLL cells was enhanced by TNFα, although the maximal response was observed after a delay of 7 days after addition of the cytokine (89). These results have been confirmed by other studies, which, however, showed variations in the proportion of B-CLL cells responsive to TNFα (97,98). Other authors reported an inhibitory function or no effect (90,95,99). Data in the literature are also conflicting on the possibility that TNFα may or may not influence the apoptotic program of B-CLL lymphocytes. Although in some reports TNFα was incapable of protecting neoplastic B-CLL lymphocytes from programmed cell death in vitro (16), Tangye et al. (53) included TNFα in the number of cytokines that may suppress B-CLL cell apoptosis through a delay in down-regulation of Bcl-2.

In addition to its direct effects on the proliferation and survival of B-CLL cells, TNFα may well play an important role in the pathophysiology of the disease through its influence on the expression and release of other cytokines. In fact, mRNAs for IL-1α, IL-1β, and IL-6 are induced in B-CLL cells treated with TNFα in vitro (11). Although IL-6 seems to inhibit TNFα-induced proliferation (see preceding), IL-1 has been reported to protect B-CLL cells from apoptotic death. Furthermore, Trentin et al. (95) also reported the ability of TNFα to up-regulate the p55 IL-2 receptor, suggesting a possible role in the regulation of the response of B-CLL cells to IL-2.

H. Transforming Growth Factor β

Transforming growth factor β (TGFβ) has been described as a potent inhibitor of various cell types, including among others primitive hematopoietic progenitors. It displays a wide range of immunoregulatory properties, as shown by its capacity of inhibiting NK and LAK cell activation, of down-regulating the proliferation and activation of mature T cells, of depressing B-cell proliferation and IgG and IgM synthesis. TGFβ has thus been suggested to be a negative autocrine regulator of normal lymphocyte growth and differentiation (100,101). Most human cells have specific cell surface TGFβ receptors. Three types of high-affinity receptors for TGFβ have been identified and termed type I, type II, and type III. Type I and II receptors are considered to be the signal-transducing TGFβ receptors, whereas type III receptor appears to promote ligand binding to type I and type II (102).

TGFβ is produced by B-CLL cells and is present in the serum of patients (103–105). B-CLL lymphocytes are sensible to TGFβ-induced inhibition of DNA synthesis, although in a variable way and in general to a lesser extent than normal B cells (106). Some investigators have proposed that TGFβ may serve as an endogenous growth inhibitor for B-CLL cells and may contribute to the slow progression of the leukemia in vivo (105). However, the inhibitory effect of TGFβ on B-CLL cells seems to depend on the nature of the stimulation used (e.g., no antiproliferative effect is reported if B-CLL cells are stimulated through the CD40 pathway) (105,107), and, in particular, it appears to vary within the patient population. In fact, about one third of B-CLL cases in the different studies are reported to be insensitive to the inhibitory effect of TGFβ or even to be stimulated toward DNA synthesis (105,106). One of the mechanisms whereby B-CLL cells escape from normal TGFβ regulation seems to be an alteration of TGFβ receptor expression (108). Indeed, DeCoteau et al. (109) showed that loss of sensitivity to TGFβ growth inhibition is associated in B-CLL lymphocytes with the absence of detectable surface type I specific receptor, whereas both sensitive and insensitive B-CLL cells express normal levels of type II receptors. The defects in TGFβ receptor expression might be associated with the clinical and biological progression of B-CLL, although no correlation between loss of TGFβ receptor surface protein expression and stage of the disease has been reported (108,109).

In addition to its inhibitory effect on B-cell proliferation, TGFβ promotes apoptosis in various cell types, including normal and leukemic B cells (110). B-CLL cells, in accordance with the pathogenesis of the disease, in which a defective apoptotic program seems to be more important than an aberrant proliferation, have consistently shown resistance to the proapoptotic effects of TGFβ (111,112). Moreover, because the proliferation of the same cells appears to be variably inhibited by TGFβ, defects in the receptor complex are unlikely responsible for this resistance. Some downstream events in the TGFβ-induced programmed cell death, such as cell cycle dysregulation or defects in signal transduction, may be altered in B-CLL lymphocytes.

In addition to its potential role in the expansion of the leukemic clone, TGFβ might be important in the genesis of some of the related defects observed in these patients. In fact, in B-CLL patients the levels of TGFβ production by bone marrow stromal cells have been found to be significantly increased compared with normal controls (113). This overproduction has been suggested to play a major role in the pathophysiology of the bone marrow failure observed in advanced-stage B-CLL and in some of the T- and B-cell defects that lead to the immunodeficiency found in most B-CLL patients. Furthermore, production of TGFβ by tumor cells has been reported to induce a shift toward Th2 cytokine production and progression of immunosuppressive states in tumor-bearing mice, both directly and through IL-10 production (114). An analogous situation is possible in B-CLL, in which a preferential expression of Th2 cytokines has been described.

III. MEMBRANE SIGNALS

A. CD30

The CD30 surface molecules in B-CLL may have important implications both for the growth and expansion of the malignant population and for the immune functions of the host. Indeed, recent observations propose a complex model of reciprocal interaction between leukemic B-CLL cells and residual T lymphocytes mediated by CD30 molecules.

The CD30 antigen is a transmembrane receptor, member of the TNF/nerve growth factor (NGF) receptor superfamily, originally described as a feature of Reed-Sternberg cells in Hodgkin's disease. Subsequently, its different expression in various T-cell subsets has been reported. In T cells, the CD30 antigen expression has been strictly associated with the ability to respond to and to produce IL-4 (115). In fact, it is highly expressed on type 2 T cells (Th2), which secrete IL-4, IL-5, and IL-10 (116,117), whereas Th1 T cells, which secrete primarily IL-2 and IFNγ, are negative for CD30 expression.

In contrast to the restricted expression of the CD30 antigen, its specific ligand, the CD30 ligand (CD30L), is a membrane glycoprotein with a wide pattern of cellular expression, including activated T cells, stimulated monocytes/macrophages, and most neoplastic and normal B cells. The interaction of the CD30L with its specific receptor is capable of inducing either cell death or proliferation, depending on the cell type and on different intracellular signaling pathways.

B-CLL lymphocytes, as many neoplasms of lymphoid and myeloid origin, have been found positive for CD30L mRNA and surface protein, although at a lower level compared with other B lymphoproliferative disorders (118,119). More controversial is the expression of the CD30 antigen on B-CLL cells and the possibility that CD30/CD30L autocrine or paracrine loops may have a role in initiating and maintaining the neoplastic process in B-CLL, as evidenced in Hodgkin's disease. Gattei and colleagues (118), in a molecular and phenotypic study of 181 patients with myeloid and lymphoid hematopoietic malignancies, failed to detect a constitutive expression of CD30 on B-CLL cells. On the other hand, Trentin et al. (119) found that B-CLL cells expressed not only the CD30L but also low levels of CD30 on their surface. Presence of the CD30 mRNA was also documented by reverse transcriptase-polymerase chain reaction (RT-PCR) analysis.

A dysregulated expression of CD30 molecules has also been described in the non-neoplastic compartment of B-CLL patients. In fact, de Totero et al. (40) reported that activated B-CLL T cells show a significant increase in the expression of CD30 compared with normal controls and that high levels of soluble CD30 can be found in B-CLL serum samples. This increased expression and release of CD30 was found to be largely due to the expansion, in the peripheral blood of B-CLL patients, of a CD3+/CD8+/CD28−

large granular lymphocyte subset capable of producing and releasing IL-4. Interestingly, a similar population of cytotoxic CD8+ T cells capable of producing IL-4 and of expressing CD30, named Tc2 cells, has recently been characterized (120). This subset, usually present in low percentages in normal individuals but detectable in significant numbers in certain disease states, can expand in vitro in excess of IL-4 and can promote a type 2 CD4 response. The excess of CD30+ CD8 T cells reported in B-CLL patients could, therefore, represent one of the aspects of the dysregulated B-CLL T-cell compartment, polarized through a Th-2–like immune response, and may reflect the expansion in B-CLL patients of chronically activated T lymphocytes. Regardless of its immunological origin, this peculiar T-lymphocyte subset might deliver a growth signal to the neoplastic clone through its interaction with the specific counter-receptor present on the CD30+ T cells and further contribute to the expansion of B-CLL tumor cells. Conversely, recent reports have suggested that CD30 may be involved in the induction of T-cell death after the resolution of an immune response (121). The CD30/CD30L interaction could then also contribute to the impairment of cell-mediated immune functions and even represent a potential mechanism of tumor escape through the induction of death of CD30+ T cells with potential antitumor activity (Fig. 2).

B. CD40

The CD40 molecule is a member of the TNFα receptor superfamily that is expressed by almost all B lymphocytes and is critical for B-cell differentiation and activity (122). Triggering of the CD40 pathway in germinal center B cells results, in fact, in inhibition of apoptosis (123), proliferation, differentiation with Ig isotype switching (124), and expression of activation antigens, including CD23 (125) and Fas (126).

The CD40 ligand (CD40L/CD154) is a 39-kDa membrane glycoprotein mainly expressed on activated T cells and is one of the costimulatory help signals offered by specific, antigen-reactive T cells to B cells presenting that antigen in the context of the histocompatibility leukocyte antigen (HLA) system (127). Normal T lymphocytes express CD40L only for a few hours after activation, but in certain diseases CD40L expression can be increased (128) and T-cell malignancies expressing CD40L have been described (129). Less established is the expression of the CD40L by human B cells, although several reports indicate that the CD40L is expressed in certain human B-cell tumors (130). In addition, the CD40L may also be released in a soluble form of approximately 18 to 20-kDa, which forms homotrimers capable of inducing B-cell activation and differentiation (131).

In B-CLL, several abnormalities of the CD40/CD40L interaction have been reported, potentially capable of contributing to many of the immune defects frequently found in these patients and to B-cell tumor growth (Fig. 3). As in most B-cell tumors, B-CLL cells express CD40 (132), and stimulation of CD40 on B-CLL cells in vitro induces a strong up-regulation of adhesion and costimulatory molecules, enhanced proliferation, and increased cytokine production (20,133,134). More contradictory are the literature data on the influence of CD40 triggering on B-CLL lymphocyte apoptosis. A decrease in spontaneous and drug-induced apoptosis with a concomitant elevation in the antiapoptotic protein Bcl-XL have been described in B-CLL cells treated in vitro with the CD40L (135). However, different authors reported that activation of CD40 on B-CLL cells using soluble anti-CD40 antibodies did not influence survival or apoptosis (136).

Native B-CLL cells are unable to function efficiently as antigen-presenting cells, and they fail to induce a relevant T-cell immune response. Therefore, the CD40 pathway

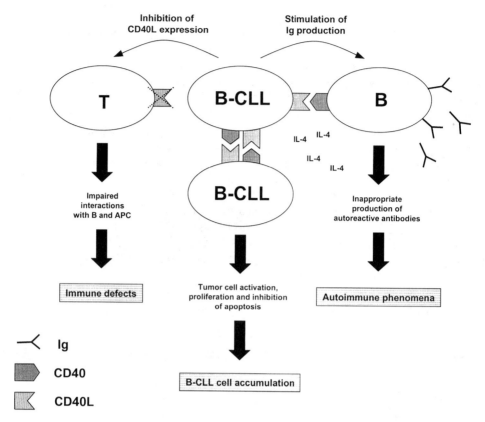

Figure 3 Potential CD40 mediated interactions in B-CLL. Expression of both CD40 and CD40L on B-CLL cells may represent an autocrine or paracrine tumor growth factor. In addition, B-CLL cells can inhibit the expression of CD40L by nonmalignant T cells, impairing their interactions with B and antigen-presenting cells (APC) and contributing to the immune defects present in B-CLL patients. In the presence of T-cell–derived factors, such as IL-4, CD40L expression on tumor cells can also mediate a stimulus to the inappropriate production of autoreactive Ig by B cells (modified from Ref. 41).

in B-CLL cells is actively investigated as a way to improve antigen presentation in the context of immunotherapeutic approaches. Allogeneic CD40 stimulated B-CLL cells have been reported to be able to activate CD8+ cytolytic T cells with activity against both native and CD40 treated B-CLL cells. The same CD40 B-CLL cells were only able, in an autologous setting, to activate CD4+ T cells that had no major cytolytic activity (134). Whether the lack of autologous CD8+ growth is due to underlying defects in the T-cell compartment of the B-CLL bearing host remains to be explained, but the future design of immunotherapy protocols for B-CLL will need to take into account the increasing amount of knowledge on the highly abnormal immune compartment in B-CLL patients.

Using a different approach, Kato et al. (137) reported the transduction of B-CLL leukemic cells with an adenovirus encoding the murine CD154 antigen. These CD154-infected B-CLL cells showed an increased expression of immune accessory molecules, such as CD80 and CD86, and allowed the generation of cytotoxic T lymphocytes specifically directed against autologous unmodified leukemia cells. Moreover, the transactivation of noninfected bystander leukemia B cells could also be demonstrated. Recently, the first results of a phase I trial of immune gene therapy were reported by the same group. Nine intermediate- or high-risk B-CLL patients were treated with escalating doses of CD154 infected autologous leukemia cells, resulting in activation of circulating bystander leukemia cells, as well as reductions in absolute lymphocyte counts and lymph node sizes (138).

Defects in the CD40 pathway have been described in the accessory compartment in B-CLL patients, in whom both B-CLL blood and splenic T cells have been found incapable of expressing the CD40L after CD3-mediated activation (139). Although normal T cells show an increase of CD40L mRNA and related surface expression of the protein within 4 hours from activation, in T cells from B-CLL patients the same induction of CD40L mRNA is not accompanied by protein expression. Furthermore, the observation that leukemic B-CLL lymphocytes can also induce a down-modulation of the CD40L on allogeneic T cells suggests that in patients with B-CLL the great excess of CD40-bearing leukemia B cells could interfere with the interactions of nonneoplastic T cells with antigen-specific B lymphocytes or other antigen-presenting cells. Again, this mechanism could provide an explanation for some of the immune abnormalities associated with B-CLL and also represent a potential mechanism of immune escape by CD40-expressing tumors. Indeed, mutations in the CD40L gene are known to be responsible for the X-linked hyper-IgM syndrome (140). The dysregulated CD40/CD40L interaction in these patients results in a syndrome of immunodeficiency and autoimmune phenomena that resembles the clinical manifestations of B-CLL.

In addition to CD40, B-CLL lymphocytes may also express the CD40L molecule. In the study of Schattner et al. (141), a subset of freshly isolated B-CLL cells constitutively expressed the CD40L, as detected by immunofluorescence flow cytometry, by RT-PCR and by immunoprecipitation. In the presence of costimulation by means of accessory molecules and of T-lymphocyte–derived cytokines, such as IL-4, the expression of both CD40 and the CD40L on tumor cells may contribute to B-CLL tumor growth in vivo through an autocrine or paracrine mechanism (142). Moreover, the CD40L expressed by B-CLL cells is functional and capable of stimulating IgG production by target, nonmalignant B cells in coculture to a degree similar to that triggered by purified T cells. This ability of the B-CLL malignant clone to mediate a costimulatory function and isotype switching, normally induced by T cells, could be implicated in the inappropriate production of autoreactive antibodies in these patients.

It has also been demonstrated that the serum of patients with B-CLL presents increased levels of soluble and functionally active CD40L compared with normal donors (143). These findings might have relevance in vivo in the autoimmune manifestations associated with B-CLL, because high level of soluble CD40L have been reported in the plasma of systemic lupus erythematosus patients, where they correlated with clinical disease activity (144). Furthermore, the high levels of serum CD40L in B-CLL patients might influence the response to chemotherapy. In fact, in the presence of the soluble anti-CD40 antibody incubation of B-CLL cells with fludarabine results in a decreased proportion of apoptotic cells (145), and the CD40/CD40L system is thought to be effective in inhibiting the apoptotic response to fludarabine (146).

C. Fas

The Fas receptor (APO-1/CD95) is a transmembrane glycoprotein of 48 kDa that belongs to the TNF/NGF receptor superfamily and is one of the principal regulators of apoptosis in normal cells, because its ligation with anti-Fas monoclonal antibodies or the Fas ligand (FasL) results in a rapid apoptotic cell death (147,148). For this reason, the role of Fas has been actively investigated in B-CLL, where a dysfunction in the B-cell apoptotic program is likely to have an important role in the pathogenesis of the disease. The Fas protein is expressed in a variety of normal and neoplastic hematopoietic cells, including activated T and B cells and is thought to be involved in the regulation of cellular homeostasis and maintenance of self-tolerance of lymphocytes (149,150). In resting naïve T cells, both the Fas antigen and the FasL are expressed at low levels but are up-regulated on activation by antigens through T-cell receptor (TCR) signaling (151). FasL expression has been also demonstrated on activated normal murine B cells (152) and on human neoplastic cells (153).

Although resting leukemic cells from B-CLL patients are either negative or weakly positive for Fas expression (154–156), they usually express both the full-length (coding the membrane isoform) and the truncated form (corresponding to the soluble isoform) of the Fas mRNA (155,156). However, different stimuli, such as IFNα, IFNγ, or *Staphylococcus aureus* Cowan I (SAC), in combination with IL-2 are known to up-regulate Fas expression in vitro on B-CLL cells. Moreover, increased levels of soluble Fas have been found in the serum of B-CLL patients (157).

Not only the actual in vivo expression of the Fas molecule on B-CLL cells remains to be explained, but their susceptibility to Fas-mediated apoptotic programs is also controversial. Although some authors reported a responsiveness to anti-Fas–induced apoptosis in B-CLL cells stimulated by SAC and IL-2 (158), both IFN (α and γ) and CD40-activated Fas-positive B-CLL cells are resistant to apoptosis induction with anti-Fas antibodies (154,159). It is possible that the FasL and the anti-Fas antibody may stimulate different signaling pathways, as suggested by some authors (160), or that the different activation systems used may influence the ability of B-CLL cells to undergo Fas-induced apoptosis. As is the case with many factors capable of affecting B-CLL cell survival and programmed cell death, the Fas-induced apoptosis in B-CLL lymphocytes has also been associated with Bcl-2 mRNA down-regulation (158). However, Mainou-Fowler et al. (38) suggested a Bcl-2–independent pathway in their study on increased spontaneous apoptosis in fresh B-CLL lymphocytes treated with an anti-Fas antibody.

These findings obtained using in vitro models might be somewhat different from what happens in vivo, where the Fas sensitivity of neoplastic B-CLL cells may also be affected by the peculiar immunological milieu. In fact, it has been shown that elevated serum levels of soluble CD40L, as those detected in B-CLL patients, protect B-CLL leukemic cells from FasL-mediated apoptosis (143). Moreover, the expression of Fas by B-CLL cells and the sensitivity to lysis by the FasL may also be differently affected by type I and type II cytokines (161). B-CLL cells cultured in media containing type I cytokines, such as IL-12 or IFNα, show an increased Fas expression and are lysed by autologous FasL-bearing T cells, whereas both effects can be abrogated by the type II cytokine IL-4. The reported shift toward a type II cytokine phenotype in T cells from B-CLL patients may confer a particular in vivo relevance to these findings (39,40).

CD19+ B-CLL cells have been found to constitutively express a functionally active FasL, because they are capable of killing target T-cell acute lymphocytic leukemia cells in vitro (162). Functional FasL expression has been demonstrated on several human neoplasms and FasL-expressing tumor cells are capable of killing target cells in vitro. This mechanism of active killing has been implicated in immune escape of tumor cells and by this mechanism T-lymphocyte subsets involved in antitumor responses may be inactivated.

In B-CLL, the Fas/FasL system might also be implicated in the pathogenesis of the cellular immune defects present in this disease, as well as in the defects of the helper compartment and the decreased CD4+/CD8+ ratio. Indeed, both CD4+ and CD8+ T cells from B-CLL patients show an increased Fas expression compared with normal donors. However, the Fas sensitivity of the two T-cell subsets to Fas-mediated killing is different and only B-CLL CD4+ cells undergo apoptosis after treatment with an agonistic Fas antibody (162). The potential clinical relevance of these observations is confirmed by the finding that the Fas sensitivity of CD4+ cells in B-CLL patients correlated with a CD4+/CD8+ ratio below the lower threshold of healthy individuals.

IV. REGULATORY MOLECULES

Most of the cytokines and membrane molecules discussed in this chapter eventually influence B-CLL tumor cells through their effects on the mechanisms regulating cell proliferation and apoptosis. In B-CLL, tumor progression is likely to be more the consequence of a progressive accumulation of small resting G0/G1 lymphoid cells than the proliferation of actively dividing cells. In fact, even in advanced disease, cell cycle analysis by [^{3}H]thymidine uptake or flow cytometry and immunocytochemistry with the Ki-67 antibody consistently showed that most malignant cells are in the G0/G1 phase, and very few or none are in the S phase (163,164). The abnormally prolonged survival of B-CLL cells in vivo is a major biological feature of this disease and is presumably related to a deregulated control of cell cycle progression and programmed cell death. Also characteristic of the disease is the great heterogeneity in the clinical behavior of patients with B-CLL. A prolonged, indolent clinical course for several months or years is experienced by many patients, whereas others present with, or rapidly develop, a more aggressive disease. The notion of the prognostic value of the lymphocyte doubling time in B-CLL (165) underscores the relevant impact that cell cycle regulatory mechanisms may have in the pathogenesis of the disease and in its heterogeneous clinical course. Many regulatory molecules and genes may have a role in B-CLL cell accumulation, and several of them, such as p53 and Bcl-2, have been intensively investigated in the last years. Some of the recent findings in this field will be reviewed in the following, with particular emphasis on the impact that cytokines and growth factors may have on the altered intracellular machinery operational in B-CLL and on the prognostic value of regulatory molecule expression.

A. Bcl-2

The 26-kDa Bcl-2 protein protects cells from the induction of apoptosis by different stimuli, including the withdrawal of survival factors, heat shock, and treatment with DNA damaging agents (166). Bcl-2 is the prototype of a family of related proteins, which includes antiapoptotic members, such as Bcl-XL, Bcl-w, MCL-1, A1, and the BAX, BAK, and BAD proapoptotic proteins (167).

Bcl-2 functions to prevent activation of the cell death proteases (caspases), apparently both by inhibiting release of protease activators from mitochondria and by sequestering through physical interactions with a cytosolic protease activator known as CED-4 (168).

The Bcl-2 gene was first discovered in follicular non-Hodgkin's lymphoma, a malignancy that shares many similarities with B-CLL, because both diseases are characterized by the accumulation of quiescent, noncycling lymphocytes (169). In most cases of follicular lymphoma, the inappropriate transcription of the Bcl-2 gene arises from its juxtaposition under the control of enhancer elements associated with the Ig heavy chain gene loci (170). By contrast, chromosomal translocations involving the Bcl-2 gene do not occur in B-CLL cells, although high levels of Bcl-2 protein can been found in most cases, and other mechanisms, such as the hypomethylation of the promoter region of the gene, may be involved (171,172).

Because most B-CLL samples constitutively express high levels of Bcl-2, Bcl-2 overexpression may play a major role in the resistance to apoptosis characteristic of this disease and thus in its pathogenesis and clinical course. However, most studies have failed to find a direct correlation between Bcl-2 levels and chemoresistance in vitro and in vivo (173–175). Relative amounts of apoptosis-related genes may be more important than individual protein levels to regulate susceptibility to a given apoptotic stimulus and the balance between Bcl-2, and another proapoptotic member of the Bcl-2 family, Bax, has been indicated as more relevant that Bcl-2 expression alone. Bcl-2 heterodimerizes with Bax to prevent apoptosis, whereas Bax homodimers accelerate cell death and counteract the survival function of Bcl-2/Bax heterodimers (176). In several reports, the Bcl-2/Bax ratio has been inversely related with drug-induced apoptosis in vitro and clinical response to chemotherapy (173–175,177,178). Recently, Pepper et al. (179) demonstrated that B-CLL cells resistant to chlorambucil in vitro failed to up-regulate Bax, as typically observed in sensitive cells. It is possible that other known and unknown genes are also important in the regulation of apoptosis in B-CLL and that the final defect arises from a pattern of expression generally skewed toward prevention of apoptosis.

Several cytokines and growth factors can modify the pattern of proliferation and survival of B-CLL cells, as well as their susceptibility to apoptotic stimuli. As discussed earlier, B-CLL cells are known to produce a number of cytokines, including IL-8, TNFα, and IL-10, and cytokine networks in vivo are thought to play a relevant role in the clinical course of the disease. Bcl-2–dependent mechanisms might be involved in the prevention of apoptosis induced by several cytokines, but different pathways could also be implicated. For instance, IL-4 has been reported to protect B-CLL cells from Fas-induced apoptosis by a mechanism that is Bcl-2 independent (38), and IL-5 seems to increase spontaneous apoptosis also in a Bcl-2 independent manner (37). However, delayed down-regulation has been proposed by others as a common mechanism for the suppression of apoptosis obtained by treatment with IFNγ, IL-2, IL-4, IL-6, IL-13, and TNFα (53). Also IL-8, a cytokine possibly implicated in a B-CLL autocrine loop, seems to protect from spontaneous and induced apoptosis through a Bcl-2–dependent mechanism (65). IFNα, which has been attempted in the treatment of patients with B-CLL, has been reported to increase Bcl-2 expression and to protect B-CLL cells from apoptotic death in vitro, suggesting that the clinical responses to IFNα observed in a proportion of patients are not due to a direct effect on the malignant cells (180). In summary, the Bcl-2 protein probably plays a central role in mediating the effect on B-CLL cells of several autocrine/paracrine "survival" loops that might operate in vivo.

The importance of Bcl-2 in the defective programmed cell death mechanisms occurring in B-CLL cells and the possible implications for the treatment of the disease have been stressed in a recent article. Using an antisense oligonucleotide, the authors were able to specifically inhibit Bcl-2 expression in B-CLL cells; this resulted in Bax overexpression and in an increase in apoptotic cell death in vitro (181). The increased expression of the Bax protein after antisense-mediated down-regulation of Bcl-2 further points to the relevant role played by the Bcl-2/Bax ratio in regulating programmed cell death in B-CLL.

B. p53

The p53 protein plays an important role in the coupling of DNA damage to cell-cycle arrest and to the induction of apoptosis. In cells with undamaged DNA, p53 protein expression is maintained at a low level as a result of rapid turnover. An increase in stability after the induction of DNA damage results in an increased level of p53, which is followed by apoptosis induction (182). Genetic studies on apoptosis induction in adriamycin-treated mouse fibroblasts suggest that Bax is an important (but not the only) effector of p53-mediated apoptosis (183,184).

The p53 tumor suppressor gene is located on chromosome 17 band p13.1. Mutations or deletions of the p53 gene make cells resistant to DNA damaging agents, such as adriamycin or radiation, and may facilitate the emergence of neoplastic clones with a survival advantage (185,186). p53 is the most frequently altered gene in human cancer, being mutated in approximately 50% of all human tumors (187,188). Gene mutations and protein detection by immunological methods are usually associated, because mutated p53 has a prolonged half-life compared with the rapid intracellular turnover of the wild-type protein (189).

In B-CLL, where the accumulation of resting lymphocytes stands for a deregulation of apoptosis in the tumor clone, p53 mutations are nevertheless relatively rare. p53 mutations are detected in 10% to 15% of B-CLL cases and are associated with poor response to therapy and shorter survival (190,191). Mutations are more frequent (about 40%) in Richter's immunoblastic transformation (192). In a recent analysis of 181 B-CLL patients followed at a single institution (193), the percentage of p53 positivity correlated with the clinical stage and the phase of the disease, showing a low expression at diagnosis (8 of 112, 7.1%) and a significantly higher expression in patients studied during the course of the disease (7 of 35, 20%) and, to a further extent, with disease progression (12 of 34, 35.3%). Moreover, the percentage of cells stained by p53 antibodies was in most cases lower than the percentage of leukemic cells and the highest percentage of p53-positive cells was observed in stages B and C and in patients with progressive disease, supporting the hypothesis that p53 dysregulation can be a late event in the progression of the disease. The expansion of an initially minor subclone with a mutated p53 during disease progression has indeed been shown in brain tumors and in acute myeloid leukemia (194,195).

Most chemotherapeutic drugs, as well as x-ray irradiation, ultimately kill tumor cells by triggering apoptosis. Therefore, it can be expected that malignant cells that possess defects in their machinery for apoptosis, such as the p53 protein, are intrinsically more resistant to the cytotoxic actions of anticancer drugs. Data in vitro on the p53 mutation impact on the sensitivity of B-CLL cells to chemotherapeutic drugs are conflicting (196,197), but it must be noted that multiple factors could affect chemosensitivity of B-CLL cells in vitro (198). In a recent article, Pettitt et al. (199) found only a small difference in fludarabine-induced cell killing between B-CLL cells with p53 dysfunction and cases with functionally intact p53. The authors concluded that the poor therapeutic response to purine analogues observed in patients with p53 defects is likely to be caused by the emergence, on a background of genomic instability, of B-CLL cell clones that are resistant to nucleoside-induced killing for reasons unrelated to p53. On the contrary, an increased resistance in vitro to drug-induced apoptosis in p53 mutant B-CLL cells has been reported by other authors (200,201). Nevertheless, the relationship in vivo between p53 mutations and treatment failure has been documented in several studies (193,202). el Rouby et al. (190) reported a remission rate of 93% in patients without p53 mutations, even after adjustment for prognostic factors (age, sex, race, and Rai stage), compared with 14% in patients with p53 mutations. In their study, patients with p53 gene mutations had a 13-fold greater risk of death than patients without p53 mutations, confirming the great impact of p53 status as a prognostic factor in B-CLL patients.

C. p27

In eukarotic cells, the progression through the different phases of the cell cycle is mainly governed by the cyclin-dependent kinase (CDK) complexes, consisting of a positive regulatory cyclin subunit and a catalytic serine/threonine kinase subunit (203). Several of these cyclin-CDK complexes are involved at different stages of the cell cycle, and their sequential and well-ordered formation, activation, and subsequent inactivation play a key role in the G1/S and G2/M transitions. Five distinct classes of mammalian cyclins (A, B, C, D, and E) and an increasing number of CDKs have been identified (204). D-type cyclins are synthesized early in the G1 phase and are likely to be regulators of the G1/S transition (205,206). Moreover, there are several protein inhibitors of cyclin-CDKs activity (CKI, cyclin-dependent kinase inhibitors) implicated in regulating cyclin-CDK activity (207,208). P27Kipl (p27) is a member of the KIP/CIP family of CKI, mainly involved in growth inhibitory processes. High levels of p27 are found in cells arrested in G0/G1, and its expression declines as cells progress toward the S phase (209,210). Growth inhibitory signals, like cell-to-cell contact and cytokines with antiproliferative action, are known to up-regulate p27 expression (211,212). Correspondingly, in vitro the overexpression of p27 has been shown to arrest cells in G0/G1 (210). p27 is able to bind tightly to cyclin E-CDK2 and to cyclin D2-CDK4, both required for entry into the S phase (211).

The key role played by the p27 protein as a link between extracellular signals and the cell cycle machinery has led to several studies investigating its expression in transformed cells. A p27 down-regulation has been demonstrated in several solid tumors, and its low levels correlate with poor survival rates, high-grade neoplasms, or both (213,214). In a recent paper, 91 of 112 cases of mantle cell lymphomas showed a loss of p27, and this was associated with a decreased overall survival (215).

Because p27 expression appears to correlate inversely with the cell proliferation index, a different pattern of expression can be expected in an accumulative disorder such as B-CLL. In fact, Vrhovac et al. (216) reported a constitutively high expression of p27 in all of the 88 B-CLL samples examined. p27 levels were independent of the absolute number of circulating lymphocytes but strongly correlated with both lymphocyte and total tumor mass doubling time, and high p27 expression was associated with a poorer overall prognosis. Moreover, high p27 expression correlated with a decreased rate of apoptosis in vitro, because cells expressing high levels of p27 survived longer in culture. Figure 4 depicts the potential implication of p27 overexpression in the pathogenesis of B-CLL.

The heterogeneous clinical picture of B-CLL has already been discussed. Particularly interesting is the evidence that some patients remain stable for many years without treatment even in the presence of a high lymphocyte count. In this category of patients, a better immunological control of the disease, as well as a different balance between tumor cell proliferation and apoptosis, may be hypothesized. Indeed, the analysis of p27 levels in a group of 75 B-CLL patients with documented stable or progressive disease, based on the clinical course and treatment requirement, showed significantly lower p27 mean values in stable compared with progressive cases (submitted). The biological relevance of cell cycle control in the clinical history of this disease and the role of p27 expression are further confirmed by these data.

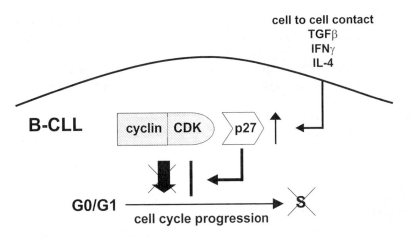

Figure 4 p27 and control of cell cycle in B-CLL. In B-CLL cells, the overexpression of p27 may contribute to the accumulation of the neoplastic clone by blocking the tumor cell in the G0 phase of the cell cycle. p27 inhibits the cyclin-CDK complexes, which are necessary to progress to the S-phase. Extracellular signals, such as cytokines, growth factors, and membrane signals, can influence p27 expression.

The key role of the p27 protein as a link between extracellular signals and the cell cycle machinery is demonstrated by the influence that cytokines and growth factors can have on p27 expression. Inhibitory cytokines such as TGFβ or IFNγ can increase p27 levels, and defects in this pathway have been reported in human solid tumors (211,212). In normal resting B cells, p27 expression is up-regulated by IL-4 (217). Correspondingly, in B-CLL cells IL-4 is reported to maintain or increase p27 levels (216), in contrast with the p27 down-modulation observed after in vitro exposure to fludarabine. Further studies are necessary to establish the effects on p27 expression of different cytokines that play a role in the process of B-CLL cell survival and proliferation.

V. CONCLUSIONS AND PERSPECTIVES

The presently available technologies have greatly contributed to unravel the cell-to-cell cross-talk that is operational in B-CLL within the leukemic clone and the different accessory nonneoplastic cell populations. On the basis of the data accumulated over the years and reviewed in this chapter, it is now evident that several cytokines, membrane signals, and regulatory molecules play an important role in both the leukemic population and in the host immune compartment of B-CLL patients. This opens new conceptual and applicative scenarios. First, it allows a better understanding of the biological mechanisms that regulate the accumulation process that takes place in B-CLL, a unique feature of this disease that appears to be largely contributed by a decreased apoptotic machinery of the leukemic B-cell populations. In addition, it enables light to be shed on the progressive immunodeficiency, which is present in patients with B-CLL, which worsens as the disease progresses and which plays a primary role in the complications, mainly infections, that are often the primary cause of death. From a clinical point of view, we are starting to appreciate that the marked heterogeneity in the clinical course of patients with apparent similar features may be contributed by a differential action exerted by both cytokines and regulatory molecules. In turn, this opens new therapeutic prospects on the basis of strategies aimed at correcting an identified defect or at interrupting a given cytokine loop. The recently activated protocols directed at transducing the CD40L into B-CLL cells represent the first example of a form of intervention that stems from a better understanding of the biology of B-CLL and accessory cells. It is foreseeable that in the near future we will succeed in identifying early in the disease B-CLL patients with a stable or progressive clinical picture and in designing more targeted therapeutic protocols according to objective biological parameters.

ACKNOWLEDGMENTS

This work was supported by Istituto Superiore di Sanità (Rome), Italy-USA project on "Therapy of Tumors," Associazione Italiana per la Ricerca sul Cancro (AIRC, Milan), and Ministero dell'Università e della Ricerca Scientifica (Rome). EO is in receipt of a fellowship from AIRC (Milan).

REFERENCES

1. Y Furutani, M Notake, M Yamayoshi, J Yamagishi, H Nomura, M Ohue, R Furuta, T Fukui, M Yamada, S Nakamura. Cloning and characterization of the cDNAs for human and rabbit interleukin-1 precursor. Nucleic Acids Res 13:5869–5882, 1985.
2. PE Auron, AC Webb, LJ Rosenwasser, SF Mucci, A Rich, SM Wolff, CA Dinarello. Nucleotide sequence of human monocyte interleukin 1 precursor cDNA. Proc Natl Acad Sci USA 81:7907–7911, 1984.
3. CA Dinarello. An update on human interleukin 1: From molecular biology to clinical relevance. J Clin Immunol 5:287–297, 1985.
4. JE Sims, CJ March, D Cosman, MB Widmer, HR MacDonald, CJ McMahan, CE Grubin, JM Wignall, JL Jacksin, SM Call. cDNA expression cloning of the IL-1 receptor, a member of the immunoglobulin superfamily. Science 241:585–589, 1988.
5. K Matsushima, G Tosato, D Benjamin, JJ Oppenheim. B-cell-derived interleukin-1 (IL-1)-like factor. II. Sources, effects, and biochemical properties. Cell Immunol 94:418–426, 1985.
6. V Pistoia, F Cozzolino, A Rubartelli, M Torcia, S Roncella, M Ferrarini. In vitro production of interleukin 1 by normal and malignant human B lymphocytes. J Immunol 136:1688–1692, 1986.
7. F Melchers, A Erdei, T Schulz, MP Dierich. Growth control of activated, synchronized murine B cells by the C3d fragment of human complement. Nature 317:264–267, 1985.
8. C Uggla, M Aguilar-Santelises, A Rosen, H Mellstedt, M Jondal. Spontaneous production of interleukin 1 activity by chronic lymphocytic leukemia cells. Blood 70:1851–1857, 1987.
9. F Morabito, EF Prasthofer, NE Dunlap, CE Grossi, AB Tilden. Expression of myelomonocytic antigens on chronic lymphocytic leukemia B cells correlates with their ability to produce interleukin 1. Blood 70:1750–1757, 1987.
10. M Aguilar-Santelises, JF Amador, H Mellstedt, M Jondal. Low IL-1 beta production in leukemic cells from progressive B cell chronic leukemia (B-CLL). Leuk Res 13:937–942, 1989.
11. HE Heslop, AC Bianchi, FT Cordingley, M Turner, W Chandima, CP De Mel, AV Hoffbrand, MK Brenner. Effects of interferon alpha on autocrine growth factor loops in B lymphoproliferative disorders. J Exp Med 172:1729–1734, 1990.
12. JM Plate, WH Knospe, JE Harris, SA Gregory. Normal and aberrant expression of cytokines in neoplastic cells from chronic lymphocytic leukemias. Hum Immunol 36:249–258, 1993.
13. H Takeuchi, I Katayama. Interleukin 1 (IL-1 alpha and IL-1 beta) induces differentiation/activation of B cell chronic lymphoid leukemia cells. Cytokine 6:243–246, 1994.

14. A Brizard, F Morel, JC Lecron, B Dreyfus, F Brizard, A Barra, JL Preud'homme. Proliferative response of B chronic lymphocytic leukemia lymphocytes stimulated with IL2 and soluble CD23. Leuk Lymphoma 14:311–318, 1994.

15. T Mainou-Fowler, JA Copplestone, AG Prentice. Effect of interleukins on the proliferation and survival of B cell chronic lymphocytic leukaemia cells. J Clin Pathol 48:482–487, 1995.

16. AP Jewell, PM Lydyard, CP Worman, FJ Giles, AH Goldstone. Growth factors can protect B-chronic lymphocytic leukaemia cells against programmed cell death without stimulating proliferation. Leuk Lymphoma 18:159–162, 1995.

17. KA Smith. Interleukin-2: Inception, impact and implication. Science 240:1169–1176, 1988.

18. D de Totero, P Francia di Celle, A Cignetti, R Foa. The IL-2 receptor complex: expression and function on normal and leukemic B cells. Leukemia 9:1425–1431, 1995.

19. O Lantz, C Grillot-Courvalin, C Schmitt, JP Fermand, JC Brouet. Interleukin 2-induced proliferation of leukemic human B cells. J Exp Med 161:1225–1230, 1985.

20. AC Fluckiger, JF Rossi, A Bussel, P Bryon, J Banchereau, T Defrance. Responsiveness of chronic lymphocytic leukemia B-cells activated via surface Igs or CD40 to B-cell tropic factors. Blood 80:3173–3181, 1992.

21. R Foa, M Giovarelli, C Jemma, MT Fierro, P Lusso, ML Ferrando, F Lauria, G Forni. Interleukin 2 (IL2) and interferon-γ production by T lymphocytes from patients with B-chronic lymphocytic leukemia: Evidence that normally released IL2 is absorbed by the neoplastic B cell population. Blood 66:614–619, 1985.

22. G Semenzato, R Foa, C Agostini, R Zambello, L Trentin, F Vinante, F Benedetti, M Chilosi, G Pizzolo. High serum levels of soluble interleukin 2 receptor in patients with B chronic lymphocytic leukemia. Blood 70:396–400, 1987.

23. LA Rubin, G Jay, DL Nelson. The released interleukin 2 receptor binds interleukin 2 efficiently. J Immunol 137:3841–3844, 1986.

24. O Ayanlar-Batuman, E Ebert, SP Hauptman. Defective interleukin-2 production and responsiveness by T cells in patients with chronic lymphocytic leukemia of B cell variety. Blood 67:279–284, 1986.

25. R Foa, MT Fierro, M Giovarelli, P Lusso, G Benetton, M Bonferroni, G Forni. Immunoregulatory T-cell defects in B-cell chronic lymphocytic leukemia: Cause or consequence of the disease? The contributory role of a decreased availability of interleukin 2 (IL2). Blood Cells 12:399–412, 1987.

26. M Alvarez de Mon, J Casas, R Laguna, ML Toribio, MO de Landazuri, A Durantez. Lymphokine induction of NK-like cytotoxicity in T cells from B-CLL. Blood 67:228–232, 1986.

27. M Howard, J Farrar, M Hilfiker, B Johnson, K Takatsu, T Hamaoka, WE Paul. Identification of a T cell-derived B cell growth factor distinct from interleukin 2. J Exp Med 155:914–923, 1982.

28. S Karray, T DeFrance, H Merle-Beral, J Banchereau, P Debre, P Galanaud. Interleukin 4 counteracts the interleukin 2-induced proliferation of monoclonal B cells. J Exp Med 168:85–94, 1988.

29. L Llorente, F Mitjavila, MC Crevon, P Galanaud. Dual effects of interleukin 4 on antigen-activated human B cells: induction of proliferation and inhibition of interleukin 2-dependent differentiation. Eur J Immunol 20:1887–1892, 1990.

30. H Zola, L Flego, H Weedon. Expression of IL-4 receptor on human T and B lymphocytes. Cell Immunol 150:149–158, 1993.

31. P Francia di Celle, A Carbone, D Marchis, D Zhou, S Sozzani, S Zupo, M Pini, A Mantovani, R Foa. Cytokine gene expression in B-cell chronic lymphocytic leukemia: evidence of constitutive interleukin-8 (IL-8) mRNA expression and secretion of biologically active IL-8 protein. Blood 84:220–228, 1994.

32. C van Kooten, I Rensink, L Aarden, R van Oers. Interleukin-4 inhibits both paracrine and autocrine tumor necrosis factor-alpha-induced proliferation of B chronic lymphocytic leukemia cells. Blood 80:1299–1306, 1992.

33. JE Reittie, AV Hoffbrand. Interleukin-4 (IL-4) inhibits proliferation and spontaneous cytokine release by chronic lymphocytic leukaemia cells. Leuk Res 18:55–60, 1994.

34. HG Drexler, MK Brenner, E Coustan-Smith, SM Gignac, AV Hoffbrand. Analysis of signal transduction in B chronic lymphocytic leukemia cells. Blood 71:1461–1469, 1988.

35. C Hivroz, B Geny, JC Brouet, C Grillot-Courvalin. Altered signal transduction secondary to surface IgM cross-linking on B-chronic lymphocytic leukemia cells. Differential activation of the phosphatidylinositol-specific phospholipase C. J Immunol 144:2351–2358, 1990.

36. M Dancescu, M Rubio-Trujillo, G Biron, D Bron, G Delespesse, M Sarfati. Interleukin 4 protects chronic lymphocytic leukemic B cells from death by apoptosis and upregulates Bcl-2 expression. J Exp Med 176:1319–1326, 1992.

37. T Mainou-Fowler, VA Craig, JA Copplestone, MD Hamon, AG Prentice. Interleukin-5 (IL-5) increases spontaneous apoptosis of B-cell chronic lymphocytic leukemia cells in vitro independently of bcl-2 expression and is inhibited by IL-4. Blood 84:2297–2304, 1994.

38. T Mainou-Fowler, VA Craig, AJ Copplestone, MD Hamon, AG Prentice. Effect of anti-APO1 on spontaneous apoptosis of B cells in chronic lymphocytic leukemia: the role of bcl-2 and interleukin 4. Leuk Lymphoma 19:301–308, 1995.

39. X Mu, NE Kay, MP Gosland, CD Jennings. Analysis of blood T-cell cytokine expression in B-chronic lymphocytic leukaemia: evidence for increased levels of cytoplasmic IL-4 in resting and activated CD8 T cells. Br J Haematol 96:733–735, 1997.

40. D de Totero, G Reato, F Mauro, A Cignetti, S Ferrini, A Guarini, M Gobbi, CE Grossi, R Foa. IL4 production and increased CD30 expression by a unique CD8+ T-cell subset in B-cell chronic lymphocytic leukaemia. Br J Haematol 104:589–599, 1999.

41. E Orsini, A Guarini, R Foa. Accessory cells, cytokine loops and cell-to-cell interactions in chronic lymphocytic leukemia. Rev Clin Exp Hamatol 4:73–98, 2000.

42. OS Frankfurt, JJ Byrnes, L Villa. Protection from apoptotic cell death by interleukin-4 is increased in previously treated chronic lymphocytic leukemia patients. Leuk Res 21:9–16, 1997.

43. K Ikebuchi, GG Wong, SC Clark, JN Ihle, Y Hirai, M Ogawa. Interleukin 6 enhancement of interleukin 3-dependent proliferation of multipotential hemopoietic progenitors. Proc Natl Acad Sci USA 84:9035–9039, 1987.

44. T Taga, M Hibi, Y Hirata, K Yamasaki, K Yasukawa, T Matsuda, T Hirano, T Kishimoto. Interleukin-6 triggers the association of its receptor with a possible signal transducer, gp130. Cell 58:573–581, 1989.

45. M Murakami, M Hibi, N Nakagawa, T Nakawaga, K Yasukawa, K Yamanishi, T Taga, T Kishimoto. IL-6-induced homodimerization of gp-130 and associated activation of a tyrosine kinase. Science 260:1808–1810, 1993.

46. D Novick, LM Shulman, L Chen, M Revel. Enhancement of interleukin-6 cytostatic effect on human breast carcinoma cells by soluble IL-6 receptor from urine and reversion by monoclonal antibody. Cytokine 4:6–11, 1992.

47. M Kalai, FA Montero-Julian, J Grotzinger, V Fontaine, P Vandenbussche, R Deschuyteneer, A Wollmer, H Brailly, J Content. Analysis of the human interleukin-6/human interleukin-6 receptor binding interface at the amino acid level: Proposed mechanism of interaction. Blood 4:1319–1333, 1997.

48. T Lavabre-Bertrand, C Exbrayat, J Liautard, JP Gaillard, PP Baskevitch, N Poujol, C Duperray, P Bourquard, J Brochier. Detection of membrane and soluble interleukin-6 receptor in lymphoid malignancies. Br J Haematol 91:871–877, 1995.

49. A Biondi, V Rossi, R Bassan, T Barbui, S Bettoni, M Sironi, A Mantovani, A Rambaldi. Constitutive expression of the interleukin-6 gene in chronic lymphocytic leukemia. Blood 73:1279–1284, 1989.

50. C van Kooten, I Rensink, L Aarden, R van Oers. Effect of IL-4 and IL-6 on the proliferation and differentiation of B-chronic lymphocytic leukemia cells. Leukemia 7:618–624, 1993.

51. D Aderka, Y Maor, D Novick, H Engelmann, Y Kahn, Y Levo, D Wallach, M Revel. Interleu-kin-6 inhibits the proliferation of B-chronic lymphocytic leukemia cells that is induced by tumor necrosis factor-alpha or -beta. Blood 81:2076–2084, 1993.

52. JE Reittie, KL Yong, P Panayiotidis, AV Hoffbrand. Interleukin-6 inhibits apoptosis and tumour necrosis factor induced proliferation of B-chronic lymphocytic leukaemia. Leuk Lymphoma 22:83–90, 1996.

53. SG Tangye, RL Raison. Human cytokines suppress apoptosis of leukaemic CD5+ B cells and preserve expression of bcl-2. Immunol Cell Biol 75:127–135, 1997.

54. T Pettersson, K Metsarinne, AM Teppo, F Fyhrquist. Immunoreactive interleukin-6 in serum of patients with B-lymphoproliferative diseases. J Intern Med 232:439–442, 1992.

55. M Aguilar-Santelises, A Loftenius, C Ljungh, SB Svenson, B Andersson, H Mellstedt, M Jondal. Serum levels of helper factors (IL-1 alpha, IL-1 beta and IL-6), T-cell products (sCD4 and sCD8), sIL-2R and beta 2-microglobulin in patients with B-CLL and benign B lymphocy-tosis. Leuk Res 16:607–613, 1992.

56. J Hulkkonen, J Vilpo, L Vilpo, M Hurme. Diminished production of interleukin-6 in chronic lymphocytic leukaemia (B-CLL) cells from patients at advanced stages of disease. Br J Haematol 100:478–483, 1998.

57. V Callea, F Morabito, F Luise, A Piromalli, M Filangeri, C Stelitano, P Iacopino, F Nobile, M Brugiatelli. Clinical significance of sIL2R, sCD23, sICAM-1, IL6 and sCD14 serum levels in B-cell chronic lymphocytic leukemia. Haematologica 81:310–315, 1996.

58. N Lahat, E Aghai, B Maroun, A Kinarty, M Quitt, P Froom. Increased spontaneous secretion of IL-6 from B cells of patients with B chronic lymphatic leukaemia (B-CLL) and autoimmu-nity. Clin Exp Immunol 85:302–306, 1991.

59. M Baggiolini, A Walz, SL Kunkel. Neutrophil-activating peptide-1/interleukin 8, a novel cytokine that activates neutrophils. J Clin Invest 84:1045–1049, 1989.

60. EJ Leonard, A Skeel, T Yoshimura, K Noer, S Kutvirt, D Van Epps. Leukocyte specificity and binding of human neutrophil attractant/activation protein-1. J Immunol 144:1323–1330, 1990.

61. K Matsushima, JJ Oppenheim. Interleukin 8 and MCAF: novel inflammatory cytokines in-ducible by IL 1 and TNF. Cytokine 1:2–13, 1989.

62. MJ Smyth, COC Zachariae, Y Norihisa, JR Ortaldo, A Hishinuma, K Matsushima. IL-8 gene expression and production in human peripheral blood lymphocyte subsets. J Immunol 146: 3815–3823, 1991.

63. RM Strieter, SW Chensue, TJ Standiford, MA Basha, HJ Showell, SL Kunkel. Disparate gene expression of chemotactic cytokines by human mononuclear phagocytes. Biochem Bio-phys Res Commun 166:886–891, 1990.

64. S Molica, G Vitelli, D Levato, L Levato, A Dattilo, GM Gandolfo. Clinico-biological impli-cations of increased serum levels of interleukin-8 in B-cell chronic lymphocytic leukemia. Haematological 84:208–211, 1999.

65. P Francia di Celle, S Mariani, L Riera, A Stacchini, G Reato, R Foa. Interleukin-8 induces the accumulation of B-cell chronic lymphocytic leukemia cells by prolonging survival in an autocrine fashion. Blood 87:4382–4389, 1996.

66. P Vieira, R de Waal-Malefyt, MN Dang, KE Johnson, R Kastelein, DF Fiorentino, JE deVries, MG Roncarolo, TR Mosmann, KW Moore. Isolation and expression of human cy-tokine synthesis inhibitory factor cDNA clones: homology to Epstein-Barr virus open reading frame BCRFI. Proc Natl Acad Sci USA 88:1172–1176, 1991.

67. TR Mosmann, KW Moore. Role of IL-10 in cross-regulation of Th1 and Th2 responses. Immunol Tod 12:A49–A53, 1991.

68. P Wang, P Wu, MI Siegel, RW Egan, MM Billah. IL-10 inhibits transcription of cytokine genes in human peripheral blood mononuclear cells. J Immunol 153:811–816, 1994.

69. G Del Prete, M De Carli, F Almerigogna, MG Giudizi, R Biagiotti, S Romagnani. Human IL-10 is produced by both type 1 helper (Th1) and type 2 helper (Th2) T cell clones and

inhibits their antigen-specific proliferation and cytokine production. J Immunol 150:353–360, 1993.

70. DF Fiorentino, A Zlotnik, P Vieira, TR Mosmann, M Howard, KW Moore, A O'Garra. IL-10 acts on the antigen-presenting cell to inhibit cytokine production by Th1 cells. J Immunol 146:3444–3451, 1991.

71. L Faulkner, G Buchan, M Baird. Interleukin-10 does not affect phagocytosis of particulate antigen by bone marrow-derived dendritic cells but does impair antigen presentation. Immunology 99:523–531, 2000.

72. J Sjoberg, M Aguilar-Santelises, AM Sjogren, EK Pisa, A Ljungdahl, M Bjorkholm, M Jondal, H Mellstedt, P Pisa. Interleukin-10 mRNA expression in B-cell chronic lymphocytic leukaemia inversely correlates with progression of disease. Br J Haematol 92:393–400, 1996.

73. J Jurlander, CF Lai, J Tan, CC Chou, CH Geisler, J Schriber, LE Blumenson, SK Narula, H Baumann, MA Caligiuri. Characterization of interleukin-10 receptor expression on B-cell chronic lymphocytic leukemia cells. Blood 89:4146–4152, 1997.

74. A Egle, I Marschitz, B Posch, M Herold, R Greil. IL-10 serum levels in B-cell chronic lymphocytic leukaemia. Br J Haematol 94:211–212, 1996.

75. EF Kamper, AD Papaphilis, MK Angelopoulou, LT Kopeikina, MP Siakantaris, GA Pangalis, JC Stavridis. Serum levels of tetranectin, intercellular adhesion molecule-1 and interleukin-10 in B-chronic lymphocytic leukemia. Clin Biochem 32:639–645, 1999.

76. WU Knauf, B Ehlers, S Bisson, E Thiel. Serum levels of interleukin-10 in B-cell chronic lymphocytic leukemia. Blood 86:4382–4383, 1995.

77. Y Levy, JC Brouet. Interleukin-10 prevents spontaneous death of germinal center B cells by induction of the bcl-2 protein. J Clin Invest 93:424–428, 1994.

78. RA Baiocchi, ME Ross, JC Tan, CC Chou, L Sullivan, S Haldar, M Monne, MV Seiden, SK Narula, J Sklar. Lymphomagenesis in the SCID-hu mouse involves abundant production of human interleukin-10. Blood 85:1063–1074, 1995.

79. AC Fluckiger, I Durand, J Banchereau. Interleukin 10 induces apoptotic cell death of B-chronic lymphocytic leukemia cells. J Exp Med 179:91–99, 1994.

80. A Kitabayashi, M Hirokawa, AB Miura. The role of interleukin-10 (IL-10) in chronic B-lymphocytic leukemia: IL-10 prevents leukemic cells from apoptotic cell death. Int J Hematol 62:99–106, 1995.

81. AP Jewell, CP Worman, PM Lydyard, KL Yong, FJ Giles, AH Goldstone. Interferon-alpha up-regulates bcl-2 expression and protects B-CLL from apoptosis in vitro and in vivo. Br J Haematol 88:268–274, 1994.

82. M Buschle, D Campana, SR Carding, C Richard, AV Hoffbrand, MK Brenner. Interferon gamma inhibits apoptotic cell death in B cell chronic lymphocytic leukemia. J Exp Med 177:213–218, 1993.

83. R Castejon, JA Vargas, Y Romero, M Briz, RM Munoz, A Durantez. Modulation of apoptosis by cytokines in B-cell chronic lymphocytic leukemia. Cytometry 38:224–230, 1999.

84. KP MacDonald, AR Pettit, C Quinn, GJ Thomas, R Thomas. Resistance of rheumatoid synovial dendritic cells to the immunosuppressive effects of IL-10. J Immunol 163:5599–5607, 1999.

85. S Sharma, M Stolina, Y Lin, B Gardner, PW Miller, M Kronenberg, SM Dubinett. T cell-derived IL-10 promotes lung cancer growth by suppressing both T cell and APC function. J Immunol 163:5020–5028, 1999.

86. MK Brenner. Tumor necrosis factor. Br J Haematol 69:149–152, 1988.

87. G Gehr, R Gentz, M Brockhaus, H Loetscher, W Lesslauer. Both tumor necrosis factor receptor types mediate proliferative signals in human mononuclear cell activation. J Immunol 149:911–917, 1992.

88. L Tartaglia, DV Goeffel. Two TNF receptors. Immunology Today 13:151–153, 1992.

89. FT Cordingley, A Bianchi, AV Hoffbrand, JE Reittie, HE Heslop, A Vyakarnam, M Turner,

A Meager, MK Brenner. Tumor necrosis factor as an autocrine tumour growth factor for chronic B-cell malignancies. Lancet 1:969–971, 1988.

90. R Foa, M Massaia, S Cardona, AG Tos, A Bianchi, C Attisano, A Guarini, PF di Celle, MT Fierro. Production of tumor necrosis factor-alpha by B-cell chronic lymphocytic leukemia cells: a possible regulatory role of TNF in the progression of the disease. Blood 76:393–400, 1990.

91. F Adami, A Guarini, M Pini, F Siviero, R Sancetta, M Massaia, L Trentin, R Foa, G Semenzato. Serum levels of tumour necrosis factor-alpha in patients with B-cell chronic lymphocytic leukaemia. Eur J Cancer 30A:1259–1263, 1994.

92. M Aguilar-Santelises, D Gigliotti, LM Osorio, AD Santiago, H Mellstedt, M Jondal. Cytokine expression in B-CLL in relation to disease progression and in vitro activation. Med Oncol 16:289–295, 1999.

93. AP Jewell, CP Worman, FJ Giles, AH Goldstone. Serum levels of TNF, IL-6 and sCD23 correlate with changes in lymphocyte count in patients with B-cell chronic lymphocytic leukaemia receiving interferon-alpha therapy. Leuk Lymphoma 24:327–333, 1997.

94. W Digel, W Schoniger, M Stefanie, H Janssen, C Buck, M Schmid, A Raghavachar, F Porzsolt. Receptors for tumor necrosis factor on neoplastic B cells from chronic lymphocytic leukemia are expressed in vitro but not in vivo. Blood 76:1607–1613, 1990.

95. L Trentin, R Zambello, C Agostini, C Enthammer, A Cerutti, F Adami, S Zamboni, G Semenzato. Expression and regulation of tumor necrosis factor, interleukin-2, and hematopoietic growth factor receptors in B-cell chronic lymphocytic leukemia. Blood 84:4249–4256, 1994.

96. A Waage, T Espevik. TNF receptors in chronic lymphocytic leukemia. Leuk Lymphoma 3: 41–46, 1994.

97. W Digel, M Stefanic, W Schoniger, C Buck, A Raghavachar, N Frickhofen, H Heimpel, F Porzsolt. Tumor necrosis factor induces proliferation of neoplastic B cells from chronic lymphocytic leukemia. Blood 73:1242–1246, 1989.

98. R Moberts, H Hoogerbrugge, T van Agthoven, B Lowenberg, I Touw. Proliferative response of highly purified B chronic lymphocytic leukemia cells in serum free culture to interleukin-2 and tumor necrosis factors alpha and beta. Leuk Res 13:973–980, 1989.

99. F Burke, D Griffin, N Elwood, C Davis, G Stamp, A Rohatiner, TA Lister, F Balkwill. The effect of cytokines on cultured mononuclear cells from patients with B cell chronic lymphocytic leukemia. Hematol Oncol 11:23–33, 1993.

100. J Massague. The transforming growth factor-β family. Ann Rev Cell Biol 6:597–641, 1990.

101. SC Wallick, IS Figari, RE Morris, AD Levinson, MA Palladino. Immunoregulatory role of transforming growth factor β (TGF-β) in development of killer cells: Comparison of active and latent TGF-β1. J Exp Med 172:1777–1784, 1990.

102. HY Lin, A Moustakas. TGF-β receptors: structure and function. Cell Mol Biol 40:337–349, 1994.

103. JP Kremer, G Reisbach, C Nerl, P Dormer. B-cell chronic lymphocytic leukaemia cells express and release transforming growth factor-beta. Br J Haematol 80:480–487, 1992.

104. M Schena, G Gaidano, D Gottardi, F Malavasi, LG Larsson, K Nilsson, F Caligaris-Cappio. Molecular investigation of the cytokines produced by normal and malignant B lymphocytes. Leukemia 6:120–125, 1992.

105. M Lotz, E Ranheim, TJ Kipps. Transforming growth factor beta as endogenous growth inhibitor of chronic lymphocytic leukemia B cells. J Exp Med 179:999–1004, 1994.

106. LG Israels, SJ Israels, A Begleiter, L Verburg, L Schwartz, MR Mowat, JB Johnston. Role of transforming growth factor-beta in chronic lymphocytic leukemia. Leuk Res 17:81–87, 1993.

107. M Schuler, T Tretter, F Schneller, C Huber, C Peschel. Autocrine transforming growth factor-beta from chronic lymphocytic leukemia-B cells interferes with proliferative T cell signals. Immunobiology 200:128–139, 1999.

108. L Lagneaux, A Delforge, D Bron, M Massy, M Bernier, P Stryckmans. Heterogenous response of B lymphocytes to transforming growth factor-beta in B-cell chronic lymphocytic leukaemia: correlation with the expression of TGF-beta receptors. Br J Haematol 97:612–620, 1997.

109. JF DeCoteau, PI Knaus, H Yankelev, MD Reis, R Lowsky, HF Lodish, ME Kadin. Loss of functional cell surface transforming growth factor β (TGF-β) type I receptor correlates with insensitivity to TGF-β in chronic lymphocytic leukemia. Proc Natl Acad Sci USA 94:5877–5881, 1997.

110. C Buske, D Becker, M Feuring-Buske, H Hannig, G Wuef, C Schofer, W Hiddemann, B Wormann. TGF-β inhibits growth and induces apoptosis in leukemic B cell precursors. Leukemia 11:386–392, 1997.

111. RS Douglas, RJ Capocasale, RJ Lamb, PC Nowell, JS Moore. Chronic lymphocytic leukemia B cells are resistant to the apoptotic effects of transforming growth factor-β. Blood 89:941–947, 1997.

112. L Lagneaux, A Delforge, M Bernier, P Stryckmans, D Bron. TGF-β activity and expression of its receptors in B-cell chronic lymphocytic leukemia. Leuk Lymphoma 31:99–106, 1998.

113. L Lagneaux, A Delforge, C Dorval, D Bron, P Stryckmans. Excessive production of transforming growth factor-beta by bone marrow stromal cells in B-cell chronic lymphocytic leukemia inhibits growth of hematopoietic precursors and interleukin-6 production. Blood 82:2379–2385, 1993.

114. H Maeda, A Shiraishi. TGF-beta contributes to the shift toward Th2-type responses through direct and IL-10 mediated pathways in tumor-bearing mice. J Immunol 156:73–78, 1996.

115. T Nakamura, RK Lee, SY Nam, BK Al-Ramadi, PA Koni, K Bottomly, ER Podack, RA Flavell. Reciprocal regulation of CD30 expression on CD4+ T cells by IL-4 and IFN-gamma. J Immunol 158:2090–2098, 1997.

116. R Manetti, F Annunziato, R Biagioth, MG Giudizi, MP Piccinni, L Giannarini, S Sampognaro, P Parronchi, F Vinante, G Pizzolo. CD30 expression by CD8+ T cells producing type 2 helper cytokines. Evidence for large numbers of CD8+CD30+ T cell clones in human immunodeficiency virus infection. J Exp Med 180:2407–2411, 1994.

117. G Del Prete, M De Carli, F Almerigogna, CK Daniel, MM D'Elios, G Zancuoghi, F Vinante, G Pizzolo, S Romagnani. Preferential expression of CD30 by human CD4+ T cells producing Th2-type cytokines. FASEB J 9:81–86, 1995.

118. V Gattei, M Degan, A Gloghini, A De Iuliis, S Improta, FM Rossi, D Aldinucci, V Perin, D Serraino, R Babare, V Zagonel, HJ Gruss, A Carbone, A Pinto. CD30 ligand is frequently expressed in human hematopoietic malignancies of myeloid and lymphoid origin. Blood 89: 2048–2059, 1997.

119. L Trentin, R Zambello, R Sancetta, M Facco, A Cerutti, A Perin, M Siviero, U Basso, M Bortolin, F Adami, C Agostini, G Semenzato. B lymphocytes from patients with chronic lymphoproliferative disorders are equipped with different costimulatory molecules. Cancer Res 57:4940–4947, 1997.

120. M Vukmanovic-Stejic, B Vyas, P Gorak-Stolinska, A Noble, DM Kemeny. Human Tc1 and Tc2/Tc0 CD8 T-cell clones display distinct cell surface and functional phenotypes. Blood 95:231–240, 2000.

121. WG Telford, SY Nam, ER Podack, RA Miller. CD30-regulated apoptosis in murine CD8 T cells after cessation of TCR signals. Cell Immunol 182:125–136, 1997.

122. I Stamenkovic, EA Clark, B Seed. A B-lymphocyte activation molecule related to the nerve growth factor receptor and induced by cytokines in carcinomas. EMBO J 8:1403–1410, 1989.

123. YJ Liu, DE Joshua, GT Williams, CA Smith, J Gordon, IC MacLennan. Mechanism of antigen-driven selection in germinal centres. Nature 342:929–931, 1989.

124. S Lederman, MJ Yellin, AM Cleary, A Pernis, G Inghirami, LE Cohn, LR Covey, JJ Lee, P Rothman, L Chess. T-BAM/CD40-L on helper T lymphocytes augments lymphokine-

induced B cell Ig isotype switch recombination and rescues B cells from programmed cell death. J Immunol 152:2163–2171, 1994.

125. S Saeland, V Duvert, T Moreau, J Banchereau. Human B cell precursors proliferate and express CD23 after CD40 ligation. J Exp Med 178:113–120, 1993.

126. TL Rothstein, JK Wang, DJ Panka, LC Foote, Z Wang, B Stanger, H Cui, ST Ju, A Marshak-Rothstein. Protection against Fas-dependent Th1-mediated apoptosis by antigen receptor engagement in B cells. Nature 374:163–165, 1995.

127. S Lederman, MJ Yellin, A Krichevsky, J Belko, JJ Lee, L Chess. Identification of a novel surface protein on activated CD4+ T cells that induces contact-dependent B cell differentiation (help). J Exp Med 175:1091–1101, 1992.

128. M Koshy, D Berger, MK Crow. Increased expression of CD40 ligand on systemic lupus erythematosus lymphocytes. J Clin Invest 98:826–837, 1996.

129. G Inghirami, S Lederman, MJ Yellin, A Chadburn, L Chess, DM Knowles. Phenotypic and functional characterization of T-BAM (CD40 ligand)+ T-cell non-Hodgkin's lymphoma. Blood 84:866–872, 1994.

130. AV Moses, SE Williams, JG Strussenberg, ML Heneveld, RA Ruhl, AC Bakke, GC Bagby, JA Nelson. HIV-1 induction of CD40 on endothelial cells promote the outgrowth of AIDS-associated B-cell lymphomas. Nat Med 3:1242–1249, 1997.

131. D Graf, S Muller, U Korthauer, C van Kooten, C Weise, RA Kroczel. A soluble form of TRAP (CD40 ligand) is rapidly released after T cell activation. Eur J Immunol 25:1749–1754, 1995.

132. JA Ledbetter, G Shu, M Gallagher, EA Clark. Augmentation of normal and malignant B cell proliferation by monoclonal antibody to the B cell-specific antigen BP50 (CDW40). J Immunol 138:788–794, 1987.

133. DH Crawford, D Catovsky. In vitro activation of leukaemic B cells by interleukin-4 and antibodies to CD40. Immunology 80:40–44, 1993.

134. R Buhmann, A Nolte, D Westhaus, B Emmerich, M Hallek. CD40-activated B-cell chronic lymphocytic leukemia cells for tumor immunotherapy: stimulation of allogeneic versus autologous T cells generates different types of effector cells. Blood 93:1992–2002, 1999.

135. S Kitada, JM, Zapata, M Andreeff, JC Reed. Bryostatin and CD40-ligand enhance apoptosis resistance and induce expression of cell survival genes in B-cell chronic lymphocytic leukaemia. Br J Heamatol 106:995–1004, 1999.

136. N Laytragoon-Lewin, E Duhony, XF Bai, H Mellstedt. Downregulation of the CD95 receptor and defect CD40-mediated signal transduction in B-chronic lymphocytic leukemia cells. Eur J Haematol 61:266–271, 1998.

137. K Kato, MJ Cantwell, S Sharma, TJ Kipps. Gene transfer of CD40-ligand induces autologous immune recognition of chronic lymphocytic leukemia B cells. J Clin Invest 101:1133–1141, 1998.

138. TJ Kipps, WG Wierda, SJ Woods, MJ Cantwell, LZ Rassenti, CE Prussak. Gene therapy for CLL. VIII International Workshop in CLL Paris, 1999, p 24.

139. M Cantwell, T Hua, J Pappas, TJ Kipps. Acquired CD40-ligand deficiency in chronic lymphocytic leukemia. Nature Med 3:984–989, 1997.

140. RC Allen, RJ Armitage, ME Conley, H Rosenblatt, NA Jenkins, NG Copeland, MA Bedell, S Edelhoff, CM Disteche, DK Simoneaux. CD40 ligand gene defects responsible for X-linked hyper-IgM syndrome. Science 259:990–993, 1993.

141. EJ Schattner, J Mascarenhas, I Reyfman. Chronic lymphocytic leukemia B cells can express CD40 ligand and demonstrate T-cell type costimulatory capacity. Blood 91:2689–2697, 1998.

142. RR Furman, Z Asgary, JO Mascrenhas, HC Liou, EJ Schattner. Modulation of NF-kappa B activity and apoptosis in chronic lymphocytic leukemia B cells. J Immunol 164:2200–2206, 2000.

143. A Younes, V Snell, U Consoli, K Clodi, S Zhao, JL Palmer, EK Thomas, RJ Armitage,

M Andreeff. Elevated levels of biologically active soluble CD40 ligand in the serum of patients with chronic lymphocytic leukaemia. Br J Haematol 100:135–141, 1998.

144. K Kato, E Santana-Sahagun, LZ Rassenti, MH Weisman, N Tamura, S Kobayashi, H Hashimoto, TJ Kipps. The soluble CD40 ligand sCD154 in systemic lupus erythematosus. J Clin Invest 104:947–955, 1999.

145. MF Romano, A Lamberti, P Tassone, F Alfinito, S Costantini, F Chiurazzi, T Defrance, P Bonelli, F Tuccillo, MC Turco, S Venuta. Triggering of CD40 antigen inhibits fludarabine-induced apoptosis in B chronic lymphocytic leukemia cells. Blood 92:990–995, 1998.

146. MF Romano, A Lamberti, MC Turco, S Venuta. CD40 and B chronic lymphocytic leukemia cell response to fludarabine: the influence of NF-kappaB/Rel transcription factors on chemotherapy-induced apoptosis. Leuk Lymphoma 36:255–262, 2000.

147. S Yonehara, A Ishii, M Yonehara. A cell-killing monoclonal antibody (anti-Fas) to a cell surface antigen co-downregulated with the receptor of tumor necrosis factor. J Exp Med 169: 1747–1756, 1989.

148. T Suda, T Takahashi, P Goldstein, S Nagata. Molecular cloning and expression of the Fas ligand, a novel member of the tumor necrosis factor family. Cell 75:1169–1178, 1993.

149. F Rieux-Laucat, F Le Deist, C Hivroz, IA Roberts, KM Debatin, A Fisher, JP de Villartay. Mutations in Fas as associated with human lymphoproliferative syndrome and autoimmunity. Science 268:1347–1349, 1995.

150. F Le Deist, JF Emile, F Rieux-Laucat, M Benkerrou, I Roberts, N Brousse, A Fisher. Clinical, immunological, and pathological consequences of Fas-deficient conditions. Lancet 348:719–723, 1996.

151. KM Latinis, LL Carr, EJ Peterson, LA Norian, SL Eliason, GA Koretzky. Regulation of CD95 (Fas) ligand expression by TCR-mediated signaling events. J Immunol 158:4602–4611, 1997.

152. M Hahne, T Renno, M Schroeter, M Irmler, L French, T Bornard, HR MacDonald, J Tschopp. Activated B cells express functional Fas ligand. Eur J Immunol 26:721–724, 1996.

153. PR Walker, P Saas, PY Dietrich. Role of Fas ligand (CD95L) in immune escape: The tumor cell strikes back. J Immunol 158:4521–4524, 1997.

154. P Panayiotidis, K Ganeshaguru, L Foroni, AV Hoffbrand. Expression and function of the FAS antigen in B chronic lymphocytic leukemia and hairy cell leukemia. Leukemia 9:1227–1232, 1995.

155. S Kamihira, Y Yamada, Y Hirakata, K Tsuruda, K Sugahara, M Tomonaga, T Maeda, K Tsukasaki, S Atogami, N Kobayashi. Quantitative characterization and potential function of membrane Fas/APO-1 (CD95) receptors on leukemic cells from chronic B and T lymphoid leukemias. Br J Haematol 99:858–865, 1997.

156. K Tsuruda, Y Yamada, Y Hirakata, K Sugahara, T Maeda, S Atogami, M Tomonaga, S Kamihira. Qualitative and quantitative characterization of Fas (APO-1/CD95) on leukemic cells derived from patients with B-cell neoplasms. Leukemia Res 23:159–166, 1999.

157. E Knipping, KM Debatin, K Stricker, B Heilig, A Eder, PH Krammer. Identification of soluble APO-1 in supernatants of human B- and T-cell lines and increased serum levels in B- and T-cell leukemias. Blood 85:1562–1569, 1995.

158. MY Mapara, R Bargou, C Zugck, H Dohner, F Ustaoglu, RR Jonker, PH Krammer, B Dorken. APO-1 mediated apoptosis or proliferation in human chronic B lymphocytic leukemia: correlation with bcl-2 oncogene expression. Eur J Immunol 23:702–708, 1993.

159. D Wang, GJ Freeman, H Levine, J Ritz, MJ Robertson. Role of the CD40 and CD95 (APO-1/Fas) antigens in the apoptosis of human B-cell malignancies. Br J Haematol 97: 409–417, 1997.

160. AR Thilenius, K Braun, JH Russell. Agonist antibody and Fas ligand mediate different sensitivity to death in the signaling pathways of Fas and cytoplasmic mutants. Eur J Immunol 27:1108–1114, 1997.

161. JF Williams, MJ Petrus, JA Wright, A Husebekk, V Fellowes, EJ Read, RE Gress,

DH Fowler. Fas-mediated lysis of chronic lymphocytic leukaemia cells: role of type I versus type II cytokines and autologous FasL-expressing T cells. Br J Haematol 107:99–105, 1999.

162. I Tinhofer, I Marschitz, M Kos, T Henn, A Egle, A Villunger, R Greil. Differential sensitivity of CD4+ and CD8+ T lymphocytes to the killing efficacy of Fas (Apo-1/CD95) ligand+ tumor cells in B chronic lymphocytic leukemia. Blood 91:4273–4281, 1998.

163. P Dormer, H Theml, B Lau. Chronic lymphocytic leukemia: A proliferative or accumulative disorder? Leuk Res 7:1–10, 1983.

164. E Kimby, H Mellstedt, B Nilsson, B Tribukait, M Bjorkholm, G Holm. S-phase lymphocytes in chronic lymphocytic leukemia (CLL) in relation to immunoglobulin isotypes on the leukemic clone and to disease activity. Leukemia 1:432–436, 1987.

165. E Montserrat, J Sanchez-Bisono, N Vinolas, C Rozman. Lymphocyte doubling time in chronic lymphocytic leukemia: Analysis of its prognostic significance. Br J Haematol 62: 567–575, 1986.

166. DL Vaux, S Cory, JM Adams. Bcl-2 gene promotes haemopoietic cell survival and cooperates with c-myc to immortalize pre-B cells. Nature 335:440–442, 1988.

167. E Yang, SJ Korsmeyer. Molecular thanatopsis. A discourse on the bcl-2 family and cell death. Blood 88:386–401, 1996.

168. C Reed. Double identity for proteins of the bcl2 family. Nature 387:773–776, 1997.

169. Y Tsujimoto, J Cossman, E Jaffe, GM Croce. Involvement of the bcl-2 gene in human follicular lymphoma. Science 228:1440–1443, 1985.

170. ML Cleary, SD Smith, J Sklar. Cloning and structural analysis of cDNAs for bcl2 and a hybrid bcl-2/immunoglobulin transcript resulting from the t(14;18) translocation. Cell 47: 19–28, 1986.

171. M Schena, LG Larsson, D Gottardi, G Gaidano, M Carlsson, K Nilsson, F Caligaris-Cappio. Growth- and differentiation-associated expression of bcl-2 in B-chronic lymphocytic leukemia cells. Blood 79:2981–2989, 1992.

172. M Hanada, D Delia, A Aiello, E Stadtmauer, JC Reed. bcl-2 gene hypomethylation and high-level expression in B-cell chronic lymphocytic leukemia. Blood 82:1820–1828, 1993.

173. C Pepper, P Bentley, T Hoy. Regulation of clinical chemoresistance by bcl-2 and bax oncoproteins in B-cell chronic lymphocytic leukemia. Br J Haematol 95:513–517, 1996.

174. M Aguilar-Santelises, ME Rottenberg, N Lewin, H Mellstedt, M Jondal. Bcl-2, Bax, and p53 expression in B-cell in relation to in vitro survival and clinical progression. Int J Cancer 69:114–117, 1996.

175. C Pepper, T Hoy, DP Bentley. Bcl-2/Bax ratios in chronic lymphocytic leukaemia and their correlation with in vitro apoptosis and clinical resistance. Br J Cancer 76:935–938, 1997.

176. ZN Oltvai, CL Milliman, SJ Korsmeyer. Bcl-2 heterodimerizes in vivo with a conserved homologue, Bax, that accelerates programmed cell death. Cell 74:609–619, 1993.

177. DJ McConkey, J Chandra, S Wright, W Plunkett, TJ McDonnell, JC Reed, M Keating. Apoptosis sensitivity in chronic lymphocytic leukemia is determined by endogenous endonuclease content and relative expression of BCL-2 and BAX. J Immunol 156:2624–2630, 1996.

178. A Thomas, S el Rouby, JC Reed, S Krajewski, M Potmesil, EW Newcomb. Drug-induced apoptosis in B-cell chronic lymphocytic leukemia: Relationship of p53 gene mutation, bcl-2/bax proteins in drug resistance. Oncogene 12:1055–1062, 1996.

179. C Pepper, A Thomas, T Hoy, P Bentley. Chlorambucil resistance in B-cell chronic lymphocytic leukaemia is mediated through failed Bax induction and selection of high Bcl-2-expressing subclones. Br J Heamatol 104:581–588, 1999.

180. AP Jewell, CP Worman, PM Lydyard, KL Yong, FJ Giles, AH Goldstone. Interferon-alpha up-regulates bcl-2 expression and protects B-CLL cells from apoptosis in vitro and in vivo. Br J Heamatol 88:268–274, 1994.

181. C Pepper, A Thomas, T Hoy, F Cotter, P Bentley. Antisense-mediated suppression of Bcl-2 highlights its pivotal role in failed apoptosis in B-cell chronic lymphocytic leukaemia. Br J Haematol 107:611–615, 1999.

182. AJ Levine. p53, the cellular gatekeeper for growth and cell division. Cell 88:323–331, 1997.

183. ME McCurrach, TMF Connor, CM Knudson, SJ Korsmeyer, SW Lowe. Bax-deficiency promotes drug resistance and oncogenic transformation by attenuating p53-dependent apoptosis. Proc Natl Acad Sci USA 94:2345–2349, 1997.

184. HJ Brady, GS Salomons, RC Bobeldijk, AJ Berns. T cells from baxalpha transgenic mice show accelerated apoptosis in response to stimuli but do not show restored DNA damage-induced cell death in the absence of p53. EMBO J 15:1221–1230, 1996.

185. AJ Levine, J Momand, CA Finlay. The p53 tumour suppressor gene. Nature 351:453–456, 1991.

186. DP Lane. p53 guardian of the genome. Nature 358:15–16, 1992.

187. M Hollstein, D Sidransky, D Vogelstein, CC Harris. p53 mutations in human cancers. Science 253:49–53, 1991.

188. M Prokocimer, V Rotter. Structure and function of p53 in normal cells and their aberrations in cancer cells: Projections on the hematologic cell lineages. Blood 84:2391–2411, 1994.

189. JV Gannon, R Greaves, R Iggo, DP Lane. Activating mutations in p53 produce a common conformational effect. A monoclonal antibody specific for the mutant form. EMBO J 9:1595–1602, 1990.

190. S el Rouby, A Thomas, D Costin, CR Rosenberg, M Potmesil, R Silber, EW Newcomb. p53 gene mutation in B-cell chronic lymphocytic leukemia is associated with drug resistance and is independent of MDR1/MDR3 gene expression. Blood 82:3452–3459, 1993.

191. E Wattel, C Preudhomme, B Hecquet, M Vanrumbeke, B Quesnel, I Dervitte, P Morel, P Fenaux. p53 mutations are associated with resistance to chemotherapy and short survival in hematologic malignancies. Blood 84:3148–3157, 1994.

192. G Gaidano, P Ballerini, JZ Gong, G Inghirami, A Neri, EW Newcomb, IT Magrath, DM Knowles, R Dalla-Favera. p53 mutations in human lymphoid malignancies: Association with Burkitt lymphoma and chronic lymphocytic leukemia. Proc Natl Acad Sci USA 88:5413–5417, 1991.

193. I Cordone, S Masi, FR Mauro, S Soddu, O Morsilli, T Valentini, ML Vegna, C Guglielmi, F Mancini, S Giuliacci, A Sacchi, F Mandelli, R Foa. p53 expression on B-cell chronic lymphocytic leukemia: A marker of disease progression and poor prognosis. Blood 91:4342–4349, 1998.

194. D Sidransky, T Mikkelsen, K Schwechheimer, ML Rosenblum, W Cavanee, B Vogelstein. Clonal expansion of p53 mutant cells is associated with brain tumour progression. Nature 355:846–847, 1992.

195. H Wada, M Asada, S Nakazawa, H Itoh, Y Kobayashi, T Inoue, K Fukumoro, LC Han, K Sugita, R Hanada, N Akuta, N Kobayashi, S Mizutani. Clonal expansion of p53 mutant cells in leukemia progression in vitro. Leukemia 8:53–59, 1994.

196. A Thomas, S el Rouby, JC Reed, S Krajewski, R Silber, M Potmesil, EW Newcomb. Drug-induced apoptosis in B-cell chronic lymphocytic leukemia: relationship between p53 gene mutation and bcl-2/bax proteins in drug resistance. Oncogene 12:1055–1062, 1996.

197. F Morabito, M Filangeri, I Callea, G Sculli, V Callea, NS Fracchiolla, A Neri, M Brugiatelli. Bcl-2 protein expression and p53 gene mutation in chronic lymphocytic leukemia: correlation with in vitro sensitivity to chlorambucil and purine analogs. Haematologica 82:16–20, 1997.

198. S Kitada, J Andersen, S Akar, JM Zapata, S Takayama, S Krajenski, HG Wang, X Zhang, F Bullrich, CM Croce, K Rai, J Hines, JC Reed. Expression of apoptosis-regulating proteins in chronic lymphocytic leukemia: Correlations with in vitro and in vivo chemoresponses. Blood 9:3379–3389, 1998.

199. AR Pettitt, PD Sherrington, JC Cawley. The effect of p53 dysfunction on purine analogue cytotoxicity in chronic lymphocytic leukaemia. Br J Haematol 106:1049–1051, 1999.

200. R Silber, B Degar, D Costin, EW Newcomb, M Mani, CR Rosenberg, L Morse, JC Drygas, ZN Canellakis, M Potmesil. Chemosensitivity of lymphocytes from patients with B-cell

chronic lymphocytic leukemia to chlorambucil, fludarabine, and camptothecin analogs. Blood 84:3440–3446, 1994.

201. JB Johnston, P Daeninck, L Verburg, K Lee, G Williams, LG Israels, MR Mowat, A Begleiter. p53, MDM-2, BAX and BCL-2 and drug resistance in chronic lymphocytic leukemia. Leuk Lymphoma 26:435–449, 1997.

202. E Wattel, C Preudhomme, B Hecquet, M Vanrumbeke, B Quesnel, I Dervite, P Morel, P Fenaux. p53 mutations are associated with resistance to chemotherapy and short survival in hematologic malignancies. Blood 84:3148–3157, 1994.

203. CJ Sherr. Gl phase progression: cycling on cue. Cell 79:551–555, 1994.

204. S Van den Heuvel, E Harlow. Distinct roles for cyclin-dependent kinases in cell cycle control. Science 262:2050–2054, 1993.

205. K Ando, F Ajchenbaum-Cymbalista, JD Griffin. Regulation of Gl/S transition by cyclins D2 and D3 in hematopoietic cells. Proc Natl Acad Sci USA 90:9571–9575, 1993.

206. F Ajchenbaum, K Ando, JA DeCaprio, JD Griffin. Independent regulation of human D-type cyclin gene expression during Gl phase in primary human T lymphocytes. J Biol Chem 268: 4113–4119, 1993.

207. T Hunter, J Pines. Cyclins and cancer II: cyclin D and CDK inhibitors come of age. Cell 79:573–582, 1994.

208. CJ Sherr, JM Roberts. Inhibitors of mammalian Gl cyclin-dependent kinases. Genes Dev 9: 1149–1163, 1995.

209. K Polyak, MH Lee, H Erdjument-Bromage, A Koff, JM Roberts, P Tempst, J Massague. Cloning of p27[Kipl], a cyclin-dependent kinase inhibitor and a potential mediator of extracellular antimitogenic signals. Cell 78:59–66, 1994.

210. H Toyoshima, T Hunter. p27, a novel inhibitor of Gl cyclin-Cdk protein kinase activity, is related to p21. Cell 78:67–74, 1994.

211. K Polyak, JY Kato, MJ Solomon, CJ Sherr, J Massague, JM Roberts, A Koff. p27Kipl, a cyclin-Cdk inhibitor, links transforming growth factor-beta and contact inhibition to cell cycle arrest. Genes Dev 8:9–22, 1994.

212. BL Harvat, P Seth, AM Jetten. The role of p27Kipl in gamma interferon-mediated growth arrest of mammary epithelial cells and related defects in mammary carcinoma cells. Oncogene 14:2111–2122, 1997.

213. RM Yang, J Naitoh, M Murphy, HJ Wang, J Philipson, JB deKernion, M Loda, RE Reiter. Low p27 expression predicts poor disease-free survival in patients with prostate cancer. J Urol 159:941–945, 1998.

214. M Loda, B Cukor, SW Tam, P Lavin, M Fiorentino, GF Draetta, JM Jessup, M Pagano. Increased proteasome-dependent degradation of the cyclin-dependent kinase inhibitor p27 in aggressive colorectal carcinomas. Nat Med 3:231–234, 1997.

215. R Chiarle, LM Budel, J Skolnik, G Frizzera, M Chilosi, A Corato, G Pizzolo, J Magidson, A Montagnoli, M Pagano, B Maes, C De Wolf-Peeters, G Inghirami. Increased proteasome degradation of cyclin-dependent kinase inhibitor p27 is associated with a decreased overall survival in mantle cell lymphoma. Blood 95:619–626, 2000.

216. R Vrhovac, A Delmer, R Tang, JP Marie, R Zittoun, F Ajchenbaum-Cymbalista. Prognostic significance of the cell cycle inhibitor p27[Kipl] in chronic B-cell lymphocytic leukemia. Blood 91:4694–4700, 1998.

217. DA Blanchard, MT Affredou, A Vazquez. Modulation of the p27kipl cyclin-dependent kinase inhibitor expression during IL-4-mediated human B cell activation. J Immunol 58:3054–3061, 1997.

8

Randomized Trials: What Do They Teach Us About Chronic Lymphocytic Leukemia Treatment?

G. DIGHIERO

Institut Pasteur, Paris, France

I. INTRODUCTION

B-cell chronic lymphocytic leukemia (CLL), the most common form of leukemia in Western countries, results from relentless accumulation of small mature, slowly dividing, monoclonal B lymphocytes (1). B-CLL cells are characterized by coexpression of pan B-cell markers CD5 and CD23, negativity for CD22 and FMC7 molecules, and low expression of the B cell receptor surface immunoglobulin and Ig associated molecule CD79b (2–4).

CLL is a heterogeneous disease, with some patients having a long survival and never requiring treatment, whereas in others the disease pursues an aggressive course that demands intensive and expensive treatment, including bone marrow transplantation (1). The development of the Rai (5,6) and Binet (7) staging systems permitted a significant advance in the comprehension of CLL prognosis and allowed the identification of patients with different risk factors and the planning of therapy accordingly.

The aim of this work is to discuss the contribution to therapeutic strategy definition of the different randomized trials carried out in CLL patients. Because an analysis of therapeutic results obtained before the advent of staging systems is almost impossible because of the heterogeneous groups of patients involved, we will limit this review to randomized trials in which patients were stratified according to their clinical stage.

II. STAGING SYSTEMS IN CLL

Although some prognostic factors including sex, age, peripheral lymphocytosis, lymph node and spleen enlargement, anemia, and thrombopenia had been reported to have prognostic value in CLL, the specific importance of each of these factors remained uncertain until the staging proposals of Rai et al. and Binet et al. were published (1,5,6,7).

The modified clinical staging of Rai et al. (5,6) segregates CLL patients into three groups: stage 0 is associated with good prognosis and is characterized by the presence of blood and bone-marrow lymphocytosis only and the absence of anemia and/or thombocytopenia; stages I and II are associated with an intermediate prognosis and are defined by hyperlymphocytosis plus either enlarged lymph nodes and/or hepatomegaly, or splenomegaly, or both and the absence of anemia and/or thombocytopenia; stages III and IV are associated with a poor prognosis and are characterized by lymphocytosis, anemia, and/or thombocytopenia (nodes, spleen or liver may or may not be enlarged). The prognostic value of this staging system has been validated by several investigators (8–10).

The Binet (7) staging system includes three groups: stage A (good prognosis) is characterized by the involvement of less than three lymphoid areas (areas include the cervical, axillary, and inguinal lymph nodes, whether unilateral or bilateral, and the spleen and liver) and no anemia or thrombocytopenia; stage B, at least three areas involved and no anemia or thrombocytopenia; stage C, anemia and/or thrombocytopenia (independent of the areas involved). The validity of this system has been confirmed in six retrospective series and in a prospective series of 973 cases (8–10).

Comparison of both systems in the French series shows that Rai's good prognosis group (stage 0) includes 31% of all CLL patients with a 10-year survival of 59%, whereas Binet's good prognosis group (stage A) includes 63% of CLL patients, with a 10-year survival of 51% (8–11). Two-thirds of Rai's stage I and one-third of Rai's stage II (considered intermediate prognosis) are also included in Binet's stage A good prognosis group. The intermediate prognosis group (stage B) in Binet's system includes 30% of patients who have a poorer prognosis (median, 57 months) than the intermediate group of Rai (stages I and II), which includes 59% of patients, with a median survival of 83 months (8). Finally, because the cutoff value for Hb is 100 g/L in Binet's staging and 110 g/L in Rai's, fewer patients are included in Binet's high-risk group (7% for stage C) than Rai's staging (11% for stages III + IV).

Clinical staging systems other than those of Rai and Binet have been proposed in CLL (9,12,13), but they have not been used extensively in clinical practice. The International Workshop in CLL (14) recommended the adoption of an integrated Binet-Rai staging system, in which the Binet stage (A, B, C) was to be further defined by adding the appropriate Rai stage (0, I, II, III, or IV).

III. TREATMENT OF INDOLENT CLL

It is not clear whether early therapy benefits patients with indolent CLL. This form of the disease includes patients with a median age of 64 years and a survival greater than 10 years.

In indolent CLL, chlorambucil given daily or intermittently, alone or in combination with corticosteroids, is the most commonly used drug. It often provides a period of relief from any symptoms, even in advanced disease. However, there has been much uncertainty as to whether such chemotherapy should be started immediately or whether this therapy could be appropriately deferred until required for symptomatic relief. Several randomized trials have been activated to address this question.

The French Cooperative Group in CLL, activated two long-term trials (CLL-80 and CLL-85) in stage A patients addressing this question (11). In the CLL-80 trial (mean follow-up > 11 years), early therapy with chlorambucil (CB) in a daily continuous schedule (dCB) was compared with a watch-and-wait policy, whereas in the CLL-85 trial (mean follow-up > 6 years) an intermittent schedule of CB and prednisone (CBPr) was compared with a watching policy. The CLL-80 and 85 trials included, respectively, 609 and 926 previously untreated CLL stage A patients randomly assigned according to a first intention to treat basis between no treatment (CLL-80, 308 patients) and (CLL-85; 466 patients) or dCB (301 patients, CLL-80) or CBPr (460 patients, CLL-85 trial). End points were overall survival, treatment response, and disease progression.

In 1990, a previous report from the same group described the initial results of the CLL-80 trial, which showed that survival of patients treated immediately after diagnosis was similar to that of patients randomly assigned to the abstention arm (15). A further expanded report of the same group provided long-term results of the CLL-80 trial and reported the results from the CLL-85 trial (11).

In the CLL-80 trial, 344 deaths were reported at the reference date; 169 in the abstention group (10-year survival of 54%) and 175 in the dCB group with a 10-year survival of 47% (relative risk 1.14 $P = 0.23$). A benefit for dCB in slowing disease progression was observed ($P = 0.02$). Progression of disease to stages B or C was significantly decreased in the dCB group; 127 patients from the first group entered stage B or C compared with only 102 patients in the second group. However, the 5-year survival of patients progressing in the dCB group was significantly shorter, 45% in the nontreated group compared with 18% in the chlorambucil group ($P < 0.0001$). At the reference date (mean follow-up > 11 years), 27% of patients randomly assigned to defer therapy had died from causes related to CLL (31% in the initially treated group), and 158 patients (51%) had been shifted to treatment during stage A (97), stage B (44), or stage C (17). There were more deaths related to CLL in the CB group, 96 versus 87, and interestingly more deaths related to neoplasia in the CB group (28 versus 22). Moreover, within the dCB group, a tendency to higher incidence of neoplasia was observed (66 versus 48 in the abstention group).

In the CLL-85 trial, 247 deaths had been recorded at the reference date, 126 in the ABS group and 121 in the CBPr group (7-year survival of 69% for both groups; relative risk = 0.96; $P = 0.74$). Patients responsive to treatment (69%) displayed better survival ($P < 0.001$) than patients who failed to respond. CBPr succeeded in slowing disease progression ($P = 0.004$), although survival of patients progressing on the CBPr was significantly shorter ($P < 0.002$). At the reference date (mean follow-up > 6 years) 189 patients from the abstention arm (41%) had been shifted to receive treatment while being in stage A ($n = 107$), stage B ($n = 63$), or stage C ($n = 19$). In conclusion, both trials demonstrate that CB either in a continuous or in an intermittent schedule accompanied by Pr is unable to prolong survival in these patients. Because deferring therapy until it is required by disease progression to stages B or C does not compromise the survival of these patients, initial therapy could have been appropriately deferred for this group of CLL patients, comprising 63% of patients afflicted with this disease. However, these results also show that 27% of stage A CLL patients will die of causes related to disease, 41% will progress to stages B and C, and more than half of these patients will need therapy during evolution. This is also true for stage 0 from Rai, in which 25% of patients will die of causes related to the disease, and 42% will require treatment during evolution.

The establishment of the International Workshop on CLL (IWCLL) group allowed the sharing of results. To further investigate the advantages of early therapy with CB compared with deferred treatment for stage A CLL patients, series from the MRC-CLL1 trial (78 patients), the MRC-CLL2 (239 patients) (16), the CALGB (45 patients) (17), the French Cooperative trials 80 (609 patients) and 85 (926 patients) (11,15), and from the PETHEMA (157 patients) (18) were pooled together (19).

The results of the treatment comparison for all deaths when collated suggest that in terms of survival there is certainly no evidence that treating patients immediately with standard chlorambucil treatments prolongs survival (11,19). Because more than 50% of early stage patients may die of other causes, patients whose cause of death was definitely not CLL have been censored. Again, this analysis clearly showed that early treatment was unable to prolong survival in indolent CLL.

When segregating patients according to the French stage A' and A", no demonstrable benefit was observed for early treatment. Although survival differed among these A' and A" patients, there is no evidence that treatment is advantageous for any one group (19).

Although these results demonstrate that chlorambucil in classical schedules fails to influence survival in indolent CLL, it has been proposed that high-dose continuous CB influences CLL survival. The IgC ICLL 01 trial (20) compared the classical intermittent chlorambucil plus prednisone schedule to high-dose chlorambucil (15 mg fixed dose daily to either complete remission or toxicity or to a maximum of 6 months). A significant difference in response, which also translated into a survival difference in favor of high-dose chlorambucil, was observed.

Altogether, these results suggest that standard therapy with chlorambucil is unable to influence survival and that treatment for these patients, whose median survival is longer than 10 years, could have been appropriately deferred.

As for the role of prednisone in CLL treatment (21,22), only limited data could be collected (120 randomized patients), and this sort of number gives very wide confidence intervals. Nevertheless, it appears that prednisone does not increase the effectiveness of chlorambucil.

Although the Rai and Binet staging systems have succeeded in identifying patients with a favorable prognosis (Rai's stage 0 and Binet's stage A), >25% of these patients still die of causes related to CLL, and about 50% of them require treatment during the course of disease (11). Thus, early identification of those patients who will not evolve, (i.e., definition of smouldering CLL) is an important goal to better define therapeutical strategies).

IV. SMOULDERING CLL

The French group proposed a classification dividing stage A into A' A" (11,23). Criteria for A' were hemoglobin level greater than 120 g/L and lymphocyte count lower than 30,000/mm^3 and for A" haemoglobin less than 120 g/L and/or lymphocytosis greater than 30,000/mm^3. The survival of these two groups was clearly different with a 5-year survival of 82% in the A' group and 62% in the A" group. Interestingly, the survival of the A' group was very close to that of a sex- and age-matched French population (11,23).

In a further step to define smouldering CLL, the 609 patients included in the CLL-80 trial were classified according to A, A′, A″, stage 0 from Rai and Montserrat's proposal (23). A′ accounted for 80% of stage A, smouldering CLL according to Montserrat 58%, and stage 0 48%. Five-year survival was, respectively, 87%, 88%, and 89%, for these three groups of patients and 5-year freedom of disease progression was, respectively, 75%, 80%, and 84% (23). In addition, the long-term results of the CLL-80 trials showed that death related to CLL was observed in 25% of Rai's stage 0 patients (including 40% of stage A patients) and 27% of A′ patients (including 80% of stage A patients). Therapy was required for 43% of patients within Rai's 0 and for 51% of A′ patients.

Although the choice between different proposals remains arbitrary, a definition of smouldering CLL appears feasible. Whatever the definition used, survival rates of patients are similar to those of the normal population. However, approximately 10% of patients with smouldering CLL will progress to stage C within 5 years, >25% of these patients will die from CLL, and 50% of these patients will need treatment. These results further emphasize the need for a better understanding of the mechanisms involved in the surveillance of the leukemic population and of the cause of this disease, which hopefully would allow the development of effective new therapeutic approaches. Recent reports indicate that cytogenetic markers (24) and the mutational pattern of Ig V_H genes (25,26) may help early identification of indolent CLL with a more aggressive disease course.

V. TREATMENT OF ADVANCED CLL

In advanced forms of the disease, single- and multiple-drug regimens have been proposed. CB alone or in association with corticosteroids in a daily or intermittent schedule has been traditionally used to treat CLL. Ten randomized trials, involving 2035 patients mostly with Binet stage B or C, although some were classified according to Rai's staging system, compared CB with polychemotherapy regimens (COP in four, CHOP in five, and CB plus epirubicin in the remaining one).

The CLL-80 trial from the French Cooperative Group compared daily continuous CB with 12-month COP regimens (one COP regimen during the first 6 months and one every 3 months during 18 months) in 291 previously untreated stage B patients. Long-term results from this trial failed to demonstrate any benefit in response and survival of the COP regimen compared with CB (27). Similar results were observed in an MRC trial, in which 234 patients were randomly allocated to receive CB or COP (18). In addition, a Spanish trial (58 patients) (28) and an Eastern Cooperative Oncology Group trial (99 patients) (29) compared intermittent CB in association with prednisone with the COP regimen and failed to find any difference in terms of survival.

Five different trials compared the CHOP regiment with chlorambucil in advanced symptomatic CLL patients (stages B and/or C and stages III and IV from Rai) and failed to find differences in terms of survival, although better responses were observed for the CHOP regimen (30–33). Only the ISCI trial found a significant difference in response, which was also translated into a survival advantage favoring high-dose CB (34). However, these results have not been reproduced as yet and need to be confirmed.

In the CLL-80 trial, the French Cooperative Group on CLL randomly assigned 70 stage C patients between COP and CHOP (COP plus doxorubicin 25 mg/m² IV day 1) (35–37). Median survival was 22 months with COP and 62 months with CHOP, supporting a beneficial effect of low-dose doxorubicin for stage C patients. However, Jaksic recently detected a better overall response in ''advanced CLL'' with high-dose CLB compared with CHOP (34), and the Eastern Cooperative Oncology Group has reported a median survival of 49 months in stage C patients treated by CLB + PRD or COP, which did not significantly differ with the survival observed in the CLL-80 CHOP arm of the French Cooperative Trial (29). The CHOP regimen has been compared with CLB + PRD in advanced CLL in randomized trials by the Danish and Swedish groups, and no difference in survival could be found (31,32). Although, higher responses with CHOP were observed in all these trials, they failed to translate into a survival advantage.

To analyze the interest of CHOP compared with standard treatments, data from these different groups were pooled for metanalysis study (19). These series had long follow-up and included advanced-stage patients, although not always defined by the same staging system. Although the initial trial from the French Cooperative Group, as well as other groups using anthracycline-containing regimens, generated the hypothesis that CHOP was a better treatment, this was not supported by the following trials. Overall, the collation of data does not show evidence that CHOP actually prolongs survival compared with standard treatment. If deaths not caused by CLL are excluded, there is a possibility that CHOP is superior, but this difference is definitely not significant. Because the French study was confined to stage C patients, subgroups were also analyzed, and again there was no evidence of a different effect. Although the French trial was correctly designed and carried out and its statistical significance clear, metaanalysis studies did not confirm these initial results. Alternatively, the possibility exists that the higher dose of cyclophosphamide used in the French CHOP compared with classical CHOP could have an influence on these results. Recent results from the CLL-90 study, where this schedule was found superior to the classical CAP regimen (37), might support this view.

In nonrandomized trials, other combinations, including MOPP (1), M2 (38), CAP (39), and POACH (40) have given results generally identical to those obtained with CLB.

During the late 1980s, purine analogs emerged as major drugs in CLL and generated a tremendous interest. They were first used in progressive and refractory CLL patients (41–46). Long-term single institution nonrandomized studies indicate that fludarabine (FDB) alone or associated with prednisone is able to induce 30% of true clinical, hematological, and bone marrow biopsy confirmed complete remission, as well as having an overall response rate of about 78%, whereas resistance to FDB is observed in 22% of cases (45). Once complete remission is obtained, the median time to progression of the patients is around 30 months. Most patients appear to relapse, but there is a small subset (10%–15%) of long-term responders, although recurrence can also be expected for them. The median survival of these patients is close to 5 years, which is not different from previous reports in CLL. With regard to relapsing patients, about 60% can be resalvaged with FDB, although the expected duration of response is in the order of 15 months compared with 30 months for initial responders.

Overall, these results indicate that FDB as a single agent or combined with corticosteroids is not curative. Combination with corticosteroids is probably disadvantageous, and combinations with other drugs, in particular cyclophosphamide, are promising (45).

The historical series of the Scripps Clinic experience on the use of 2-chlorodeoxyadenosine (CDA) in the treatment of alkylator failure CLL showed that 4% of these patients obtained a complete remission, and 50% of patients had a partial remission, with an overall response rate of 54% (47). In previously untreated patients, an overall response rate of 85%, with 60% achieving complete remission, was observed (48). Pooling together the different nonrandomized studies, there were 102 patients, 37% of which obtained complete remission using the NCI criteria and 39% of which showed a partial response (49).

CDA has potent activity in CLL. Myelosuppression and infection are the major adverse effects, the long-term impact on progression-free and overall survival remains to be explained. Determination of the relative effectiveness of CDA compared with FDB in the front-line therapy of CLL will ultimately require a randomized study.

These initial results derived from nonrandomized trials indicate that purine analogs may play an important role in CLL treatment, either in front-line therapy or in salvage therapy. To determine whether these drugs improve survival in CLL, two randomized trials compared FDB with anthracyclin-containing regimens, two compared FDB with a classical schedule of CB, and two trials compared FDB with high-dose CB.

A European trial (50) compared FDB therapy with the CAP regimen for treatment of CLL in a randomized, multicenter prospective trial, including 100 previously untreated stage B + C patients and 96 pretreated patients with CB or similar nonanthracycline-containing regimens. Patients were randomly assigned to either fludarabine (25 mg/m^2 per day on days 1–5) or CAP (cyclophosphamide 750 mg/m^2 per day and doxorubicin 50 mg/m^2 per day on day 1, and prednisone 40 mg/m^2 per day on days 1–5), both given for six courses. Remission rates were significantly higher after fludarabine than CAP, with overall response rates of 60% and 44%, respectively ($P = 0.023$). A higher response rate to fludarabine was observed in both untreated (71% vs 60%, $P = 0.26$) and pretreated (48% vs 27%, $P = 0.036$) cases, although the difference was statistically significant only in pretreated cases. In the latter group, remission duration and survival did not differ between treatment groups, with a median remission duration of 324 days after fludarabine and 179 days after CAP ($P = 0.22$) and median survival times of 728 days and 731 days, respectively. In untreated cases, on the other hand, fludarabine induced significantly longer remissions than CAP ($P < 0.001$) although this difference did not translate into a survival advantage. Treatment-associated side effects in both regimens consisted predominantly of myelosuppression and in particular granulocytopenia. CAP-treated patients had a higher frequency and severity of nausea and vomiting (25% vs 5%, $P < 0.001$) and alopecia (65% vs 2%, $P < 0.001$). These results indicate that FDB compared favorably with CAP in terms of response, although this difference did not induce a survival improvement.

In 1990, the French Cooperative Group (37) activated a trial in which previously untreated patients with stage B or C CLL were randomly allocated to receive six monthly courses of either FDB (25 mg/m^2 IV daily for 5 days) or cyclophosphamide (750 mg/m^2 IV day 1), doxorubicin (50 mg/m^2 IV day 1), and prednisone (40 mg/m^2 orally on days 1–5) (CAP), or to the French CHOP regimen consisting of IV vincristin 1 mg/m and doxorubicin 25 mg/m^2 on day 1, plus cyclophosphamide (300 mg/m^2) and prednisone (40 mg/m^2) given orally on days 1 to 5. End points were treatment response, overall survival, and tolerance.

As of January 1, 1999, 938 patients (stage B, 651; stage C, 287) had been enrolled in this trial. Randomization was stratified according to Binet's classification. Main outcomes were overall survival, six-course response, and toxicity-defined secondary end points. In a previous interim analysis (9-02-96), it was found that CAP compared with CHOP and FDB induced lower rates of response, resulting in the discontinuation of accrual in this group.

On January 1, 1999, 350 deaths were recorded and 16 patients lost to follow-up. As expected, median survival was better for stage B (81 months) than for stage C patients (60 months). Causes of death were related to CLL in 75% of cases, and overall survival did not differ between the three arms ($P = 0.32$). Compared with CHOP and fludarabine, CAP was associated with lower rates of response (73%, 73%, 59%, respectively), notably clinical and hematological response (30%, 40%, 15%). The incidence of infections (<5%) and autoimmune hemolytic anemia (<2%) were similar in the randomized groups. Fludrabine induced protracted thrombocytopenia and neutropenia more frequently than CHOP and CAP but was associated with a lower incidence of nausea and vomiting ($P = 0.005$) and hair loss ($P = 0.0001$). Although no survival difference was found between CHOP and FDR, FDB was found to obtain more complete hematological remissions than CHOP and tended to delay recurrent progression and treatment rescue.

A CALGB, SWOG, CTG/NC1-C, and ECOG Inter-group randomized study aimed to compare FDB and CB for patients with previously untreated CLL with active disease (51). The eligibility criteria were all high-risk patients or those intermediate-risk patients who had active disease; all were previously untreated with a performance status of <3. Between October 1990 and December 1994, 544 previously untreated CLL patients with active disease were randomly assigned to receive FDB (25 mg/m^2 IV daily for 5 days) or CB (40 mg/m^2 PO on day 1), or a combination of FDB + CB (20 mg/m^2 of each drug) q4wk for up to 12 months. Nonresponders or responders to FDB or CB alone whose CLL progressed within 6 months of treatment were crossed over to the other arm.

Survival analysis for this report was based on 385 patients. A significantly higher overall response rate was obtained among 167 evaluable patients on FDB (70%) (27% CR + 43% PR) compared with 45% (3% CR + 42% PR) among 173 patients on CB ($P = 0.0001$). Among 119 patients on FDB + CB, 65% responses were noted overall (25% CR + 40% PR). Response duration after FDB was significantly longer than with CB: 117 patients on FDB with either CR or PR had a median duration of response of 32 months versus 18 months among 73 patients on CB ($P = 0.0002$). Similarly, the median progression-free survival time (from study entry to disease progression or death from any cause) was 27 months for patients receiving FDB versus 17 months for patients on CB ($P < 0.0001$).

With a median follow-up of 30 months, there was no difference in overall survival ($P = 0.49$), although this comparison is complicated by the crossover design of the study. An estimated 62% of patients on both arms survived at least 4 years. Seventy-four patients initially treated with CB were transferred to FDB; however, there were only 29 crossovers from FDB to CB. Both drugs were well tolerated with similar toxicity profiles except for a 20% incidence of grade 3 + grade 4 leukopenia with FDB versus 7% with CB ($P = 0.001$). However, toxicities were significantly worse for the combination arm, with a 42% and 45% incidence of thrombocytopenia and neutropenia (grade 3 and grade 4) and approximately twice the frequency of serious grade 3 and 4 infections than the individual one-arm protocols. These results led to the discontinuation of the combination arm somewhat sooner than the total protocol.

An Italian trial (52) compared FDB (classical schedule) with intermittent CB combined with prednisone in 150 advanced CLL patients. Response rates were very close in both arms, which could be explained by the higher dosage of CB used in this study than in the American trial. Response duration was longer in the FDB arm, and toxicity was found to be comparable.

The EORTC started a randomized trial aiming to compare high-dose continuous CB (10 mg/m^2) with FDB at a classical dosage (25 mg/m^2 day 1 to 5 q3wk). This treatment was administered over 18 weeks (53). Eighty-four patients have been enrolled so far in this trial and response evaluation available for 74 patients with a median follow-up of 33 months. Response rates, overall survival, and progression-free survival were comparable in both arms. The German CLL Study Group (54), in a study of younger patients resistant to alkylating agents compared high-dose CB (0.2 mg/kg/day) given continuously during 6 months with FDB (25 mg/m² day 1–3 every 28 days) plus cyclophosphamide (250 mg/m² day 1–3 every 28 days). A higher response rate (88% versus 67%) and lower toxicity was observed for combined FDB and cyclophosphamide.

The Polish Leukemia Study Group (55) compared CDA plus prednisone (CDA at 0.12 mg/kg/day and prednisone at 30 mg/m² during 5 consecutive days each month) with a classical intermittent CB plus prednisone schedule in 229 previously untreated advanced CLL patients. Although the CDA-containing regimen obtained a significantly higher response rate (86% overall response compared with 59% for the CB containing regimen; $P < 0.002$), better response did not translate into survival advantage.

VI. CONCLUSIONS

One of the major advances achieved in CLL treatment is the better identification of patients who should be considered for immediate treatment. The long-term results of the two French Cooperative group trials (11,15) clearly demonstrate that cytotoxic treatment can be appropriately deferred for indolent CLL patients (stage A). These include 65% of CLL patients with a median age of 64 years who have a survival expectancy of >10 years, which is close to the life expectancy of a normal sex- and age-matched population. The meta-analysis study pooling patients from these two large trials plus results from several smaller studies definitively confirm this notion (11,19). The French series also demonstrates that deferring therapy until it is required by disease progression to stages B or C does not compromise survival of these patients, thus reinforcing the notion that therapy should be deferred for these patients until progression is observed (11). This attitude may be reconsidered in the case that new drugs or treatment modalities able to introduce significant improvement in survival of these patients become available. This is particularly important, because the long-term results of the CLL-80 trial with a median follow-up >11 years show that about >25% of patients with indolent disease forms (stage A from Binet or stage 0 from Rai) will die of causes related to CLL, in about 40% the disease will progress to a more advanced stage, and about half of these patients will require treatment during their evolution. However, 50% of these patients will not show any evolution and will die of causes unrelated to CLL. Although both Rai and Binet staging systems succeed well in identifying indolent CLL, they are not able to predict disease progression or disease-related mortality. Recent work on genetic markers like cytogenetic abnormalities (24) and the mutational pattern of immunoglobulin V_H genes seem to be strong prognostic predictors. Although the prognostic significance of the chromosome 13 deletion remains unclear and there is controversy related to the prognosis significance of trisomy 12, chromosome 11 deletion appears to be correlated with tumoral and aggressive forms of the disease (24). Evidence from three different and independent studies shows that the expression of unmutated V_H genes in CLL may correspond to the malignant transformation of a naïve less-differentiated B cell, which is associated with a more aggressive disease form (25,26,56). Although these results require further confirmation, these markers appear to identify those stage A patients who will progress rapidly.

In contrast to indolent CLL, there is consensus that patients belonging to stages B and C of the Binet staging system, whose median survival is, respectively, 81 and 60 months, should be considered for early treatment with cytotoxic drugs. This is also applicable to patients belonging to stages III and IV from Rai and patients with Rai's stages I and II displaying progressive disease as defined by the NCI criteria (57). Results from the different randomized trials activated for this group of patients suggest that combination chemotherapy or purine analogs confer no survival benefit compared with CB with or without steroids. Although the better results observed in the French CHOP compared with classical CHOP and CAP could be attributed to the higher cyclophosphamide dosage, it is possible that this apparent superiority is due to chance. It is important to remember that this trial only included 70 patients, because on the basis of an interim analysis showing a significant difference between the two arms of the study, a decision to stop accrual in the COP group was made.

Despite obtaining higher response rates, chemotherapy regimens like CHOP and purine analogs do not improve survival. It is currently unclear whether the benefit obtained from these treatments is negated by the emergence of complications related to treatment or even by the emergence of resistant clones. In keeping with the latter possibility are the results from the CLL-80 trial of the French Cooperative Group showing that untreated patients evolving to stage B had a 9-year survival after initial randomization of 54% compared with 21% for patients initially randomly assigned to receive CB and evolving to stage B (11). Similar results were found in the CLL-85 trial, which compared survival of patients failing to respond either with CB prednisone or with French CHOP. Patients failing to initially respond to CHOP had a poorer survival than patients failing to respond to the CB schedule (30), which could be compensated for by the higher response rate and better survival observed for those patients initially responding to CHOP.

Alternatively, the absence of a correlation between higher response rate and survival improvement could be the consequence of subsequent treatment regimens received, which may obscure the interpretation of the survival curves. The absence of a survival advantage for FDB in the CALGB, WWOG, CTG/NCI-C, and ECOG Inter-group trials could be explained by unequal response after drug crossover after treatment failure; a significantly higher response rate was observed in patients failing to respond to CB who were subsequently transferred to FDB than for patients transferred from FDR to CB. However, in the French trial in which FDB and CHOP achieved closer response rates, a consistent number of patients was salvaged by the crossing over of CHOP to FDB and vice versa (37).

Another interesting point emerging from the comparison of older and more recent series of patients is the observation of a consistent prolongation of median survival time. For stage C patients, our group of previously untreated patients displayed a median survival of 2 years (7,35,36). It is of interest to note that the same survival patterns were observed in initial Rai's (5) and Hansen (58) initial series. In comparison, current results indicate a survival close to 60 months for these patients in most series. For stage B patients, results from initial French Cooperative Group trials (27,30) showed a median survival of 58 months, whereas in the more recent trial of this group (37), median survival was 81 months. The availability of new drugs like purine analogs or polychemotherapy regimens able to salvage patients failing to respond to initial therapy may explain at least in part this improvement of overall survival in CLL patients.

In these conditions, the prescription of front-line treatment for advanced CLL patients largely depends on the therapeutic strategy. In the case of young patients considered to undergo autologous transplantation and to achieve a complete molecular remission, purine analogs with or without other drugs like cyclophosphamide are the best candidates because of the higher remission rate. In the case of older patients for whom the aim is palliation, CB seems the better solution. For patients not included in the aforementioned categories, the optimal front-line therapy is currently unclear. Some physicians prefer CB as front-line therapy, with the possibility of transferring to CHOP or purine analogs in the case of treatment failure, whereas others, based on the superior response, the longer remission duration, and the better quality of life associated with purine analogs, prefer these drugs as front-line, treatment.

REFERENCES

1. G Dighiero, P Travade, S Chevret, P Fenaux, C Chastang, JL Binet. B-cell chronic lymphocytic leukemia: present status and future directions. French Cooperative Group on CLL. Blood 78: 1901–1914, 1991.

2. E Matutes, K Owusu-Ankomah, R Morilla, et al. The immunological profile of B-cell disorders and proposal of a scoring system for the diagnosis of CLL. Leukemia 8:1640–1645, 1994.

3. AP Zomas, E Matutes, R Morilla, K Owusu-Ankomah, BK Seon, D Catovsky. Expression of the immunoglobulin-associated protein B29 in B cell disorders with the monoclonal antibody SN8 (CD79b). Leukemia 10:1966–1970, 1996.

4. T Ternynck, G Dighiero, J Follezou, JL Binet. Comparison of normal and CLL lymphocyte surface Ig determinants using peroxidase-labeled antibodies. I. Detection and quantitation of light chain determinants. Blood 43:789–795, 1974.

5. KR Rai, A Sawitsky, EP Cronkite, AD Chanana, RN Levy, BS Pasternack. Clinical staging of chronic lymphocytic leukemia. Blood 46:219–234, 1975.

6. KR Rai, T Han. Prognostic factors and clinical staging in chronic lymphocytic leukemia. Hematol Oncol Clin North Am 4:447–456, 1990.

7. JL Binet, A Auquier, G Dighiero, et al. A new prognostic classification of chronic lymphocytic leukemia derived from a multivariate survival analysis. Cancer 48:198–206, 1981.

8. French Cooperative Group on CLL. Prognostic and therapeutic advances in CLL management: the experience of the French Cooperative Group. French Cooperative Group on Chronic Lymphocytic Leukemia. Semin Hematol 24:275–290, 1987.

9. F Mandell, G De Rossi, P Mancini, et al. Prognosis in chronic lymphocytic leukemia: a retrospective multicentric study from the GIMEMA group. J Clin Oncol 5:398–406, 1987.

10. C Rozman, E Montserrat. Chronic lymphocytic leukemia [published erratum appears in N Engl J Med 1995 Nov 30;333(22):1515]. N Engl J Med 333:1052–1057, 1995.

11. G Dighiero, K Maloum, B Desablens, et al. Chlorambucil in indolent chronic lymphocytic leukemia. French Cooperative Group on Chronic Lymphocytic Leukemia [see comments]. N Engl J Med 338:1506–1514, 1998.

12. RW Rundles, JO Moore. Chronic lymphocytic leukemia. Cancer 42:941–945, 1978.

13. B Jaksic, B Vitale. Total tumour mass score (TTM): a new parameter in chronic lymphocyte leukaemia. Br J Haematol 49:405–413, 1981.

14. International Workshop on Chronic Lymphocytic Leukemia. Chronic lymphocytic leukemia: recommendations for diagnosis, staging, and response criteria. Ann Intern Med 110:236–238, 1989.

15. French Cooperative Group on Chronic Lymphocytic Leukemia. Effects of chlorambucil and therapeutic decision in initial forms of chronic lymphocytic leukemia (stage A): results of a randomized clinical trial on 612 patients. Blood 75:1414–1421, 1990.

16. D Catovsky, J Fooks, S Richards. The UK Medical Research Council CLL trials 1 and 2. Nouv Rev Fr Hematol 30:423–427, 1988.

17. C Shustik, R Mick, R Silver, A Sawitsky, K Rai, L Shapiro. Treatment of early chronic lymphocytic leukemia: intermittent chlorambucil versus observation. Hematol Oncol 6:7–12, 1988.

18. Spanish Cooperative Group Pethema. Treatment of Chronic Lymphocytic Leukemia: a preliminary report of Spanish (Pethema) trials. Leuk Lymphoma 5:89–91, 1991.

19. CLL Trialists' Collaborative Group. Chemotherapeutic options in chronic lymphocytic leukemia: a meta-analysis of the randomized trials. CLL Trialists' Collaborative Group. J Natl Cancer Inst 91:861–868, 1999.

20. B Jaksic, M Brugiatelli. High dose continuous chlorambucil vs intermittent chlorambucil plus prednisone for treatment of B-CLL—IGCI CLL-01 trial. Nouv Rev Fr Hematol 30:437–442, 1988.

21. AG Bosanquet, SR McCann, GM Crotty, MJ Mills, D Catovsky. Methylprednisolone in advanced chronic lymphocytic leukaemia: rationale for, and effectiveness of treatment suggested by DiSC assay. Acta Haematol 93:73–79, 1995.

22. S Molica. High-dose dexamethasone in refractory B-cell chronic lymphocytic leukemia patients [letter]. Am J Hematol 47:334, 1994.

23. French Cooperative Group on Chronic Lymphocytic Leukaemia. Natural history of stage A chronic lymphocytic leukaemia untreated patients. Br J Haematol 76:45–57, 1990.

24. H Dohner, S Stilgenbauer, K Dohner, M Bentz, P Lichter. Chromosome aberrations in B-cell chronic lymphocytic leukemia: reassessment based on molecular cytogenetic analysis. J Mol Med 77:266–281, 1999.

25. TJ Hamblin, Z Davis, DG Oscier, FK Stevenson. Unmutated Ig V(H) genes are associated with a more aggressive form of chronic lymphocytic leukemia. Blood 94:1848–1854, 1999.

26. RN Damle, T Wasil, F Fais, et al. Immunoglobulin V gene mutation status and CD38 expression as novel prognostic indicators in chronic lymphocytic leukemia. Blood 1999. In press.

27. French Cooperative Group on Chronic Lymphocytic Leukemia. A randomized clinical trial of chlorambucil versus COP in stage B chronic lymphocytic leukemia. Blood 75:1422–1425, 1990.

28. E Montserrat, A Alcala, R Parody, et al. Treatment of chronic lymphocytic leukemia in advanced stages. A randomized trial comparing chlorambucil plus prednisone versus cyclophosphamide, vincristine, and prednisone. Cancer 56:2369–2375, 1985.

29. B Raphel, JW Andersen, R Silber, et al. Comparison of chlorambucil and prednisone versus cyclophosphamide, vincristine, and prednisone as initial treatment for chronic lymphocytic leukemia: long-term follow-up of an Eastern Cooperative Oncology Group randomized clinical trial. J Clin Oncol 9:770–776, 1991.

30. French Cooperative Group on Chronic Lymphocytic Leukemia. Is the CHOP regimen a good treatment for advanced CLL? Results from two randomized clinical trials. Leuk Lymphoma 13:449–456, 1994.

31. MM Hansen, E Andersen, H Birgens, BE Christensen, TG Christensen, C Geisler. CHOP versus chlorambucil + prednisone in chronic lymphocytic leukemia. Leuk Lymphoma 4:93–96, 1991.

32. E Kimby, H Mellstedt. Chlorambucil/prednisone versus CHOP in symptomatic chronic lymphocytic leukemia of B-cell type. Leuk Lymphoma 4:93–96, 1991.

33. D Catovsky, T Hamblin, S Richards. Preliminary results of the UK medical research council trial in chronic lymphocytic leukaemia-CLL3. Br J Haematol 102:278, 1998.

34. B Jaksic, M Brugiatelli, I Krc, et al. High dose chlorambucil versus Binet's modified cyclophosphamide, doxorubicin, vincristine, and prednisone regimen in the treatment of patients with advanced B-cell chronic lymphocytic leukemia. Results of an international multicenter randomized trial. International Society for Chemo-Immunotherapy, Vienna. Cancer 79:2107–2114, 1997.

35. French Cooperative Group on CLL. Effectiveness of "CHOP" regimen in advanced untreated chronic lymphocytic leukaemia. French Cooperative Group on Chronic Lymphocytic Leukaemia. Lancet 1:1346–1349, 1986.

36. French Cooperative Group on CLL. Long-term results of the CHOP regimen in stage C chronic lymphocytic leukaemia. French Cooperative Group on Chronic Lymphocytic Leukaemia. Br J Haematol 73:334–340, 1989.

37. M Leporrier, S Chevret, B Cazin, et al. Randomized clinical trial comparing two anthracyclin-

containing regimens (ChOP and CAP) and fludarabine (FDR) in advanced Chronic Lymphocytic Leukaemia (CLL) (abstract n. 2682). Blood 94:603a, 1999.

38. S Kempin, BJd Lee, HT Thaler, et al. Combination chemotherapy of advanced chronic lymphocytic leukemia: the M-2 protocol (vincristine, BCNU, cyclophosphamide, melphalan, and prednisone). Blood 60:1110–1121, 1982.

39. JP Hester, EA Gehan. Cytoxan, adriamycin, prednisone (CAP) chemotherapy for chronic lymphocytic leukemia. Proc Am Soc Clin Oncol 19:214, 1978.

40. MJ Keating, M Scouros, S Murphy, et al. Multiple agent chemotherapy (POACH) in previously treated and untreated patients with chronic lymphocytic leukemia. Leukemia 2:157–164, 1988.

41. MR Grever, KJ Kopecky, CA Coltman, et al. Fludarabine monophosphate: a potentially useful agent in chronic lymphocytic leukemia. Nouv Rev Fr Hematol 30:457–459, 1988.

42. LD Piro, CJ Carrera, E Beutler, DA Carson. 2-Chlorodeoxyadenosine: an effective new agent for the treatment of chronic lymphocytic leukemia. Blood 72:1069–1073, 1988.

43. MJ Keating, H Kantarjian, M Talpaz, et al. Fludarabine: a new agent with major activity against chronic lymphocytic leukemia. Blood 74:19–25, 1989.

44. S O'Brien, H Kantarjian, M Beran, et al. Results of fludarabine and prednisone therapy in 264 patients with chronic lymphocytic leukemia with multivariate analysis-derived prognostic model for response to treatment. Blood 82:1695–1700, 1993.

45. MJ Keating, S O'Brien, S Lerner, et al. Long-term follow-up of patients with chronic lymphocytic leukemia (CLL) receiving fludarabine regimens as initial therapy. Blood 92:1165–1171, 1998.

46. JC Byrd, KR Rai, EA Sausville, MR Grever. Old and new therapies in chronic lymphocytic leukemia: now is the time for a reassessment of therapeutic goals. Semin Oncol 25:65–74, 1998.

47. A Saven, LD Piro. 2-Chlorodeoxyadenosine: a potent antimetabolite with major activity in the treatment of indolent lymphoproliferative disorders. Hematol Cell Therap 38:S93–101, 1996.

48. A Saven, RH Lemon, M Kosty, E Beutler, LD Piro. 2-Chlorodeoxyadenosine activity in patients with untreated chronic lymphocytic leukemia. J Clin Oncol 13:570–574, 1995.

49. G Dighiero. Chronic lymphocytic leukemia treatment. Hematol Cell Therap 39:S31–40, 1997.

50. French Cooperative Group on CLL, S Johnson, AG Smith, et al. Multicentre prospective randomised trial of fludarabine versus cyclophosphamide, doxorubicin, and prednisone (CAP) for treatment of advanced-stage chronic lymphocytic leukaemia. Lancet 347:1432–1438, 1996.

51. KR Rai, B Peterson, L Elias, al e. A randomized comparison of Fludarabine and chlorambucil for patients with previously untreated chronic lymphocytic leukemia. A CALGB, SWOG, CTG/NCI-C and ECOG inter-group study (abstract). Blood 88:552a, 1996.

52. M Spriano, F Chiurazzi, V Liso, P Mazza, S Molica, M Gobbi. Multicentre prospective randomized trial of fludarabine versus chlorambucil and prednisone in previously untreated patients with active B-CLL, International Workshop on CLL, Paris, France, 29–31 October, 1999.

53. B Jaksic, A Delmer, M Brugiatelli, et al. Interim analysis of a randomised EORTC study comparing high dose chlorambucil (HD-CLB) vs fludarabine (FAMP) in untreated B-cell chronic lymphocytic leukaemia (CLL). Hematol Cell Therap 39:S87, 1997.

54. M Hallek, M Wilhelm, B Emmerich, et al. Fludarabine plus cyclophosphamide, and dose-intensified chlorambucil for the treatment of advanced CLL-results of a phase II study (CLL2 protocol) of the German CLL Study Group, International Worshop on CLL, Paris, France, 29–31 October, 1999.

55. T Robak, JZ Blonski, M Kasznicki, et al. Cladribine with prednisone versus chlorambucil with prednisone as first-line therapy in B-CLL, International Workshop on CLL, Paris, France, 1999.

56. K Maloum, O Pritsch, C Magnac, et al. Expression of unmutated VH genes is a detrimental prognostic factor in chronic lymphocytic leukemia. Blood 96:377–379, 2000.
57. BD Cheson, JM Bennett, M Grever, et al. National Cancer Institute-sponsored Working Group guidelines for chronic lymphocytic leukemia: revised guidelines for diagnosis and treatment. Blood 87:4990–4997, 1996.
58. MM Hansen. Chronic lymphocytic leukaemia. Clinical studies based on 189 cases followed for a long time. Scand J Haematol Suppl 18:3, 1973.

9

Genetic Approaches to the Therapy of Chronic Lymphocytic Leukemia

THOMAS J. KIPPS

University of California San Diego, San Diego, California

I. INTRODUCTION

Somatic gene therapy refers to methods that insert an exogenous gene into somatic cells to provide the recipient cells with a desired new property. A new gene either may be taken up into the cell, a process referred to as *transfection*, or may be delivered into the cell by way of a virus vector, a process referred to as *transduction*. Delivery of genes to somatic cells could complement and thereby correct a genetic defect, provide the transduced cell with a missing or novel function, modulate the immune response, or initiate cell suicide in the presence of certain drugs. In any case, the end result is to permute the genetic makeup of somatic cells by adding new genes that direct desired changes in the cell's phenotype.

Advances in vector design, genetic engineering, and vector production have provided for new opportunities for gene therapy (1). Several vectors have been devised to introduce genes into somatic cells. The most commonly used vectors will be discussed along with their noted relative ability to transfer genes into chronic lymphocytic leukemia (CLL) cells or for their ability to induce cellular immune responses against CLL-associated antigens.

II. VIRUS VECTORS FOR GENE TRANSFER

A. Retrovirus Vectors

Retroviruses are RNA viruses based on Moloney murine leukemia virus (2). Like other virus vectors, retrovirus vectors lack genes required for successful replication and production of progeny virus in the transduced cells. Propagation of the virus vector requires "packaging" cell lines that previously are transfected to express three virus genes, namely *gag, pol*, and *env*. The products of these genes are necessary for the replication of the virus genome, assembly, and packaging of the virus particles. Such lines allow for production of retrovirus particles that are only composed of the transgene and required *cis*-acting elements, such as the retrovirus long-terminal repeat (LTR) or psi (Ψ) packaging element (Fig. 1). These *cis*-acting elements are responsible for driving high-level expression of the transgene or for packaging of the retrovirus genome into particles, respectively. Development of improved nonmurine packaging cell lines has lowered the risk for recovery or replication-competent retrovirus (RCR) and allowed for production of recombinant vector at titers of 10^8 plaque-forming units (PFU)/mL in crude samples and 10^{10} pfu/mL in concentrated purified preparations.

Retrovirus vectors have several features that make them well-suited for somatic gene therapy: (1) they are small and relatively easy to manipulate; (2) they integrate in the host chromosome, allowing for sustained expression of an inserted transgene in daughter cells of the originally transduced cell; (3) amphotropic retroviruses can infect a wide variety of cell types from many different species; and (4) retroviruses deleted of essential genes encoding RNA polymerase and/or viral coat proteins can accommodate foreign transgenes ranging from 1 to 7 kb in size. Finally, another major advantage to retrovirus vectors is that the transfected cell does not necessarily express retroviral genes other than that of the desired transgene. In part, because of these advantages, retroviruses have been favored for many gene therapy applications.

Retroviruses, however, have limitations that mitigate their overall usefulness for gene transfer. A major disadvantage is that retroviruses cannot transduce nonreplicating cells. Because most cells in the body are not engaged in cell replication, retroviruses generally are poorly suited to deliver genes to cells in vivo. This problem is compounded by the fact that retroviruses often are produced to titers of greater than 10^5 to 10^6 virus particles/mL. Because most retroviruses cannot withstand ultracentrifugation or other concentrating procedures, it is difficult to increase the titer of such viral preparations. Thus, large volumes of retroviral preparations may be required to provide sufficient numbers of virus particles for gene therapy of human patients. For these and other reasons, many gene therapy protocols use retrovirus for gene transfer to somatic cells that are manipulated (and often cultured and selected) in vitro (3,4).

Improvements in vector design have enhanced the usefulness of retroviruses for use in gene transfer studies. One development is the generation of pseudotyped retroviruses,

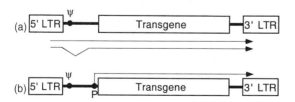

Figure 1 Examples of retrovirus vectors that each possess only the psi (ψ) packaging sequence and two long terminal repeats (LTR). Located between the two LTR is a transgene. Expression of the transgene either can be driven by the promoter activity of the LTR (a) or by an endogenous promoter (P) that flanks the 5′ end of the transgene (b). The fine arrows indicate the RNA transcripts that can be produced in either case.

such as those encapsulated with the vesicular stomatitis virus G protein (5). These vectors are more resilient than standard amphotropic retroviruses to the shearing forces of ultracentrifugation, making it easier to concentrate the virus vector to higher titer (6). Pseudotyped retroviruses also can infect proliferating lymphocytes, such as activated T cells, more efficiently than standard amphotropic retrovirus vectors, making them better candidates for use in gene therapy of hematological neoplasms (7). In addition, vectors based on Lentivirus, such as human immune deficiency virus (HIV), have been developed that also can be pseudotyped and that have the ability to transduce nondividing cells (8). As such, these vectors may be used to transduce resting lymphocytes, and possibly CLL cells, without having to induce cell proliferation before transfection.

B. Adenovirus

Adenovirus is a 36-kb double-stranded DNA virus that can infect many different types of cells efficiently and with low pathogenicity (9). This broad tissue tropism makes adenovirus an attractive vehicle for gene therapy (10). In addition, adenovirus vectors have several advantages over those derived from retroviruses: (1) unlike retrovirus vectors, adenovirus vectors can transfect genes into nonreplicating cells; (2) adenovirus infection generally is not associated with malignant transformation of the infected cells; and (3) adenovirus vectors are relatively stable and can be produced and concentrated to relatively high titers of approximately 10^{12} pfu/mL.

Current adenovirus vectors generally carry deletions in the immediate-early genes E1A, E1B, and/or E3, or E4, making it impossible for these vectors to replicate in cells that do not express such essential virus genes in *trans* (Fig. 2). Such replication defective adenovirus vectors can be propagated in the human kidney cell line, 293, a cell line that constitutively expresses the E1 genes and that also can be transfected to express E3 or E4 (11). Deletion of these essential viral genes allows for the adenovirus vectors to carry transgene inserts of up to 7.5 kb in size.

The major disadvantage of adenovirus vectors is that the transgene does not become incorporated into the chromosomal DNA of the transfected cell. Therefore, expression of the transgene is transient in actively replicating cells. Another disadvantage is the immunogenicity of adenovirus vectors, making it difficult to repeatedly transduce cells with adenovirus vectors in vivo. ''Gutless'' adenovirus vectors have been developed that lack all the adenovirus genes and thus do not induce significant immune responses. However, such vectors only can be grown in the presence of a helper virus and generally are produced to significantly lower titers.

However, some of the ''disadvantages'' of adenovirus vectors actually can be construed as advantages, particularly for gene transfer strategies intended to generate cellular vaccines for immune therapy. First, because the virus does not integrate into the infected cell's genome, there is no risk of insertional mutagenesis, in which insertion of virus DNA causes disruption of essential genes, such as tumor suppressor genes. Moreover, if the transfected cell does survive infection, it will not pass on the adenovirus genome to successive generations of daughter cells. This provides for finite expression of the transgene. Second, the adenovirus proteins expressed by the infected cell may provide for ''adjuvant'' activity, enhancing the ability to develop an immune response against the transfected cell. This could be an advantage in strategies intended to induce an immune response against the transfected cell and/or the transgene product.

Although it is claimed that adenovirus is directly cytotoxic for CLL B cells (12),

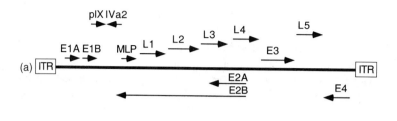

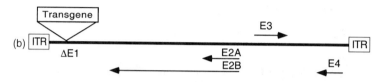

Figure 2 Adenovirus type 5 (Ad5) and an Ad5-derived vector. (a) The map of the adenovirus is depicted showing the inverted-terminal repeat (ITR) sequences and the different transcription units for wild-type virus, as indicated by the arrows. Alternate splicing generates RNA for the early (E), intermediate (pIX and IVa2), and late (L) genes from the primary transcript. (b) Deletion of the E1 region (E1Δ) generates a crippled first generation adenovirus vector that is unable to replicate in cells that cannot supply the E1 genes in trans. Transgenes can be inserted in the deleted region. The resulting vector expresses the transgene but cannot efficiently express the other early genes, because the E1 gene is important for the induction of the E2, E3, and E4 promoters. Second-generation adenovirus vectors have been developed that have deletions or inactivating mutations in another early gene, namely E4, thus reducing further the expression of virus genes and hence the immunogenicity of infected cells.

CLL cells are relatively resistant to infection with adenovirus. The initial attachment of adenovirus to the target cell membrane is by means of a 46-kDa cell surface protein designated as CAR, for "*cytomegalovirus-a*denovirus *r*eceptor" (13,14) in a process that apparently depends on heparan sulfate-glycosaminoglycans (15). Attached virus then is internalized by the cell in a second step process that is facilitated by expression of $\alpha_v\beta_3$ and/or $\alpha_v\beta_5$ integrins (16). CLL cells do not express CAR at significant levels. Nevertheless, CLL cells can be transduced with adenovirus vectors at high virus concentration (17), by means of a CAR-independent pathway of adenovirus infection (18). Moreover, infection of CLL cells in our experience does not cause CLL cells to undergo apoptosis at a higher rate than that observed in nontransfected leukemia cells. Instead, transgene expression in transfected CLL cells is sustained for several days at high levels and without significant loss of cell viability (17,19). Because adenovirus can be made to high titer, it is feasible to use adenovirus vectors for transduction of large numbers of CLL cells ex vivo with culture conditions that allow for high reactant concentrations of virus particles and leukemia cells (20).

C. Adeno-Associated Virus

Adeno-associated virus (AAV) is a defective human parvovirus that can infect many different types of mammalian cells (21). It is a single-strand DNA virus carrying a 4680

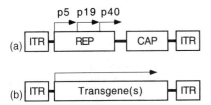

Figure 3 Structure of adeno-associated virus (AAV). (a) Depicts the wild-type adeno-associated virus that contains the *REP* gene and *CAP* gene, encoding the proteins responsible for virus replication and the virus capsid, respectively. These genes are situated between the inverted terminal repeats (ITR). The fine arrows indicate the transcription units for Rep proteins p5, p19, and p40, respectively. (b) Shows a representative adeno-associated virus vector. The essential *REP* and *CAP* genes are deleted, making room for one or more transgenes that collectively cannot be larger than approximately 4 kb. These vectors still require a helper virus and to have the products of the two essential deleted genes provided in trans. The arrow indicates the transcription unit of the transgene(s).

base long DNA molecule (Fig. 3). Replication of AAV requires coinfection of the cell with a helper virus, usually an adenovirus. Without a helper virus, AAV establishes latency by integrating its genome into the chromosomes of the infected cell. AAV has two large open reading frames that constitute a gene encoding the *Rep* proteins required for replication (Rep) and a capsid gene. In addition, at each end of the AAV genome there are 145 base-inverted terminal repeat (ITR) sequences that serve as viral origins of replications. The ITRs are the only elements that are required in *cis* for packaging of the AAV genome or viral integration into the infected cell's chromosome. Deletion of the intervening sequences allows for insertion of up to 4.5 kb of foreign DNA.

These viruses have several advantages that have stimulated interest in AAV as a potential vehicle for human gene therapy (1) AAV can infect a large variety of mammalian cells; (2) AAV can integrate into the host cell's genome, potentially allowing for long-term expression in cells descendant from the originally infected host cell; (3) AAV supposedly can infect postmitotic cells, allowing for possible in vivo gene delivery; (4) AAV particles are very stable, allowing for concentration of virus to more than 10^{12} particles/mL; and (5) cells transduced with AAV vectors lacking the Rep and Cap genes are not likely to be immunogenic, because the integrated AAV-vector generates no viral antigens. To date, AAV has not been associated with any human diseases, even though more than 80% of the adult population has evidence for prior exposure and/or infection to AAV. Because of these features, AAV seems well suited for use in human gene therapy (22).

Again, however, as with any current vector, AAV does have some drawbacks that limit its use at present. First, the size of the foreign DNA that can be accommodated into the AAV genome is relatively small ($\leq$4.5 kb). Second, good packaging cell lines that can express high levels of the Rep protein to complement Rep-deficient AAV do not exist, owing to the toxicity of the AAV Rep protein. This makes it difficult to produce AAV consistently at titers greater than 10^6 particles/mL. Furthermore, AAV vectors apparently do not infect lymphocytes or CLL cells efficiently, making it necessary to consider ex vivo transduction strategies that use AAV vectors at high concentration. Nonetheless, AAV vectors can transfer genes encoding antigens to cells in skin or muscle efficiently, allowing for their potential use in vaccine strategies intended to elicit immune responses against tumor-associated antigens.

D. Herpes Simplex Virus

1. Herpes Simplex Virus, Type I

Herpes simplex virus-1 (HSV-1) is an icosahedral-enveloped double-stranded DNA virus that has a wide host range (reviewed in Ref. 23). HSV-1 may be modified for use as a vehicle for gene delivery to mammalian cells (23,24). Because the HSV-1 genome is approximately 150 kb in size, it may accept relatively large DNA inserts of up to 30 kb without interfering with viral function (Fig. 4). Gene inserts containing exons under the control of a strong heterologous promoter (e.g., that of cytomegalovirus) are expressed at high levels in infected cells (25).

Possessing a feature common to other DNA animal viruses, HSV-1 has a set of "immediate early (IE) genes" that are expressed first after infection. These genes may act in *trans* to support viral expression and replication (24,26,27). To study the function of these IE gene products, mutant strains lacking a particular IE gene have been developed (28,29). Propagation of these mutant strains requires cell lines that are transfected with the IE gene deleted from the mutant virus. Cells expressing the deleted HSV-1 IE gene permit the IE gene product to function on the HSV-1 genome in *trans*. The mutant HSV-1 virus is defective in its ability to form infectious units in cells lacking the essential transgene (28).

Recent advances have reduced the cytotoxicity of HSV-1 type vectors dramatically. One form of HSV-based vector is the HSV amplicon (30). Transgene DNA first is amplified in prokaryotic cells along with the HSV-1 origin and packaging signal. After transfection, the cells are superinfected with a helper HSV to produce an HSV-amplicon. More recently, a helper-free HSV amplicon system was developed that provides all the *trans* viral function on a set of cosmids (31). The use of such amplicons simplifies the vector construction and minimizes the adverse effects caused by infection with live HSV.

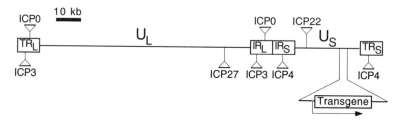

Figure 4   Structure of the herpes simplex virus-I (HSV-1) vectors. The unique long (U$_L$) region and the unique short (U$_S$) region of the virus are indicated. The U$_L$ region is flanked by a terminal repeat for U$_L$ (TR$_L$) and an internal repeat for U$_L$ (IR$_L$), whereas the U$_S$ region is flanked by an internal repeat for U$_S$ (IR$_S$) and a terminal repeat for U$_S$ (TR$_S$) as indicated. Highlighted are the immediate early genes, which include ICP0, ICP4, ICP6, ICP22, and ICP27. The first generation HSV-1 vectors had inactivating mutations in ICP4, resulting in a virus that was unable to replicate in cells that could not supply this gene in trans. Second-generation vectors also have inactivating mutations in other immediate early genes, such as ICP22 and/or ICP27, in addition to the mutation in ICP4. These vectors are more attenuated than the first-generation vectors and have a delayed cytopathic effect on infected cells. Located in the U$_S$ is a representative transgene. Because of its large size, HSV-1 vectors can accommodate large payloads of one or more transgenes. A bar in the top left-hand corner indicates the scale for 10 kb.

HSV-1 has broad host range and, like other DNA viruses such as adenovirus, can infect resting, postmitotic cells. Attachment of the virus apparently is facilitated by cationic molecules, such as heparan sulfate. Infection is mediated by the binding of HSV-1 envelope glycoproteins B and/or C to the glycosaminoglycan chains of cell surface proteoglycans (32–34), followed by entry by means of the herpes virus entry-mediators (Hve), HveA, or HveC (35–40). In addition, the HSV-1 glycoprotein D has been shown to bind to cell surface receptors directly, designated herpesvirus-entry-mediator (Hve) A and HveC (38,41). In many cell types, HveC appears to be the prominent receptor for HSV-1.

We found that CLL B cells are highly sensitive to infection with vectors derived from replication-defective herpes simplex virus-1 (rdHSV-1) (42). Similarly, we noted that normal B cells, T cells, precursor B cell lines, and acute lymphocytic leukemia cells also are highly sensitive to infection with vectors derived from HSV-1. We found that CLL B cells express high-levels of HveA but not HveC, the other known receptor for HSV-1. HveA, otherwise called HVEM (43), TR2 (44), or ATAR (45), is a type I transmembrane protein that is a member of the tumor necrosis factor receptor superfamily. Transfection of Chinese hamster ovarian (CHO) cells with HveA cDNA derived from CLL cells renders these ordinarily HSV-resistant cells highly sensitive to infection by HSV-1. Antibodies to HveA block HSV-1 infection of CLL cells and HveA-transfected CHO cells with similar efficiencies in vitro. As such, it appears that HveA is the primary receptor for HSV-1 on CLL B cells.

In some cases, all the CLL cells can be made to express a transgene at multiplicity of infection (MOI) ratios of ≤0.3. Moreover, in all cases, nearly all of the CLL cells could be made to express an HSV-1–encoded transgene at a MOI ratio of 1. The MOI ratio is the number of pfu of virus divided by the number of cells transduced. The number of pfu/mL for HSV-1–based vectors is determined by testing each rdHSV-1 preparation for its ability to form plaques in vitro on confluent monolayers of Vero cells that had been transfected with the essential genes required to complement the defective rdHSV-1 vector. Vero cells are derived from green monkey kidney cells and are highly sensitive to infection with HSV-1. Because MOI ratios of less than 1 could infect virtually all leukemia cells, CLL cells seem to be more sensitive to infection with rdHSV-1 than E5, HeLa, or Vero cells. Consistent with this, we noted that proportions of CLL cells that expressed the transgene were significantly greater than that of HeLa cells at any given MOI ratio. In contrast, the relative sensitivity for infection of CLL cells for adenovirus vectors is significantly less than that noted for HeLa cells, or even 293 cells, the cells used to propagate adenovirus vectors in vitro (17). As such, HSV-1–derived vectors are relatively efficient vehicles for effecting gene transfer into CLL cells.

Once inside the cell, wild-type HSV-1 translocates to the cell nucleus, where it undergoes replication. Twenty-four hours after infection, the infected cell undergoes cytolysis (the so-called cytopathic effect), thereby releasing infectious virus particles. In contrast to B cells of normal donors, CLL B cells are resistant to the cytopathic effects of infection by rdHSV-1 and maintain high-level expression of the transgene for several days after infection. The resistance of CLL cells to the cytopathic effect of HSV-1 is probably due to the high-level expression of the antiapoptotic protein, bcl-2. Consistent with this, we found that transduction of HeLa cells with a retrovirus expression vector encoding bcl-2–rendered HeLa cells resistant to the cytopathic effects of rdHSV-1 (42). As such, HSV-1–derived vectors should be excellent vehicles with which to transfer genes into CLL B cells.

2. Herpes Simplex Virus, Type II

Herpes simplex virus type 2 (HSV-2) belongs to the same virus family as HSV-1 and shares many biological and structural features. Despite belonging to the same family as HSV-1, HSV-2 uses different receptors to mediate cell entry. HveB (Prr2) seems to serve as a predominant receptor for HSV-2–type virus (39). Hematopoietic cells appear highly sensitive to infection with this virus (46). Indeed, high proportions of CD34$^+$ marrow cells or acute leukemia cells can be made to express a transgene at MOI ratios of less than 1. Because such virus vectors also are propagated on modified Vero cells, the ability to infect such cells at MOI <1 reflects the high sensitivity of hematopoietic cells for infection by HSV-2 relative to that of other cell types. Collectively, the data suggest that in general HSV vectors have potential for use in transferring genes into normal hematopoietic or leukemia cells.

E. Other Virus Vectors

Several other viruses are being investigated for their potential use in human gene therapy. Vaccinia, for example, has been used since the nineteenth century for vaccination against smallpox. Because of the familiarity with it use, broad tissue tropism, ease of delivery, and ability to direct high levels of transgene expression, it is being evaluated for its ability to direct synthesis of transgenes encoding selected antigens and/or immunomodulatory cytokines (47–49).

Interest has focused recently on alpha viruses, such as the Sindbis virus (50) or Semliki Forest virus (SFV) (51). These vectors have several potential advantages, namely (1) broad tissue tropism; (2) the ability to direct high levels of mRNA and protein expression within the infected cell; (3) the ability to inhibit the infected host cell's synthesis of protein; and (4) their relative small size, allowing for it to be manipulated easily to direct expression of desired transgenes (51,52). As much as 25% of the protein synthesized by cells infected with SFV vectors, for example, can be the product of the inserted transgene. Despite their broad host range, however, alpha viruses do not appear to infect CLL cells or other types of neoplastic B cells at high efficiency (unpublished observations).

Nonetheless, because of the high-level expression of transgene in infected cells, injection of these vectors into skin or muscle can induce vigorous immune responses against the vector-encoded transgene product (53,54). Moreover, dendritic cells transduced with SFV vectors containing transgenes encoding the immunoglobulin variable region could induce cytotoxic T lymphocytes reactive specific for lymphoblastoid cells expressing the same immunoglobulin variable regions, indicating that SFV vectors can be used to generate anti-idiotypic cellular immune responses (55). As such, these vectors may be well suited to induce immune responses against idiotypic determinants expressed by B cell lymphomas and leukemias, such as CLL.

F. Nonvirus Vectors

DNA plasmid expression vectors can be used for gene transfer. Generally, the transgene is place downstream of a strong promoter, such as the heterologous cytomegalovirus promoter/enhancer region and upstream of a polyadenylation signal sequence to allow for appropriate RNA processing and transport from the nucleus. Transfection of cells with such plasmid DNA can effect high-level expression of the transgene, provided the RNA has appropriate Kozak sequences for initiating effective translation of the RNA into protein

(56). DNA plasmid expression vectors are easy to construct and do not have virus genes or proteins that might induce unwanted toxicity or immunity against transfected cells. Despite this elegance, however, plasmid DNA cannot transfect CLL cells effectively using any one of a variety of techniques, such as lipofection, electroporation, or calcium phosphate precipitation. Moreover, stable transgene expression requires cell division and integration of the plasmid into the nucleus of the transfected cell. Because most CLL cells are in G_1 and are noncycling, DNA plasmid expression vectors generally cannot effect stable gene transfer into CLL cells.

G. Oligonucleotides

Oligonucleotides are short pieces of synthetic, generally single-stranded DNA. These short stretches of DNA have proven invaluable for use as probes or polymerase-chain-reaction primers for desired segments of DNA. Improvements in chemistry have provided for oligonucleotides with advantageous physical properties. For example, oligonucleotides can be generated in which the nucleotide bases are linked together by means of a phosphorothioate backbone that resists degradation by nucleases that otherwise rapidly metabolize standard, single-stranded DNA. This enhances the half-life of the oligonucleotide both outside and inside the cell, allowing the oligonucleotide to achieve higher intracellular concentrations that favor binding to complementary RNA or DNA molecules.

"Gene interference" is the term given to antisense oligonucleotides that can block or inhibit expression of aberrant or undesired genes (57). Several hematological malignancies result from certain genetic alterations that can be targeted by this approach (58). One major example of such an aberrant or aberrantly expressed gene is the overexpression of *BCL-2* in indolent B cell lymphomas and in CLL. Over-expression of *BCL-2* results in resistance to apoptosis, either spontaneously (59) or in response to ordinarily cytotoxic drugs (60). Antisense oligonucleotides targeted at the open reading frame of the *BCL-2* mRNA can cause specific down-regulation of *BCL-2* in cells that express this gene, thus reducing the cell's resistance to undergoing apoptosis (61,62). A phase I clinical trial was performed in which nine lymphoma patients were given daily subcutaneous injections of an 18-base phosphorothioate antisense oligonucleotide for 2 weeks. One patient had a complete response, and three had stable disease after therapy (63). Conceivably, coadministration of such antisense oligonucleotides with chemotherapy could achieve higher rates of complete responses.

III. THE IMMUNE RESPONSE AND GENE THERAPY

A. Overview

Gene therapy may be used to elicit or alter the host immune response. In fact, this form of human gene therapy was first introduced the nineteenth century, when Jenner used a viral vector, *Vaccinia*, to induce immunity to variola. The success of this strategy is underscored by the fact that this once-feared scourge of humanity that was responsible for smallpox has now been virtually eliminated.

The basic premise underlying this approach is that tumors express antigens that can be recognized by the host immune system. Indeed, cancer is a genetic disease, generally resulting from acquired mutations in genes that ordinarily encode proteins necessary for the orderly differentiation and/or growth of somatic cells. These mutations can cause qualitative and/or quantitative differences between cancer and normal cells in their expressed intracellular and/or surface membrane proteins that may be recognized by the host immune system. In addition, the protein product of the mutated gene represents a neoantigen that also could be targeted by the immune system. For B cell malignancies such as CLL, the clone of neoplastic cells also possesses unique antigen determinants of the immunoglobulin receptor molecules that generally are shared by all members of the neoplastic B cell clone. Because of hypervariable regions and somatic mutations, the immunoglobulin antigen receptor molecules have unique antigenic epitopes, called idiotypes (Id). The Id is an unique antigenic determinant that is generated through genetic recombination or mutational change within the immunoglobulin variable region genes. Because the Id generally is exclusively expressed by all the cells of a neoplastic B cell population, it represents a tumor-specific antigen that is an attractive target for immunotherapy.

B. DNA Vaccines

Direct injection of naked DNA plasmid expression vectors into skin or muscle can transfect somatic cells in vivo. Early studies, investigating the use of liposomal-mediated gene transfer, discerned that the naked plasmid DNA used in control samples also was taken up and expressed by cells in injected mouse skeletal muscle (64). Injection of naked plasmid DNA into muscle can result in expression of a reporter gene, driven either by the long terminal repeat (LTR) of Rous sarcoma virus (RSV) or the promoter/enhancer of the human cytomegalovirus (CMV), for up to 60 days. The transgene product encoded by the plasmid generally can be detected after the first day and sometimes for a long as 1.5 years in mice (65). DNA also can be affixed onto gold particles, allowing for injection into the skin by use of a "gene gun" (66). Alternatively, skin cells can be transfected with DNA delivered into the skin by means of direct injection or through use of a Tyne device that ordinarily is used for allergy testing (67).

Injection of plasmid DNA expression vectors can induce an immune response against the transgene product (reviewed in Ref. 68). Moreover, injection of plasmid DNA encoding immunoglobulin variable regions can induce an anti-Id immune response (69).

Molecular engineering and improvements in our understanding of DNA vaccine technology have provided for DNA vaccines that have enhanced activity. Synthetic oligodeoxynucleotides containing CpG motifs (immunostimulatory sequences, or ISS) have been described as potent adjuvants of type 1 immune responses when coadministered with protein or peptide vaccines (70). In addition, DNA vaccines have been generated that encode chimeric antigens that, in some regards, follow a hapten-carrier paradigm. Because of the ease in manipulating DNA, it is readily feasible to construct genes encoding both antigen and carrier in a single polypeptide.

Chimeric idiotype/adjuvant constructs have been generated to induce immunity against nonimmunogenic idiotypes (Ids). Tao and Levy generated strongly immunogenic Id vaccines by linking a weakly immunogenic Id protein to the immune-stimulatory cytokine, granulocyte-macrophage colony-stimulating factor (GM-CSF) (71). The fusion protein retained the biological activity of native GM-CSF. Unlike immunization with Id alone, immunization with this fusion cytokine-antigen could induce Id-specific antibodies without other carrier proteins or adjuvants and thereby generate protective immunity from challenge with an otherwise lethal dose of Id-bearing tumor cells. Similarly, King and colleagues showed enhanced immunity to Ids from myeloma and lymphoma tumors when genetically linked to fragment C (FrC) of tetanus toxin (72). This chimeric construct, when injected into mouse muscle, was able to enhance both humoral and cellular immunity against the tumor Id. Although immunization with DNA constructs encoding Id alone failed to induce anti-Id antibodies, a vector driving expression of a fusion gene encoding both Id and FrC could elicit antibodies and immunity against Id and TT-derived epitopes. Furthermore, tumor challenge experiments with mice prevaccinated with the Id-FrC expression plasmid showed an inhibition of tumor growth from injected myeloma cells.

Similarly, Biragyn and colleagues demonstrated that a nonimmunogenic Ig variable region (sFv) could elicit a strong anti-idiotype immune response when fused with either interferon inducible protein-10 (IP-10) or monocyte chemotactic protein-3 (MCP-3) that retained functional activity (73). IP-10 and MCP-3 belong to a growing number of chemokines, or *chemotactic cytokines*. These factors are small, secreted proteins of 8–15 kDa that can attract leukocytes bearing the relevant chemokine receptor (e.g., CCR1, CCR2, or CCR3). Monocytes exposed to interferon-gammma (IFN-γ) produce high levels of IP-10, a chemokine that can attract T cells, neutrophils, and other monocytes. Similarly, MCP-3 has the capacity to attract a broad range of cells, such as monocytes and dendritic cells, T lymphocytes, natural killer cells, basophils, and eosinophils (reviewed in Ref. 74 and 75). Chemokine-sFv fusion proteins that retained chemokine activity could induce anti-Id antibodies and protective cellular immunity against an otherwise lethal challenge of syngeneic Id-bearing lymphoma cells. On the other hand, fusion proteins possessing a truncated and inactive chemokine or a standard carrier protein were not effective. Coinjection of DNA encoding Id and chemokine on separate plasmids also was not effective in inducing anti-Id immunity. Moreover, detectable antibody responses to Id apparently were induced only when the sFv antigen was correctly folded and linked with chemokine that retained its biological activity. Collectively, these data indicate that the antigenicity of a protein can be improved significantly when conjugated to a biologically active chemokine or immunogenic carrier protein.

C. Cellular Vaccines

Tumors that ordinarily are poorly immunogenic can be modified through gene therapy to become effective tumor cell vaccines (76). For this, genes encoding immunostimulatory cytokines such as interleukins 2 or 4, GM-CSF, tumor necrosis factor, or interferon are inserted into tumor cells or host cells that may home to the tumor's microenvironment in vivo (77–83). Tumor cells genetically altered to express accessory surface molecules used by antigen-presenting cells to stimulate T cell immunity (84–86) also have been generated. Such modified tumors may induce host cellular immunity against the genetically altered tumor cell population. An exciting aspect of this immunity is that it also may cross-react against unmodified parent tumor cells and induce protective immunity against otherwise lethal tumors in experimental animals.

CLL cells also may express distinctive proteins that potentially could be targeted by the immune system. CLL is a neoplasm of well-differentiated appearing, slowly dividing B lymphocytes that express specific differentiation antigens and surface immunoglobulin. Several studies have found that the immunoglobulins expressed in CLL have features that distinguish them from the antibodies made by normal nonmalignant B cells (87–89). Furthermore, CLL B cells often harbor cytogenetic abnormalities responsible for the pathogenesis (90) or progression (91–93) of the disease. Moreover, the number of cytogenetic abnormalities present in the leukemia B cells of any one patient can increase over time. Any of these genetic alterations may encode "altered-self" antigens that potentially could be targeted by the patient's immune system. Considering the slow growth kinetics of CLL cells and the expression of proteins that distinguish such cells from other somatic cells, including normal B lymphocytes, CLL should be amenable to immune therapy.

However, patients with CLL generally acquire an immune deficiency that could mitigate attempts to induce active immunity against CLL cells. Patients with CLL have an increased susceptibility to infection as a result of acquired defects in both antibody and cellular immune function (94). Furthermore, patients with CLL often do not respond to vaccines, such as those intended to protect against pneumonia or influenza. Often patients will have profound hypogammaglobulinemia and impaired delayed-type hypersensitivity to test antigens, making them nonresponsive or weakly responsive to skin tests for mumps or tuberculosis despite having had prior infection. This may be due in part to leukemia-cell elaboration of immunosuppressive cytokines, such as transforming growth factor-beta (TGF-β) (95), or suppressive factors, such as soluble CD27 (96).

Moreover, leukemia cells are stealthlike in their ability to evade immune detection, even by allogeneic T cells of normal healthy donors. This is in large part secondary to the surface phenotype of the leukemic cell (97). Indeed, despite expressing abundant amounts of class II major histocompatibility antigens, CLL B cells cannot stimulate normal allogeneic T cells in mixed lymphocyte reactions, even in the presence of neutralizing antibodies to immunosuppressive cytokines, such as TGF-β.

Recent advances in our understanding of how lymphocytes interact with one another have provided insight into the mechanisms that contribute to the immune incompetence of patients with CLL (98). Accessory molecules expressed by T cells and antigen-presenting B cells can influence whether the interaction leads to T cell activation and proliferation versus T cell anergy. The latter is the term provided for T cells that no longer respond to antigen even though they express antigen-specific receptors. The leukemia B cells lack expression of important costimulatory molecules that can lead to T cell activation. In addition, leukemic B cells can down-modulate T cell surface molecules that are required to induce expression of such molecules on antigen-presenting cells (97). As a consequence, the leukemic B cell has a tolerogenic influence on T cells, even on those isolated from normal allogeneic donors. For these reasons, it may be necessary to change the stealthlike phenotype of the leukemia cell toward one that can stimulate T cells to generate immune responses against the leukemia B cell population.

We found that the stealthlike phenotype of leukemia B cells can be reversed. Exposure of the CLL B cells to sufficient numbers of activated T cells, for example, can effect dramatic changes in the surface phenotype of CLL B cells within 48 to 72 hours (98). The signals are mediated largely by the TNF family of ligands and receptors expressed on activated T cells and leukemic B cells (98,99). A critical component to this reaction is the ligand for CD40 (CD154). This molecule is expressed on activated T cells within hours after T cell activation (100), allowing activated T cells to engage CD40 on the leukemia B cell surface. This, along with signals derived from other members of the TNF family, triggers a cascade of events that ultimately can result in the leukemia cell expressing significantly higher levels of immune costimulatory surface accessory molecules, such as CD54 (ICAM-1), CD80, and CD86. These molecules are critical for inducing a proliferative T-cell response to presented antigens (101,102). Moreover, these changes allow the leukemic cell to engage nonactivated autologous T cells to respond to leukemia-associated antigens.

Although methods exist for inducing such changes in the leukemia cells in vitro, such methods require that the leukemia cells be cultured ex vivo for prolonged periods with foreign stimulator cells or proteins. Because of this, we generated a crippled adenovirus that carried the gene encoding a recombinant form of CD40-ligand, designated Ad-CD154. Infection of CLL B cells with Ad-CD154 induces dramatic changes in the leukemia cell phenotype (19). Within 18 hours of infection, the CLL B cells express immune costimulatory molecules that are critical for inducing a vigorous immune response. Also, factors that render the leukemia B cells tolerogenic are down-modulated by infection with Ad-CD154. Such modified leukemia cells are highly effective simulators in autologous mixed lymphocyte reactions and can induce the generation of cytotoxic T lymphocytes (CTL) specific for autologous noninfected leukemia cells in vitro (19).

Because Ad-CD154–infected CLL B cells could induce autologus T cells to generate CTL against the patient's leukemia cells in vitro, we conceived a phase I clinical trial for gene therapy of CLL (20). Leukemia cells were harvested by pheresis and then infected ex vivo with Ad-CD154 in a good-manufacturing practice (GMP) facility. The cells were examined for expression of the CD154 and immune-costimulatory molecules. After sterility testing, some of the modified leukemia cells were administered back to the same patient as a single intravenous injection given over a few minutes. This strategy allowed us to conduct a dose-escalation study, in which we infused defined numbers of leukemia cells that expressed CD154-transgene (103).

The biological effects of this treatment were encouraging. Within 24 to 48 hours after receiving the modified cells, nearly all of the patients who received the lowest dose of Ad-CD154–infected autologous cells ($\geq 3 \times 10^8$) had measurable increases in plasma cytokines, such as interleukin (IL)-12, interferon gamma (IFN-γ). Furthermore, noninfected CLL B cells were noted to express low levels of immune costimulatory molecules 1 to 2 days after treatment and lasted for several days, if not longer. The expression of such molecules on noninfected CLL cells may be due to a bystander effect in which noninfected CLL cells are stimulated by contact with CD154-expressing cells. Such immune costimulatory molecules were not induced on noninfected CLL B cells that were incubated in plasma from the treated patients, indicating that a soluble factor was not responsible for this effect.

The clinical effects of this treatment were encouraging. Most patients experienced acute falls in the blood leukemia cell counts within the first few days after treatment. Subsequently the lymphocyte count tended to return to approximately 60% of pretreatment levels. However, not all the blood lymphocytes that returned were CLL B cells. In nearly all treated patients we noted significant increases in the absolute numbers of both CD4$^+$ T cells and CD8$^+$ T cells at 1 week after treatment, sometimes to more than four times that of pretreatment levels. After the first week or two, many patients experienced stabilization in absolute lymphocyte counts. The CLL B cell counts of many of the treated patients remained at or below treatment levels for several weeks, if not longer. One to two weeks after gene therapy, nearly all of the treated patients experienced significant reductions in lymph node size lasting for more than several weeks. As such, this strategy may have activity even in patients who have advanced disease with high leukemia cell counts and diffuse adenopathy. More pronounced clinical effects are anticipated with repeat dosing, which will be examined in a phase II study.

IV. CONCLUSION

Advances in vector technology have provided new tools with which to transfer genes into normal or neoplastic cells. These tools allow for novel therapeutic strategies with which to treat neoplastic disease. Because of the accessibility of neoplastic cells, slow growth kinetics, relative ease in monitoring tumor cells, and improvements in our understanding of the biology and immunology of CLL, this leukemia is an excellent target disease for application of these new technologies. Indeed, gene therapy may provide effective new treatment strategies for patients with CLL or related hematological malignancies.

REFERENCES

1. N Wu, MM Ataai. Production of viral vectors for gene therapy applications. Curr Opin Biotechnol 11:205–208, 2000.
2. EM Gordon, WF Anderson. Gene therapy using retroviral vectors. Curr Opin Biotechnol 5: 611–616, 1994.
3. IM Verma, RK Naviaux. Human gene therapy. Curr Opin Genet Dev 1:54–59, 1991.
4. T Friedmann, L Xu, J Wolff, JK Yee, A Miyanohara. Retrovirus vector-mediated gene transfer into hepatocytes. Mol Biol Med 6:117–125, 1989.
5. JK Yee, T Friedmann, JC Burns. Generation of high-titer pseudotyped retroviral vectors with very broad host range. Methods Cell Biol 43(Pt A):99–112, 1994.
6. A Miyanohara, JK Yee, K Bouic, P LaPorte, T Friedmann. Efficient in vivo transduction of the neonatal mouse liver with pseudotyped retroviral vectors. Gene Ther 2:138–142, 1995.
7. S Sharma, M Cantwell, TJ Kipps, T Friedmann. Efficient infection of a human T-cell line and of human primary peripheral blood leukocytes with a pseudotyped retrovirus vector. Proc Natl Acad Sci USA 93:11842–11847, 1996.
8. L Naldini, U Blomer, P Gallay, D Ory, R Mulligan, FH Gage, IM Verma, D Trono. In vivo gene delivery and stable transduction of nondividing cells by a lentiviral vector. Science 272: 263–267, 1996.
9. MA Rosenfeld, W Siegfried, K Yoshimura, K Yoneyama, M Fukayama, LE Stier, PK Paakko, P Gilardi, LD Stratford-Perricaudet, M Perricaudet. Adenovirus-mediated transfer of a recombinant alpha 1-antitrypsin gene to the lung epithelium in vivo. Science 252:431–434, 1991.
10. BC Trapnell, M Gorziglia. Gene therapy using adenoviral vectors. Curr Opin Biotechnol 5: 617–625, 1994.
11. FL Graham, J Smiley, WC Russell, R Nairn. Characteristics of a human cell line transformed by DNA from human adenovirus type 5. J Gen Virol 36:59–74, 1977.
12. DJ Medina, W Sheay, L Goodell, P Kidd, E White, AB Rabson, RK Strair. Adenovirus-mediated cytotoxicity of chronic lymphocytic leukemia cells. Blood 94:3499–3508, 1999.
13. JM Bergelson, JF Modlin, W Wieland-Alter, JA Cunningham, RL Crowell, RW Finberg. Clinical coxsackievirus B isolates differ from laboratory strains in their interaction with two cell surface receptors. Journal of Infectious Diseases 175:697–700, 1997.
14. MC Bewley, K Springer, YB Zhang, P Freimuth, JM Flanagan. Structural analysis of the mechanism of adenovirus binding to its human cellular receptor, CAR. Science 286:1579–1583, 1999.
15. MC Dechecchi, A Tamanini, A Bonizzato, G Cabrini. Heparan sulfate glycosaminoglycans are involved in adenovirus type 5 and 2-host cell interactions. Virology 268:382–390, 2000.
16. TJ Wickham, P Mathias, DA Cheresh, GR Nemerow. Integrins alpha v beta 3 and alpha v beta 5 promote adenovirus internalization but not virus attachment. Cell 73:309–319, 1993.
17. MJ Cantwell, S Sharma, T Friedmann, TJ Kipps. Adenovirus vector infection of chronic lymphocytic leukemia B cells. Blood 88:4676–4683, 1996.
18. C Hidaka, E Milano, PL Leopold, JM Bergelson, NR Hackett, RW Finberg, TJ Wickham, I Kovesdi, P Roelvink, RG Crystal. CAR-dependent and CAR-independent pathways of adenovirus vector-mediated gene transfer and expression in human fibroblasts. J Clin Invest 103: 579–587, 1999.

19. K Kato, MJ Cantwell, S Sharma, TJ Kipps. Gene transfer of CD40-ligand induces autologous immune recognition of chronic lymphocytic leukemia B cells. J Clin Invest 101:1133–1141, 1998.

20. TJ Kipps, MJ Cantwell, S Sharma, K Kato. Gene therapy of chronic lymphocytic leukemia. Cancer Res Ther Control 7:37–41, 1998.

21. N Muzyczka. Use of adeno-associated virus as a general transduction vector for mammalian cells. Curr Top Microbiol Immunol 158:97–129, 1992.

22. RM Kotin. Prospects for the use of adeno-associated virus as a vector for human gene therapy. Hum Gene Ther 5:793–801, 1994.

23. JG Stevens. Human herpesviruses: a consideration of the latent state. Microbiol Rev 53:318–332, 1989.

24. AI Geller. Herpesviruses: expression of genes in postmitotic brain cells. Curr Opin Genet Dev 3:81–85, 1993.

25. PA Johnson, K Yoshida, FH Gage, T Friedmann. Effects of gene transfer into cultured CNS neurons with a replication-defective herpes simplex virus type 1 vector. Brain Res Mol Brain Res 12:95–102, 1992.

26. RD Everett. The products of herpes simplex virus type 1 (HSV-1) immediate early genes 1, 2 and 3 can activate HSV-1 gene expression in trans. J Gen Virol 67:2507–2513, 1986.

27. NA DeLuca, PA Schaffer. Physical and functional domains of the herpes simplex virus transcriptional regulatory protein ICP4. J Virol 62:732–743, 1988.

28. PA Johnson, MG Best, T Friedmann, DS Parris. Isolation of a herpes simplex virus type 1 mutant deleted for the essential UL42 gene and characterization of its null phenotype. J Virol 65:700–710, 1991.

29. PA Johnson, A Miyanohara, F Levine, T Cahill, T Friedmann. Cytotoxicity of a replication-defective mutant of herpes simplex virus type 1. J Virol 66:2952–2965, 1992.

30. RR Spaete, N Frenkel. The herpes simplex virus amplicon: a new eucaryotic defective-virus cloning-amplifying vector. Cell 30:295–304, 1982.

31. Y Saeki, T Ichikawa, A Saeki, EA Chiocca, K Tobler, M Ackermann, XO Breakefield, C Fraefel. Herpes simplex virus type 1 DNA amplified as bacterial artificial chromosome in Escherichia coli: rescue of replication-competent virus progeny and packaging of amplicon vectors. Hum Gene Therapy 9:2787–2794, 1998.

32. BC Herold, RJ Visalli, N Susmarski, CR Brandt, PG Spear. Glycoprotein C-independent binding of herpes simplex virus to cells requires cell surface heparan sulphate and glycoprotein B. J Gen Virol 75:1211–1222, 1994.

33. F Tufaro. Virus entry: two receptors are better than one. Trends Microbiol 5:257–258; discussion 258–259, 1997.

34. PG Spear, MT Shieh, BC Herold, D WuDunn, TI Koshy. Heparan sulfate glycosaminoglycans as primary cell surface receptors for herpes simplex virus. Adv Exp Med Biol 313:341–353, 1992.

35. F Eberlé, P Dubreuil, MG Mattei, E Devilard, M Lopez. The human PRR2 gene, related to the human poliovirus receptor gene (PVR), is the true homolog of the murine MPH gene. Gene 159:267–272, 1995.

36. M Lopez, F Eberlé, MG Mattei, J Gabert, F Birg, F Bardin, C Maroc, P Dubreuil. Complementary DNA characterization and chromosomal localization of a human gene related to the poliovirus receptor-encoding gene. Gene 155:261–265, 1995.

37. RJ Geraghty, C Krummenacher, GH Cohen, RJ Eisenberg, PG Spear. Entry of alphaherpesviruses mediated by poliovirus receptor-related protein 1 and poliovirus receptor. Science 280:1618–1620, 1998.

38. C Krummenacher, AV Nicola, JC Whitbeck, H Lou, W Hou, JD Lambris, RJ Geraghty, PG Spear, GH Cohen, RJ Eisenberg. Herpes simplex virus glycoprotein D can bind to poliovirus receptor-related protein 1 or herpesvirus entry mediator, two structurally unrelated mediators of virus entry. J Virol 72:7064–7074, 1998.

39. MS Warner, RJ Geraghty, WM Martinez, RI Montgomery, JC Whitbeck, R Xu, RJ Eisenberg, GH Cohen, PG Spear. A cell surface protein with herpesvirus entry activity (HveB) confers susceptibility to infection by mutants of herpes simplex virus type 1, herpes simplex virus type 2, and pseudorabies virus. Virology 246:179–189, 1998.

40. F Cocchi, L Menotti, P Mirandola, M Lopez, G Campadelli-Fiume. The ectodomain of a novel member of the immunoglobulin subfamily related to the poliovirus receptor has the attributes of a bona fide receptor for herpes simplex virus types 1 and 2 in human cells. J Virol 72:9992–10002, 1998.

41. JC Whitbeck, C Peng, H Lou, R Xu, SH Willis, M Ponce de Leon, T Peng, AV Nicola, RI Montgomery, MS Warner, AM Soulika, LA Spruce, WT Moore, JD Lambris, PG Spear, GH Cohen, RJ Eisenberg. Glycoprotein D of herpes simplex virus (HSV) binds directly to HVEM, a member of the tumor necrosis factor receptor superfamily and a mediator of HSV entry. J Virol 71:6083–6093, 1997.

42. DJ Eling, PA Johnson, S Sharma, F Tufaro, TJ Kipps. Chronic lymphocytic leukemia B cells are highly sensitive to infection by herpes simplex virus-1 via herpesvirus-entry-mediator A. Gene Therapy 7:1210–1216, 2000.

43. RI Montgomery, MS Warner, BJ Lum, PG Spear. Herpes simplex virus-1 entry into cells mediated by a novel member of the TNF/NGF receptor family. Cell 87:427–436, 1996.

44. BS Kwon, KB Tan, J Ni, KO Lee, KK Kim, YJ Kim, S Wang, R Gentz, GL Yu, J Harrop, SD Lyn, C Silverman, TG Porter, A Truneh, PR Young. A newly identified member of the tumor necrosis factor receptor superfamily with a wide tissue distribution and involvement in lymphocyte activation. J Biol Chem 272:14272–14276, 1997.

45. H Hsu, I Solovyev, A Colombero, R Elliott, M Kelley, WJ Boyle. ATAR, a novel tumor necrosis factor receptor family member, signals through TRAF2 and TRAF5. J Biol Chem 272:13471–13474, 1997.

46. D Dilloo, D Rill, C Entwistle, M Boursnell, W Zhong, W Holden, M Holladay, S Inglis, M Brenner. A novel herpes vector for the high-efficiency transduction of normal and malignant human hematopoietic cells. Blood 89:119–127, 1997.

47. GR Peplinski, K Tsung, JA Norton. Vaccinia virus for human gene therapy. Surgical Oncology Clinics of North America 7:575–588, 1998.

48. M Sivanandham, SD Scoggin, RG Sperry, MK Wallack. Prospects for gene therapy and lymphokine therapy for metastatic melanoma. Ann Plast Surg 28:114–118, 1992.

49. GW Wilkinson, LK Borysiewicz. Gene therapy and viral vaccination: the interface. Br Med Bull 51:205–216, 1995.

50. FW Johanning, RM Conry, AF LoBuglio, M Wright, LA Sumerel, MJ Pike, DT Curiel. A Sindbis virus mRNA polynucleotide vector achieves prolonged and high level heterologous gene expression in vivo. Nucleic Acids Res 23:1495–1501, 1995.

51. P Liljestrom, H Garoff. A new generation of animal cell expression vectors based on the Semliki Forest virus replicon. Biotechnology (NY) 9:1356–1361, 1991.

52. JJ Wahlfors, SA Zullo, S Loimas, DM Nelson, RA Morgan. Evaluation of recombinant alphaviruses as vectors in gene therapy. Gene Therapy 7:472–480, 2000.

53. SP Mossman, F Bex, P Berglund, J Arthos, SP O'Neil, D Riley, DH Maul, C Bruck, P Momin, A Burny, PN Fultz, JI Mullins, P Liljeström, EA Hoover. Protection against lethal simian immunodeficiency virus SIVsmmPBj14 disease by a recombinant Semliki Forest virus gp160 vaccine and by a gp120 subunit vaccine. J Virol 70:1953–1960, 1996.

54. P Colmenero, P Liljeström, M Jondal. Induction of P815 tumor immunity by recombinant Semliki Forest virus expressing the P1A gene. Gene Therapy 6:1728–1733, 1999.

55. F Osterroth, A Garbe, P Fisch, H Veelken. Stimulation of cytotoxic T cells against idiotype immunoglobulin of malignant lymphoma with protein-pulsed or idiotype-transduced dendritic cells. Blood 95:1342–1349, 2000.

56. M Kozak. Structural features in eukaryotic mRNAs that modulate the initiation of translation. J Biol Chem 266:19867–19870, 1991.

57. AR Yuen, BI Sikic. Clinical studies of antisense therapy in cancer. Front Biosci 5:D588–593, 2000.

58. N Agarwal, AM Gewirtz. Oligonucleotide therapeutics for hematologic disorders. Biochim Biophys Acta 1489:85–96, 1999.

59. D Hockenbery, G Nunez, C Milliman, RD Schreiber, SJ Korsmeyer. Bcl-2 is an inner mitochondrial membrane protein that blocks programmed cell death. Nature 348:334–336, 1990.

60. JC Reed, S Kitada, S Takayama, T Miyashita. Regulation of chemoresistance by the bcl-2 oncoprotein in non-Hodgkin's lymphoma and lymphocytic leukemia cell lines. Ann Oncol 5:61–65, 1994.

61. FE Cotter, P Johnson, P Hall, C Pocock, N al Mahdi, JK Cowell, G Morgan. Antisense oligonucleotides suppress B-cell lymphoma growth in a SCID-hu mouse model. Oncogene 9:3049–3055, 1994.

62. MJ White, J Chen, L Zhu, S Irvin, A Sinor, MJ DiCaprio, K Jin, DA Greenberg. A Bcl-2 antisense oligonucleotide increases alpha-amino-3-hydroxy-5-methylisoxazole-4-propionic acid (AMPA) toxicity in cortical cultures. Annals of Neurology 42:580–587, 1997.

63. A Webb, D Cunningham, F Cotter, PA Clarke, F di Stefano, P Ross, M Corbo, Z Dziewanowska. BCL-2 antisense therapy in patients with non-Hodgkin lymphoma. Lancet 349:1137–1141, 1997.

64. JA Wolff, RW Malone, P Williams, W Chong, G Acsadi, A Jani, PL Felgner. Direct gene transfer into mouse muscle in vivo. Science 247:1465–1468, 1990.

65. JA Wolff, JJ Ludtke, G Acsadi, P Williams, A Jani. Long-term persistence of plasmid DNA and foreign gene expression in mouse muscle. Hum Mol Genet 1:363–369, 1992.

66. DC Tang, M DeVit, SA Johnston. Genetic immunization is a simple method for eliciting an immune response. Nature 356:152–154, 1992.

67. E Raz, DA Carson, SE Parker, TB Parr, AM Abai, G Aichinger, SH Gromkowski, M Singh, D Lew, MA Yankauckas, SM Baird, GH Rhodes. Intradermal gene immunization: The possible role of DNA uptake in the induction of cellular immunity to viruses. Proc Natl Acad Sci USA 91:9519–9523, 1994.

68. S Gurunathan, DM Klinman, RA Seder. DNA vaccines: immunology, application, and optimization. Annu Rev Immunol 18:927–974, 2000.

69. A Watanabe, E Raz, H Kohsaka, H Tighe, SM Baird, TJ Kipps, DA Carson. Induction of antibodies to a kappa variable region by gene immunization. J Immunol 151:2871–2876, 1993.

70. H Tighe, M Corr, M Roman, E Raz. Gene vaccination: plasmid DNA is more than just a blueprint. Immunol Today 19:89–97, 1998.

71. MH Tao, R Levy. Idiotype/granulocyte-macrophage colony-stimulating factor fusion protein as a vaccine for B-cell lymphoma [see comments]. Nature 362:755–758, 1993.

72. CA King, MB Spellerberg, D Zhu, J Rice, SS Sahota, AR Thompsett, TJ Hamblin, J Radl, FK Stevenson. DNA vaccines with single-chain Fv fused to fragment C of tetanus toxin induce protective immunity against lymphoma and myeloma [see comments]. Nat Med 4:1281–1286, 1998.

73. A Biragyn, K Tani, MC Grimm, S Weeks, LW Kwak. Genetic fusion of chemokines to a self tumor antigen induces protective, T-cell dependent antitumor immunity [see comments]. Nat Biotechnol 17:253–258, 1999.

74. BJ Rollins. Chemokines. Blood 90:909–928, 1997.

75. AD Luster. Chemokines—chemotactic cytokines that mediate inflammation. N Engl J Med 338:436–445, 1998.

76. D Pardoll. Immunotherapy with cytokine gene-transduced tumor cells: the next wave in gene therapy for cancer. Curr Opin Oncol 4:1124–1129, 1992.

77. B Gansbacher, K Zier, B Daniels, K Cronin, R Bannerji, E Gilboa. Interleukin 2 gene transfer into tumor cells abrogates tumorigenicity and induces protective immunity. J Exp Med 172:1217–1224, 1990.

78. Immunization of cancer patients using autologous cancer cells modified by insertion of the gene for interleukin-2. Hum Gene Ther 3:75–90, 1992.

79. A Uchiyama, DS Hoon, T Morisaki, Y Kaneda, DH Yuzuki, DL Morton. Transfection of interleukin 2 gene into human melanoma cells augments cellular immune response. Cancer Res 53:949–952, 1993.

80. MP Colombo, G Ferrari, A Stoppacciaro, M Parenza, M Rodolfo, F Mavilio, G Parmiani. Granulocyte colony-stimulating factor gene transfer suppresses tumorigenicity of a murine adenocarcinoma in vivo. J Exp Med 173:889–897, 1991.

81. G Dranoff, E Jaffee, A Lazenby, P Golumbek, H Levitsky, K Brose, V Jackson, H Hamada, D Pardoll, RC Mulligan. Vaccination with irradiated tumor cells engineered to secrete murine granulocyte-macrophage colony-stimulating factor stimulates potent, specific, and long-lasting anti-tumor immunity. Proc Natl Acad Sci USA 90:3539–3543, 1993.

82. SE Karp, A Farber, JC Salo, P Hwu, G Jaffe, AL Asher, E Shiloni, NP Restifo, JJ Mule, SA Rosenberg. Cytokine secretion by genetically modified nonimmunogenic murine fibrosarcoma. Tumor inhibition by IL-2 but not tumor necrosis factor. J Immunol 150:896–908, 1993.

83. A Belldegrun, CL Tso, T Sakata, T Duckett, MJ Brunda, SH Barsky, J Chai, R Kaboo, RS Lavey, WH McBride, et al. Human renal carcinoma line transfected with interleukin-2 and/ or interferon alpha gene(s): implications for live cancer vaccines. J Natl Cancer Inst 85:207– 216, 1993.

84. RF James, S Edwards, KM Hui, PD Bassett, F Grosveld. The effect of class II gene transfection on the tumourigenicity of the H-2K-negative mouse leukaemia cell line K36.16. Immunology 72:213–218, 1991.

85. SE Townsend, JP Allison. Tumor rejection after direct costimulation of CD8+ T cells by B7-transfected melanoma cells [see comments]. Science 259:368–370, 1993.

86. L Chen, S Ashe, WA Brady, I Hellstrom, KE Hellstrom, JA Ledbetter, P McGowan, PS Linsley. Costimulation of antitumor immunity by the B7 counterreceptor for the T lymphocyte molecules CD28 and CTLA-4. Cell 71:1093–1102, 1992.

87. TA Johnson, LZ Rassenti, TJ Kipps. Ig VH1 genes expressed in B-cell chronic lymphocytic leukemia exhibit distinctive molecular features. J Immunol 158:235–246, 1997.

88. LZ Rassenti, TJ Kipps. Lack of allelic exclusion in B cell chronic lymphocytic leukemia. J Exp Med 185:1435–1445, 1997.

89. F Fais, F Ghiotto, S Hashimoto, B Sellars, A Valetto, SL Allen, P Schulman, VP Vinciguerra, K Rai, LZ Rassenti, TJ Kipps, G Dighiero, H Schroeder, M Ferrarini, N Chiorazzi. Chronic lymphocytic leukemia B cells express restricted sets of mutated and unmutated antigen receptors. J Clin Invest 102:1515–1525, 1998.

90. G Meinhardt, CM Wendtner, M Hallek. Molecular pathogenesis of chronic lymphocytic leukemia: factors and signaling pathways regulating cell growth and survival. J Mol Med 77: 282–293, 1999.

91. D Lens, PJ De Schouwer, RA Hamoudi, M Abdul-Rauf, N Farahat, E Matutes, T Crook, MJ Dyer, D Catovsky. p53 abnormalities in B-cell prolymphocytic leukemia. Blood 89: 2015–2023, 1997.

92. JB Johnston, P Daeninck, L Verburg, K Lee, G Williams, LG Israels, MR Mowat, A Begleiter. P53, MDM-2, BAX and BCL-2 and drug resistance in chronic lymphocytic leukemia. Leuk Lymphoma 26:435–449, 1997.

93. F Bullrich, D Rasio, S Kitada, P Starostik, T Kipps, M Keating, M Albitar, JC Reed, CM Croce. ATM mutations in B-cell chronic lymphocytic leukemia. Cancer Res 59:24–27, 1999.

94. VA Morrison. The infectious complications of chronic lymphocytic leukemia. Semin Oncol 25:98–106, 1998.

95. M Lotz, E Ranheim, TJ Kipps. Transforming growth factor beta as endogenous growth inhibitor of chronic lymphocytic leukemia B cells. J Exp Med 179:999–1004, 1994.

96. MH Van Oers, ST Pals, LM Evers, CE van der Schoot, G Koopman, JM Bonfrer, RQ Hintzen,

AE von dem Borne, RA van Lier. Expression and release of CD27 in human B-cell malignancies. Blood 82:3430–3436, 1993.

97. MJ Cantwell, T Hua, J Pappas, TJ Kipps. Acquired CD40-ligand deficiency in chronic lymphocytic leukemia. Nature Medicine 3:984–989, 1997.

98. EA Ranheim, TJ Kipps. Activated T cells induce expression of B7/BB1 on normal or leukemic B cells through a CD40-dependent signal. J Exp Med 177:925–935, 1993.

99. EA Ranheim, TJ Kipps. Tumor necrosis factor-alpha facilitates induction of CD80 (B7-1) and CD54 on human B cells by activated T cells: complex regulation by IL-4, IL-10, and CD40L. Cell Immunol 161:226–235, 1995.

100. C van Kooten, J Banchereau. CD40-CD40 ligand: a multifunctional receptor-ligand pair. Adv Immunol 61:1–77, 1996.

101. LL Lanier, S O'Fallon, C Somoza, JH Phillips, PS Linsley, K Okumura, D Ito, M Azuma. CD80 (B7) and CD86 (B70) provide similar costimulatory signals for T cell proliferation, cytokine production, and generation of CTL. J Immunol 154:97–105, 1995.

102. U Matulonis, C Dosiou, G Freeman, C Lamont, P Mauch, LM Nadler, JD Griffin. B7-1 is superior to B7-2 costimulation in the induction and maintenance of T cell-mediated antileukemia immunity. Further evidence that B7-1 and B7-2 are functionally distinct. J Immunol 156:1126–1131, 1996.

103. WG Wierda, MJ Cantwell, LZ Rassenti, CE Prussak, TJ Kipps. CD40-ligand (CD154) gene therapy for chronic lymphocytic leukemia. Blood 96:2917–2924, 2000.

10

Combination Strategies for Purine Nucleoside Analogs

VARSHA GANDHI and WILLIAM PLUNKETT

The University of Texas M. D. Anderson Cancer Center, Houston, Texas

I. INTRODUCTION

The clinical development of ara-C as the most effective agent for treatment of acute myeloid leukemias interested chemists in synthesizing new nucleoside analogs. The plethora of analogs generated from the chemical pharmacopoeia provides an opportunity to understand the structure-based differences in the metabolic and mechanistic aspects. At the same time, we are faced with a challenge of identifying the selective target and/or diseases for each of these newer nucleoside analogs.

The metabolic commonality among nucleoside analogs that have been used in the preclinical or clinical settings is their phosphorylation to the respective triphosphates. These are the proximal active metabolites, which after incorporation into DNA elicit cytotoxicity. Nucleoside analogs have been used effectively and intensively in hematological malignancies, assuming that the common mechanistic feature among these agents is their incorporation into DNA during replication, followed by inhibition of DNA synthesis, which initiates drug-induced programmed cell death. Hence, classically for the past 40 years, the major target that has been identified for nucleoside analogs is DNA replication. Thus, it has been something of a paradox that this class of agents is active in indolent malignancies that are characterized by a low growth fraction. Clearly, it is important to evaluate ancillary metabolic pathways for nucleoside analogs to become incorporated into DNA, such excision DNA repair processes that require unscheduled DNA synthesis in replacing excised single strands of DNA. In addition, leads are now emerging that suggest that some analogs may interfere directly with RNA synthesis. Finally, it is possible that other targets exist that are susceptible to nucleotide analog-induced activation of cell death without the need for incorporation into DNA. The evaluation of such pathways holds substantial promise for understanding the actions of nucleotide analogs and for applying this knowledge to the design of combination therapies.

II. METABOLISM AND ACTIONS

If ara-C serves as a paradigm for pyrimidine nucleoside analogs, arabinosyladenine (ara-A) may be considered a prototype for purine analogs. However, the rapid deamination of this agent made it impossible for further development of this agent for cancer chemotherapy (1). As an alternative, Montgomery (2) synthesized a congener of ara-A that is resistant to deamination by virtue of the presence of a halogen on the nucleobase. Arabinosyl-2-fluoroadenine (F-ara-A) not only provided a deamination-resistant deoxyadenosine analog that served as a model purine nucleoside analog but also generated interest that resulted in other congeners such as cladribine (2-chlorodeoxyadenosine, Ortho Biotech) and clofarabine (2-chloro-2′-fluoro-arabinosyladenine, Bioenvision), a newer agent that combines both halogen groups. Because of its low solubility, in the clinic F-ara-A was formulated as its monophosphate, which is designated as fludarabine. Solubility problems also hindered the use of arabinosylguanine (ara-G) in the clinic until a relatively soluble pro-drug nelarabine (Compound GW506U78) was synthesized (3) at Burroughs Wellcome (Fig. 1).

   The enzyme, dCyd kinase, phosphorylates all these nucleoside analogs to the respective monophosphates. The fact that the affinity of the enzyme is vastly different for these nucleosides, as evident by the kinetic values (3–7, Table 1), is one of the determinants of the effective doses defined in clinical trials. In addition to this kinase, dGuo kinase has also been indicated for phosphorylation of cladribine (8) and ara-G (3,9). Although kinetic constants for dCyd kinase may be helpful to identify the optimal doses, generally maximum tolerated dose is achieved far below the optimal level needed for saturation of the kinase. This limitation stresses the opportunity for biochemical modulation strategies for enhancement of phosphorylation of the available substrate, as discussed later. Although not formally identified, the kinases that phosphorylate the analog monophosphates to the respective diphosphates (monophosphate kinase) and triphosphates (nucleoside diphosphate kinase) may be assumed to have higher efficiencies for converting their respective substrates to product than does deoxycytidine kinase or deoxyguanosine kinase. This is probably true for fludarabine and ara-G. For both these analogs, the triphosphates serve as the major metabolite while the free drug, monophosphate and diphosphate, make up

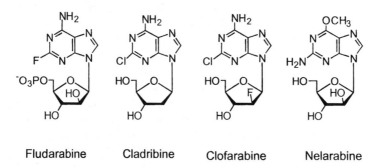

Fludarabine   Cladribine   Clofarabine   Nelarabine

Figure 1 Structures of purine nucleoside analogs.

Table 1 Metabolic Properties of Purine Nucleoside Analogs

	Fludarabine	Cladribine	Clofarabine	Nelarabine
Deamination				
ADA	No	No	No	Demethoxylation to ara-G
Phosphorylation				
Nucleoside kinase	dCyd	dCyd and dGuo	dCyd	dCyd and dGuo
Km, µM	200–400	5 and 40	14	900 and 7
Major cellular metabolite	Triphosphate	Monophosphate	Monophosphate	Triphosphate
Triphosphate elimination				
Property	Monophasic	Monophasic	Biphasic	Monophasic
Half-life	slow	slow	slow	slow

less than 20% of the total metabolites in the cell (10–12). For nucleoside analogs with adenine bases containing a chlorine atom (cladribine and clofarabine), the monophosphate has been consistently shown as the major metabolite both in cultured cells (13,14) and in clinical samples (15). The monophosphate, in this instance, may serve as a depot form for generating the triphosphate even after the end of drug infusion, although the regulation of such an equilibrium is unknown.

The slow elimination kinetics of the triphosphate is common among all these purine nucleoside analogs. The increased residence time of the triphosphate is evident in the cells in culture but is much more demonstrable in circulating leukemia cells during therapy. This may be one of the reasons for success of purine analogs in indolent diseases, which may require a chronic presence of analog triphosphate to combat these disorders. Furthermore, the prolonged retention of the purine nucleotides stands in contrast to pyrimidine nucleoside analogs, which are retained at one-half to one-tenth as effectively (16–18).

The mechanistic similarities among the dAdo analogs fludarabine, cladribine, and clofarabine are striking (Table 2). The triphosphate of each is inhibitory to ribonucleotide reductase (13,19–22). It is assumed that the mechanism of this inhibition involves the interaction of the analog triphosphates with the global allosteric inhibitory site of the

Table 2 Mechanistic Aspects of Purine Nucleoside Analogs

	Fludarabine	Cladribine	Clofarabine	Nelarabine
Ribonucleotide reductase				
Inhibition	Yes	Yes	Yes	No
Metabolite for inhibition	Triphosphate	Triphosphate	Triphosphate	
Actions on DNA				
Dominant site in DNA	Terminal	Internal	Internal	N/A
Affinity for incorporation[a]	2.1	1.9	N/A	10
Resistance to excision	Strong	None	N/A	Strong[b]
Self-potentiation actions	Yes	Yes	Yes	No

[a] Ratio of Km values for analog TP and dATP or dGTP.
[b] Unpublished data.
N/A Not available.

enzyme. Such inhibition has resulted in a decrease in the deoxynucleotide pools during in vitro experiments using whole cells and during therapy in circulating leukemia cells. As such, the relative concentrations of deoxynucleotides in cells serve as surrogate end points for measuring drug-induced inactivation of the enzyme. Importantly, this action would change the ratio of the concentrations of the analog triphosphate to dATP. Because the triphosphates of fludarabine, cladribine, and clofarabine compete with dATP for incorporation into DNA, such a change in the ratio of the concentrations of these nucleotides would favor the likelihood of analog selection for incorporation. Thus, the pharmacodynamic action of lowering the concentrations of endogenous deoxynucleotides by analog triphosphate inhibition of ribonucleotide reductase could increase the use of the same analog for incorporation into DNA without actually changing its concentration in the cells. This interaction is known as self-potentiation (23). Furthermore, as repair of DNA damage induced by other agents draws on endogenous pools of cellular deoxynucleoside triphosphates, this mechanism applies equally well to analog incorporation into replicating and repairing DNA. In contrast to the dAdo analogs, the inhibitory activity on ribonucleotide reductase has not been demonstrated for the triphosphate of ara-G. The multiplicity of sites of action of deoxyadenosine analogs and the regulatory aspects of their metabolism predispose these drugs to self-potentiation. As a result, the designs of several therapeutic strategies have attempted to take advantage of the potential for self-potentiation that is a feature of this class of antimetabolites.

In addition, lowering of deoxynucleotide pools also has implications for the use of deoxyadenosine analogs in biochemical modulation strategies. As discussed later in detail, the activity of deoxycytidine kinase is regulated by dCTP. Decreased cellular dCTP concentrations could effectively activate deoxycytidine kinase and thereby facilitate phosphorylation of analogs that use this key enzyme for activation (24). This is a second example of a self-potentiating mechanism of action.

In whole cell systems in culture, it has been established that the purine nucleoside antimetabolites are incorporated into DNA to elicit cytotoxicity (22,25–28). In vitro DNA synthesis model systems have demonstrated that this incorporation could halt further incorporation with the analog residing mainly at the 3′-terminus of DNA, as is the case with fludarabine (28) and ara-G (29). Alternatively, the ability of polymerase to add deoxynucleotide to the analog results in the partial internalization of the drug in DNA, as is the case with cladribine (21,25) and clofarabine (13,22). These observations have also been duplicated in whole cells for dAdo analogs (13,28). Demonstrating the incorporation of each analog into DNA and the inhibition of DNA synthesis in clinical samples is a daunting issue, because in indolent diseases only a small portion of the tumor cell population is involved in DNA synthesis.

Proof-reading enzymes, such as the $3′ \rightarrow 5′$ exonucleases associated with DNA polymerases delta, epsilon, and gamma excise mismatched deoxynucleotides in a proof-reading function that enhances the fidelity of DNA replication. Recent studies have demonstrated that these polymerase-associated exonucleases are capable of recognizing misincorporated nucleotide analogs and, to a limited degree, of excising them (28,30,31). In addition to being a poor substrate for elongation by DNA polymerases, the stability of F-ara-AMP in 3′-termini suggests that it is resistant to removal by proofreading activities (30). Furthermore, it appears that when a DNA polymerase attempts to excise terminal F-ara-AMP, a mechanism-based reaction occurs that inactivates both the exonuclease and polymerase functions of the enzyme. In contrast, internally localized cladribine monophosphate is highly susceptible for excision by such exonucleases (31). Although not completely resistant to excision, ara-GMP is difficult to remove from the 3′-terminus by Klenow fragment (Gandhi, unpublished).

In addition to the DNA-directed actions of nucleoside analogs, incorporation into RNA has been demonstrated uniquely for F-ara-ATP (32,33). This was associated with a decrease in transcription of genomic DNA and also in new proteins. This is likely to arise from the incorporation of F-ara-AMP into the nascent transcript, because the signals from exon-specific probes were decreased in portions of the transcript distal to the promoter of the dihydrofolate reductase gene (32). In primary CLL cells, the inhibition of RNA transcription correlated significantly with the cytotoxic action of fludarabine in CLL cells. Furthermore, inhibition of RNA synthesis by fludarabine led to a specific depletion of certain cellular proteins from CLL cells. These actions not only provide a new target for fludarabine in these quiescent leukemia cells but also suggest strategies for combinations of this agent with other RNA or protein inhibitors such as actinomycin D or puromycin (33).

The hallmark feature of apoptosis is internucleosomal cleavage of genomic DNA, a process activated by caspases. Caspase-3 is a critical component of the caspase cascade that is common to both the pathway initiated by membrane receptors and the mitochondrial pathway. With regard to the latter, it has been demonstrated that caspase-3 activation in the cytosol is induced by the addition of dATP and cytochrome c. Three protein factors, designated apoptotic protease activating factors (Apafs) are sufficient to result in dATP-dependent activation of caspase-3. Caspase-3 activation begins when procaspase-9 (also known as Apaf-3) binds to Apaf-1 in a reaction activated by cytochrome c (Apaf-2) released from mitochondria and dATP (34). Because of their structural similarities, purine nucleoside analogs may also function as activators of dATP-dependent caspase activation and apoptosis. Indeed, recent data suggest that chlorodeoxyadenosine triphosphate (35), fludarabine triphosphate, clofarabine triphosphate, and ara-GTP (36) result in the induction of such an apoptotic program both in cell-free systems and in primary CLL cells. These findings suggest an additional mechanism by which these purine analogs might induce cell death in quiescent cells in the absence of their incorporation into DNA.

III. CLINICAL USE OF ANALOGS

At present, it appears that each nucleoside analog is effective against a specific subset of adult leukemias. Fludarabine is most effective for indolent diseases such as CLL (37) and low-grade non-Hodgkin's lymphomas (38). Cladribine has established activity for hairy cell leukemia (39,40), whereas at this early stage, nelarabine appears to be selective for T-ALL (41), T-PLL, and B-CLL (42). Although phase I investigations with clofarabine have been initiated, it is too early to identify its selectivity (43). The specificity and activity of these analogs are so potent that each has been effective in achieving objective clinical responses even when used as a single agent for the aforementioned leukemias. It is not clear, at present, why and how the specificity is generated, and this is a challenge that the biochemists and clinicians face. Nonetheless, these observations demonstrate the need for evaluation of new nucleoside analogs in the preclinical and clinical settings.

The first responsibility that we face now is to identify and maximize the selectivity of these newer nucleoside analogs in the clinic. A paradigm for such efforts is establishment of cladribine for treatment of hairy cell leukemia (39,40). The second formidable task that we face now is to optimize single-agent chemotherapy on the basis of the metabolic and mechanistic aspects of these newer nucleoside analogs. Initial knowledge of pharmacokinetics and pharmacodynamics will aid in this process. Such studies may provide a target cellular concentration and the residence time for the cytotoxic metabolites.

The last confronting issue is to develop and implement combination strategies that include metabolic rationales for maximal accumulation/modulation of cytotoxic metabolites. Such approaches are being achieved by using biochemical modulators such as fludarabine (44,45) or cladribine (21) to increase accumulation of nucleoside analog triphosphate (for example ara-C 5′-triphosphate, ara-CTP). An additional strategy that is being exploited is based on mechanistic interactions for increasing the target and opportunity for drug action. Mechanistic strategies combine agents that induce DNA damage, which initiates incision DNA repair processes that require the resynthesis of a single-strand DNA into which nucleoside analogs may be incorporated by otherwise nonreplicating cells (46).

IV. COMBINATION STRATEGIES WITH NUCLEOSIDE ANALOGS

Although nucleoside analogs are clearly active in CLL and low-grade non-Hodgkin's lymphoma, both as initial treatment and for disease that has become refractory to treatment with alkylating agents, it is apparent that any analog alone is unlikely to generate a significant population of long-term survivors. Thus, rationales are needed for the design and evaluation of nucleoside analog-based therapies that feature combinations with other effective antileukemia agents. New knowledge of the varied mechanisms of action of nucleoside analogs and an appreciation of the biology of tumor cells provides an opportunity to develop metabolism-based and mechanism-based strategies in the design of combination therapies.

A. Metabolism-Based Strategies

Deoxycytidine kinase is the rate-limiting step for the phosphorylation of most nucleoside analogs to their active triphosphates, albeit some use deoxyguanosine kinase as well. (3–9, Table 1) Studies of the pharmacokinetics of analogs such as ara-C 5′-triphosphate (ara-CTP) in leukemia cells during therapy demonstrated strong correlations between the ability of cells to accumulate and retain ara-CTP and clinical response of AML to both high-dose and continuous infusion ara-C therapies (47,48). Similarly, cellular pharmacokinetic investigations during therapy suggested a strong association of peak levels of ara-GTP in target leukemia cells and response to nelarabine therapy, stressing the need for enhancement of triphosphate concentrations in cells (18). It is well known that activity of these kinases is feedback inhibited by the respective end products, dCTP and dGTP (9,49–51). Studies using a leukemia cell line demonstrated that decreased cellular deoxynucleotide concentrations caused by the inhibition of ribonucleotide reductase by F-ara-ATP were associated with an increase in the rate of ara-C phosphorylation by deoxycytidine kinase (24,52,53). These results contributed to the design of clinical trials to test the biochemical modulation of ara-C metabolism by fludarabine (44,45).

Cellular pharmacokinetic studies during a clinical trial specifically designed to test the biochemical modulation demonstrated that the area under the concentration times time curve for ara-CTP in AML blasts was increased nearly twofold after fludarabine infusion (45). A consistent, but somewhat smaller, increase was observed in CLL lymphocytes when a similar strategy was used (44). Analyses of both studies demonstrated that augmented intracellular exposure to ara-CTP was due to an acceleration in the rate of ara-CTP accumulation rather than an decrease in its elimination rate or an alteration of the plasma pharmacokinetics of either ara-C or its deamination product ara-U (45). Because the selected dose rate of ara-C generates plasma ara-C concentrations (>10 µM) that maximize ara-CTP accumulation in leukemia cells, the enhancement of ara-CTP accumulation by fludarabine should be viewed as a strategy that increases the intracellular ara-CTP dose intensity.

The successful biochemical modulation that was demonstrated in leukemia cells during therapy was also accompanied by clinical benefit for patients with AML (54,55) and MDS (56,57). To overcome the toxicity of prolonged neutropenia, granulocyte-colony stimulating factor (G-CSF) was added to this regimen resulting in the fludarabine/ara-C/ G-CSF (FLAG) therapy. Because of its success in AML, the regimen was extended to other leukemia types such as ALL (58) and CML (59). In addition to the adult leukemias, the fludarabine and ara-C combination with or without growth factor has been successfully used for pediatric acute leukemias (60–62). More recently, this regimen has been used as preparative therapy to nonmyeloablative bone marrow transplantation in myeloid disease (63).

Although fludarabine has been used most extensively for biochemical modulation, because cladribine and clofarabine triphosphates also inhibit ribonucleotide reductase these purine nucleoside analogs are perfect candidates for such strategies. In fact, cladribine has been demonstrated to be effective modulator for ara-CTP accumulation in leukemia blasts during therapy of adult (21,64) and pediatric (65) patients with AML. Clofarabine has been shown to increase ara-CTP accumulation in leukemia cell lines and primary CLL cells (66), and its use during therapy is warranted.

By use of a similar approach for indolent leukemias, fludarabine was administered just before nelarabine to biochemically modulate the cellular metabolism of ara-G generated from nelarabine (42). This was based on initial studies in a leukemia cell line (52) and in primary leukemia cells (67) that demonstrated greater accumulation of ara-GTP in cells after treatment with F-ara-A in vitro. These investigations suggested the feasibility of a biochemical modulation approach to intracellular dose-intensification of ara-GTP. A pilot study of this strategy has been initiated in patients with indolent B-cell malignancies refractory to treatment with fludarabine or alkylating agents (68). The treatment design features nelarabine infusions on day 1, 3, and 5, which are preceded by fludarabine treatment on days 3 and 5. Investigations of the cellular pharmacology again demonstrated the association of significantly higher concentrations in the leukemic lymphocytes of responding patients, several of whom were resistant to prior fludarabine therapy. Interestingly, the prolonged retention of ara-GTP (t1/2 of elimination, >24 hr) limited a full evaluation of the biochemical modulation activity of fludarabine on cellular pharmacology of ara-GTP. However, the clinical effectiveness of this combination for alkylator and fludarabine refractory or relapsed B-CLL patients strongly suggest that nelarabine may use metabolic pathways (e.g., deoxyguanosine kinase) and action mechanisms that confer sensitivity to cells that are resistant to fludarabine. Thus, further investigations for the combination of these two agents are warranted (42,68).

B. Mechanism-Based Strategies

The most prevalent action of purine nucleoside analogs associated with cell death requires the incorporation of these drugs into DNA. Once incorporated, some nucleotide analogs then serve as relatively poor substrates for the addition of subsequent nucleotides by DNA polymerases, and the process of DNA replication thereby becomes inhibited. The current hypothesis stipulates that cells sense analog-induced delays in DNA replication and that these sensing mechanisms signal for additional processes responsible for removal of the analog. If the cell is unable to remove the analog by proofreading DNA repair mechanisms that would permit resumption of DNA replication, the stalled replication fork will eventually generate a signal initiating cell death, either by apoptosis or mitotic catastrophe. Thus, incorporation into DNA is the best characterized mechanism for nucleotide analog–induced cell death (26,27). A major limitation to the potential effectiveness of nucleoside analogs is the fact that only a small fraction of most tumors are actively in cycle, and yet fewer are in S phase when the drugs are administered. Therefore, therapeutic strategies are needed to expand the fraction of the tumor population that is synthesizing DNA.

One approach to increasing the number of cells engaged in DNA synthesis has focused on conditions that induce the various forms of excision DNA repair. These mechanisms, including base, nucleotide, and cross-link repair, act by incision on either side of nucleotides and adjacent nucleotides that have been damaged and then excise this as a single strand of oligonucleotides. This is followed by resynthesis of the single strand of DNA in the excision patch. Because these repair processes share many of the same DNA polymerizing and metabolizing enzymes that are required for DNA replication, it has been hypothesized that incorporation of a nucleotide analog into a patch of repairing DNA by these enzymes would prevent the repair of damaged DNA. In addition, it is possible that the incorporated analog would be sensed by mechanisms similar to those that monitor the progress of DNA replication, an action that might also activate the apoptosis signal. Thus, combinations of nucleosides with alkylating agents or platinum derivatives, which are known to initiate excision DNA repair processes, might act to sensitize cells that are otherwise kinetically resistant to nucleoside analogs.

An additional mechanism that will result in synergy between DNA damaging agents and dAdo analogs acts through ribonucleotide reductase. This enzyme is activated by DNA-damaging agents to fulfil the requirement of dNTP synthesis needed for a successful DNA repair (69–73). This is more so in the case of DNA-damaging agents that initiate repair of a long patch of DNA such as nucleotide excision repair or recombinational repair. Triphosphates of analogs such as fludarabine, cladribine, and clofarabine are potent inhibitors of ribonucleotide reductase. It can be postulated that these analogs would inhibit this enzyme ready for synthesis of repair dNTPs. As a consequence of this action, the repair process will either halt or slow down.

Combining nucleotide analogs with agents that initiate excision DNA repair will form new sites for incorporation of the analogs that did not exist in quiescent cells. To this end, the synergistic activity of fludarabine and ionizing radiation has been demonstrated in tumor-bearing mice (74,75). In a second approach to generating targets for the action of fraudulent nucleotides, fludarabine was combined with chemotherapeutic agents, which either produce cross-links or adducts that signal DNA repair. An example of this tactic is the combination of fludarabine with cisplatin. Together, these drugs produce synergistic cytotoxicity in growing cells in culture, the mechanism of which involves the inhibition of the repair of cisplatin-induced cross-links in the DNA (76).

Cyclophosphamide is an alkylating agent that shows activity against a wide variety of hematopoietic neoplasms, some solid tumors, and in the context of bone marrow transplantation. The cytotoxic lesion is thought to result from the formation of interstrand DNA cross-links, which are found after incubation with the activated prodrug 4-hydroperoxy-cyclophosphamide (4-HC) in vitro (77) and after in vivo cyclophosphamide administration (78). Although the precise mechanism of repair by removal of DNA interstrand cross-links caused by bifunctional alkylating agents such as phosphoramide mustard, melphalan, busulfan, or cisplatin has not been explained, in vitro studies with human CLL lymphocytes indicate a kinetic process that varies among individuals (79–82). DNA base alkylation by cyclophosphamide will activate base excision repair, nucleotide excision repair, and the removal of interstrand DNA cross-links. Nevertheless, the results obtained with 4-HC are qualitatively similar to ultraviolet light (UV) light, which was chosen originally because it activates nucleotide excision repair almost exclusively.

As seen after UV irradiation, treatment with 4-HC for 15 minutes also elicited induction of unscheduled DNA synthesis as measured by [^{3}H]thymidine incorporation in quiescent lymphocytes. There was also a dose-dependent response when fludarabine triphosphate was loaded in cells by incubation with 0.1 to 30 μM F-ara-A followed by a 15-minute exposure to 20 μM 4-HC (83). As was the case after UV induction of nucleotide excision repair, this was accompanied by inhibition of unscheduled DNA synthesis and incorporation of [^{3}H] F-ara-A into the DNA of the lymphocytes, which remained in G_0. When the induction of DNA repair by 4-HC was evaluated by the single-cell gel electrophoresis (comet) assay, it was clear that F-ara-A alone had no effect on comet formation. In lymphocytes treated with 4-HC alone, the significant increase in tail moment that was observed initially (zero hour) diminished rapidly after washing into fresh media, suggesting rapid completion of the processes requiring DNA incision/ligation. However, when cells were first loaded with fludarabine triphosphate and then treated with 4-HC and washed into fresh medium, the original comet signal was greater than after 4-HC alone and failed to recover to control values. Both MTT assays of cell viability and pulsed-field gel electrophoresis of high-molecular weight DNA fragmentation, which accompanies apoptosis, indicated that the effect of the combination was greater than the sum of each drug alone.

These results support the hypothesis that initiation of DNA repair in quiescent cells will permit the incorporation of a nucleotide analog into the DNA of these cells. The fact that combining what are essentially nontoxic levels of agents (cisplatin, cyclophosphamide) or modalities (UV or ionizing radiation) that initiate DNA repair with nucleoside analogs such as fludarabine resulted in substantially greater killing than the sum of either agent alone suggests that the combination is acting by a mechanism different from that of either agent alone. This is consistent with the working hypothesis, which postulates that agents that induce DNA repair in quiescent cells will enable the incorporation of nucleotide analogs into the DNA of quiescent cells, thereby initiating signals for cell death. Recent clinical studies designed to implement this rationale have proved effective in the treatment of indolent hematological diseases (84).

In summary, during the past decade, fludarabine has had a major impact in increasing the effectiveness of treatment of indolent B-cell malignancies. However, the use fludarabine as a single agent is on the decline. One reason for this is the realization that fludarabine as monotherapy is unlikely to produce sustained disease-free survival. Nevertheless, this has not discouraged the development of a second generation of purine nucleoside analogs (nelarabine and clofarabine) that use metabolic pathways and exert actions that are distinct from fludarabine. A second impetus for the move away from single-agent treatment comes from the emergence of new strategies for combination therapies. Prominent among these is the rationale for combining nucleotide analogs with clinically active therapeutic agents that initiate excision repair processes. The activities of several of these mechanism-based strategies have now been validated in clinical trials. Also, biochemical modulation strategies that use fludarabine or cladribine in combination with ara-C have been validated with cellular pharmacology investigations. These treatments are effective in acute myelogenous leukemias and form the nucleus for combinations with cisplatin and mitoxantrone for the treatments of Richter's transformed CLL and low-grade lymphoma, respectively.

The development of monoclonal antibodies that target surface antigens highly expressed in lymphoid malignancies, CD20 and CD52, has provided a second area of new opportunities. Because Rituximab and Campath 1H are active in fludarabine-resistant disease as single agents, new regimens that combine either of these antibodies with fludarabine are under current investigation. Finally, the immunosuppression associated with purine nucleoside analog therapy has been a continued concern for clinical investigators. Recently, the same combination regimens of fludarabine with either ara-C or cyclophosphamide that have been used as intensive chemotherapy for treatment of AMLs or CLLs, respectively, have been used to advantage to reduce immunological function. This approach facilitates the subsequent transplantation of allogeneic donor lymphocytes or stem cells and, in so doing, has given rise to the field of nonmyeloablative transplantation.

Clearly, understanding of the cellular pharmacology and mechanisms of action of fludarabine has been essential to the conceptualization of mechanism-based combination strategies. It is somewhat ironic, however, that the mechanisms by which fludarabine acts alone in the successful treatment of indolent lymphocytic diseases have not yet been clearly established and may differ from those defined in cell culture models.

The present review has sought to bring together the current state of understanding of the plasma pharmacokinetics and cellular pharmacodynamics of fludarabine and the newly emerging purine nucleosides, nelarabine and clofarabine, with the hope that this may be useful in the design and evaluation of future combinations.

ACKNOWLEDGMENTS

Supported in part by grants CA 32839 and CA 57629 from the National Cancer Institute, Department of Health and Human Services.

REFERENCES

1. GA LePage, A Khaliq, JA Gottleib. Studies of 9-β-D-arabinofuranosyladenine in man. Drug Metab Dispos 1:756–759, 1973.
2. JA Montgomery, K Hewson. Synthesis of potential anticancer agents. X. Fluoroadenosine. J Am Chem Soc 79:4559, 1957.
3. CU Lambe, DR Averett, MT Paff, et al. 2-Amino-6-methoxypurine arabinoside: an agent for T-cell malignancies. Cancer Res 55:3352–3356, 1995.
4. DS Shewach, KK Reynolds, L Hertel. Nucleotide specificity of human deoxycytidine kinase. Mol Pharmacol 42:518–524, 1993.
5. TA Krenitsky, JV Tuttle, GW Koszalka, et al. Deoxycytidine kinase from calf thymus: substrate and inhibitor specificity. J Biol Chem 251:4055–4061, 1976.
6. DA Carson, DB Wasson, J Kaye, et al. Deoxycytidine kinase-mediated toxicity of deoxyadenosine analogs toward human lymphoblasts in vitro and toward murine L1210 leukemia in vivo. Proc Nat Acad Sci USA 77:6865–6869, 1980.
7. WB Parker, SC Shaddix, LM Rose et al. Comparison of the mechanism of cytotoxicity of 2-chloro-9-(2-deoxy-2-fluoro-β-D-arabinofuranosyl)adenine, 2-chloro-9-(2-deoxy-2-fluoro-β-D-ribofuranosyl)adenine, and 2-cholor-9-(2-doxy-2,2-difluoro-β-D-ribofuranosyl)adenine in CEM cells. Mol Pharmacol 55:515–520, 1999.
8. L Wang, A Karlsson, ES Arner, et al. Substrate specificity of mitochondrial 2′-deoxyguanosine

kinase. Efficient phosphorylation of 2-chlorodeoxyadenosine. J Biol Chem 268:22847–22852, 1993.

9. RA Lewis, L Link. Phosphorylation of arabinosyl guanine by a mitochondrial enzyme of bovine liver. Biochem Pharmacol 38:2001–2006, 1989.

10. DS Shewach, PE Daddona, E Ashcraft, et al. Metabolism and selective cytotoxicity of 9-β-D-arabinofuranosylguanine in human lymphoblasts. Cancer Res 45:1008–1014, 1985.

11. V Verhoef, A Fridland. Metabolic basis of arabinonucleoside selectivity for human leukemic T- and B-lymphoblasts. Cancer Res 45:3646–3650, 1985.

12. W Plunkett, S Chubb, L Alexander, et al. Comparison of the toxicity and metabolism of 9-β-D-arabinofuranosyl-2-fluoroadenine and 9-β-D-arabinofuranosyladenine in lymphoblastoid cells. Cancer Res 40:2349–2355, 1980.

13. WB Parker, SC Shaddix, CH Chang, et al. Effects of 2-chloro-9-(2-deoxy-2-fluoro-β-D-arabinofuranosyl)adenine on K562 cellular metabolism and the inhibition of human ribonucleotide reductase and DNA polymerases by its 5′-triphosphate. Cancer Res 51:2386–2394, 1991.

14. C Xie, W Plunkett. Metabolism and actions of 2-chloro-9-(2-deoxy-2-fluoro-β-D-arabinofuranosyl)adenine in human lymphoblastoid cells. Cancer Res 55:2847–2852, 1995.

15. J Liliemark, G Juliusson. Cellular pharmacokinetics of 2-chloro-2′-deoxyadenosine nucleotides: comparison of intermittent and continuous intravenous infusion and subcutaneous and oral administration in leukemia patients. Clin Cancer Res 1:385–390, 1995.

16. V Gandhi, A Kemena, MJ Keating, W Plunkett. Cellular pharmacology of fludarabine triphosphate in chronic lymphocytic leukemia cells during fludarabine therapy. Leuk Lymph 10:49, 1993.

17. F Albertioni, S Lindemalm, V Reichelova, et al. Pharmacokinetics of cladribine in plasma and its 5′-monophosphate and 5′-triphosphate in leukemic cells of patients with chronic lymphocytic leukemia. Clin Cancer Res 4:653–658, 1998.

18. V Gandhi, W Plunkett, CO Rodriguez, et al. Compound GW506U78 in refractory hematologic malignancies: relationship between cellular pharmacokinetics and clinical response. J Clin Oncol 16:3607–3615, 1998.

19. EL White, SC Shaddix, RW Brockman, et al. Comparison of the actions of 9-β-D-arabinofuranosyl-2-fluoroadenine and 9-β-D-arabinofuranosyladenine on target enzymes form mouse tumor cells. Cancer Res 42:2260–2266, 1982.

20. WB Parker, AK Bapat, J-X Shen, et al. Interaction of 2-halogenated dATP analogs (F, Cl, and Br) with human DNA polymerases, DNA primase, and ribonucleotide reductase. Mol Pharmacol 34:485–492, 1988.

21. V Gandhi, E Estey, MJ Keating, et al. Chlorodeoxyadenosine and arabinosylcytosine in patients with acute myelogenous leukemia: pharmacokinetic, pharmacodynamic, and molecular interactions. Blood 87:256–264, 1996.

22. KC Xie, W Plunkett. Deoxynucleotide pool depletion, and sustained inhibition of ribonucleotide reductase and DNA synthesis after treatment of human lymphoblastoid cells with 2-chloro-9-(2-deoxy-2-fluoro-β-D-arabinofuranosyl)adenine. Cancer Res 56:3030–3037, 1996.

23. W Plunkett, P Huang, V Gandhi. Metabolism and action of fludarabine. Sem Oncol 17(suppl, 5):3–17, 1990.

24. V Gandhi, W Plunkett. Modulation of arabinosylnucleoside metabolism by arabinosylnucleotides in human leukemia cells. Cancer Res 48:329–334, 1988.

25. P Hentosh, R Koob, RL Blakley. Incorporation of 2-halogeno-2′-deoxyadenosine 5′-triphosphates into DNA during replication by human polymerases alpha and beta. J Biol Chem 265: 4033–4039, 1990.

26. CO Rodriguez, Jr, V Gandhi. Arabinosylguanine-induced apoptosis of T-lymphoblastic cells: Incorporation into DNA is a necessary step. Cancer Res 59:4937–4943, 1999.

27. P Huang, W Plunkett. Fludarabine- and gemcitabine-induced apoptosis: Incorporation of analogs into DNA is a criticial event. Cancer Chemther Pharmacol 36:181–188, 1995.

28. P Huang, S Chubb, W Plunkett. Termination of DNA synthesis by 9-β-D-arabinofuranosyl-

2-fluoroadenine 5′-triphosphate. A mechanism of toxicity. J Biol Chem, 265:16617–16623, 1990.

29. V Gandhi, S Mineishi, P Huang, AJ Chapman, Y Yang, F Chen, B Nowak, S Chubb, LW Hertel, W Plunkett. Cytotoxicity, metabolism, and mechanisms of action of 2′,2′-difluoro-deoxyguanosine in Chinese hamster ovary cells. Cancer Res 55:1517–1524, 1995.

30. K Kamiya, P Huang, W Plunkett. Inhibition of the 3′ → 5′ exonuclease of human DNA polymerase ε by fludarabine-terminated DNA. J Biol Chem 271:19428–19435, 1996.

31. P Hentosh, P Grippo. 2-chloro-2′-deoxyadenosine monophosphate residues in DNA enhance susceptibility to 3′ → 5′ exonuclease. Biochem J 302:567–571, 1994.

32. P Huang, W Plunkett. Action of 9-β-D-arabinofuranosyl-2-fluoroadenine on RNA metabolism. Molec Pharmac 39:449–55, 1991.

33. P Huang, A Sandoval, E Van Den Neste, et al. Inhibition of RNA transcription: A biochemical mechanism of fludarabine-induced apoptosis in chronic lymphocytic leukemia cells. Leukemia 14:1405–1413, 2000.

34. X Liu, H Zou, C Slaughter, et al. DFF, a heterodimeric protein that functions downstream of caspase-3 to trigger DNA fragmentation during apoptosis. Cell 89:175–184, 1997.

35. LM Leoni, Q Chao, HB Cottam, et al. Induction of an apoptotic program in cell-free extracts by 2-chloro-2′-deoxyadenosine 5′-triphosphate and cytochrome c. Proc Nat Acad Sci USA 95:9567–9571, 1998.

36. D Genini, I Budihardjo, W Plunkett, et al. Nucleotide requirement for the in vitro activation of Apaf-1-mediated caspase pathway. J Biol Chem 275:29–34, 2000.

37. MJ Keating, S O'Brien, S Lerner, et al. Long-term follow-up of patients with chronic lymphocytic leukemia (CLL) receiving fludarabine regimens as initial therapy. Blood 92:1165, 1998.

38. P McLaughlin, FB Hagemeister, JE Romaguera, et al. Fludarabine, mitoxantrone, and dexamethasone: an effective new regimen for indolent lymphoma. J Clin Oncol 14:1262–1268, 1996.

39. BD Cheson, JM Sorensen, DA Vena, et al. Treatment of hairy cell leukemia with 2-chloro-deoxyadenosine via the Group C protocol mechanism of the National Cancer Institute: a report of 979 patients. Clin Oncol 16:3007–3017, 1998.

40. A Saven, C Burian, JA Koziol, et al. Long-term follow-up of patients with hairy cell leukemia after cladribine treatment. Blood 92:1918–1926, 1998.

41. J Kurtzberg, MJ Keating, JO Moore, et al. 2-amino-9-β-D-arabinosyl-6-methoxy-9H-guanine (GW 506: Compound 506U) is highly active in patients with T-cell malignancies: Results of a phase I trial in pediatric and adult patients with refractory hematological malignancies. Blood 88:669a, 1996.

42. S O'Brien, D Thomas, H Kantarjian, et al. Compound 506 has activity in mature lymphoid leukemia. Blood 92:490a, 1998.

43. P Kozuch, N Ibrahim, F Khuri, P Hoff, E Estey, V Gandhi, M Du, MB Rios, W Plunkett, MJ Keating, H Kantarjian. Phase I clinical and pharmacological study of clofarabine. Blood 94:127a, 1999.

44. V Gandhi, A Kemena, MJ Keating, et al. Fludarabine infusion potentiates arabinosylcytosine metabolism in lymphocytes of patients with chronic lymphocytic leukemia. Cancer Res 52:897–905, 1992.

45. V Gandhi, E Estey, MJ Keating, et al. Fludarabine potentiates metabolism of arabinosylcytosine in patients with acute myelogenous leukemia during therapy. J Clin Oncol 11:116–124, 1993.

46. W Plunkett, Y Kawai, A Sandoval, et al. Mechanism-based rationales for combination therapies of lymphoid malignancies. Haematologica 84(Suppl 10):73–77, 1999.

47. W Plunkett, S Iacoboni, E Estey, L Danhauser, JO Liliemark, MJ Keating. Pharmacologically-directed ara-C therapy for refractory leukemia. Sem Oncol 12 (suppl 3):20–30, 1985.

48. EH Estey, MJ Keating, KB McCredie, EJ Freireich, W Plunkett. Cellular ara-CTP pharmacokinetics, response, and karyotype in newly diagnosed acute myelogenous leukemia. Leukemia 4:95–99, 1990.

49. S Grant. Biochemical modulation of cytosine arabinoside. Pharmac Ther 48:29–44, 1990.
50. RL Momparler, GA Fischer. Mammalian deoxynucleoside kinase: I. Deoxycytidine kinase: purification, properties and kinetic studies with cytosine arabinoside. J Biol Chem 243:4298–4304, 1968.
51. NS Datta, DS Shewach, MC Hurley, et al. Human T-lymphoblast deoxycytidine kinase: Purification and properties. Biochemistry 28:114–123, 1989.
52. V Gandhi, W Plunkett. Interaction of arabinosyl nucleotides in K562 human leukemia cells. Biochem Pharmacol 38:3551–3558, 1989.
53. V Gandhi, B Nowak, MJ Keating, W Plunkett. Modulation of arabinosylcytosine metabolism by arabinosyl-2-fluoroadenine in lymphocytes from patients with chronic lymphocytic leukemia: implications for combination therapy. Blood 74:2070–2075, 1989.
54. E Estey, W Plunkett, V Gandhi, MB Rios, H Kantarjian, MJ Keating. Fludarabine and arabinosylcytosine therapy of refractory and relapsed acute myelogenous leukemia. Leukemia Lymphoma 4:343–350, 1993.
55. M Montillo, S Mirto, MC Petti, R Latagliata, S Magrin, A Pinto, V Zagonel, G Mele, A Tedeschi, F Ferrara, Fludarabine, cytarabine, and G-CSF (FLAG) for the treatment of poor risk acute myeloid leukemia. Am J Hematol 58:105–109, 1998.
56. EH Estey, HM Kantarjian, S O'Brien, S Kornblau, M Andreeff, M Beran, S Pierce, M Keating. High remission rate, short remission duration in patients with refractory anemia with excess blasts (RAEB) in transformation (RAEB-t) given acute myelogenous leukemia (AML)-type chemotherapy in combination with granulocyte-CSF (G-CSF). Cytokines Mol Ther 1:21–28, 1995.
57. TJ Nokes, S Johnson, D Harvey, AH Goldstone. FLAG is a useful regimen for poor prognosis adult myeloid leukaemias and myelodysplastic syndromes. Leuk Lymphoma 27:93–101, 1997.
58. M Montillo, A Tedeschi, R Centurioni, P Leoni. Treatment of relapsed adult acute lymphoblastic leukemia with fludarabine and cytosine arabinoside followed by granulocyte colony-stimulating factor (FLAG-GCSF). Leuk Lymphoma 25:579–583, 1997.
59. A Tedeschi, M Montillo, F Ferrara, A Nosari, G Mele, C Copia, P Leoni, E Morra. Treatment of chronic myeloid leukemia in the blastic phase with fludarabine, cytosine arabinoside and G-CSF. Eur J Haematol 64:182–187, 2000.
60. G Fleischhack, C Hasan, N Graf, G Mann, U Bode. IDA-FLAG (idarubicin, fludarabine, cytarabine, G-CSF), an effective remission-induction therapy for poor-prognosis AML of childhood prior to allogeneic or autologous bone marrow transplantation: experiences of a phase II trial. Br J Haematol 102:647–655, 1998.
61. VI Avramis, S Wiersma, MD Krailo, LV Ramilo-Torno, A Sharpe, W Liu-Mares, R Kowck, GH Reaman, JK Sato. Pharmacokinetic and pharmacodynamic studies of fludarabine and cytosine arabinoside administered as loading boluses followed by continuous infusions after a phase I/II study in pediatric patients with relapsed leukemias. The Children's Cancer Group. Clin Cancer Res 4:45–52, 1998.
62. A Leahey, K Kelly, LB Rorke, B Lange. A phase I/II study of idarubicin (Ida) with continuous infusion fludarabine (F-ara-A) and cytarbine (ara-C) for refractory or recurrent Pediatric acute myeloid leukemia (AML). J Pediatr Hematol Oncol 19:304–308, 1997.
63. S Giralt, E Estey, M Albitar, K van Besien, G Rondon, P Anderlini, S O'Brien, I Khouri, J Gajewski, R Mehra, D Claxton, B Andersson, M Beran, D Przepiorka, C Koller, S Kornblau, M Korbling, M Keating, H Kantarjian, R Champlin. Engraftment of allogeneic hematopoietic progenitor cells with purine analog-containing chemotherapy: harnessing graft-versus-leukemia without myeloablative therapy. Blood 89:4531–4536, 1997.
64. SM Kornblau, V Gandhi, M Andreeff, M Beran, H Kantarjian, CA Koller, S O'Brien, W Plunkett, E Estey. Clinical and laboratory studies of 2-chlorodeoxyadenosine ± cytosine arabinoside for relapsed or refractory acute myelogenous leukemia in adults. Leukemia 10:1563–1569, 1996.
65. KM Radomski, V Gandhi, DK Srivastava, BI Razzouk, FG Behm, W Plunkett, C-H Pui, JE

Rubnitz, RC Ribeiro. Interim analyssi of cytarabine (ara-C) and cladribine (2-CDA) combination therapy in acute myeloid leukemia. Blood 96:327a, 2000.

66. V Gandhi, LE Robertson, W Plunkett. 2-chloro-2′-fluoro-arabinosyladenine: Pharmacokinetics and action in chronic lymphocytic leukemia cells. Proc Am Assoc Cancer Res 34:414, 1993.

67. CO, Jr Rodriguez, JK Legha, E Estey, MJ Keating, V Gandhi. Pharmacological and biochemical strategies to increase the accumulation of arabinofuranosylguanine triphosphate in primary human leukemia cells. Clin Cancer Res 3:2107–2113, 1997.

68. V Gandhi, W Plunkett, S Weller, M Du, M Ayres, Jr CO Rodriguez, P Ramakrishna, GL Rosner, JP Hodge, S O'Brien, MJ Keating. Evaluation of the combination of nelarabine and fludarabine in leukemias: Clinical response, pharmacokinetics and pharmacodynamics in leukemia cells. J Clin Oncol Submitted.

69. SJ Elledge, Z Zhou, JB Allen. Ribonucleotide reductase: regulation, regulation, regulation. Trends Biochem Sci 17:119–123, 1992.

70. RAR Hurta, JA Wright. Alterations in the activity and regulation of mammaliam ribonucleotide reducase by chlorambucil. A DNA damaging agent. J Biol Chem 267:7066–7071, 1992.

71. ML Kuo, TJ Kinsella. Expression of ribonucleotide reductase after ionizing radiation in human cervical carcinoma cells. Cancer Res 58:2245–2252, 1998.

72. M Rodriguez, V Gandhi. Relationship between unscheduled DNA synthesis and increase in the expression of ribonucleotide reductase protein in chronic lymphocytic leukemia cells. Proc Am Assoc Cancer Res 40:402, 1999.

73. H Tanaka, H Arakawa, T Yamaguchi et al. A ribonucleotide reductase gene involved in a p53-dependent cell-cycle checkpoint for DNA damage. Nature 404:42–49, 2000.

74. V Gregoire, N Hunter, L Milas, WA Brock, W Plunkett, WN Hittleman. Potentiation of radiation-induced regrowth delay in murine tumors by fludarabine. Cancer Res 54:468–474, 1994.

75. V Gregoire, NT Van, C Stephens, WA Brock, L Milas, W Plunkett, WN Hittleman. The role of fludarabine-induced apoptosis and cell cycle synchronization in enhanced murine tumor radiation response in vivo. Cancer Res 54:6201–6209, 1994.

76. L-Y Yang, L Li, MJ Keating, W Plunkett. Arabinosyl-2-fluoroadenine augments cisplatin cytotoxicity and inhibits cisplatin-DNA cross-link repair. Mol Pharmacol 47:1072–1079, 1995.

77. J Hilton. Deoxyribonucleic acid cross-linking by 4-hydroperoxycyclophosphamide in cyclophosphamide sensitive and resistant L1210 cells. Biochem. Pharmacol 33:1867–1872, 1984.

78. JA Skare, KR Schrotel. Alkaline elution of rat testicular DNA: detection of DNA cross-links after in vivo treatment with chemical mutagens. Mutat Res 130:295–303, 1984.

79. A Eastman, N Schulte. Enhanced DNA repair as a mechanism of resistance to cis-diamminedichloroplatinum. Biochemistry 27:4730–4734, 1988.

80. L Panasci, D Henderson, SJ Torrres-Garcia. Transport, metabolism and DNA interaction of melphalan in lymphocytes form patients with chronic lymphocytic leukemia. Cancer Res 48: 1972–1976, 1988.

81. SJ Torres, L Cousineau, S Caplan. Correlation of resistance to nitrogen mustards in chronic lymphocytic leukemia with enhanced removal of melphalan-induced DNA cross-links. Biochem Pharmacol 38:3122–3128, 1989.

82. R Geleziunas, A McQuillan, A Malapetsa, M Hutchinson, D Kopriva, MA Wainberg, J Hiscott, J Bramson, L Panasci. Increased DNA synthesis and repair-enzyme expression in lymphocytes form patients with chronic lymphocytic leukemia resistant to nitrogen mustards. J Nat Cancer Inst 83:557–564, 1991.

83. Y Kawai, W Plunkett. DNA repair induced by 4-hydroperoxycyclophosphamide permits fludarabine nucleotide incorporation and is associated with synergystic induction of apoptosis in quiescent human lymphocytes. Blood 94:655a, 1999.

84. S O'Brien, H Kantarjian, M Beran, El Freireich, S Kornblau, S Lerner, J Gilbreath, M Keating. Fludarabine and cyclophosphamide therapy in chronic lymphocytic leukemia. Blood 88(suppl 1):480, 1996.

11

Differential Diagnosis of the Chronic B-Cell Lymphoid Leukemias

RANDY D. GASCOYNE

British Columbia Cancer Agency, Vancouver, British Columbia, Canada

I. INTRODUCTION

In the recent past, most chronic leukemias were diagnosed under the rubric of chronic lymphocytic leukemia (CLL) if blast cells were not a feature and the neoplastic cells resembled mature lymphocytes. The advent of flow cytometric immunophenotypic analysis has revolutionized our approach to this category of disease, because many distinctive B- and T-cell leukemias are now recognized (1,2). In most instances, rendering an accurate diagnosis is clinically important, because a specific therapy may be indicated. The approach to diagnosis often involves a multiparameter analysis, including careful morphological assessment, flow cytometrical immunophenotypical analysis, cytochemistry, cytogenetic, and molecular genetic studies. Major advances in diagnostic techniques, in particular the correlation of peripheral blood morphology with histopathology of biopsy sections and improved molecular/cytogenetic knowledge has made it necessary to revise both the approach and the classification of the CLLs. This chapter will first list the reactive disorders characterized by a peripheral blood lymphocytosis, followed by a discussion of the chronic B-cell lymphocytic leukemias. A detailed discussion of B-cell prolymphocytic leukemia (PLL) and the group of T-cell chronic leukemias will not be included, because these are discussed elsewhere.

II. METHODOLOGY

A variety of laboratory techniques are required for the accurate study of CLLs. Although many regard peripheral blood smear morphology as the ''gold standard'' for diagnosis and classification, the vagaries of blood smear preparation render many samples suboptimal for

209

detailed morphological assessment. In vitro storage artifacts and technical differences in blood smear preparation can produce suboptimal smears. Moreover, subtle distinctions between peripheral blood morphology and well-described histological findings in certain subtypes of lymphoproliferative disorders result in confusing diagnostic criteria. For example, most cases of mantle cell lymphoma have indistinct nucleoli when assessed with hematoxylin and eosin (H & E)–stained histological sections but may have quite prominent nucleoli when the cells are found in the peripheral blood (3,4). Similarly, B-cell PLL cells are much larger than the cells found in classic CLL and have very prominent, typically central nucleoli when viewed in peripheral blood smear; but in H & E stained sections are imperceptibly larger than the small lymphocytes of CLL and have small, barely visible nucleoli (5). It is important to be aware of these subtle morphological distinctions when comparing histological findings with peripheral blood morphology.

Nevertheless, peripheral blood films are the method of choice for the initial evaluation of virtually all cases of CLL (1). Currently, however, more emphasis is placed on ancillary studies used to determine the lineage and molecular characteristics of these disorders. These data are integrated with the morphology to accurately subtype a chronic leukemia. Cytochemistry and serum protein electrophoresis studies are still used in selected cases to help distinguish between subtypes of chronic lymphoid leukemia. The single most important technique for distinguishing benign from neoplastic lymphocytosis and further delineating the specific subtype of chronic leukemia is flow cytometric immunophenotypical analysis. Differences in the frequency of antigen expression reported for different subtypes of chronic leukemia using flow cytometry can largely be accounted for by (1) differences in equipment; (2) different antibody reagents; (3) variable antibody labeling techniques; (4) different fluorochrome combinations; (5) lack of standardized instrument calibration and methods (two-color vs three-color vs four-color analysis), and (6) differences in the subjective interpretation of histogram data. These factors should be considered when interpreting the distribution and frequency of antigen expression in chronic leukemias. A good example of the impact of these factors is revealed by the published frequency for CD11c coexpression in typical CD5$^+$ B-cell CLL, which varies between 5% and 90% of cases (6). Some of this variability may be real but is more likely explained by the factors listed earlier.

Molecular and cytogenetic data are sometimes used to aid in the diagnosis of chronic leukemias. The association of characteristic cytogenetic findings and specific subtypes of lymphoid neoplasms is well established. These include the t(14;18)(q32;q21) of follicular lymphoma (FL), the t(11;14)(q13;q32) of mantle cell lymphoma (MCL), and the t(11;18)(q21;q21) of extranodal marginal zone lymphomas (MZL) (7). Molecular techniques can also be used to substitute for classical cytogenetic studies, including Southern blot analysis, polymerase chain reaction (PCR), and fluorescence in situ hybridization (FISH) studies. These techniques can be used to establish both clonality and lineage and are particularly useful for the determination of specific oncogene rearrangements that may be helpful in difficult cases. More complex diagnostic tests such as Fiber-FISH, 5' bcl-6 gene mutations and immunoglobulin heavy chain (IgH) sequencing are not routinely used in the differential diagnosis of these disorders but are currently considered research tools.

III. BENIGN LYMPHOCYTOSIS

The causes of reactive lymphocytosis are listed in Table 1, separated into B-cell and T-cell types. The initial approach to any case of lymphocytosis begins with the distinction

Table 1   Reactive Lymphocytosis

B-cell
   Postsplenectomy state
   Persistent polyclonal B-cell lymphocytosis
T-cell
   Viral infections (EBV, CMV, etc.)
   Bordetella pertussis
   Syphilis
   Tuberculosis
   Serum sickness
   Thyrotoxicosis
   Addison's disease
   Postsplenectomy state

between benign and malignant disorders. After careful morphological review, flow cytometry is typically required to determine the lineage and resolve the differential diagnosis, with the goal of arriving at a specific diagnosis. A detailed discussion of the reactive disorders is beyond the scope of this chapter. However, one of these entities is discussed below, principally because it may be confused with a CLL.

IV.   PERSISTENT POLYCLONAL B-CELL LYMPHOCYTOSIS

Originally described in 1982, this is an uncommon disorder characterized by a mild, polyclonal B-cell lymphocytosis occurring in middle-aged women with a history of smoking (8). The patients may be asymptomatic or complain of fatigue and nonspecific upper respiratory tract symptoms. Lymphadenopathy is not a feature, but mild splenomegaly is seen

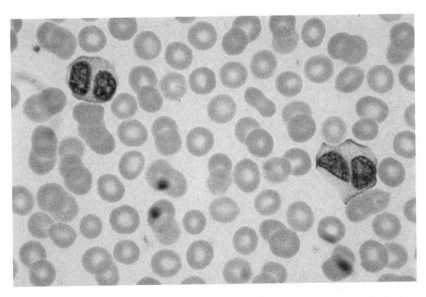

Figure 1   Peripheral blood smear of polyclonal B-cell lymphocytosis showing reactive lymphocytes with bilobed nuclei.

in a small number of patients (9). The peripheral blood smear reveals a mild elevation of the white blood cell (WBC) count and characteristic mature lymphocytes with bilobed nuclei (see Fig. 1). The lymphocyte morphology is variable, and may in some cases resemble B-CLL or the atypical lymphocytes found in viral infections. It is important to recognize this disorder and to distinguish it from malignant lymphoproliferative diseases that share similar features. Persistent polyclonal B-cell lymphocytosis (PBCL) is chronic but appears clinically benign. There is some suggestion that the disorder may be reversible if the patients stop smoking (10). Associated findings include polyclonal gammopathy with elevated IgM and borderline or low IgG and IgA levels, a strong association with HLA-DR7, a possible association with Epstein Barr virus infection and isochromosome 3q abnormalities (9). Molecular studies of PBCL are scant, but some have revealed either a germline configuration or oligoclonal pattern for immunoglobulin heavy chain (IgH), whereas others using more sensitive tests report multiple, minor bcl-2 oncogene rearrangements (11). The recognition of the disorder is facilitated by the finding of increased polyclonal B-cells (normal kappa/lambda distribution) with characteristic nuclear features and absent coexpression of CD5. There are few causes of benign B-cell lymphocytosis, although mild increases in B lymphocytes can rarely be seen in connective tissue diseases, post bone marrow transplant and following splenectomy.

V. CLASSIFICATION OF B-CELL LEUKEMIAS

The following is a discussion of the chronic B-cell lymphoid leukemias but does not include lymphoblastic disorders. The primary distinction of subtypes is based on first dividing the cases into B-cell vs T-cell disorders. Included in this discussion are several primary non-Hodgkin's lymphomas (NHL) because of the frequent occurrence of a leukemic phase in these neoplasms. The main subtypes are listed in Table 2, some of which will be discussed in greater detail later. PLL of B-cell type and the entire group of chronic

Table 2 Chronic Lymphoid Leukemias

B-cell
  Chronic lymphocytic leukemia (CLL)
  CLL variants (atypical CLL and CLL/PL)
  Prolymphocytic leukemia
  Hairy cell leukemia
  Hairy cell leukemia-variant
  Splenic lymphoma with villous lymphocytes (SLVL)
  Unclassifiable chronic B-cell leukemias
  Follicular lymphoma in leukemic phase
  Mantle cell lymphoma in leukemic phase
  Lymphoplasmacytic lymphoma in leukemic phase
  MALT/monocytoid B-cell lymphoma in leukemic phase
T-cell
  True T-cell CLL
  Prolymphocytic leukemia
  Sézary syndrome
  Adult T-cell leukemia/lymphoma (HTLV-I)
  Large granular lymphocytosis (T-cell and NK types)
  Peripheral T-cell lymphoma in leukemic phase

T-cell leukemias are covered elsewhere in this book, so will be discussed only briefly in the context of a differential diagnosis. Emphasis will be placed on the approach to diagnosis.

VI. B-CHRONIC LYMPHOCYTIC LEUKEMIA

B-CLL is a common disorder, accounting for most CLLs. Although previously defined by a persistent lymphocytosis of $>10 \times 10^9$, a clinical diagnosis of CLL now requires an absolute lymphocytosis with a lower limit of $>5 \times 10^9/L$ (12). Clearly, cases can be detected earlier in disease evolution by either flow cytometry or gene rearrangement studies. The threshold of $>5 \times 10^9/L$ is used to distinguish CLL from small lymphocytic lymphoma (SLL), a disease that shares virtually identical characteristics, except significant peripheral blood involvement (13).

In classic CLL, the lymphocytes are small with regularly shaped nuclear and cytoplasmic outlines; mature, clumped chromatin, and nucleoli that are either inconspicuous or not visible (see Fig. 2). The nuclear/cytoplasmic ratio is high, and the cytoplasm is homogeneous and weakly basophilic. The thin rim of visible cytoplasm in typical CLL is a useful distinguishing feature from follicular lymphomas in leukemic phase, in which the cytoplasm may be difficult to discern (14). Smudge cells are characteristic of CLL but in fact can be found in any disorder leading to lymphocytosis. They represent an artifact of blood smear preparation. Typically, this finding is most easily seen when the WBC is significantly elevated.

The bone marrow aspirate in CLL is usually hypercellular, whereas the bone marrow biopsy specimen shows a variable pattern of infiltration. The degree of infiltration, which may be interstitial, nodular, mixed, or diffuse, tends to correlate with the clinical stage but has been shown to have independent prognostic significance in CLL (15). Not uncommonly, growth centers, the characteristic pale-staining structures containing prolympho-

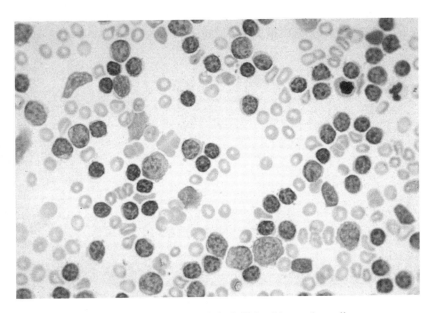

Figure 2   Peripheral blood smear of typical CLL with smudge cells.

cytes and paraimmunoblasts, may be found in bone marrow biopsy specimens. The lymph node histological findings in CLL are disease-specific and identical to SLL (16). The infiltrate is diffuse, but a pseudo-follicular pattern is well described, with alternating pale and light zones imparting nodularity to the sections. The pale zones represent the growth centers, the site of cellular proliferation, and contain characteristic cell types (outlined earlier), brighter CD20 expression and rare mitotic figures (13). An interfollicular pattern of nodal infiltration is also occasionally seen and may have bone marrow involvement with an unusual pattern of associated germinal center formation (17).

B-CLL has a signature phenotype and is characteristically CD19$^+$, CD5$^+$, dim CD20, CD22 dim, and surface Ig dim with light chain restriction for either kappa or lambda (18). The IgH subtype is typically IgM +/− IgD. CD23 is moderate to bright, and FMC-7 is either negative or only partially expressed. CD11c, CD25, and CD38 are variably expressed. CD79b, also known as Ig-β, a component of the B-cell receptor complex, is typically negative or dim in CLL (19,20). A comparison of the major immunophenotypical characteristics of the B-CLLs is listed in Table 3. The determination of a B-cell phenotype distinguishes this disorder from the chronic T-cell leukemias.

B-CLL is morphologically heterogeneous, with several variants now described. These include so-called CLL of mixed type and "atypical" CLL (1). The latter subtype has variable cytological findings, with more abundant, flowing cytoplasm. The nuclear outlines tend to be irregular, and there are admixed larger cells reminiscent of prolymphocytes, accounting for >10% of the cells in the blood smear (see Fig. 3). Characteristically, the heterochromatin is still clumped, as is typical of CLL. This peripheral blood finding may have a histological correlate as evidenced by a degree of nuclear irregularity unusual for classic CLL/SLL, and has been referred to in the past as "SLL with cleaved cells" (21). On the basis of peripheral blood morphology alone, this subtype may be very difficult to distinguish from MCL (see below). However, atypical CLL characteristically lacks blast-like cells and demonstrates co-expression of CD11c.

The other form of CLL of mixed-cell type has a dimorphic picture with both small lymphocytes and prolymphocytes, the latter being >10%, but <55% of the cells (see Fig. 4). This subtype is referred to as CLL/PL and tends to be associated with more aggressive

Table 3 Immunophenotypic Features of Chronic B-Cell Leukemias

Marker	CLL	PLL	HCL	HCL-V	SLVL	FL	MCL
CD19	++	++	+++	+++	++	++	++
CD20	Dim	+++	+++	+++	++	++	++
sIg	Dim	+++	+++	+++	++	++	++
CD5	++	−/+	−	−	−/+	−	++
CD10	−	−/+	−	−	−/+	++	−
CD11c	−/+ Dim	−/+	++	++	+/−	−	−ᵃ
CD22	−/+ Dim	++	+++	+++	++	++	++
CD23	++	−/+	−	−	−/+	−	−
CD25	−/+	+/−	+++	−	+/−	−	−
CD38	−/+	+/−	−/+	−/+	−/+	−/+	−
CD79b	−	++	++	++	++	++	++
CD103	−	−	+++	+++	+/−	−	−

ᵃ MCL rarely expresses CD11c.

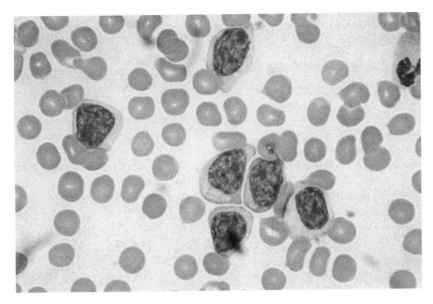

Figure 3 Peripheral blood smear of atypical CLL with cells demonstrating more abundant flowing cytoplasm and irregular nuclear outlines.

clinical behavior (1). It is likely that CLL/PL represents a form of disease progression in CLL but importantly may be found at initial presentation in some patients. Although not well established, this peripheral blood morphology may be associated with histological findings described as ''sheeting-out'' of growth centers, which can be seen in some lymph node biopsy specimens from patients with CLL/SLL (22).

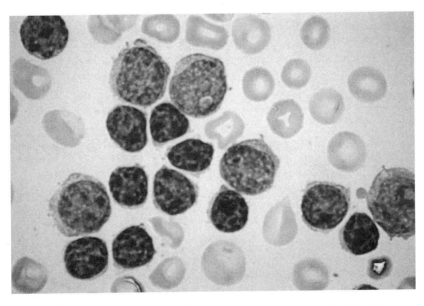

Figure 4 Blood smear of a case of CLL/PL with many admixed prolymphocytes.

The immunophenotype of atypical CLL is indistinguishable from classic CLL, although more frequent expression of CD11c may be seen. CLL/PL can have a composite immunophenotype, with about half the cases reportedly lacking CD5 (2). Typically, the expression of surface Ig is brighter, and the cells may be CD22$^+$ and FMC-7$^+$. A table highlighting the distinctive features of the CD5$^+$ B-cell leukemias including MCL is provided (Table 4).

Cytogenetic and molecular genetic testing have a place in the diagnostic workup of chronic lymphoid leukemias, but presently the usefulness of this approach is limited. CLL cells have clonal IgH rearrangements and were previously thought to lack evidence of exposure to the germinal center milieu. Earlier studies had shown that IgH variable-region (V_H) gene segments in CLL were lacking somatic mutations, consistent with a pregerminal center cell of origin. However, recent studies have clearly shown that CLL cases possess molecular heterogeneity, a finding that appears to be associated with several features, including morphology, immunophenotype, and survival (23–26). B-CLL can be grouped into two, and possibly three, molecular groups on the basis of a combined analysis of V_H and *bcl-6* genes (27,28). The cases with germline configuration of the V_H genes tend to be associated with typical morphology and the presence of 13q14 deletions (25). A putative tumor suppressor gene, *CLL1*, is thought to reside at this chromosomal location and may play a role in the pathogenesis of CLL (29,30). Mutations of the 5′ noncoding region of the *bcl-6* gene on chromosome 3q27 represent a histogenetic marker of B-cell transit through the germinal center and occur frequently in B-cell lymphomas derived from the germinal center or post-germinal center B-cells. CLL cases with germline V_H genes tend to have non-mutated *bcl-6* genes (28). This molecular profile is associated with expression of CD38 and frequently portends an inferior survival. The second group of B-CLL patients have nonmutated V_H genes and lack *bcl-6* mutations, but the clinical significance of this finding is unclear. The third group has somatic mutations of both V_H and *bcl-6* genes, tends to lack expression of CD38, and is associated with an atypical morphology, trisomy 12, and a better survival (27,28).

B-CLL cases lack typical *bcl-2* oncogene rearrangements, however, rare cases with variant translocations involving the immunoglobulin light chain genes (lambda) have been described (31). Similarly, CLL was thought to be associated in some cases with t(11;14)(q13;q32), the characteristic karyotypic alteration of MCL that results in deregu-

Table 4 Diagnostic Features of CD5$^+$ Chronic B-Cell Leukemias

Feature	CLL	Atypical CLL	CLL/PL	MCL
Nuclear	Clumped	Clumped	Mixed	Homogeneous
Nucleoli	Absent	−/+	+/−	++
Cytoplasm	Thin rim	Moderate, lightly basophilic	++	++
CD23	++	++	−/+	−
CD11c	−/+	+/−	+/−	−[a]
FMC-7	−	−	+/−	++
CD79b	−/+ Dim	−/+ Dim	++	++
+12	−/+	++	+	−
Del 13q14	++	−/+	+	+
V_H genes	Germline	Mutated	−/+	Germline

[a] MCL rarely expresses CD11c.

lated expression of the *bcl-1* or cyclin D1 gene (32). However, careful review of these cases suggests that most more likely represent MCL in leukemic phase. Thus, absent *bcl-1* and *bcl-2* oncogene rearrangements favor a diagnosis of CLL in difficult cases.

Cytogenetic alterations in CLL are variable but include trisomy 12, del 13q14, and del 11q (22–23), the latter being associated with mutations of the ataxia-telangiectasia (*ATM*) gene (33). Rearrangement of the *bcl-3* gene is associated with t(14;19)(q32;q13) and occurs uncommonly in CLL. It appears to be associated with atypical morphology, younger age at diagnosis, and inferior survival (34). More recently, additional chromosomal rearrangements have been described in CLL, including 6p24–25, 12p12–13, 4q21, and monosomy 21 (35). The relevance of these cytogenetic alterations is untested. *Bcl-6* mutations involving the 5' noncoding region are present in approximately 22% of cases. IgH V_H region mutations are found in a subset of cases as described earlier (36).

VII. PROLYMPHOCYTIC LEUKEMIA

B-cell prolymphocytic leukemia (PLL) is a rare disease, the existence of which as a distinct lymphoproliferative disorder is fraught with controversy. Originally described in 1974, this chronic leukemia is typically associated with a high WBC, marked splenomegaly and absent lymphadenopathy (37). It will only be discussed briefly here because it is adequately covered in Chapter 24.

The neoplastic cells of PLL, by definition, account for >55% of the peripheral blood lymphocytes. They are characterized by large cell size, round or oval nucleus with a prominent central nucleolus, relatively well-condensed nuclear chromatin, and a lower nuclear/cytoplasmic ratio than the small lymphocyte of CLL. The immunophenotype of PLL differs from CLL, as shown in Tables 3 and 4. Remote publications had suggested an association of t(11;14)(q13;q32) and B-PLL, but careful review suggests that many of these cases were in fact MCL with a pronounced leukemic component. In contrast to PLL, the nuclear outline of cells in the peripheral blood of patients with MCL tends to be irregular, and the morphology reveals a cytological spectrum in most cases, including the presence of occasional blast cells (see later). Cytogenetic reports of PLL are scant in the literature but appear to show similar aberrations to those seen in CLL, including deletions of 13q and 11q (38).

VIII. HAIRY CELL LEUKEMIA

Hairy cell leukemia (HCL) is an uncommon disorder, accounting for approximately 2% of leukemias. It is much more common in men, occurs most often in middle age, and typically is seen with splenomegaly and pancytopenia (1). Elevation of the WBC at diagnosis is uncommon (only 10%–20% of patients have leukemic cells $>5 \times 10^9$), but circulating cells can be identified in most cases, and thus careful attention to morphological detail is a prerequisite for diagnosis. Monocytopenia is a consistent peripheral blood finding.

HCL in most cases demonstrates a unique morphology, classic bone marrow biopsy histological findings, and a signature immunophenotype and thus is easily distinguished from other chronic leukemias (39). The neoplastic cells are larger than CLL cells with nuclei that are round, oval, or kidney shaped. The nuclear/cytoplasmic ratio is low, and the nucleus is often eccentrically placed. The nuclear chromatin is quite distinct, described as "sievelike," often with a relatively inconspicuous or single, small nucleolus. The cytoplasm is abundant, pale blue, and typically has irregular cytoplasmic projections. Importantly, the cytoplasmic features of HCL are not consistent, and although some suggest that cytoplasmic features should serve as the primary basis for recognition of HCL, others believe that the diagnosis of HCL is best made by use of nuclear criteria. A rare blastic variant of HCL has been described (40).

The bone marrow aspirate may produce a dry tap because of reticulin fibrosis, but the bone marrow biopsy is always involved. The histopathological findings of the bone marrow are characteristic in HCL and thus are important diagnostic features useful for differential diagnosis (39). Most often, the infiltrate is diffuse and blends imperceptibly with the surrounding normal haematopoietic elements. Focal involvement occurs but is uncommon. The cells are widely separated because of abundant cytoplasm and produce a "chicken-wire" or "fried-egg" appearance. Cytoplasmic projections are not visible in paraffin sections. A background of reticulin fibrosis is often apparent with silver staining. Immunohistochemistry is particularly useful for delineating the infiltrate in HCL, especially when trying to determine the presence of residual disease after therapy. A panel including any of the following reagents; CD20, CD75, MB2 and DBA.44, is useful for this purpose (41). The splenic histological findings in HCL are characteristic, producing a red pulp infiltrate with marked diminution of the white pulp and associated red blood cell lakes. Cytochemical studies are performed less frequently in this era, but tartrate-resistant acid phosphatase (TRAP) remains a useful test for the diagnosis of HCL. Although many of the aforementioned chronic leukemias are weakly positive using this cytochemical technique, HCL is typically strongly positive.

The immunophenotype of HCL is characteristic, and thus flow cytometric analysis has for the most part replaced other diagnostic strategies such as cytochemistry and electron microscopy (18). Forward-angle light scatter is usually higher than other chronic leukemias, facilitating the recognition of HCL and the determination of minimal residual disease. Hairy cells express bright CD19, CD20, and CD22. These cells also express CD11c, CD25, CD103 and bright FMC-7. The expression of CD11c is bright, in contrast to dim co-expression in CLL and the leukemic cells of many lymphomas (see later). Hairy cells do not express CD5, CD10, or CD23.

Cytogenetic studies in HCL are not performed routinely. Recurrent abnormalities are not well recognized, but structural and numerical abnormalities involving chromosomes 2, 5, and 7 have been described (42). Molecular genetic studies are uncommonly required for diagnosis. The neoplastic cells have clonal IgH rearrangements, 25% of cases have 5' bcl-6 gene mutations, and little is known about the mutation frequency of the V_H genes (36).

IX. HAIRY CELL LEUKEMIA-VARIANT

A variant form of HCL (HCL-V) has been described with features intermediate between HCL and B-PLL, however, it remains controversial whether HCL-V represents a distinct clinicopathological entity (43). These patients share clinical features with HCL, including male predominance and splenomegaly but, in contrast to patients with HCL, have an elevated WBC and lack both neutropenia and monocytopenia. The circulating cells have abundant villous cytoplasm and a round nucleus but, in contrast to typical HCL, have a single prominent nucleolus (see Fig. 5). The nuclear chromatin is more heterochromatic than usual HCL. The cells are characteristically TRAP-negative, and the bone marrow histological findings are distinct from HCL, both in the lack of reticulin fibrosis and the

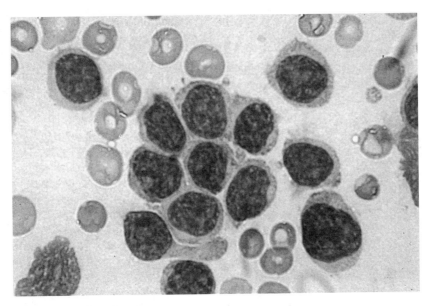

Figure 5 Peripheral blood smear of a case of HCL-V with cells showing morphological features intermediate between prolymphocytes and classic hairy cells.

pattern of infiltration. In HCL-V, the infiltrates are not diffuse, rather focal interstitial nodules predominate. The splenic histological findings are identical to usual HCL (2).

The immunophenotype of HCL-V is similar to HCL but with distinct differences. The cells show bright expression of CD19, CD20, FMC-7, CD11c, and CD22. They are CD103$^{+/-}$ but are characteristically CD25-negative. The cells lack CD5 and CD10. The main implications of this diagnosis are related to the variable response of HCL-V to treatment modalities usually reserved for classic HCL (44). Some have questioned the existence of HCL-V as a distinct disorder, instead suggesting a relationship with splenic lymphoma with villous lymphocytes (SLVL) (45). This raises the question of whether both SLVL and HCL-V are in any way related to each other, and perhaps both related to marginal zone lymphomas (MZL). These issues remain unresolved, but clarity may be brought to the question through the continued use of classical cytogenetics with or without gene expression profiling.

X. SPLENIC LYMPHOMA WITH VILLOUS LYMPHOCYTES

Splenic lymphoma with villous lymphocytes (SLVL) was first proposed as a distinct disorder in 1987 and described as a chronic leukemia with features overlapping those of HCL (46,47). The recognition of this disorder can be traced back to 1979. A series of cases of suspected HCL patients were treated by splenectomy, revealing an atypical splenic histological finding. White pulp infiltration was seen in these cases in contrast to the typical red pulp pattern characteristic of HCL.

SLVL is more common in men (2:1), with a reported mean age at diagnosis of 72 years (48). The spleen is typically enlarged, and the degree of splenomegaly may be marked, but the spleen is not invariably palpable. The WBC is moderately increased but typically does not exceed $25 \times 10^9/L$. Slightly more than half of the patients have a small monoclonal serum protein, usually of IgM type. The disease is considered indolent and best treated with splenectomy.

The neoplastic cells of SLVL are larger than CLL cells, but usually smaller than typical hairy cells. The nucleus is either round or oval, has moderately clumped chromatin a relatively high nuclear/cytoplasmic ratio. Approximately half of the cases have a visible nucleolus, but it is much less conspicuous in comparison to PLL cells (2). The cytoplasm is more basophilic then hairy cells and characteristically has numerous short villi or cytoplasmic projections. These may appear as one longer projection, concentrated at one pole of the cell (see Fig. 6). Unlike HCL, monocytopenia is not a feature.

The bone marrow findings in SLVL are variable. The marrow aspirate may be only minimally involved, often showing <30% lymphocytes. The bone marrow biopsy is more frequently positive but demonstrates variable histological findings (39). There may be numerous, small interstitial lymphoid aggregates or scant interstitial, diffuse infiltration. Occasional cases reveal paratrabecular localization, mimicking follicular lymphoma. An intrasinusoidal pattern has also been described (49).

The splenic histological findings of SLVL have only been recently described, in contrast to the well-documented peripheral blood morphological features of SLVL. In well-characterized cases of SLVL, the splenic histological findings are identical to splenic marginal zone lymphoma (SMZL) (50–52). SLVL/SMZL are characterized by involvement of the white pulp follicles with an infiltrate that surrounds naked follicle centers. The red pulp is frequently involved as well and may demonstrate small clusters of B cells associated with epithelioid histiocytes, or may invade diffusely with a sinusoidal pattern. The cytology of the cells may vary, and in typical cases may reveal a bi-phasic cytology with a central zone of small lymphocytes surrounded by a peripheral zone of larger marginal zone-like cells. Nodal involvement by SMZL is distinct, because the neoplastic cells

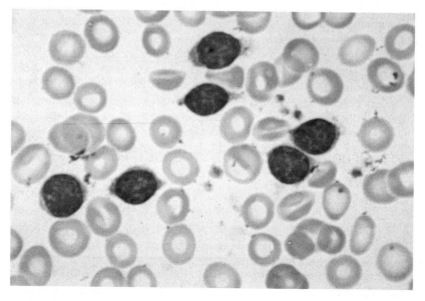

Figure 6   Blood smear of a typical case of SLVL with many lymphocytes demonstrating unipolar cytoplasmic projections.

tend to surround germinal centers, leaving an attenuated or absent mantle cuff. A primary nodal form of SMZL has recently been described without splenomegaly (53). The immunophenotype of SMZL is unique and differs from extranodal lymphomas of mucosal-associated lymphoid tissue (MALT) type.

SMZL cells express both IgM and IgD but typically lack expression of CD43. The immunophenotype of SMZL is similar to SLVL, but important differences may occur, suggesting that the immunophenotype may be affected by the compartment in which the cells are found. Flow cytometric analysis of the peripheral blood in SLVL cases reveals the cells to be CD19$^+$, CD20$^+$, CD22$^+$, FMC-7$^+$, CD79b$^+$ with variable expression of CD11c$^{+/-}$. Some cases appear to express CD25 and CD103, suggesting an overlap with HCL-V. CD5, CD10, and CD23 are usually negative. The cells lack expression of cyclin D1 (Table 3) (52).

Cytogenetic findings in SLVL and SMZL have been both controversial and enlightening. Initial studies failed to disclose any unique cytogenetic abnormalities in SLVL. Trisomy 3 was not shown to be present in SLVL by use of classical cytogenetics, but more recent studies using FISH on interphase nuclei have shown trisomy 3 in 17% of cases (54). The characteristic abnormality of MCL, t(11;14)(q13;q32), was reported to be seen in SLVL by two separate groups. However, most of the cases did not have histological documentation and were classified using peripheral blood morphology and immunophenotypic analysis alone. In both series, some of these cases were reported to be CD5$^+$ and CD23$^-$, a finding in keeping with a diagnosis of MCL. Although it remains possible that SLVL cases may involve an alternate breakpoint site on chromosome 11q13, the more likely explanation is that these cases were MCL and shared morphological features with SLVL (55). The same maybe true for trisomy 12, as "atypical" CLL may be morphologically difficult to distinguish from SLVL. These data suggest that SLVL as currently defined may include several distinct lymphoma entities, including SMZL, MCL, HCL-V, nodal MZL, and the leukemic manifestation of extranodal low-grade MALT lymphoma.

Cytogenetic studies in SMZL are now beginning to emerge (56). A concept was developed many years ago proposing that lymphomas derived from marginal zone B cells could be grouped into three clinical entities, including extranodal (MALT), nodal (monocytoid B-cell), or primary splenic (SMZL) marginal zone lymphomas. These lymphoma subtypes were morphologically similar and shared phenotypical features. In 1996, a report suggested that MZLs from different sites also shared cytogenetical features, including +3, +18, and structural rearrangements of chromosomes 1q21 and 1p34, supporting the concept that they were of a common biological derivation (57). Recent data have challenged this concept and provided insights into the fundamental genetic differences between the different types of MZLs as defined by current classification schemes. MALT lymphomas commonly harbor +3, but frequently also have a unique translocation, t(11;18)(q21;q21), resulting in a novel fusion protein called AP12-MLT (58). This translocation is found in low-grade B-cell MALT lymphomas from different mucosal sites but has not been found in either nodal MZL or primary SMZL. Moreover, the AP12-MLT rearrangement is not found in extranodal diffuse large B-cell lymphomas (DLBCL), suggesting that low-grade MALT lymphomas with this abnormality do not commonly transform, and that many primary extranodal DLBCL likely have a different histogenesis (59). The molecular hallmark of the t(11;18), the AP12-MLT fusion product, can be detected by use of reverse transcriptase-polymerase chain reaction (RT-PCR). Primary SMZL frequently demonstrates isolated deletions of chromosome 7q31-32, or more proximal rearrangements involving band 7q22, and may be associated with a higher incidence of del(10)(q22q24)

(56). No recurrent cytogenetic abnormalities have yet been associated with nodal MZL. In aggregate, these data suggest that the three lymphoma subtypes currently included under the rubric of MZL may in fact be distinct biological entities, despite relatively similar morphological, and immunophenotypical features.

The apparent heterogeneity of many of the chronic B-CLLs may be in part due to imprecise diagnostic criteria based solely upon peripheral blood morphology and immunophenotype. Histological correlation may help to resolve some of the apparent overlap but is not available in most cases. Molecular and cytogenetic data derived from peripheral blood or bone marrow samples may prove useful for this purpose. Two recent reports of cytogenetic abnormalities in HCL suggested that interstitial loss of chromosomal material at 7q22-q35 is found in some cases. One report included a case described as HCL, with del(7)(q32) as the sole cytogenetic abnormality (42). Interestingly, this case was CD25⁻. One could speculate that the later case would be best classified as HCL-V, given the lack of CD25 expression. The cytogenetic result suggests that this case likely represents the leukemic manifestation of SMZL. Systematic study of these uncommon CLLs using modern molecular and cytogenetic approaches may help to bring clarity to many of the issues surrounding the heterogeneity of these disorders.

XI. UNCLASSIFIABLE CHRONIC B-CELL LEUKEMIAS

Occasional cases of chronic B-cell leukemia are encountered that defy accurate classification. Such cases often resemble typical CLL, except that the cells have slightly less clumped chromatin, indistinct nucleoli, and more abundant pale blue cytoplasm. Typically these cases are CD5⁻, but express CD19, CD20, and CD11c. Most lack expression of CD10, CD25, or CD103 and may have variable TRAP staining (39). Molecular genetic studies are usually negative for both *bcl-1* and *bcl-2* gene rearrangements. If significant peripheral lymphadenopathy is present, consideration should be given to a lymph node biopsy, as this may provide insights into the underlying diagnosis. However, many of these patients have only slight splenomegaly and are without additional clues as to the diagnosis. It is preferable to classify such cases as small B-cell lymphoproliferative disorder, unclassifiable. In the authors' experience, the clinical pace of these cases is similar to otherwise typical CLL.

XII. FOLLICULAR LYMPHOMA

Follicular lymphoma (FL), grades 1, 2, and 3, represents the most common histological subtype of NHL in North America, accounting for approximately 31% of all cases of lymphoma (60). Although grade 3 FL is a rare tumor, FL of grades 1 and 2 are common, and bone marrow involvement may be seen in 25%–60% of patients at diagnosis. The peripheral blood is less commonly involved, but the precise frequency is difficult to ascertain, because more sensitive methods are now available to accurately determine the presence of leukemic cells (14). Some cases may have a markedly elevated WBC, causing confusion with CLL, but more typically the diagnosis is made by lymph node biopsy and subsequent staging reveals involvement of the bone marrow with or without peripheral blood.

The morphology of the cells in the peripheral blood is distinctly different from CLL cells. FL, grade 1 (small cleaved cells), is the most commonly encountered subtype. The cells are approximately the same size as CLL cells, but the nuclear chromatin is smooth, not clumped as in CLL. The chromatin is mature, and nucleoli are typically indistinct. The nuclei are often irregular, and may have characteristic nuclear clefts or indentations. The cells have almost no visible cytoplasm, giving a very distinct appearance (see Figure 7). Occasional large cells (noncleaved cells or centroblasts) may also be seen but are uncommon (39).

The bone marrow histology in FL is varied, but most cases demonstrate a classic paratrabecular pattern of infiltration with small-cleaved cells that appear to "hug" the endosteal surface of the bone. Often there is a relatively hypocellular appearance of the infiltrate immediately adjacent to the bony spicules. Independent of the histological grade of FL, most cases are predominantly small-cleaved lymphocytes. Occasional admixed large noncleaved cells and histiocytes are also present. The bone marrow aspirate may reveal the same typical FL cells, but not uncommonly the aspirate is both morphologically and phenotypically negative for lymphoma, while the biopsy specimen shows significant infiltration. Foci of transformation to DLBCL or a blastic phase is rare but may be seen on occasion. Lymph node histology in FL is well described. Often a component of marginal zone differentiation is evident, imparting a biphasic morphology to the neoplastic follicles. The cells in the marginal zone are part of the malignant clone but usually have a different immunophenotype in accordance with this compartment (Bcl-6$^-$/CD10$^-$). In some cases, these cells may preferentially circulate and will mimic SLVL cells both for morphology and immunophenotype. The differential diagnosis can be resolved by lymph node biopsy, or by demonstrating the presence of the characteristic *bcl-2* oncogene translocation of FL.

Most cases of leukemic FL have a characteristic immunophenotype. The cells are CD19$^+$, CD20 bright, with sIg moderate to bright. The cells are strongly FMC-7$^+$ but lack

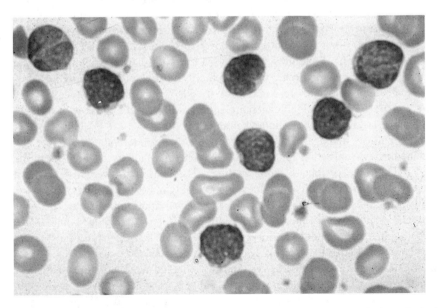

Figure 7 Blood smear from a patient with grade 1 FL showing the typical cytological features of the leukemic phase of this lymphoma. Note the typical buttock cells with clefted nuclei.

CD23 in most cases. The cells are CD5$^-$, CD11c$^-$, but are typically CD10$^+$ (Table 3) (18). As indicated earlier, some cases of FL with prominent marginal zone differentiation may circulate cells that are CD10$^-$ and will be indistinguishable from SLVL.

The cytogenetic abnormalities of FL and the corresponding molecular derangements are well described (61). Approximately 85%–90% of FL cases are characterized by a t(14;18), most of which can be detected by molecular methods, including Southern blot hybridization and PCR for *bcl-2* oncogene rearrangements. However, false negative results may occur. Moreover, not all FL cases possess a t(14;18)(q32;q21) abnormality. *Bcl-6* mutations in the 5′ noncoding region of the gene are seen in 60% of cases, and virtually all FL cases express *Bcl-6* protein (36,62). Mutational analysis of the V$_H$ genes reveals frequent somatic mutations and intraclonal diversity, the latter finding being characteristic of an antigen-driven process.

XIII. MANTLE CELL LYMPHOMA

MCL accounts for approximately 6%–7% of NHL cases in North America (60). It is more common in men than women, and the median age at diagnosis is 63 years. Most patients are first seen with advanced stage disease, with 65% of patients having involvement of bone marrow and 33% having a leukemic component (3). Common extranodal sites of disease include the spleen and gastrointestinal tract. Importantly, peripheral blood involvement in MCL has been shown by several groups to be of prognostic importance (3,63).

As indicated earlier, a leukemic component in MCL is not infrequent. Occasional cases are seen with a significant elevation of the WBC and minimal lymphadenopathy. Such cases may be difficult to distinguish from CLL. The peripheral blood morphology of the cells in MCL is distinctly different from both FL and CLL. The disease is characterized by a cytological spectrum, including small, mature-appearing lymphocytes reminiscent of CLL, small, irregular cells suggestive of FL, and larger cells with more prominent nucleoli, suggestive of prolymphocytes (see Fig. 8). The larger cells in MCL usually have irregular nuclear outlines, but some cases may have cells with round or oval nuclei and resemble the cells of PLL[4]. In contrast, cases of PLL and CLL/PL lack this cytologic spectrum, and are either monomorphic or dimorphic, respectively. In virtually all cases of MCL, a small number of cells resembling blast cells (L2 blasts) are typically seen. Rarely cases may be seen with a significant number of these latter cells and may be difficult to distinguish from acute lymphoblastic leukemia (ALL) (64).

The bone marrow findings in MCL are variable. Most often, both the aspirate and biopsy specimen show infiltration in contrast to FL. The morphology of the cells in the aspirate is similar to the peripheral blood findings. The bone marrow biopsy shows a diffuse, interstitial pattern most often, but focal interstitial lymphoid aggregates and classic paratrabecular infiltrates are also seen (3). The histological appearance is similar to the lymph node and demonstrates a monomorphic infiltrate of small, irregular lymphocytes with scattered epithelioid histiocytes, mitoses, and a virtual lack of large, transformed cells (centroblasts). *De novo* blastoid MCL may resemble ALL.

The immunophenotype of MCL is not on its own diagnostic, but features that allow discrimination from CLL are usually present (see Table 3). The cells of MCL are CD20, CD19, and FMC-7 bright. These cells express bright sIg of IgM and IgD subtype, with either kappa or lambda light chains ($\lambda > \kappa$). The cells are CD5$^+$ and lack expression of CD10 and CD23 (18). Rare cases are encountered with cells expressing dim CD11c. Similarly, CD5$^-$ MCL can be found in 3% of cases (unpublished observations, manuscript in

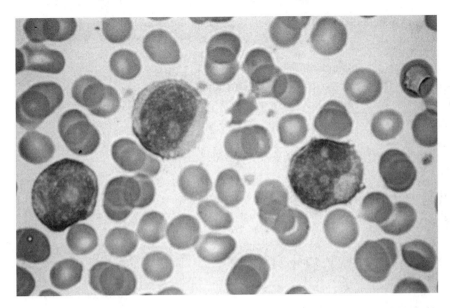

Figure 8 Peripheral blood smear of the leukemic phase of MCL with a spectrum of lymphocytes. Many of the cells are larger than classic CLL cells, with some cells demonstrating nucleoli.

preparation). With paraffin sections, the cells can be shown to express CD20 and to stain strongly for both *Bcl-2* and cyclin D1. The latter antibody is useful for distinguishing MCL from most other lymphoproliferative disorders. Only myeloma and HCL have been shown to express cyclin D1, and neither disease entity poses a problem of differential diagnosis with MCL in most cases. The neoplastic cells in MCL express CD43 and may have a moderate proliferative fraction as assessed using MIB-1 (paraffin Ki-67). Blastoid MCL cases can be distinguished from ALL by use of antibodies to CD34 and terminal deoxynucleotidyl transferase (TdT). A list of the features that allow distinction of MCL from CLL can be found in Table 5.

The molecular and cytogenetic features of MCL are well described. Most cases demonstrate a t(11;14)(q13;q32) karyotype with some degree of clonal evolution present at diagnosis. Although most breakpoints on chromosome 11q13 are located within the major translocation cluster (MTC), many others can be found widely scattered over a large stretch of genomic DNA. Thus, a PCR approach utilizing a single primer pair will be

Table 5 Features Distinguishing CLL from MCL

Feature	CLL	MCL
Dim CD20	Yes	No
Bright sIg	No	Yes
CD23	Positive	Negative
CD11c	Dim positive	Negative[a]
FMC-7	Negative	Positive
CD79b	Negative or dim	Positive

[a] MCL rarely expresses CD11c.

associated with many false negative results. Additional Southern blot probes are available. Their use will result in an increased frequency of positive cases (65). The reported association of t(11;14) and SLVL has been discussed. It is likely that most of the cases of SLVL with this translocation would be reclassified as MCL (55). Blastoid MCL may be associated with a near-tetraploid karyotype, or specific alterations of either the p53 tumor suppressor gene at chromosome 17p13, or deletions of the tumor suppressor gene p16 on chromosome 9p21 (66,67).

XIV.   LYMPHOPLASMACYTIC LYMPHOMA

Lymphoplasmacytic lymphoma (LPL) is an uncommon neoplasm, accounting for 1.2% of all lymphomas in a recent international study (60). Classification of this subtype of NHL is problematic, because there is a recognized poor intraobserver reproducibility for this subtype (only 56% agreement between experts). In Europe, similar cases may be found within the category of immunocytoma. The problems arise because of a perceived overlap with B-CLL on one hand and MZL on the other. The term ''lymphoplasmacytoid lymphoma'' was abandoned in favor of including such cases within the category of B-CLL/SLL, because it is appreciated that some cases of CLL have plasmacytoid differentiation, cytoplasmic Ig, and a small serum monoclonal protein band. Cases meeting these criteria are typically CD5$^+$. Cases of MZL including extranodal, nodal, and primary splenic types may have a degree of plasmacytic differentiation, resulting in confusion with LPL (16).

Peripheral blood involvement occurs in approximately 40% of cases, but presentation with a high WBC is uncommon. The bone marrow is involved in 75% of cases. The peripheral blood morphology characteristically reveals a spectrum of mature-appearing lymphocytes and plasmacytoid lymphocytes. The latter cells have eccentric nuclei and moderate amounts of basophilic cytoplasm. Most cases are associated with a monoclonal serum protein of IgM, IgG, or IgA subtype and thus may also have rouleaux formation. When the serum protein is IgM type and the level is sufficient to produce hyperviscosity (usually >20 g/L), the disorder is known as Waldenström's macroglobulinemia. Importantly, not all patients with LPL have a detectable serum monoclonal protein, and not all lymphoma patients with a serum protein have histological findings diagnostic of LPL. Not surprisingly, there is overlap between LPL and SLVL. Many of the latter cases have a monoclonal serum protein, often of IgM type, and the cells in the peripheral blood may resemble LPL. Therefore, distinction between these two entities may be problematic, although SLVL typically has a lower level of monoclonal serum protein. The bone marrow in LPL usually shows a nodular, interstitial pattern of infiltration and is frequently associated with many mast cells (39). Lymph node involvement is often diffuse but may reveal an interfollicular pattern. Preserved and dilated sinuses may be present.

The immunophenotype of LPL is not unique. The cells are CD19$^+$, CD20$^+$, CD22$^+$, and CD79a$^+$. They have both surface and cytoplasmic Ig, usually IgM type, lack IgD, and fail to express CD5 or CD10. They may express CD43 and dim CD11c and CD25. The neoplastic cells often express CD38. The lack of CD5 helps to distinguish LPL from CLL (see Table 3).

Few reports of cytogenetic results in LPL have appeared. An uncommon balanced translocation has recently been described, t(9;14)(p24;q32) involving a novel oncogene, *PAX-5* (68). Cases of LPL have been reported to harbor +12 and del 13q14, highlighting the overlap with CLL. *Bcl-6* gene mutations involving the 5' noncoding region occur in 40% of cases. IgH gene V_H mutations are common (36).

XV. MALT/MONOCYTOID B-CELL LYMPHOMA

Rare cases of extranodal MZL of MALT-type and so-called monocytoid B-cell lymphoma (MBCL) with a leukemic component have been reported (69). The distinction between these disorders and SLVL is problematic. Use of cytogenetic data, including molecular analyses of AP12-MLT rearrangements, may prove useful in helping to resolve the apparent morphological and immunophenotypical overlap. A subtype of MALT lymphoma with coexpression of CD5 may be associated with a predilection to involve the peripheral blood and bone marrow (70).

REFERENCES

1. JM Bennett, D Catovsky, MT Daniel, et al. Proposals for the classification of chronic (mature) B and T lymphoid leukaemias. French-American-British (FAB) Cooperative Group. J Clin Pathol 42:567–84, 1989.
2. D Catovsky, R Foa. The Lymphoid Leukemias. Cambridge: Butterworths, 1990, p. 320.
3. LH Argatoff, JM Connors, RJ Klasa, DE Horsman, RD Gascoyne. Mantle cell lymphoma: a clinicopathologic study of 80 cases. Blood 89:2067–78, 1997.
4. PL Cohen, PJ Kurtin, KA Donovan, CA Hanson. Bone marrow and peripheral blood involvement in mantle cell lymphoma. British Journal of Haematology 101:302–10, 1998.
5. AG Stansfeld, J Diebold, H Noel, et al. Updated Kiel classification for lymphomas [letter] [published erratum appears in Lancet 1988 Feb 13;1(8581):372]. Lancet 1:292–3, 1988.
6. G Marotta, D Raspadori, C Sestigiani, G Scalia, C Bigazzi, F Lauria. Expression of the CD11c antigen in B-cell chronic lymphoproliferative disorders. Leuk Lymphoma 37:145–9, 2000.
7. IA Auer, RD Gascoyne, JM Connors, et al. t(11;18)(q21;q21) is the most common translocation in Malt lymphomas. Ann Oncol 8:979–85, 1997.
8. DS Gordon, BM Jones, SW Browning, TJ Spira, DN Lawrence. Persistent polyclonal lymphocytosis of B lymphocytes. N Engl J Med 307:232–6, 1982.
9. H Mossafa, H Malaure, M Maynadie, et al. Persistent polyclonal B lymphocytosis with binucleated lymphocytes: a study of 25 cases. Groupe Francais d'Hematologie Cellulaire. Br J Haematol 104:486–93, 1999.
10. KC Carstairs, WH Francombe, JG Scott, EW Gelfand. Persistent polyclonal lymphocytosis of B lymphocytes, induced by cigarette smoking? [letter]. Lancet 1:1094, 1985.
11. R Delage, J Roy, L Jacques, V Bernier, JM Delage, A Darveau. Multiple bcl-2/Ig gene rearrangements in persistent polyclonal B-cell lymphocytosis. Br J Haematol 97:589–95, 1997.
12. BD Cheson, JM Bennett, M Grever, et al. National Cancer Institute-sponsored Working Group guidelines for chronic lymphocytic leukemia: revised guidelines for diagnosis and treatment. Blood 87:4990–7, 1996.
13. ES Jaffe. Surgical pathology of the lymph nodes and related organs. In: VA Livolsi, (ed.) Major problems in pathology. Vol. 16. Philadelphia: W. B. Saunders Company, 1995, p. 659.
14. K Foucar, RW McKenna, G Frizzera, RD Brunning. Bone marrow and blood involvement by lymphoma in relationship to the Lukes–Collins classification. Cancer 49:888–97, 1982.
15. C Rozman, E Montserrat, JM Rodriguez-Fernandez, et al. Bone marrow histologic pattern– the best single prognostic parameter in chronic lymphocytic leukemia: a multivariate survival analysis of 329 cases. Blood 64:642–8, 1984.
16. NL Harris, ES Jaffe, H Stein, et al. A revised European-American classification of lymphoid

neoplasms: a proposal from the International Lymphoma Study Group. Blood 84:1361–92, 1994.

17. YS Kim, RJ Ford Jr., JA Faber, RH Bell, KS Elenitoba-Johnson, LJ Medeiros. B-cell chronic lymphocytic leukemia/small lymphocytic lymphoma involving bone marrow with an interfollicular pattern. Am J Clin Pathol 114:41–6, 2000.

18. MJ Borowitz, R Bray, R Gascoyne, et al. U.S.-Canadian Consensus recommendations on the immunophenotypic analysis of hematologic neoplasia by flow cytometry: data analysis and interpretation. Cytometry 30:236–44, 1997.

19. KF McCarron, JP Hammel, ED Hsi. Usefulness of CD79b expression in the diagnosis of B-cell chronic lymphoproliferative disorders. Am J Clin Pathol 113:805–13, 2000.

20. EJ Moreau, E Matutes, RP A'Hern, et al. Improvement of the chronic lymphocytic leukemia scoring system with the monoclonal antibody SN8 (CD79b). Am J Clin Pathol 108:378–82, 1997.

21. MS De Oliveira, ES Jaffe, D Catovsky. Leukaemic phase of mantle zone (intermediate) lymphoma: its characterisation in 11 cases [see comments]. J Clin Pathol 42:962–72, 1989.

22. FR Dick, RD Maca. The lymph node in chronic lymphocytic leukemia. Cancer 41:283–92, 1978.

23. DG Oscier, A Thompsett, D Zhu, FK Stevenson. Differential rates of somatic hypermutation in V(H) genes among subsets of chronic lymphocytic leukemia defined by chromosomal abnormalities. Blood 89:4153–60, 1997.

24. RN Damle, T Wasil, F Fais, et al. Ig V gene mutation status and CD38 expression as novel prognostic indicators in chronic lymphocytic leukemia [see comments]. Blood 94:1840–7, 1999.

25. TJ Hamblin, Z Davis, A Gardiner, DG Oscier, FK Stevenson. Unmutated Ig V(H) genes are associated with a more aggressive form of chronic lymphocytic leukemia [see comments]. Blood 94:1848–54, 1999.

26. K Maloum, F Davi, H Merle-Beral, et al. Expression of unmutated VH genes is a detrimental prognostic factor in chronic lymphocytic leukemia [letter]. Blood 96:377–9, 2000.

27. SS Sahota, Z Davis, TJ Hamblin, FK Stevenson. Somatic mutation of bcl-6 genes can occur in the absence of V(H) mutations in chronic lymphocytic leukemia. Blood 95:3534–40, 2000.

28. D Capello, F Fais, D Vivenza, et al. Identification of three subgroups of B cell chronic lymphocytic leukemia based upon mutations of BCL-6 and IgV genes. Leukemia 14:811–5, 2000.

29. AG Brown, FM Ross, EM Dunne, CM Steel, EM Weir-Thompson. Evidence for a new tumour suppressor locus (DBM) in human B-cell neoplasia telomeric to the retinoblastoma gene. Nat Genet 3:67–72, 1993.

30. LA Hawthorn, R Chapman, D Oscier, JK Cowell. The consistent 13q14 translocation breakpoint seen in chronic B-cell leukaemia (BCLL) involves deletion of the D13S25 locus which lies distal to the retinoblastoma predisposition gene. Oncogene 8:1415–9, 1993.

31. M Adachi, Y Tsujimoto. Juxtaposition of human bcl-2 and immunoglobulin lambda light chain gene in chronic lymphocytic leukemia is the result of a reciprocal chromosome translocation between chromosome 18 and 22. Oncogene 4:1073–5, 1989.

32. Y Tsujimoto, J Yunis, L Onorato-Showe, J Erikson, PC Nowell, CM Croce. Molecular cloning of the chromosomal breakpoint of B-cell lymphomas and leukemias with the t(11;14) chromosome translocation. Science 224:1403–6, 1984.

33. T Stankovic, P Weber, G Stewart, et al. Inactivation of ataxia telangiectasia mutated gene in B-cell chronic lymphocytic leukaemia [see comments]. Lancet 353:26–9, 1999.

34. L Michaux, J Dierlamm, I Wlodarska, V Bours, H Van den Berghe, A Hagemeijer. t(14;19)/ BCL3 rearrangements in lymphoproliferative disorders: a review of 23 cases. Cancer Genet Cytogenet 94:36–43, 1997.

35. A Cuneo, MG Roberti, R Bigoni, et al. Four novel non-random chromosome rearrangements

in B-cell chronic lymphocytic leukaemia: 6p24-25 and 12p12-13 translocations, 4q21 anomalies and monosomy 21. Br J Haematol 108:559–64, 2000.

36. D Capello, U Vitolo, L Pasqualucci, et al. Distribution and pattern of BCL-6 mutations throughout the spectrum of B-cell neoplasia. Blood 95:651–9, 2000.
37. DA Galton, JM Goldman, E Wiltshaw, D Catovsky, K Henry, GJ Goldenberg. Prolymphocytic leukaemia. Br J Haematol 27:7–23, 1974.
38. D Lens, E Matutes, D Catovsky, LJ Coignet. Frequent deletions at 11q23 and 13q14 in B cell prolymphocytic leukemia (B-PLL). Leukemia 14:427–30, 2000.
39. RD Brunning, RW McKenna. Atlas of Tumor Pathology. In: J Rosai, (ed.) Tumors of the Bone Marrow. Vol. 9. Washington, D.C.: AFIP, 1993, p. 496.
40. JL Diez Martin, CY Li, PM Banks, Blastic variant of hairy-cell leukemia. Am J Clin Pathol 87:576–83, 1987.
41. H Hounieu, SM Chittal, T al Saati, et al. Hairy cell leukemia. Diagnosis of bone marrow involvement in paraffin-embedded sections with monoclonal antibody DBA.44. Am J Clin Pathol 98:26–33, 1992.
42. F Sole, S Woessner, L Florensa, et al. Cytogenetic findings in five patients with hairy cell leukemia. Cancer Genet Cytogenet 110:41–3, 1999.
43. JC Cawley, GF Burns, FG Hayhoe. A chronic lymphoproliferative disorder with distinctive features: a distinct variant of hairy-cell leukaemia. Leuk Res 4:547–59, 1980.
44. L Sainati, E Matutes, S Mulligan, et al. A variant form of hairy cell leukemia resistant to alpha-interferon: clinical and phenotypic characteristics of 17 patients. Blood 76:157–62, 1990.
45. T Sun, K Dittmar, P Koduru, M Susin, S Teichberg, J Brody. Relationship between hairy cell leukemia variant and splenic lymphoma with villous lymphocytes: presentation of a new concept. Am J Hematol 51:282–8, 1996.
46. JV Melo, U Hegde, A Parreira, I Thompson, IA Lampert, D Catovsky. Splenic B cell lymphoma with circulating villous lymphocytes: differential diagnosis of B cell leukaemias with large spleens. J Clin Pathol 40:642–51, 1987.
47. JV Melo, DS Robinson, C Gregory, D Catovsky. Splenic B cell lymphoma with "villous", lymphocytes in the peripheral blood: a disorder distinct from hairy cell leukemia. Leukemia 1:294–8, 1987.
48. X Troussard, F Valensi, E Duchayne, et al. Splenic lymphoma with villous lymphocytes: clinical presentation, biology and prognostic factors in a series of 100 patients. Groupe Francais d'Hematologie Cellulaire (GFHC). Br J Haematol 93:731–6, 1996.
49. M Parrens, P Dubus, P Agape, et al. Intrasinusoidal bone marrow infiltration revealing intravascular lymphomatosis. Leuk Lymphoma 37:219–23, 2000.
50. PG Isaacson, E Matutes, M Burke, D Catovsky. The histopathology of splenic lymphoma with villous lymphocytes. Blood 84:3828–34, 1994.
51. M Mollejo, J Menarguez, E Lloret, et al. Splenic marginal zone lymphoma: a distinctive type of low-grade B-cell lymphoma. A clinicopathological study of 13 cases. American Journal of Surgical Pathology 19:1146–57, 1995.
52. MA Piris, M Mollejo, E Campo, J Menarguez, T Flores, PG Isaacson. A marginal zone pattern may be found in different varieties of non-Hodgkin's lymphoma: the morphology and immuno-histology of splenic involvement by B-cell lymphomas simulating splenic marginal zone lymphoma. Histopathology 33:230–9, 1998.
53. E Campo, R Miquel, L Krenacs, L Sorbara, M Raffeld, ES Jaffe. Primary nodal marginal zone lymphomas of splenic and MALT type. American Journal of Surgical Pathology 23:59–68, 1999.
54. AM Gruszka-Westowood, E Matutes, LJ Coignet, A Wotherspoon, D Catovsky. The incidence of trisomy 3 in splenic lymphoma with villous lymphocytes: a study by FISH. Br J Haematol 104:600–4, 1999.

55. D Catovsky, E Matutes. Splenic lymphoma with circulating villous lymphocytes/splenic marginal-zone lymphoma. Semin Hematol 36:148–84, 1999.

56. MM Ott, A Rosenwald, T Katzenberger, et al. Marginal zone B-cell lymphomas (MZBL) arising at different sites represent different biological entities. Genes Chromosomes Cancer 28:380–6, 2000.

57. J Dierlamm, S Pittaluga, I Wlodarska, et al. Marginal zone B-cell lymphomas of different sites share similar cytogenetic and morphologic features [see comments]. Blood 87:299–307, 1996.

58. J Dierlamm, M Baens, I Wlodarska, et al. The apoptosis inhibitor gene AP12 and a novel 18q gene, MLT, are recurrently rearranged in the t(11;18)(q21;q21) associated with mucosa-associated lymphoid tissue lymphomas [In Process Citation]. Blood 93:3601–9, 1999.

59. J Dierlamm, M Baens, M Stefanova-Ouzounova, et al. Detection of t(11;18)(q21;q21) by interphase fluorescence in situ hybridization using AP12 and MLT specific probes. Blood 96: 2215–8, 2000.

60. Anonymous. A clinical evaluation of the international lymphoma study group classification of non-Hodgkin's lymphoma. Blood 89:3909–3918, 1997.

61. DE Horsman, RD Gascoyne, RW Coupland, AJ Coldman, SA Adomat. Comparison of cytogenetic analysis, southern analysis, and polymerase chain reaction for the detection of t(14;18) in follicular lymphoma. Am J Clin Pathol 103:472–8, 1995.

62. BF Skinnider, DE Horsman, B Dupuis, RD Gascoyne. Bcl-6 and Bcl-2 protein expression in diffuse large B-cell lymphoma and follicular lymphoma: correlation with 3q27 and 18q21 chromosomal abnormalities [In Process Citation]. Hum Pathol 30:803–8, 1999.

63. F Bosch, A Lopez-Guillermo, E Campo, et al. Mantle cell lymphoma: presenting features, response to therapy, and prognostic factors. Cancer 82:567–75, 1998.

64. DS Viswanatha, K Foucar, BR Berry, RD Gascoyne, HL Evans, CP Leith. Blastic mantle cell leukemia: an unusual presentation of blastic mantle cell lymphoma [In Process Citation]. Mod Pathol 13:825–33, 2000.

65. H Fan, ML Gulley, RD Gascoyne, DE Horsman, SA Adomat, CG Cho. Molecular methods for detecting t(11;14) translocations in mantle-cell lymphomas. Diagn Mol Pathol 7:209–14, 1998.

66. G Ott, J Kalla, MM Ott, et al. Blastoid variants of mantle cell lymphoma: frequent bcl-1 rearrangements at the major translocation cluster region and tetraploid chromosome clones. Blood 89:1421–9, 1997.

67. MH Dreyling, L Bullinger, G Ott, et al. Alterations of the cyclin D1/p16-pRB pathway in mantle cell lymphoma. Cancer Research 57:4608–14, 1997.

68. S Iida, PH Rao, P Nallasivam, et al. The t(9;14)(p13;q32) chromosomal translocation associated with lymphoplasmacytoid lymphoma involves the PAX-5 gene. Blood 88:4110–7, 1996.

69. A Carbone, A Gloghini, A Pinto, V Attadia, V Zagonel, R Volpe. Monocytoid B-cell lymphoma with bone marrow and peripheral blood involvement at presentation [see comments]. Am J Clin Pathol 92:228–36, 1989.

70. JA Ferry, WI Yang, LR Zukerberg, AC Wotherspoon, A Arnold, NL Harris. CD5$^+$ extranodal marginal zone B-cell (MALT) lymphoma. A low grade neoplasm with a propensity for bone marrow involvement and relapse [see comments]. Am J Clin Pathol 105:31–7, 1996.

12

Prognostic Factors in Chronic Lymphocytic Leukemia

STEFANO MOLICA

Azienda Ospedaliera "Pugliese-Ciaccio," Catanzaro, Italy

Recent advances in our understanding of biology and natural history of chronic lymphocytic leukemia (CLL), accompanied by the emergency of new therapeutic options pose a continuous challenge to physicians treating CLL patients (1–4). Many patients are now being diagnosed while asymptomatic and at a much younger age than previously, thus resulting in a longer overall survival (5,6). However, it is not clear whether the aforementioned changes have represented a true modification in the natural history of disease or more realistically are epiphenomena of other conditions. Whatever the explanation might be, different therapeutical philosophies, mainly inspired by the patients' age, should be taken into account when making treatment decisions (7). As a prerequisite for an optimal choice of therapy, prognostic assessment at the time of diagnosis should be as accurate as possible.

At present, CLL patients are staged according to The Rai or Binet stagings (8,9). However, these classification schemes, which reflect the spreading pattern of disease from nodal sites to bone marrow (BM), are not accurate enough to identify subgroups of patients with progressive CLL (10). Moreover, criteria used to define clinical stages do not necessarily parallel tumor mass, because mechanisms underlying cytopenia are not considered separately. Investigators have attempted to identify clinical parameters that would improve the prognostic discriminant power of clinical stages (10–12). These clinical characteristics are representative of two basic features: (1) the neoplasia's growth and invasive potential of leukemic cells [lymphocyte doubling time (LDT), pattern of BM involvement]; (2) the host and tumor–host relationship (age, performance status, comorbidity caused by cardiovascular or metabolic diseases) (Table 1).

Table 1 Factors Associated with a Poor Prognosis in CLL

Disease related and reflecting:	*Tumor mass*: Anemia, thrombocytopenia, high PB lymphocytosis, diffuse BM histology, increased serum levels of LDH, β2m, sCD23, sCD25, sCD27, atypical morphology, atypical immunophenotype, expression of My antigens, cytogenetic abnormalities.
	Rate of progression and spreading pattern: Rapid LDT, high TK activity, p27 expression, increased angiogenesis (i.e., high serum levels of VEGF), increased cellular expression, and release of adhesion molecules (sCD54, sCD44, sVCAM-1).
	Pathogenesis of disease: increased serum levels of TNF-α, IL-4, IL-8, IL-10, high *bcl-2* expression, CD38-expression, unmutated VH gene.
	Resistance to chemotherapy: p53 expression, high levels of Mcl-1 protein, high *bcl2/bax* ratio, high levels of b-FGF.
Host and tumor-host relationship related:	Increased age
	Poor performance status
	Comorbidity caused by host's disease (i.e., cardiovascular, metabolic, HCV infections)
	Qualitative and quantitative alterations of T-cell counterpart
	Autoimmune phenomena

For references see text.

In recent years, cellular and molecular features, including tumor cell proliferation, immunophenotype, adhesion molecule expression and release, karyotypic abnormalities, and biological findings of increased angiogenesis, have been linked with survival (1,4,10–13). However, it is not clear whether the newly identified prognostic parameters will eventually replace, or more likely integrate, clinical variables, thus forming the basis for unique approaches of therapy in specific subsets of patients.

I. CLINICAL STAGING

On the basis of variables known to adversely affect the outcome, different staging systems have been proposed. A modern CLL staging system for clinical use was introduced by Rai et al., who identified five different prognostic groups (from stage 0 to IV) (8). More recently, a modified version of such a staging was proposed under the assumption that the original stages segregate naturally into three risk groups: low (stage 0), intermediate (stage I and II), and high (stage III and IV) (14). The three categories account for 30%, 60%, and 10% of newly diagnosed CLL patients and are associated with median survival times of 10, 7, and 1.5 years, respectively. The proposal by Binet et al. (9), derived from a multivariate survival analysis, distinguishes three stages (A, B, and C) with different prognosis. Binet stage A, B, and C include 60%, 30%, and 10% of newly diagnosed CLL patients with median survival times of 9, 5, and 2 years, respectively (Table 2). Both Rai and Binet staging systems contain relevant prognostic information on either BM or lymph

Table 2 The Rai and Binet Staging System

Staging system	Stage	Modified three-stage system	Clinicohematological features	Median survival (yr)
Rai	0	Low-risk	Lymphocytes in PB and BM	>10
	I		Lymphocytosis + lymphoadenopathy	7
		Intermediate-risk		
	II		Lymphocytosis + splenomegaly and/or hepatomegaly ± lymphoadenopathy	7
	III		Lymphocytosis + anemia (hemoglobin < 110 g/L) ± lymphoadenopathy ± splenomegaly ± hepatomegaly	1.5
		High-risk		
	IV		Lymphocytosis + thrombocytopenia (platelets < 100×10^9/L) ± anemia ± lymphoadenopathy ± splenomegaly ± hepatomegaly	
Binet	A		Lymphoid areas involved <3	>10
	B		Lymphoid areas involved ≥ 3	5
	C		Anemia (hemoglobin < 100 g/L) and/or thrombocytopenia (platelets < 100×10^9/L	2

node area involvements; however, they fail to identify specific subsets of patients. In an attempt to overcome this problem, the International Workshop on CLL (IWCLL) proposed an integration of two stagings, thus creating Rai substages of the Binet system (15). Unfortunately, the IWCLL system has not obtained widespread acceptance, and investigators have continued to use either the Rai (more frequently in United States) or the Binet (more frequently in Europe) classification.

In addition to the Rai and Binet staging systems, several other classification methods have been proposed in the last two decades. The total tumor mass (TTM) score, a quantitative staging system described by Jaksic and Vitale (16), is based on the clinical assessment of disease involvement within all major body compartments. However, this approach does not take into account BM failure, a feature not consistently correlated with tumor burden. The analysis of a large retrospective series, including 1777 CLL performed by the GI-MEMA study group, identified four parameters associated with a poor prognosis: lymphocytosis ($>60 \times 10^9$/L), anemia (Hb < 10 g/dL), number of enlarged lymph nodes (>2 cm), or palpable hepatosplenomegaly (>3 cm below costal margin) (17). The extent of lymphadenopathy in addition to age (>60 years) and some serum parameters (LDH > 325 U/L, APH > 80 U/L, uric acid > 7 mg/dL) were variables entering at a significant level in a multivariate survival analysis carried out by Lee et al. (18). Although all these systems make it possible to better appreciate clinicoprognostic heterogeneity of CLL, they add relatively little information to either Rai or Binet schemes, which continue to represent, more than two decades after their introduction, the reference systems for separating CLL patients with different outcomes who may possibly require different therapeutic approaches.

II. SMOLDERING CLL

Although CLL is the quintessential example of an indolent lymphoid neoplasm, about 30% to 40% of patients with early disease progress to a more advanced clinical stage and finally die of their leukemia (Fig. 1) (19). This observation is clearly reflected in the significantly shorter survival of patients with early-stage compared with an age- and sex-matched control population (Fig. 2) (19). Clinicohematological features identifying subsets of patients with a particularly favorable clinical outcome were sought by several investigators. Han et al. (20) coined the term "benign monoclonal lymphocytosis" to describe the clinical course of a small but interesting series of 20 patients whose disease did not show progressive changes after a follow-up time, ranging from 6.4 to 24 years. Tura et al. (21) and Oscier et al. (22) analyzed their series of Rai stage 0 patients to identify factors affecting the time to disease progression. Parameters correlated with an increased risk of disease progression included LDT in the former study and the initial lymphocyte count, surface immunoglobulin phenotype, and some complex karyotype abnormalities in the latter. These observations were further extended by Montserrat et al. (23), who first proposed the definition of "smoldering" CLL for a subset of stage A patients, accounting for 30% of patients with CLL, whose life expectancy was not different from that of an age- and sex-matched control population. Clinicohematological features identifying "smoldering" CLL were hemoglobin level greater than 13 g/dL, a low absolute lymphocyte count ($<30 \times 10^9$/L), a nondiffuse pattern of BM involvement, and LDT > 12 months. The French Cooperative Group on CLL analyzed a large prospective series of stage A CLL randomized to early versus delayed therapy, thus providing a definition

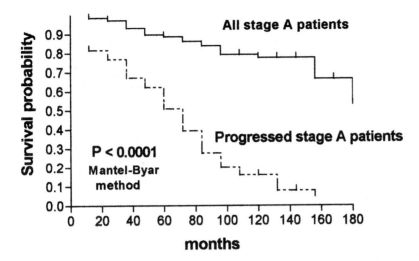

Figure 1 Survival probability of stage A patients according to the disease-progression. (From Ref. 177.)

of smoldering CLL that differs from that of Montserrat for the exclusion of LDT and BM histology; the method used for assessing the degree of BM involvement relied on percentage of lymphocytes on BM smears (24,25) (Table 3).

Molica et al. (26) in a series of patients followed up in a single institution demonstrated that whatever criteria used all proposals succeeded in defining a subset of patients with low rate of progression (about 15% at 5 years) and long life expectancy (greater than 80% at 10 years). Recent studies tried to investigate whether novel prognostic factors may assist in the identification of high-risk categories of early CLL. Three serum parameters

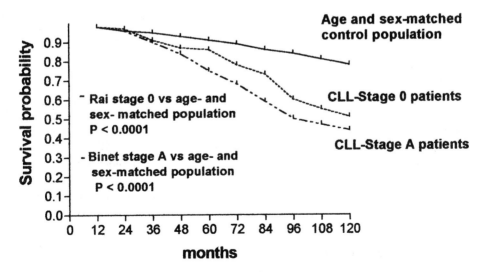

Figure 2 Survival probability of Binet stage A and Rai stage 0 patients in comparison to age- and sex-matched healthy controls. (From Ref. 177.)

Table 3   Criteria for Defining Smoldering
CLL

Montserrat et al.
  Binet stage A
  Nondiffuse bone marrow histology
  Hb > 13 g/dL
  Blood lymphocytes < 30 × 10^9/L
  Lymphocyte doubling time > 12 mo
French Cooperative Group on CLL
  A$'_1$
    Binet stage A
    Hb ≥ 12 g/dL
    Lymphocytes count < 30 × 10^9/L
  A$'_2$
    Binet stage A
    Hb ≥ 12 g/dL
    Lymphocytes count < 30 × 10^9/L
    <2 involved lymphoid areas[a]
    Bone marrow infiltration <80%
  A$'_1$
    Binet stage A
    Hb < 12 g/dL
    Lymphocytes count ≥ 30 × 10^9/L
  A$'_2$
    Binet stage A
    Hb < 12 g/dL
    Lymphocytes count ≥ 30 × 10^9/L
    2 involved lymphoid areas, or
    Bone marrow infiltration ≥ 80%

---

[a] Cervical, axillary, inguinal limph nodes (unilateral or
bilateral), spleen, liver.

(β_2-microglobulin, s-TK, and sCD23) may add prognostic information to the subclassification of patients in stage A (27–29). It is warranted, therefore, that studies carried out on large series of patients might confirm the potential prognostic value of these parameters.

How these results translate into the timing of therapy is still a complex issue. A recent meta-analysis of 2048 patients with early disease enrolled in six trials of immediate versus deferred chemotherapy (chlorambucil or chlorambucil plus prednisone) demonstrated that the 10-year survival rate was slightly worse, even though not significant, with immediate chemotherapy (44% versus 47%), thus supporting a conservative treatment strategy for patients with early CLL (30). Nonetheless, this approach should be reconsidered as soon as results of trials based on newer chemotherapy become available.

III. CLL IN YOUNGER PATIENTS

CLL is usually considered a disease of the elderly. However, about 10% to 15% of patients reported in different clinical trials are less than 50 years of age, and this proportion likely will increase in the next few years because of early diagnosis, increasing pressure of new treatment strategies, and more accurate prognostic assessment of this subgroup (31). Generally, younger and older patients display a similar distribution of clinical features (32,33). However, a different distribution of causes of deaths is found (33,34). CLL-unrelated deaths and secondary primary nonlymphoid malignancies predominate in the older age group, whereas the direct effects of leukemia are prevalent in the younger age group. As a consequence, survival advantage of younger CLL patients compared with older patients disappear when only CLL-related deaths (i.e., leukemia-progression, infections) are considered in the survival analyses (33). Furthermore, criteria of smoldering CLL apply also to young CLL patients who should not be treated unless progression of disease occurs, age not being, by itself, a criterion for intensifying therapy (32,33).

IV. CLL IN OLDER PATIENTS

Older age has consistently been shown to confer a poorer prognosis, although the reason for these differences has not been analyzed thoroughly. Older patients have an increased incidence of interacting diseases (35). The presence of this degree of comorbidity generally not seen in younger population has a major impact on the patients' survival and on the ability to tolerate treatment. Catovsky et al. (35) in the analysis of prognostic factors of patients who entered in the first Medical Research Council trial in CLL confirmed that age is an adverse prognostic factor. In fact, unrelated illnesses were particularly relevant in decreasing the survival of patients older than 70 years of age. The prevalence of CLL-unrelated competing causes of death was high in patients with early disease in the Call et al. (36) study. In such a survey, CLL was reported as the underlying cause of death only in 38% of Rai stage 0 patients. Finally, Keating et al. (37) found that age > 70 years was an adverse prognostic feature for patients treated with fludarabine, with a median survival of 32 months compared with a median of 67 months in patients aged 60 to 69 years.

In conclusion, caution should be used for prognostic parameters derived from studies that do not separate CLL- from non-CLL–related deaths. Either assessing or understanding the interactions between comorbidity, CLL and its treatment is a major challenge in the management of CLL.

V. BONE MARROW INVOLVEMENT

Although BM aspiration and biopsy are not required to diagnose CLL, they can evaluate a major site of involvement of disease (38). The pattern of BM involvement (diffuse versus nondiffuse) was the strongest predictor of survival in the study performed by Rozman et al.(39), who devised an integrated clinicopathological staging, thus separating patients of intermediate risk into two different prognostic categories. Pangalis et al. (40) observed an increased rate of disease progression among stage A or B patients who were seen with a diffuse pattern of BM involvement; however, they failed to identify different prognostic subgroups in single clinical stages. These results were in keeping with those of Han et al. (41), Desablens et al. (42), and Mauro et al. (43), who concluded that histological pattern of BM involvement does not add prognostic information to clinical stage.

Some investigators evaluated the prognostic value of BM biopsy in patients with early CLL, thus trying to clarify the relative merits of BM biopsy and lymphocyte infiltration (LI) in the evaluation of BM involvement (44–46). Montserrat et al. (44) pointed out that interobservers' reproducibility was higher for BM biopsy than for LI evaluated on BM smears. Although both BM biopsy and LI are useful in the clinical management of disease, only BM biopsy is an independent parameter predicting the risk of disease progression of stage A patients. In a prospective multicenter study carried out by Geisler et al. (45), the impact of timely therapy given to most patients at the time of progression to stage B or C might explain the lack of prognostic value of BM histology. Thus, it seems that effective and prolonged therapy may reduce the prognostic value of BM histology (45).

In conclusion, BM biopsy and LI on BM smears can be considered complementary methods for assessing BM infiltration in CLL. However, BM biopsy is a more suitable method, and its serial evaluation provides information for assessing response to therapy; absence of lymphoid nodules is compatible with a complete response (38,44,46).

Finally, the potential role for BM magnetic resonance (MR) imaging in the assessment of BM involvement of CLL patients was proposed by Lecouvet et al. (47). BM abnormalities were detected with quantitative MR imaging in 7 (33%) of 21 patients with early-stage B-cell CLL. Interestingly, in patients with abnormal quantitative MR imaging findings, treatment-free survival was significantly shorter than in patients with normal MR imaging findings (47). These results should be considered as preliminary; nonetheless, MR images enable noninvasive assessment of the BM in CLL, and this technology deserves further evaluation.

VI. LYMPHOCYTE MORPHOLOGY

Although some morphological variants have been described, results are controversial with respect to prognosis. Size of lymphocytes, number of prolymphocytes, presence of cleaved and/or lymphoplasmocytic cells have been associated with poor prognosis (48–51). Melo et al. (48) showed that the presence of $>15 \times 10^9$/L or $>10\%$ prolymphocytes was associated with a poor prognosis. Such an observation was confirmed by Vallespi et al. (50), who demonstrated that increased numbers of both prolymphocytes and cleaved cells were associated with shorter survival, but in a multivariate analysis only an increased prolymphocyte count retained prognostic significance.

On the basis of these findings, two variants of CLL have been recognized in addition to typical CLL by the French-American-British (FAB) group: (1) CLL/PLL in which there are more than 10% but less than 55% prolymphocytes in peripheral blood; (2) mixed cell type CLL characterized by a spectrum of small to large lymphocytes with occasional ($<10\%$) prolymphocytes (52). In the comprehensive study published by Criel et al. (53), cases were subclassified as morphologically typical and atypical according to the FAB proposal (52). Atypical CLL, accounting for 23% of all CLL cases, was diagnosed more frequently in advanced clinical stages, was more likely associated with trisomy 12, and had a shorter survival. Moreover, Rai's clinical staging lost its prognostic significance when applied to atypical cases (53). Oscier et al. (54) analyzed the cytomorphology of 270 stage A patients looking for factors adversely affecting disease progression. In univariate analysis the presence of either trisomy 12 or atypical morphology correlated with a more rapid progression of disease. However, such a finding was a consequence of the association between trisomy 12 and atypical morphology. Indeed, in multivariate analysis only atypical lymphocyte morphology, more than two karyotypic abnormalities, absolute lymphocyte count $>30 \times 10^9$/L, LDT $<$ 12 months, and lymph node enlargment entered the regression model at a significant level (54).

In conclusion, subclassifying CLL by morphology enables the identification of two different patient groups with typical and atypical cytological features. This separation reflects peculiar clinical presentations, cytogenetic findings, and a different prognosis.

VII. IMMUNODEFICIENCY

CLL patients have an increased risk for bacterial infections developing (55,56). Such a risk, especially in patients not receiving therapy with purine analogs, closely reflects the degree of hypogammaglobulinemia (55). Rozman et al. (57) investigated the prognostic impact and natural history of hypogammaglobulinemia in 247 CLL patients. Although a cutoff level of 700 mg/dL of IgG identified subsets of patients at different risk of death, the significance was lost in the multivariate analysis (57). On the other hand, it does not appear clearly that the observed shortened survival of patients with low IgG levels reflected an excess of life-threatening infectious episodes. Accordingly, other investigators, were unable to demonstrate a relationship between hypogammaglobulinemia and reduced overall survival (17,18,58). More recently, a correlation between disease progression and immunological abnormalities was reported. Everaus et al. (59) suggested that progressive disease more typically is associated with a marked decline of serum IgA levels and to a lesser extent with a suppression of T-cell function.

Serum evaluation of complement activation and total complement hemolytic activity (CH50) were correlated with occurrence of bacterial infections and short overall survival in Rai stage II and III patients (60,61).

Qualitative and quantitative alterations of nonneoplastic T-cell counterpart have been correlated with prognosis (62–64). An increased number of CD4- and CD8-positive and a reduced proportion of T-suppressor/effector (CD11b+) cells was correlated by Totterman et al. with more advanced clinical stages (63). According to the results of Apostopoulos et al. (64), it seems that CD4/CD8 ratio and proportion of NK cells are features of advanced disease and are associated with hypogammaglobulinemia and increased incidence of infections of respiratory tract. Finally, some soluble molecules may have an impact on the immune system. Leukemic B cells through the elaboration of suppressive cytokines, such as transforming growth factor beta (TGF-beta) and release of soluble CD27 down-modulate expression of CD40-ligand (CD154), originarily expressed by CD4-positive T-cells after immune activation (65–69). Such down-modulation has been considered responsible, at least in part, for the immune deficiency that is acquired in CLL (70).

VIII. PROLIFERATION MARKERS AND CELL-CYCLE REGULATORY MOLECULES

Several methods have been used to evaluate tumor cell proliferation and to correlate kinetic parameters with clinical outcome. Cordone et al. (71), using the monoclonal antibody Ki67, found a close correlation between the number of leukemic cells expressing such a marker and a more advanced clinical stage. However, the study did not qualify Ki67 as an independent prognostic parameter. Del Giglio et al. (72) focused on the expression of proliferating cell nuclear antigen (PCNA), a cell-cycle dependent protein, which correlated with either clinical stages or LDT. Interestingly, low PCNA levels could predict response to therapy with fludarabine. Orfao et al. (73) evaluated the proliferation rate of peripheral blood (PB) lymphocytes, as expressed by the absolute count of PB S-phase leukocytes in 80 B-cell CLL patients. Multivariate analysis revealed that the S-phase leukocyte count, although related to other clinical and biological factors, displayed an important independent value in predicting early deaths in patients with B-CLL.

The identification of p27^k, a cyclin-dependent kinase inhibitor that contributes to the cell cycle arrest, prompted Vrhovac et al. (74) to study p27 protein in the lymphocytes from 83 B-cell CLL patients and 32 patients with other chronic lymphoproliferative disorders. The expression of p27 protein was higher in B-CLL. Independently of absolute PB lymphocytosis, increased levels of p27 protein positively correlated with LDT. Interestingly, the overall survival from date of sampling was shorter in patients with high p27 expression (median survival, 24.4 months) than in patients with low p27 expression (median not reached; $P = 0.016$) (74).

The demonstration of cyclin-D1 overexpression generally indicates a diagnosis of mantle cell lymphoma (MCL) (75). However, overexpression of cyclin-D1 has been reported in various chronic lymphoproliferative disorders, namely prolymphocytic leukemia, atypical CLL, or even typical CLL (75,76). Interestingly, Levy et al. demonstrated that cyclin-D1 overexpression allows identification among the unclassified chronic lymphoproliferative disorders a subset of aggressive disorders that represents a leukemic counterpart of MCL (77).

To improve the prognostic stratification of CLL patients with "early" disease, Hallek et al. (29) evaluated serum level of thymidine kinase (s-TK), an enzyme reflecting cellular transformation to a dividing condition, in 122 B-cell CLL patients in early disease. Serum levels of s-TK added independent prognostic information to the definitions of smoldering and nonsmoldering CLL. Indeed, increased levels of s-TK (i.e., >7.0 U/L) were able to identify a subset of patients with nonsmoldering stage A disease who had a significantly shorter progression-free survival (PFS) than patients with low s-TK levels (29). Interestingly, prognostic implications of kinetic parameters are exemplified by clinical studies based on lymphocyte doubling time (LDT) (78,79). LDT, defined as the time needed to double the peripheral blood lymphocyte count, is a simple parameter particularly useful in early disease. Although not directly available at diagnosis, LDT is easy to calculate by extrapolation shortly after diagnosis. Additional clinical parameters of potential prognostic value are the lymphocyte accumulation rate (i.e., the initial lymphocyte count divided by LDT) and the assessment of static versus progressive disease; however, the semplicity and easy use makes LDT a largely accepted parameter for assessing the pace of disease (26,80).

IX. IMMUNOPHENOTYPIC CHARACTERISTICS

Detailed immunophenotypical analysis of chronic lymphoid leukemias permits specific classification, thus allowing the identification of subsets of patients clinically relevant. To better differentiate "immunologically typical CLL" from other chronic B-cell disorders a scoring system based on the immunophenotypic analysis of a panel of five membrane markers (i.e., CD5, CD22, CD23, FMC7, SmIg) has been proposed (81). More recently, it has been found that the monoclonal antibody CD79b, which recognizes the immunoglobulin-associated membrane protein B29, may further improve the diagnostic accuracy of other B-cell markers (82). However, attempts to correlate the immunophenotype with prognosis have yielded inconclusive results (58,83,84). It should be pointed out that most studies rely on the presence or absence of a given antigen, little attention being paid to its density on the cell surface. In a series of patients fulfilling strict immunological criteria of B-cell CLL (i.e., CD5+, CD23+) a bright CD20 expression significantly correlated with "atypical" morphology and to a lesser extent with survival (85). Quantitative immunophenotyping makes it possible to better appreciate the biological heterogeneity of disease; however, results are difficult to be transferred into prognosis (85).

Clinicoprognostic implications of expression of non-B lineage–related antigens have been analyzed in several studies (86–88). The presence of myelomonocytic antigens on the surface of B-neoplastic cells was frequently associated with poor prognostic features. A close association between diffuse pattern of BM infiltration and expression of myelomonocytic antigens (i.e., CD13, CD33) has been identified in otherwise typical CLL (86,88). This observation is of interest in view of the structural relationship of CD33 to the family of neural cell adhesion molecules (89).

Ikematsu et al. (90) reported that CD13- and CD11b-expression is restricted to patients with CD5-negative B-CLL. Finally, Callea et al. (91) investigated the expression of CD14 in 128 previously untreated CLL patients. Median survival was 63 months for patients with a CD14+ cell count $>5 \times 10^9$/L and 136 months for those with CD14+ cell count $< 5 \times 10^9$/L. In the multivariate regression model, Rai stage, age, and CD14+ cell count were independent factors predicting overall survival (91).

Mulligan et al. (92) analyzed a series of 10 B-cell CLL patients expressing CD8-antigen on leukemic B cells. They concluded that CD8-expression in B-CLL is probably underrecognized but is not a marker of disease progression. The CD8 on the B-CLL surface was immunochemically identical to the antigen on T cells but is unlikely to be a functionally active receptor.

CD36 is a membrane-bound glycoprotein receptor for thrombospadin expressed on a variety of hematopoietic cells; however, the expression of such an antigen was not conclusively associated with B lymphocytes. Rutella et al. (93) assessed CD36-expression in 24 B-cell CLL patients. CD36 could be detected on 45% (range, 30%–75%) of neoplastic CD19-positive cells. Clinicohematological features identifying aggressive disease such as advanced clinical stage and diffuse BM histology were associated with higher CD36 expression. These findings strongly support the view that CD36 might favor tumor cell spreading.

X. CELLULAR EXPRESSION AND SERUM RELEASE OF SOLUBLE CD23

CD23 is a functionally relevant molecule in B-cell CLL; however, studies dealing with its prognostic role have yielded inconclusive results (13,83,84). The membrane instability of CD23, which is rapidly cleaved from the cell surface into a stable form, has important clinicoprognostic implications (28,94,95). Soluble CD23 (sCD23) is a reliable and disease-specific marker that provides information on overall survival and freedom from progression in early-stage patients (28). According to Sarfati et al. (28) results of a doubling time of sCD23 level during the follow-up was associated with a 3.2-fold increased risk of death. However, there is no definitive evidence that sCD23 may replace well-recognized clinical parameters in CLL; more likely it can be incorporated into the Binet staging system, therefore leading to the separation of intermediate risk group (i.e., Binet stage B) into two subgroups that differ with respect to prognosis (94).

XI. β₂-MICROGLOBULIN

β_2-microglobulin is an extracellular protein that is noncovalently associated with alpha-chain of the class I major histocompatibility complex (MHC) gene, which is detectable in the serum. A number of studies suggest that it may have prognostic value in CLL. Hallek et al. (96) analyzed a prospective series of 113 CLL patients with early disease and found that serum β_2-microglobulin in addition to sTK, performance status, and platelet count are independent prognostic factors affecting the progression-free survival (PFS). Keating et al. (27) reported results concerning 622 patients followed up at M. D. Anderson Cancer Center. In this patient population high serum levels of β_2-microglobulin predicted prognosis also within single Rai stages. Furthermore, β_2-microglobulin predicted response to fludarabine (27).

An attractive option is that of including in prognostic models different serological markers that contribute individually to prognosis of CLL under the speculative assumption that their combined use, integrating different clinical and biological aspects of CLL, provides prognostic information superior to that of a single marker. In a single institution study, serum levels of β_{-2} microglobulin and LDH were two strong independent prognostic variables, and their combination clearly determined three prognostic groups (97). Similarly, a combination of β_{-2} microglobulin and sCD23 added independent prognostic information to the clinical parameters currently used for assessing prognosis (i.e., BM histology, LDT) and could be incorporated into the Binet system, therefore leading to the formulation of clinicobiological staging (98).

XII. CYTOGENETICS AND MOLECULAR BIOLOGY

In B-cell CLL, clonal chromosome aberrations are detected in approximately 35% to 50% of cases by conventional chromosome banding analysis (99). Comprehensive data from chromosomal banding analyses collected within the first and second meeting of the International Working Party on Chromosome in CLL identified clonal chromosome aberrations in 51% of cases. The most common aberrations diagnosed include trisomy 12 (19%), structural abnormalities of chromosome bands 13q14 (10%) and 14q32, and deletion of the long arm 11 (11q) (8%) (100,101). In the first IWCLL analysis it was found that patients with clonal abnormalities had a poorer survival compared with those with normal karyotype. Patients with 13q-deletions as the sole abnormality had a better prognosis than patients with other single abnormalities, in particular trisomy 12. The prognosis of patients with 13q-deletions was similar to that of patients with normal karyotype (102).

More recently, the development of molecular cytogenetic techniques has significantly increased our capacity to detect chromosome aberrations in tumor cells. Using fluorescence in situ hybridization (FISH), chromosome aberrations can be detected not only in dividing cells but also in interphase nuclei. Therefore, the prevalence of specific aberrations in B-cell CLL is being reassessed on the basis of results obtained using interphase cytogenetics (103). The most common structural abnormalities in B-cell CLL are deletions on the long arm of chromosome 13 at band q14, distal to the retinoblastoma (RB) gene, which occur in up to 50% of cases analyzed in interphase FISH (103,104). It is generally thought the deletions at 13q14 result in inactivation of a tumor suppressor gene (104). Although the retinoblastoma gene (RB1) was initially thought to be inactivated by 13q14 deletions in B-CLL, several lines of evidence indicate that the putative tumor suppressor gene differ from RB (105). The suggestion that the breast cancer–related gene

2 (BRCA-2) deletion is involved has not been confirmed in different studies (106,107). Despite the efforts by different groups, the specific gene involved has so far not been identified.

The cases with 13q14 deletions show heavy somatic mutations of Ig genes (108). Furthermore, patients with 13q14 abnormalities characteristically have a benign disease that usually manifests as an isolated, stable, or slowly progressive disease. Actually, they survive as long as their age-matched controls (108). The prognostic significance of 13q deletions was recently reevaluated by a study showing that such a cytogenetic abnormality is associated with a more aggressive behavior among patients with early-stage disease (low β_2-microglobulin, or Rai stage 0–II) (109).

Deletions at 11q22–23 occur in 13% to 19% of B-CLL cases (103). Like 13q14 allelic loss, 11q loss is thought to result in inactivation of a tumor suppressor gene (105). Inactivation of the ATM in cases of sporadic T-cell leukemias and finding that the absence of the ATM protein correlates with a poor outcome in B-CLL suggested that 11q deletions also result in ATM gene inactivation (110). The frequency and clinical impact of 11q23 deletions in B-CLL by interphase cytogenetics using FISH have been recently analyzed in a consistent series of patients (111). Forty-three of 214 (20%) patients exhibited 11q23 deletions, which affected the prognosis of patients less than 55 years of age (111). Given the conflicting data concerning clinical risk factors in young patients with CLL, this biological finding may be of great relevance in selecting candidates for intensive treatment approaches. Trisomy 12 occurs in up to 20% by using interphase FISH (103). A significant association between trisomy 12 and CLL with atypical morphological and/or immunological features, unmutated V_H genes, high proliferative activity, advanced disease, and poor prognosis have been reported (108). Interestingly, trisomy 12 is an early cytogenetic event in the history of CLL and is not acquired during disease evolution (112).

Another recurring chromosome abnormality involves the short arm of chromosome 6 (113). One study reported an association between CLL and particular alleles of the gene encoding TNF-alpha, designed TNF1, and located on 6q (114). Patients with aggressive disease had a particular allele of a continuous gene encoding lymphotoxin-alpha, designed TNFB*2, more often than control sujects (114).

In an attempt to identify different cytogenetic prognostic subgroups Dohner et al. (115) studied 338 B-cell CLL patients by interphase cytogenetics using a disease-specific set of diagnostic DNA probes. Patients with deletion 13q as a single cytogenetic abnormality had the longest median survival (>15 years), followed by those with 6q deletion and trisomy 12 (median survival, 11 and 10.9 years, respectively). In contrast, 17p and 11q deletions were associated with rapid disease progression and inferior survival (median survival times, 3.6 and 6.6 years, respectively).

B-CLL cells have been shown in some cases to have somatically mutated Ig variable region genes, indicating that the cells have passed through the germinal center (116). Oscier et al. (108) observed that cases with trisomy 12 and atypical morphology expressed IgV$_H$ genes that had not undergone significant somatic mutation, whereas cases with 13q14 gene lesions expressed IgV$_H$ genes that had incurred somatic mutations. These observations were further extended by Hamblin et al. (117), who identified a germ line configuration of V_H genes in 38 of 84 (45.2%) of patients, whereas 46 cases (54.8%) showed >2% somatic mutation. Unmutated V_H genes were significantly associated with VI-69 and D3-3 use, with atypical morphology, isolated trisomy 12, advanced stage, and progressive disease. In contrast, patients showing mutation of V_H genes had stable disease with typical morphology. Survival was significantly shorter for patients with unmutated V_H genes irrespective of stage. For instance, median survival for stage A patients with unmutated V_H

genes was 95 months compared with 293 months for patients whose tumors had mutated V_H genes (P = 0.0008) (114). Damle et al. (118) evaluated cell surface markers (CD38-expression) and clinical course of two groups of B-cell CLL patients stratified on the basis of the number of IgV gene mutations. Mutated forms were identified on the basis of more than 2% of IgV mutations and unmutated forms included patients with less than 2% of IgV mutations. Unmutated cases were characterized for a higher CD38 expression. When correlation with the outcome of disease was sought, it was found that unmutated cases had a higher treatment requirement and shorter overall survival. Similar results were obtained after stratifying patients according to the expression of CD38; the median survival for the CD38-high (unmutated) patients was 10 years, whereas the survival for CD38-low (mutated) patients was not reached (P = 0.0001). Given the strong association between mutation and the numbers of CD38 + B-CLL cells, they propose to use CD38 expression as a reliable assay for differing two groups that sensibly differ with respect to their natural history (118).

In addition to surface immunoglobulin, the B-cell receptor complex contains two accessory proteins, called CD79a (Ig-α) and CD79b (Ig-β), that are required for intracellular assembly, surface expression, and signal transduction of surface immunoglobulin (13). Thompson et al. (119) reported that most cases studied had somatic mutations of CD79b on leukemic B cells. They claimed that such a finding may explain the low-level expression of immunoglobulin on the surface of B-CLL cells. Alfarano et al. (120) suggest a role for the alternative splicing of CD79b in causing the reduced expression of B-cell receptor complex on the surface of B-CLL cells. However, attempts to correlate CD79b-expression with clinicohematological features did not succeed, thus supporting a limited role for CD79b as a prognostic marker (120).

p53 is a tumor suppressor gene acting as an inductor of apoptosis in genetically damaged cells. Structural alterations and point mutations of the p53 gene have been shown in 10% to 15% of CLL and have been associated with advanced disease, including Richter's syndrome, poor survival, and nonresponse to therapy (121,122). Dohner et al. (122) identified p53 deletion to be the strongest predictor of survival in multivariate analysis. In addition, deletion of p53 predicted resistance to treatment with fludarabine or pentostatine. Cordone et al. (123) evaluated p53 protein expression by immunoperoxidase in 181 B-CLL patients and found expression of protein in 15% of cases. p53-positive patients had a significantly higher percentage of prolymphocytes, more advanced clinical stage, poorer response to therapy, and shorter overall survival. Association between p53 protein expression with mutations in the gene was confirmed in 15 of the 18 (88%) immunocytochemistry-positive cases tested (123).

Lens et al. (124) studied the possible involvement of p53 in the pathogenesis of CLL/PLL; to this purpose they selected 17 patients with typical morphology and 15 CLL/PLL. Overall, 11 cases (30%) had p53 abnormalities, of which 8 cases had CLL/PLL. CLL cases with p53 and were characterized by a higher incidence of stage C, higher proliferative rate, short survival, and resistance to first-line therapy. Interestingly, trisomy 12 was more frequent in cases without p53 abnormalities, suggesting that trisomy 12 and p53 may represent different pathway of transformation in CLL (124).

XIII. CELLULAR EXPRESSION AND SERUM RELEASE OF ADHESION MOLECULES

Adhesion molecule expression has been reported in CLL and may be relevant either to understand the clinical behavior of the disease or to define distinct subsets of patients

(125–132). Low levels of β_2-integrin were associated with a diffuse pattern of BM infiltration, 11q deletion, and poor prognosis (128,133). In another study the increased expression of β_2-integrin has been related to the presence of a higher number of leukemic cells in patients with more advanced disease (125). From a biological point of view, the in vitro interaction of B-CLL cells with stromal BM cells by means of β_1- and β_2-integrins protects leukemic cells from apoptosis (134).

Leukemic B-CLL cells from most patients constitutively express ligand for LFA-1, namely ICAM-2 (CD102) and ICAM-3 (CD50) (135). Although the surface cellular expression of ICAM-1 (CD54) is generally low, ICAM-1 serum levels are increased in B-cell CLL, such a finding reflecting clinicobiological parameters of either tumor mass (i.e., clinical stages, BM histology) or disease progression (i.e., LDT, thymidine kinase activity) (130,136). When investigated in relation to clinical outcome, serum levels of ICAM-1 were able to predict life expectancy of patients (136,137) (Fig. 3).

Elevated serum levels of soluble vascular cell adhesion molecule-1 (sVCAM-1) have been reported in B-cell CLL and positively correlated with tumor burden (127). Although only ICAM-1 was an independent prognostic factor, circulating levels of sVCAM-1 could be useful for estimating risk of progression in early-stage patients (127).

Results concerning the expression of CD44 are controversial and mainly reflect differences of methods used for detecting such an antigen (immunocytochemistry versus flow cytometry) and the specificity of anti-CD44 monoclonal antibody used (125,129). Estimation of CD44 density may also be relevant, because it seems that CLL patients with intermediate and high CD44 surface density have longer survival than cases with "dim" CD44 pattern (126). More recently, the interest of investigators was attracted by the soluble form of CD44, which is elevated in approximately half of B-CLL patients and reflects tumor burden (138). In contrast, CD44 "variant isoforms" v5 and v6 were detected in normal levels in the serum of most CLL cases (138). The predictive and prognostic value of serum levels of standard CD44 was recently analyzed by Molica et al. (139), who assessed the impact on disease outcome in 68 patients with early CLL. In the stepwise multiple regression analysis only two parameters provided independent prognostic infor-

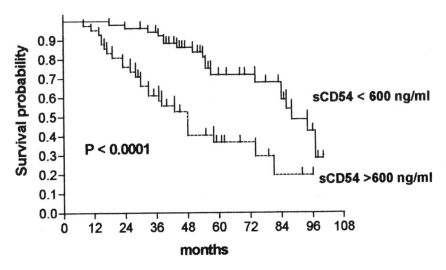

Figure 3 Survival probability of CLL patients statified on the basis of serum levels of soluble CD54. (Adapted from Ref. 137.)

mation about progression-free survival: Rai substages and levels of sCD44 higher than median value (642 ng/ml). Furthermore, sCD44 could be added to the Rai subclassification of stage A, thus providing a better prognostic stratification of patients in Rai stage I–II (139).

XIV. ABNORMAL ANGIOGENESIS IN CLL

Evidence for abnormal angiogenesis in BM of patients with B-cell CLL has been demonstrated in a recent study (140). The degree of angiogenesis measured by the microvessel density in the BM was significantly higher in CLL patients compared with normal controls. Interestingly, such a finding correlated with levels in the urine of basic fibroblastic growth factor (bFGF), a pleiotropic cytokine also playing a role in apoptosis (140). Menzel et al. (141) measured intracellular bFGF in 36 patients with CLL by use of an enzyme-linked immunoassay. In cells derived from patients with high-risk disease, the median level of intracellular b-FGF correlated with Rai clinical stages. Immunofluorescent stains of peripheral blood mononuclear cells confirmed CLL as a cellular source of b-FGF. Furthermore, the proapoptotic effect induced by fludarabine was reduced after in vitro exposure to exogenous bFGF (141). The delayed apoptosis induced by b-FGF was obtained in B-CLL cell lines by way of a up-regulation of *bcl*-2 expression (142).

Cellular levels of vascular endothelial growth factor (VEGF), a potent angiogenic growth factor, were evaluated in 232 B-cell CLL patients observed at M. D. Anderson Cancer Center. Investigators concluded that this angiogenic factor can be considered a reliable indicator of prognosis, especially in patients with low β_2-microglobulin (143). Molica et al. (144) found that independently of tumor mass, serum levels of VEGF correlate with progression-free survival (PFS) of patients in early disease. Stage A patients whose serum levels of VEGF were above the median value (i.e., 194.8 pg/mL) had an increased risk of disease progression compared with those with S-VEGF below the median value (P = 0.01) (144). Chen et al. (145) wondered whether angiogenically functional VEGF is produced by CLL cells. RT-PCR and Slot-blot analysis demonstrated that CLL cells express VEGF m-RNA; furthermore, analysis of nucleotide sequence confirmed that two smaller VEGF m-RNAs, VEGF 121 and VEGF 165, are the predominantly expressed isoforms. Although these results need to be validated in prospective studies, measurements of either cellular or circulating levels of VEGF could be informative in view of a possible application of antiangiogenetic therapies, on the basis of anti-VEGF antibodies.

XV. BIOLOGICAL MARKERS REFLECTING THE PATHOGENESIS OF DISEASE

B-cell CLL represents a neoplastic disorder caused primarily by defective programmed cell death (PCD) as opposed to increased cell proliferation (13). Defects in the PCD pathway play a pivotal role in the pathogenesis of disease, thus creating a selective survival advantage for CLL clone. Nonetheless, unstimulated B-CLL cells spontaneously undergo apoptosis on isolation from the patient in whole blood culture and in culture media (13). Although molecular events responsible for the initiation of PCD in unstimulated B-CLL cells are not completely known, a correlation with temporary induction of p53 and p21[CIPI] gene expression has been demonstrated (146).

Most B-CLLs have been reported to contain high levels of antiapoptotic protein *bcl*-2 in absence of rearrangement of *bcl*-2. Although the reason for this is unclear, some preliminary data suggest hypomethylation as a possible cause (147). Interestingly, *bcl*-2 overexpression did not correlate with main clinicohematological features but did correlate with survival, suggesting an independent prognostic value (148–150). More interesting was the pattern of *bcl*-2 protein expression after drug exposure. Gottardi et al. (151) found that fludarabine down-regulated the expression of *bcl*-2 in 5 of 12 CLL samples treated in vitro. These authors suggest that the susceptibility of leukemic cells to fludarabine-induced down-modulation of *bcl*-2 correlated with the sensitivity to this drug in vivo (151).

Bcl-2 belongs to a family of genes whose other known members are *bcl*-$_{XL}$, *bcl*-$_{XS}$, and *bax*, and either act synergistically or counteract its activity (13). Because quantitative changes of intracellular levels of *bcl*-2 and *bax* may have a relevant impact on clinical outcome during the treatment-free period and response to therapy, it could be of interest to explore clinical implications of combining information of these markers (152–153). Bcl-2 and *bax* can form homodimers and heterodimers that influence susceptibility to apoptosis. A low *bcl*-2/*bax* ratio identifies a subset of previously untreated patients with relatively indolent and stable disease; on the other hand this finding also characterizes CLL patients who are likely to respond to therapy (149–153). Pepper et al. (153) evaluated B-CLL cells for their apoptotic response to drug treatment in vitro and found that cells with high *bcl*-2/*bax* ratio were more resistant to apoptosis than cells with low *bcl*-2/*bax* ratio. Furthermore, they monitored the in vitro viability of B-CLL cells in relation to *bcl*-2 and *bax* expression over 48 hours after exposure to chlorambucil. The results showed that *bax* up-regulation was essential for chlorambucil-induced apoptosis in B-CLL (154).

Kitada et al. (155) analyzed the expression of several apoptosis-regulating proteins, including the *bcl*-2 family proteins *bcl*-2, *bcl*-x$_L$, *Mcl*-1, *Bax, Bak*, and *BAD*; the *bcl*-2-binding protein BAG-1; and the cell death protease Caspase-3 (CPP32) by immunoblotting in 58 previously untreated CLL patients. Apoptotic-regulating proteins were not associated with Rai stage, hemoglobin concentration, and lymph node involvement, although higher levels of *bcl*-2 and high *bcl*-2/*bax* ratio were correlated with high peripheral blood lymphocyte count, whereas higher levels of *bak* were weakly associated with loss of allelic heterozigosity at 13q14. Finally, higher levels of antiapoptotic protein Mcl-1 reflected a low response rate to either chlorambucil or fludarabine (155).

Bellosillo et al. (156) used antibodies specific for *bcl*-2, *bax, bcl*-$_x$ and *Mcl*-1 to verify whether the combinations of fludarabine with mafosfamide (the active form of cyclophosphamide) and/or mitoxantrone produced changes in the levels of these apoptosis-regulatory proteins. Although no modifications of *bcl*-2 and *bax* levels were observed, a significant decrease of Mcl-1 protein was obtained when cells were incubated with a combination of three drugs or with different fludarabine associations (fludarabine plus mitoxantrone or fludarabine plus mafosfamide). The timing of the decrease in Mcl-1 protein paralleled the decrease of cell viability (156).

In vitro studies have shown that several cytokines play a role in prolonging survival of B-CLL cells (157–160). Interleukin-4 (IL-4) can inhibit apoptosis of leukemia cells in vitro. However, it is controversial whether IL-4 enhances or reduces drug sensitivity or contributes to acquired drug resistance (157,161). Interleukin-8 (IL-8) is a multifactorial chemokine constitutively expressed by B-CLL cells and released in the serum, which contributes in an autocrine fashion to the cell accumulation characteristic of this disease (158,159). The close correlation between serum levels of IL-8 and intracellular amount of bcl-2, suggests that the antiapoptotic effect of IL-8 can be exerted through a *bcl*-2–dependent pathway (159,162). From a clinical point of view, IL-8 offers an additional tool for predicting the pace of disease in early clinical stages. Given the lack of correlation between serum levels of IL-8 and clinicobiological features of disease activity, a possible independent prognostic role for IL-8 can be conceived (162).

Some reports suggest that there is a constitutive cellular expression and serum release of IL-6 in B-CLL, thus playing a role in the regulation of growth and death of leukemic B cells (163,164). According to a recent published study, production of soluble IL-6 after mitogenic stimulation is high in CLL patients with early disease (164).

CLL B cells express approximately 50 to 130 functional receptors for interleukin-10 (IL-10), and studies of the activity of IL-10 on CLL B-cells have revealed that this cytokine can inhibit leukemia B cell proliferation and induce differentiation but not apoptosis in vitro (165). Using RNA polymerase chain reaction, Sjoberg et al. (166) documented increased levels of IL-10 transcript in patients with progressive disease. More recently, investigators at M. D. Anderson evaluated serum levels of IL-6 and IL-10 in 114 B-cell CLL patients, thus demonstrating that increased levels of such cytokines correlate with advanced disease but are independent prognostic factors for survival (167).

XVI. MOLECULES BELONGING TO THE NERVE GROWTH FACTOR RECEPTOR (NGFr) SUPERFAMILY

The tumor necrosis factor (TNF)/NGF receptor superfamily presently contains 10 different types of I membrane glycoprotein (168). The expression of NGFR p75, TNFR p60, TNFR p8, CD40, and CD95 show a broad tissue distribution, whereas CD27, CD30, 4-IBB, and OX-40 are mainly restricted to cells of the hematopoietic system (168). B-CLL cells are a putative source of alpha-TNF, whose serum levels progressively increase in relation to disease stage (169,170). In addition, circulating levels of alpha-TNF inversely correlated with hemoglobin concentration, thus raising the possibility that such a cytokine may contribute to the pathogenesis of anemia in B-cell CLL (171). Finally, serum levels of alpha-TNF matched those of soluble CD27, another molecule belonging to the NGFr superfamily (171). CD27 is generally expressed on B-CLL cells and released in a soluble form. The correlation between circulating levels of sCD27 and tumor load implies such a molecule as a useful disease marker (172).

CD95 (APO-1/Fas) is a membrane antigen that induces apoptosis when cross-linked by anti-Fas antibody (168). CD95 cellular expression is virtually absent on B-CLL cells; this finding together with high bcl-2 expression is consistent with resistance to apoptosis (173). Nonetheless, about 20% of B-CLL patients have increased levels of soluble CD95 (sCD95) in the serum with no correlation with tumor mass (171). This observation lends support to the idea that increased levels of sCD95 reflect T-cell activation status secondary to neoplasia. As a matter of fact, conditions for production of sCD95 by neoplastic or accessory cells need to be characterized to understand clinicobiological implications, if any, of such a finding (172).

CD40+ leukemic cells have been shown to down-regulate the expression of CD40-ligand (CD154) on the surface of normal and donor-activated CD4+ T-cells, thus resulting in severe immunodeficiency states (69). The extent to which in vitro experiments reproduce what occurs in vivo remains to be proved; meanwhile, therapeutic strategies that target these molecules are being developed (174,175). Finally, expression of CD30 on expanded CD8+ T cells is increased by IL-4 production. Because most CLL cells express CD30-ligand, this interaction may affect cell environment and immune function (176).

Taken together, these results suggest that molecules belonging to NGFr superfamily may play a role in clinical manifestation of disease; however, their prognostic value should be better assessed in future studies.

XVII. CHANGES IN THE NATURAL HISTORY OF CLL

When comparing the more recent CLL cohorts with the older ones, the two most striking differences are a longer survival and a higher proportion of patients initially seen in an early clinical stage in recent series (5,177,178). Studies derived from tumor registries of general population or including patients referred to single institutions have addressed such an issue. Call et al. (36) analyzed the incidence of CLL in Olmsted Country, Minnesota, from 1935 through 1989, thus finding a higher proportion of patients at an early stage of disease among those patients diagnosed in more recent years. A survey carried out by EUROCARE Working Group in Europe between 1985 and 1989 from 39 cancer registries in 17 countries registered significant changes of life expectancy in CLL (178). Compared with the 1978–79 period, the relative 5-year survival improved in 1987–89 period [relative risk (RR) of death for CLL, 0.65] in Europe in general and in Eastern Europe in particular. A trend for a better survival of patients diagnosed in more recent times was confirmed in the study carried out by Rozman et al. (5), who analyzed two cohorts observed at a single institution over a 30-year period. Diehl et al. (6) on the basis of data obtained from National Cancer Data Base (NCDB) analyzed age, gender, race, income, treatment, and overall survival according to the time period of diagnosis (1985–1990 and 1991–1995). In this cohort which reflects a hospital-based patient population from a broad spectrum of hospitals in the United States, the risk of developing CLL increased progressively with age without plateauing. An increasing trend toward no treatment in more recent years was observed. Finally, CLL is a more fatal disease among older patients because of disease itself, not because of comorbid conditions (6).

In conclusion, the natural history of CLL is changing, although the reasons (potential changes of biology of disease, pattern of clinical presentation, treatment, or referral) are unclear.

XVIII. ISSUES IN THE DEVELOPMENT OF NEW PROGNOSTIC FACTORS IN CHRONIC LYMPHOCYTIC LEUKEMIA

Although evaluation of new drugs is supported by an "infrastructure" of rules that permit a rapid evaluation of toxicity (phase I), activity (phase II), and definitive clinical use (phase III), structures in which performing prognostic marker studies are lacking. As far as solid tumors are concerned, a tumor marker utility grading system (TMUGS) has been proposed, in which a semiquantitative scale is used to determine whether a given marker should be incorporated into clinical practice (179). Practical guidelines for establishing prognostic markers to be used in the day-by-day practice have been developed for CLL by the National Cancer Institute–Sponsored Working Group (38). To place tumor markers in their appropriate context, separate recommendations are given for patients included in clinical trials and for patients treated in the general practice. For instance, cytogenetic analyses provide useful prognostic information either at the time of diagnosis or later in evaluating the evolution of disease. However, cytogenetic studies are expensive, time-consuming, and need highly qualified people, so they should be restricted to a research setting (38).

Future investigations of prognostic markers in CLL should be designed on a prospective basis so that clinical usefulness can be determined more rapidly than in the past.

What should be kept in mind is that although one marker can not be definitive, more accurate prognostic information can be obtained incorporating into prognostic models different makers reflecting different clinicobiological aspects of disease. Whether clinicians in the future will substitute biological variables for clinical features is matter of debate.

More likely, biological parameters might be integrated into clinicoprognostic models, thus leading to the formulation of a clinicobiological system for CLL.

REFERENCES

1. G Dighiero, P Travade, S Chevret, C Fenaux, C Chastang, JL Binet. B-cell chronic lymphocytic leukemia: present status and future directions. Blood 78:1901–1914, 1991.
2. IF Kouri, MJ Keating, R Champling. Hematopoietic stem cell transplantation for chronic lymphocytic leukemia. Curr Opin Hematol 5:454–459, 1998.
3. IF Kouri, MI Keating. High-dose chemotherapy for chronic lymphocytic leukemia: Eligibility, timing and benefit? Ann. Oncol 9:131–132, 1998.
4. E. Montserrat. Chronic lymphoproliferative disorders. Curr Opin Oncol 9:34–41, 1997.
5. C Rozman, F Bosch, E Montserrat. Chronic lymphocytic leukemia: A changing natural history? Leukemia 11:775–778, 1997.
6. LF Diehl, LH Karnell, HR Menck. The American College of Surgeons Commission on Cancer and the American Cancer Society. The National Cancer Data Base report on age, gender, treatment and outcomes of patients with chronic lymphocytic leukemia. Cancer 86:2684–2692, 1999.
7. JC Byrd, KR Rai, EA Sansville, MR Grever. Old and new therapies in chronic lymphocytic leukemia: Now is the time for a reassessment of therapeutic goals. Semin, Oncol, 25:65–74, 1998.
8. KR Rai, A Sawitsky, EP Cronkite, A Chanana, R Levy, B Pasternak. Clinical staging of chronic lymphocytic leukemia. Blood 46:219–234, 1975.
9. JL Binet, A Auquier, G Dighiero, C Chastang, H Piguet, J Goasguen, G Vaugier, G Potron, P Colona, F Oberling, M Thomas, G Tchernia, P Boivin, C Lesty, M Duault, M Monconduit, S Belabbes, F Gremy. A new prognostic classification of chronic lymphocytic leukemia derived from a multivariate survival analysis. Cancer 48:198–206, 1981.
10. S Molica. Prognostic value of biological variables in B-cell chronic lymphocytic leukemia. Can we improve upon clinical parameters? Haematologica 82:705–709, 1997.
11. M Hallek, I Kuhn-Hallek, B Emmerich. Prognostic factors in chronic lymphocytic leukemia. Leukemia 11(suppl 2):4–13, 1997.
12. JA Zwiebel, BD Cheson. Chronic lymphocytic leukemia: Staging and prognostic factors. Semin, Oncol, 25:42–59, 1998.
13. F Caligaris Cappio, TJ Hamblin. B-cell chronic lymphocytic leukemia: A bird of different feather. J Clin Oncol 17:399–408, 1999.
14. KR Rai. A critical analysis of staging in CLL. In: RP Gale, KR Rai, eds. Chronic Lymphocytic Leukemia: Recent Progress and Future Directions. New York: Alan R. Liss, 1987, pp, 252–264.
15. International Workshop on CLL. Chronic lymphocytic leukaemia: proposals for a revised prognostic system. Br J Haematol 48:365–367, 1981.
16. B Jaksic, B Vitale. Total tumor mass score (TTM): a new parameter in chronic lymphocytic leukaemia. Br J Haematol 49:405–413, 1981.
17. F Mandelli, G De Rossi, P Mancini, A Alberti, A Cajozzo, F Grignani, P Leoni, V Liso, M Martelli, A Neri, L Resegotti, G Torlontano. Prognosis in chronic lymphocytic leukemia: retrospective multicentric study from the GIMEMA Group. J Clin Oncol 5:398–406, 1987.
18. JS Lee, DO Dixon, HM Kantarjian, MJ Keating, M Talpaz. Prognosis of chronic lymphocytic leukemia: a multivariate regression analysis of 325 untreated patients. Blood 69:929–936, 1987.
19. S Molica, G Vitelli, D Levato, L Levato, A Dattilo, GM Gandolfo. Clinico-biological implications of increased serum levels of interleukin-8 in B-cell chronic lymphocytic leukemia. Haematologica 84:210–213, 1999.

20. J Han, ES Henderson, LJ Emrich, AA Sanberg. Prognostic significance of karyotypic abnormalities in B cell chronic lymphocytic leukemia: An update. Semin Hematol 24:257–263, 1987.

21. S Tura, M Cavo, M Baccarani. Stage 0 chronic lymphocytic leukemia. In: RP Gale, KR Rai, eds. Chronic Lymphocytic Leukemia: Recent Progress and Future Directions. New York: Alan R. Liss, 1987, pp 265–275.

22. DG Oscier, J Stevens, TJ Hamblin, RM Pickering, M Fitchett. Prognostic factors in stage A0 B-cell chronic lymphocytic leukemia. Br J Haematol 76:348–351, 1990.

23. E Montserrat, N Vinolas, JC Reverter, C Rozman. Natural history of chronic lymphocytic leukemia: On the progression and prognosis of early stages. Nouv Rev Fr Hematol 30:359–361, 1988.

24. French Cooperative Group on Chronic Lympocytic Leukemia. Natural history of stage A chronic lymphocytic leukaemia untreated patients. Br J Haematol 76:45–57, 1990.

25. French Cooperative Group on Chronic Lymphocytic Leukemia. Effects of chlorambucil and therapeutic decision in initial forms of chronic lymphocytic leukemia (stage A) results of a randomized clinical trial on 612 patients. Blood 75:1414–1421, 1990.

26. S Molica. Survival and disease progression studies in early chronic lymphocytic leukemia. Blood 78:895–899, 1991.

27. MJ Keating, S Lerner, H Kantarjian, EJ Freireich, S O'Brien. The serum β2-microglobulin level is more powerful than stage in predicting response and survival in chronic lymphocytic leukemia. Blood 86(suppl 1):606a, 1995.

28. M Sarfati, S Chevret, C Chastang, C Biron, P Stryckmans, G Delpesse, JL Binet. Prognostic importance of serum levels of CD23 in chronic lymphocytic leukemia. Blood 88:4259–4264, 1996.

29. M Hallek, I Langnmayer, C Nerl, W Knauf, H Dietzfebinger, D Adorf, M Ostwald, R Busch, I Kuhn-Hallek, E Thiel, B Emmerich. Elevated serum thymidine kinase levels identify a subgroup at high risk of disease progression in early, non-smoldering chronic lymphocytic leukemia. Blood 93:1732–1737, 1999.

30. CLL Trialists' Collaborative Group. Chemotherapeutic options in chronic lymphocytic leukemia: a metanalysis of randomized trials. J Natl Cancer Inst 91:861–868, 1999.

31. M de Lima, S O'Brien, S Lerner, MJ Keating. Chronic lymphocytic leukemia in the young patient. Sem Oncol 25:107–116, 1998.

32. E Montserrat, F Gomis, T Vallespi, A Rios, A Romero, J Soler, A Alcala, M Morey, C Ferran, J Diaz-Mediavilla, A Flores, S Woessner, J Battle, C Gonzales-Aza, M Rovira, JC Reverter, C Rozman. Presenting features and prognosis of chronic lymphocytic leukemia in younger adults. Blood 78:1545–1551, 1991.

33. S Molica, M Brugiatelli, V Callea, F Morabito, D Levato, F Nobile, A Alberti. Comparison of younger versus older B-cell chronic lymphocytic leukemia patients for clinical presentation and prognosis. A retrospective study of 53 cases. Eur J Haematol 52:216–21, 1994.

34. FR Mauro, R Foa, D Giannarelli, I Cordone, S Crescenzi, E Pescarmona, R Sala, R Cerretti, F Mandelli. Clinical characteristics and outcome of young chronic lymphocytic leukemia patients: A single institution study of 204 cases. Blood 94:448–454, 1999.

35. D Catovsky, J Fooks, S Richards. Prognostic factors in chronic lymphocytic leukemia: The importance of age, sex and response to treatment in survival. Br J Haematol 72:141–147, 1989.

36. TG Call, RL Phyliky, P Noel, TM Habermann, CM Beard, WM O'Fallon, LT Kurland. Incidence of chronic lymphocytic leukemia in Olmsted Country, Minnesota, 1935 through 1989, with emphasis on changes in initial stage at diagnosis. Mayo Clinic Proc 69:323–328, 1994.

37. P Kozuch, S O'Brien, H Kantarajian, S Lerner, K-A Do, MJ Keating. The M.D. Anderson

Cancer Center experience in CLL patients aged 70 year and older. VIII International Workshop on CLL, 29–31 October, 1999; Paris. Programme and Abstract Book, p 61.

38. BD Cheson, JM Bennett, M Grever, N Kay, MJ Keating, S O'Brien, KR Rai. National Cancer Institute Sponsored Working Group guidelines for chronic lymphocytic leukemia: Revised guidelines for diagnosis and treatment. Blood 87:4990–4997, 1996.

39. C Rozman, E Montserrat, JM Rodriguez Fernandez, R Ayats, T Vallespi, A Parody, A Rios, D Prados, M Morey, F Gomis, A Alalà, M Gutiérrez, J Maldonado, C Gonzales, M Giralt, L Hernandez-Nieto, A Cabrera, JM Fernandez-Ranana. Bone marrow pattern. The best single prognostic parameter in chronic lymphocytic leukemia: a multivariate analysis of 329 cases. Blood 64:642–648, 1984.

40. GA Pangalis, VA Boussiotis, C Kittas. B-chronic lymphocytic leukemia. Disease progression in 150 untreated stage A and B patients as predicted by bone marrow patterns. Nouv Rev Fr Hematol 30:373–375, 1988.

41. T Han, M Minowa, ML Bloom, N Samadori, AA Sandberg, ES Henderson. Bone marrow infiltration patterns and their prognostic significance in chronic lymphocytic leukemia: Correlation with clinical, immunologic, phenotypic, and cytogenetic data. J Clin Oncol 2:562–570, 1984.

42. B Desablens, JF Claisse, C Piprot-Choffat, MF Gontier. Prognostic value of bone marrow biopsy in chronic lymphocytic leukemia. Nouv Rev Fr Hematol 31:179–182, 1989.

43. FR Mauro, G De Rossi, VL Burgio, R Caruso, D Giannarelli, B Monarca, C Romani, CD Baroni, F Mandelli. Prognostic value of bone marrow histology in chronic lymphocytic leukemia. A study of 335 untreated cases from a single institution. Haematologica 79:334–41, 1994.

44. E Montserrat, N Villamor, JC Reverter, RM Brugues, D Tassies, F Bosch, JL Aguilar, JL Vives-Corrons, M Rozman, C Rozman. Bone marrow assessment in B-cell chronic lymphocytic leukemia: Aspirate or biopsy? A comparative study in 258 patients. Br J Haematol 93: 111–116, 1996.

45. CH Geisler, K Hou-Jensen, OM Jensen, N Tinggaard, M Mork Hansen, NE Hansen, M Holm, B Egeland Christensen, A Drivsholm, J Boye Nielsen, K Thorling, E Andersen, JK Larsen, K Andersen. The bone marrow infiltration pattern in B-cell chronic lymphocytic leukemia is not an important prognostic factor. Danish CLL Study Group. Eur J Haematol 57:292–300, 1996.

46. S Molica, L Tucci, D Levato, C Docimo. Clinical and prognostic evaluation of bone marrow infiltration (biopsy versus aspirate) in early chronic lymphocytic leukemia. A single center study. Haematologica 82:286–290, 1997.

47. FE Lecouvet, B Vande Bergh, L Michaux, PJ Schmitz, J Malghem, J Jamart, BE Maldague, A Ferrant, JL Michaux. Early chronic lymphocytic leukemia: Prognostic value of quantitative bone marrow MR imaging findings and correlation with hematologic variables. Radiology 204:813–818, 1997.

48. JV Melo, D Catovsky, WM Gregory, DAG Galton. The relationship between chronic lymphocytic leukemia and prolymphocytic leukemia. IV. Analysis of survival and prognostic features. Br J Haematol 65:23–29, 1987.

49. LC Peterson, CD Bloomfield, RD Brunning. Relationship of clinical staging and lymphocyte morphology to survival in chronic lymphocytic leukaemia. Br J Haematol 54:563–567, 1980.

50. T Vallespi, E Montserrat, MA Sanz. Chronic lymphocytic leukaemia: prognostic value of lymphocyte morphological subtypes. A multivariate survival anaysis of 146 patients. Br J Haematol 77:478–485, 1991.

51. S Molica, A Alberti. Investigation of nuclear clefts as a prognostic parameter in chronic lymphocytic leukemia. Eur J Haematol 41:62–65, 1988.

52. JM Bennett, D Catovsky, MT Daniel, G Fladrin, DAG Galton, HR Gralnick, C Sultan. The French-Americam-British (FAB) proposal for the classification of chronic (mature) B and T lymphoid leukaemias. J Clin Pathol 42:567–584, 1898.

53. A Criel, G Verhoef, R Vlietinck, C Mecucci, J Billiet, L Michaux, P Meeus, A Louwagie, A Van Orshoven, A Van Hoof, M Boogaerts, Van den Berghe, C Wolf-Peeters. Further characterization of morphologically defined typical and atypical CLL: a clinical, immunophenotypic, cytogenetic and prognostic study on 390 cases. Br J Haematol 97:383–391, 1997.

54. DG Oscier, E Matutes, A Copplestone, RM Pickering, R Chapman, R Gillingham, D Catovsky, TJ Hamblin. Atypical lymphocyte morphology: An adverse prognostic factor for disease progression in stage A CLL independent of trisomy 12. Br J Haematol 98:934–939, 1997.

55. S Molica. Infections in chronic lymphocytic leukemia: Risk factors, and impact on survival, and treatment. Leuk & Lymphoma 13:203–214, 1994.

56. DP Kontoyianis, EJ Anaissie, GP Bodey. Infection in chronic lymphocytic leukemia: A reappraisal. In: BD Cheson, ed. Chronic Lymphocytic Leukemia, Scientific Advances and Clinical Developments. New York: Marcel Dekker, Inc., 1993, pp 399–417.

57. C Rozman, E Montserrat, N Vinolas. Serum Immunoglobulins in B- chronic lymphocytic leukemia. Natural history and prognostic significance. Cancer 61:279–283, 1988.

58. A Orfao, M Gonzales, JR San Miguel, A Rios, MC Canizo, J Hernandez, ML Maricato, AL Borasca. B-cell chronic lymphocytic leukemia: Prognostic value of the immunophenotype and the clinico-hematological features. Am J Hematol 31:26–31, 1989.

59. H Everaus, E Luik, J Lehtmaa. Active and indolent chronic lymphocytic leukemia–immune and hormonal peculiarities. Cancer Immunol Immunother 45:109–114, 1997.

60. ME Heath, BD Cheson. Defective complement activity in chronic lymphocytic leukemia. Am J Hematol 19:63–73, 1985.

61. L Varga, E Czink, Z Miszlai, K Paloczi, A Benyai, G Szegedi, G Fust. Low activity of the classical complement pathway predicts short survival of patients with chronic lymphocytic leukemia. Clin Exp Immunol 99:112–116, 1995.

62. R Foà, D Catovsky, M Brozovic, G Marsh, T Ooyirilangkumaran, M Cherchi, DAG Galton. Clinical staging and immunological findings in chronic lymphocytic leukemia. Cancer 44: 483–487, 1979.

63. TH Totterman, M Carlsson, B Simonsson, M Bengtsson, K Nilsson. T-cell activation and subset patterns are altered in B-CLL and correlate with the stage of disease. Blood 74:786–792, 1989.

64. A Apostopulos, A Symeonidis, N Zoumbvos. Prognostic significance of immune function parameters in patients with chronic lymphocytic leukemia. Eur J Haematol 44:39–44, 1990.

65. M Lotz, E Ranheim, TJ Kipps. Trasforming growth factor beta as endogenous growth inibitor of chronic lymphocytic leukemia B cells. J Exp Med 179:999–1004, 1994.

66. L Lagneaux, A Delforge, D Bron, M Massy, M Bernier, P Stryckmans. Heterogenous response of B lymphocytes to trasforming growth factor-beta in B-cell chronic lymphocytic leukemia: correlation with the expression of TGF-beta receptors. Br J Haematol 97:612–620, 1997.

67. EA Ranheim, MJ Cantwell, TJ Kipps. Expression of CD27 and its ligand, CD70, on chronic lymphocytic leukemia B cells. Blood 85:3556–3565, 1995.

68. K Kato, MJ Cantwell, S Sharma, TJ Kipps. Gene transfer of CD40-ligand induces autologous immune recognition of chronic lymphocytic leukemia B cells. J Clin Invest 101:1133–1141, 1998.

69. MJ Cantwell, T Hua, J Pappas, TJ Kipps. Acquired CD40-ligand deficiency in patients with chronic lymphocytic leukemia. Nature Med 3:984–989, 1997.

70. IS Grewal, RA Flavell. The CD40 ligand. At the center of the immune universe? Immunol Res 16:59–70, 1997.

71. I Cordone, E Matutes, D Catowsky. Monoclonal antibody Ki-67 identifies B and T cells in cycle in chronic lymphocytic leukemia: Correlation with disease activity. Leukemia 6:902–906, 1992.

72. A Del Giglio, S O'Brien, RJ Ford Jr, J Manning, H Saya, M Keating, D Johnston, FD Chamone, AB Deisseroth. Proliferating cell nuclear antigen (PCNA) expression in chronic lymphocytic leukemia (CLL). Leuk Lymph 10:265–271, 1993.

73. A Orfao, J Ciudad, M Gonzales, JF San Miguel, AR Garcia, MC Lopez Berges, F Ramos, MC Del Canizo, M Sanz. Prognostic value of S-phase white blood cell count in B-cell chronic lymphocytic leukemia. Leukemia 20:47–51, 1992.

74. R Vrhovac, A Delmer, R Tang, J Pierre-Marie, R Zittoun, F Ajchenbau-Cymbalista. Prognostic significance of cell cycle inhibitor p27^{kip1} in chronic lymphocytic leukemia. Blood 91: 4694–4700, 1998.

75. F Bosch, A Lopez-Guillermo, E Campo, JM Ribera, E Conde, MA Piris, T Vallespi, S Woesssner, E Montserrat. Mantle cell lymphoma: presenting features, response to therapy, and prognostic factors. Cancer 82:567–575, 1998.

76. C Dascalescu, R Gressin, M Callanan, JL Sotto, D Leroux. t(11;14)(q13;q32): Chronic lymphocytic leukaemia or matle cell leukaemia? Br J Haematol 95:572–573, 1996.

77. V Levy, V Ugo, A Delmer, R Tang, S Ramond, JY Perrot, R Vrhovac, JP Marie, R Zittoun, F Ajchenbaum-Cymbalista. Cyclin D1 overexpression allows the identification of an aggressive subset of leukemic lymphoproliferative disorder. Leukemia 13:1343–1351, 1999.

78. E Montserrat, J Sanchez-Bisono, N Vinolas, JC Reverter, C Rozman. Lymphocyte doubling time in chronic lymphocytic leukaemia: analysis of its prognostic significance. Br J Haematol 62:567–575, 1986.

79. S Molica, A Alberti. Prognostic value of lymphocyte doubling time in chronic lymphocytic leukemia. Cancer 60:2712–2716, 1987.

80. S Molica, JC Reverter, A Alberti, E Montserrat. Timing of diagnosis and lymphocyte accumulation pattern in chronic lymphocytic leukemia: Analysis of their clinical significance. Eur J Haematol 44:277–281, 1990.

81. E Matutes, K Owusu-Ankomah, R Morilla, J Garcia Marco, A Houlihan, TH Que, D Catovsky. The immunological profile of B-cell disorders and proposal of a scoring system for the diagnosis of CLL. Leukemia 8:1640–1645, 1994.

82. EJ Moreau, E Matutes, RP A'Hern, AM Morilla, RM Morilla, KA Owusu-Ankomah, BK Seon, D Catovsky. Improvement of the chronic lymphocytic leukemia scoring system with the monoclonal antibody SN8 (CD79b). Am J Clin Pathol 108:378–382, 1997.

83. AR Newman, B Peterson, FR Davey, C Brabyn, H Collins, VL Brunetto, DB Duggan, RB Weiss, I Royston, FE Millard, AA Miller, CD Bloomfield. Phenotypic markers and bcl-1 gene rearrangements in B-cell chronic lymphocytic leukemia: A Cancer and Leukemia Group B Study. Blood 82:1239–1246, 1993.

84. CH Geisler, JK Larsen, NE Hansen, MM Hansen, BE Christensen, B Lund, H Nielsen, T Plesner, K Thorling, E Andersen, PK Andersen. Prognostic importance of flow cytometric immunophenotyping of 540 consecutive patients with B-cell chronic lymphocytic leukemia. Blood 78:1795–1802, 1991.

85. S Molica, D Levato, A Dattilo, A Mannella. Clinico-prognostic relevance of quantitative immunophenotyping in B-cell chronic lymphocytic leukemia with emphasis on the expression of CD20 antigen and surface immunoglobulins. Eur J Haematol 60:47–52, 1998.

86. A Pinto, V Zagonel, A Carbone, D Serraino, G Marotta, R Volpe, A Colombatti, L Del Vecchio. CD13 expression in B-cell chronic lymphocytic leukemia is associated with the pattern of bone marrow infiltration. Leuk Lymphoma 6:209–218, 1992.

87. D Tassies, E Montserrat, JC Reverter, C Rozman. Myelomonocytic antigens in B-cell chronic lymphocytic leukemia. Leuk Res 19:841–848, 1995.

88. S Molica, A Dattilo, A Alberti. Myelomonocytic associated antigens in B-chronic lymphocytic leukemia: Analysis of clinical significance. Leuk Lymphoma 5:139–144, 1991.

89. C Peiper, RD Leboeuf, CB Highes, FE Prasthofer, MJ Borowitz, C Dewutter-Dambuyant, WS Walker, RA Ashmum, AT Lood. Report on the CD33 cluster Workshop: biochemical

and genetic characterization of gp67. In: W Knapp, ed. New York: Leukocyte Typing IV. Oxford University Press 1989, pp 814–816.

90. W Ikematsu, H Ikematsu, S Okamura, T Otsuka, M Harada, O Niwa. Surface phenotype and Ig heavy chain gene usage in chronic B-cell leukemias: expression of myelomonocytic surface markers in CD5-negative chronic B-cell leukemia. Blood 83:2602–2610, 1994.

91. V Callea, P Morabite, BM Oliva, C Stelitano, D Levato, A Dattilo, F Gangemi, A Iorfida, P Iacopino, F Nobile, S Molica, M Brugiatelli. Surface CD14 positivity in B-cell chronic lymphocytic leukaemia is related to clinical outcome. Br J Haematol 107:347–352, 1999.

92. SP Mulligan, LP Dao, SE Francis, ME Thomas, J Gibson, MF Cole-Sinclair, M Wolf. B-cell chronic lymphocytic leukaemia with CD8 expression: report of 10 cases and immuno-chemical analysis of the CD8 antigen. Br J Haematol 103:157–162, 1998.

93. S Rutella, C Rumi, P Puggioni, T Barberi, A Di Mario, LM Larocca, G Leone. Expression of thrombospondin receptor (CD36) in B-cell chronic lymphocytic leukemia as an indicator of tumor cell dissemination. Haematologica 84:419–424, 1999.

94. S Molica, D Levato, M Dell'Olio, R Matera, M Minervini, A Dattilo, M Carotenuto, M Carotenuto. Cellular expression and serum circulating levels of CD23 in B-cell chronic lymphocytic leukemia. Implications for prognosis. Haematologica 81:428–433, 1996.

95. W Reinisch, M Willheim, M Hilgarth, C Gasche, R Mader, S Szepfasuli, G Steger, R Berger, K Lechner, G Boltz-Nitulescu, JD Schwarzmeier. Soluble CD23 reliably reflects disease activity in B-cell chronic lymphocytic leukemia. J Clin Oncol 12:2146–2152, 1994.

96. WU Knauf, I Langenmayer, B Ehlers, B Mohr, D Adorf, CH Nerl, M Hallek, TH Zwingers, B Emmerich, E Thiel. Serum levels of soluble CD23, but not soluble CD25, predict disease progression in early stage B-cell chronic lymphocytic leukemia. Leuk Lymphoma 27:523–532, 1997.

97. B Desablens, JC Capiod, V Gouilleaux. Are sCD23, sCD25, LDH and beta-2 microglobulin efficient to evaluate prognosis of B-CLL? Br J Haematol 102(suppl 1):194a, 1998.

98. S Molica, D Levato, N Cascavilla, L Levato, P Musto. Clinico-prognostic implications of simultaneous increased serum levels of soluble CD23 and β2-microglobulin in B-cell chronic lymphocytic leukemia. Eur J Haematol 62:117–122, 1999.

99. JM Hernandez, C Mecucci, A Criel, P Meeus, L Michaux, A Van Hoof, G Verhoef, A Louwagie, JM Scheiff, JL Michaux, M Boogarts, H Van den Berghe. Cytogenetic analysis of B cell chronic lymphocytic leukemias classified according to morphological and immunophenotypic (FAB) criteria. Leukemia 9:2140–2146, 1995.

100. G Juliusson, D Oscier, G Gahrton. Cytogenetic findings and survival in B-cell chronic lymphocytic leukemia. Second WCLL compilation of data on 662 patients. Leuk & Lymphoma 5(suppl 1):21–25, 1991.

101. G Juliusson, G Gahrton. Cytogenetics in CLL and related disorders. In: C Rozman, ed. Chronic Lymphocytic Leukaemia and Related Disorders. Vol. 6. London: Bailliere's, 1993, pp 821–848.

102. G Juliusson, DG Oscier, M Fitchett, FM Ross, G Stockdill, MJ Mackie, AC Parker, GL Castoldi, A Cuneo, S Knuutila, E Elonen, G Gahrton. Prognostic subgroups in B-cell chronic lymphocytic leukemia defined by specific chromosomal abnormalities. N Engl J Med 323:720–724, 1990.

103. H Dohner, S Stilgenbauer, K Dohner, M Bentz, P Lichter. Chromosome aberrations in B-cell chronic lymphocytic leukemia: reassessment based on molecular cytogenetic analysis. J Mol Med 77:266–281, 1999.

104. R Bigoni, A Cuneo, MG Roberti, A Bordi, GM Rigolin, N Piva, G Scapoli, R Spanedda, M Negrini, F Bullrich, ML Veronese, CM Croce, G Castoldi. Chromosome aberrations in atypical chronic lymphocytic leukemia: a cytogenetic and interphase cytogenetic study. Leukemia 11:1933–1940, 1997.

105. F Bullrich, M Negrini, CM Croce. Molecular genetics of chronic lymphocytic leukemia.

Hematology 1999. American Society of Hematology Educational Program Book; New Orleans, December 3–7, 1999, pp 255–258.

106. JA Garcia Marco, C Caldas, CM Price, LM Wiedemann, A Ashworth, D Catovsky. Frequent somatic deletion of the 13q12.3 locus encompassing BRCA2 in chronic lymphocytic leukemia. Blood 88:1568–1575, 1996.

107. MM Corcoran, O Rasool, Y Liu, A Iyengar, D Grander, RE Ibbotson, M Merun, X Wu, V Brodyansky, AC Gradiner, G Juliusson, RM Chapman, G Ivanova, M Tiller, G Gahrton, N Yankovsky, E Zabarovsky, DG Oscier, S Einhorn. Detailed molecular delineation of 13q14.3 loss in B-cell chronic lymphocytic leukemia. Blood 91:1382–1390, 1998.

108. DG Oscier, A Thompsett, D Zhu, FK Stevenson. Differential rates of somatic hypermutation in V(H) genes among subsets of chronic lymphocytic leukemia defined by chromosomal abnormalities. Blood 89:4153–4160, 1997.

109. O Starostik, S O'Brien, CY Chung, M Haidar, T Manshouri, H Kantarajian, E Freireich, M Keating, M Albitar. The prognostic significance of 13q14 deletions in chronic lymphocytic leukemia. Leuk Res 23:795–801, 1999.

110. T Stankovic, P Weber, G Stewart, T Bedenham, J Murray, PJ Byrd, PAH Moss, A Malcom, R Taylor. Inactivation of ataxia teleangectasia mutated gene in B-cell chronic lymphocytic leukemia. Lancet 353:26–29, 1999.

111. H Dohner, S Stilgenbauer, MR James, A Benner, T Weilgum, M Bentz. 11q deletions identify a new subset of B-cell chronic lymphocytic leukemia characterized by extensive nodal involvement and inferior prognosis. Blood 89:2616–2522, 1997.

112. A Cuneo, R Bigoni, GL Castoldi. Towards a clinically relevant classification of chronic lymphocytic leukemia and related disorders. Haematologica 83:577–579, 1998.

113. K Offit, DC Louie, NZ Parsa, D Filippa, M Gangi, R Siebert, RS Chaganti. Clinical and morphological features of B-cell small lymphocytic lymphoma with del(6)(q21q23). Blood 83:2611–2618, 1994.

114. J Demeter, F Porzsolt, S Ramisch, D Schmidt, G Messer. Polymorphism of the tumor necrosis factor-alpha and lymphotoxin-alpha genes in chronic lymphocytic leukemia. Br J Haematol 97:107–112, 1997.

115. H Dohner, S Stilgenbauer, A Krober, K Dohner, E Leupolt, M Bentz, AD Ho, A Benner, P Lichter. Chromosome aberrations identify prognostic subgroups of B-cell chronic lymphocytic leukemia. Blood 92(suppl 1):429a, 1998.

116. M Naylor, D Capra. Mutational status of Ig V_H genes provides clinically valuable information in B-cell chronic lymphocytic leukemia. Blood 94:1937–1839, 1999.

117. TJ Hamblin, Z Davis, A Gardiner, DG Oscier, FK Stevenson. Unmutated Ig V_H genes are associated with a more aggressive form of chronic lymphocytic leukemia. Blood 94:1848–1854, 1999.

118. RN Damle, T Wasil, F Fais, F Ghiotto, A Valetto, SL Allen, A Bucbinder, D Budman, K Dittmar, J Kolitz, SM Lichtman, P Schulman, VP Vinciguerra, KR Rai, M Ferrarini, N Chiorazzi. Ig V gene mutation status and CD38 expression as novel prognostic indicators in chronic lymphocytic leukemia. Blood 94:1840–1847, 1999.

119. AA Thompson, JA Talley, HN Do, HL Kagan, L Kunkel, J Berenson, MD Cooper, A Saxon, R Wall. Aberrations of B-cell receptor B29 (CD79b) gene in chronic lymphocytic leukemia. Blood 90:1387–1394, 1997.

120. A Alfarano, S Indraccolo, P Circosta, S Minuzzo, A Vallario, R Zamarchi, A Fregonese, F Calderazzo, A Faldella, M Aragno, C Camaschella, A Amadori, F Caligaris-Cappio. An alternatively spliced form of CD79b gene may account for altered B-cell receptor expression in B-cell chronic lymphocytic leukemia. Blood 93:2327–2335, 1999.

121. P Fenaux, C Preudhomme, JL Lai, I Quiquandon, P Jonveaux, M Vanrumbeke, C Sartiaux, P Morel, MH Loucheaux-Lefevre, F Bauters, R Berger, P Kerkaert. Mutations of p53 gene in B-cell chronic lymphocytic leukemia: A report of 39 cases with cytogenetic analysis. Leukemia 6:246, 1992.

122. H Dohner, K Fischer, M Bentz, K Hansen, A Benner, G Cabot, D Diehl, R Schlenk, J Coy, S Stilgenbauer, M Volkmann, P Galle, A Poustka, W Hunstein, P Lichter. p53 gene deletion predicts poor survival and non-response to therapy with purine analogs in chronic B-cell leukemias. Blood 85:1580–1588, 1995.

123. I Cordone, S Masi, FR Mauro, S Soddu, O Morsilli, T Valentini, ML Vegna, C Guglielmi, F Mancini, S Giuliacci, A Sacchi, F Mandelli, R Foa. p53 expression in B-cell chronic lymphocytic leukemia: A marker of disease progression and poor prognosis. Blood 91:4342–4349, 1998.

124. D Lens, MJS Dyer, J Garcia-Marco, JJC De Schower, RA Hamoudi, D Jones, N Farahat, E Matutes, D Catovsky. p53 abnormalities in CLL are associated with excess of prolymphocytes and poor prognosis. Br J Haematol 99:848–857, 1997.

125. G De Rossi, D Zarcone, FR Mauro, G Cerruti, C Tenca, A Puccetti, F Mandelli, CE Grossi. Adhesion molecule expression on B-cell chronic lymphocytic leukemia cells: Malignant cell phenotypes define distinct disease subsets. Blood 81:2679–2687, 1993.

126. G De Rossi, C Tenca, G Cerruti, D Zarcone, CE Grossi. Adhesion molecule expression on B-cells from acute and chronic lymphoid leukemias. Leuk Lymphoma 16:31–36, 1994.

127. I Christiansen, C Sundstrom, TH Totterman. Elevated serum levels of soluble cell adhesion molecule-1 (sVCAM-1) closely reflect tumour burden in chronic B-lymphocytic leukaemia. Br J Haematol 103:1129–1137, 1998.

128. A Domingo, E Gonzales-Barca, X Castellsague, A Fernandez-Sevilla, A Grafiena, N Crespo, C Ferran. Expression of adhesion molecules in 113 patients with B-cell chronic lymphocytic leukemia: relationship with clinico-prognostic features. Leuk Res 21:67–73, 1997.

129. W Eisterer, W Hilbe, R Stauder, O Bechter, F Frend, J Thaler. An aggressive subtype of B-CLL is characterized by strong CD44 expression and lack of CD11c. Br J Haematol 93:661–669, 1996.

130. S Molica, A Dattilo, A Mannella, D Levato, L Levato. Expression on leukemic cells and serum circulating levels of intercellular adhesion molecule-1 (ICAM-1) in B-cell chronic lymphocytic leukemia. Implications for prognosis. Leuk Res 19:573–580, 1995.

131. G Csanaky, E Matutes, JA Vass, R Morilla, D Catovsky. Adhesion receptors on peripheral blood leukemic B cells. A comparative study on B cell chronic lymphocytic leukemia and related lymphoma/leukemias. Leukemia 11:408–415, 1997.

132. MK Angelopoulou, FN Kontopidou, GA Pangalis. Adhesion molecules in B-chronic lymphoproliferative disorders. Sem Hematol 36:178–197, 1999.

133. S Sembries, H Pahl, S Stilgenbauer, H Dohner, F Schriever. Reduced expression of adhesion molecules and cell signaling receptors by chronic lymphocytic leukemia cells with 11q deletion. Blood 93:624–631, 1999.

134. P Panayiotidis, D Jones, K Ganeshaguru, L Foroni, AV Hoffbrand. Human bone marrow stromal cell prevent apoptosis and support the survival of chronic lymphocytic leukaemia cells in vitro. Br J Haematol 92:97–103, 1996.

135. S Molica, A Dattilo, A Mannella, D Levato. Intercellular adhesion molecules (ICAMs) 2 and 3 are frequently expressed in B cell chronic lymphocytic leukemia. Leukemia 10:907–908, 1996.

136. I Christiansen, C Gidlof, AC Wallgren, B Simonsson, TH Totterman. Serum levels of soluble intercellular adhesion molecule 1 are increased in chronic B-lymphocytic leukemia and correlate with clinical stage and prognostic markers. Blood 84:3010–3016, 1994.

137. S Molica, D Levato, M Dell'Olio, N Cascavilla, R Matera, M Minervini, A Dattilo, M Carotenuto, P Musto. Clinico-prognostic implications of increased levels of soluble CD54 in the serum of B-cell chronic lymphocytic leukemia patients: results of multivariate survival analysis. Haematologica 82:148–151, 1997.

138. G De Rossi, P Marroni, M Paganuzzi, FR Mauro, C Tenca, D Zarcone, A Velardi, S Molica, CE Grossi. Increased serum levels of soluble CD44 standard, but not of variant isoforms v5 and v6, in B cell chronic lymphocytic leukemia. Leukemia 11:134–141, 1997.

139. S Molica, G Vitelli, D Giannarelli, GM Gandolfo, V Liso. Circulating levels of serum CD44 (sCD44) is an independent prognostic factor predicting the risk of disease-progression in early B-cell chronic lymphocytic leukemia. Blood 94(suppl 1):538a, 1999.

140. AR Kini, LC Peterson, NE Kay. Evidence for abnormal angiogenesis in the bone marrow of patients with B-cell chronic lymphocytic leukemia. Blood 92(suppl 1):717a, 1998.

141. T Menzel, Z Rahman, E Calleja, K White, EL Wilson, R Wieder, J Gabrilove. Elevated intracellular level of basis fibroblastic growth factor correlates with stage of chronic lympho-cytic leukemia and is associated with resistance to fludarabine. Blood 87:1056–1063, 1996.

142. A Konig, T Menzel, S Lynen, L Wrazel, A Rosen, A Al-kabit, E Raveche, JL Gabrilove. Basic fibroblastic growth factor (b-FGF) upregulates the expression of bcl-2 in B-cell chronic lymphocytic leukemia cell lines resulting in delaying apoptosis. Leukemia 11:258–265, 1997.

143. A Aguayo, H Kantarajia, T Manshouri, C Gidel, B Barlogie, C Koller, S O'Brien, M Albitar, M Keating. Low levels of vascular endothelial growth factor (VEGF) in cells of patients with chronic lymphoid leukemia (CLL) correlate with survival, particularly in patients with low beta-2 microglobulin levels. Blood 92(suppl 1):226a, 1998.

144. S Molica, G Vitelli, D Levato, GM Gandolfo, V Liso. Increased serum levels of vascular endothelial growth factor predict risk of progression in early B-cell chronic lymphocytic leukaemia. Br J Haematol 107:605–610, 1999.

145. HJ Chen, AT Treweeke, KJ Till, JC Cawley, CH Toh. Vascular endothelial growth factor (VEGF) is produced by CLL cells and stimulates angiogenesis within lymphoreticular tissues. VIII International Workshop on CLL, 29–31 October 1999, Paris. Programme and Abstract Book, pp 43.

146. J Jurlander, N Abrahamsen, P Norgaard, C Geisler, H Skovgaard Poulsen. The spontaneous initiation of aptosis in B-cell chronic lymphocytic leukemia cells cultured in vitro is related to temporary upregulation of p21^{CIP1} and p53 gene expression. Blood 92(suppl 1):266b, 1998.

147. M Hanada, D Delia, A Aiello, E Stadtmauer, JC Reed. Bcl-2 gene hypomethylation and high-level expression in B-cell chronic lymphocytic leukemia. Blood 82:1820–1828, 1993.

148. MY Mapara, K Bommert, R Bargou. Prognostic significance of bcl-2 expression in chronic lymphocytic leukemia. Blood 90(suppl 1):91a, 1997.

149. LE Robertson, K Plunkett, K McConnell, MJ Keating, TJ McDonnell. Bcl-2 expression in chronic lymphocytic leukemia and its correlation with the induction of apoptosis and clinical outcome. Leukemia 10:456–459, 1996.

150. S Molica, A Dattilo, G Crispino, D Levato, L Levato. Increased bcl-2/bax ratio in B-cell chronic lymphocytic leukemia is associated with a progressive pattern of disease. Haemato-logica 83:1122–1124, 1998.

151. D Gottardi, AM De Leo, A Alfarano, A Stacchini, P Circosta, MG Gregoretti, MG Bergui, M Aragno, F Caligaris-Cappio. Fludarabine ability to down-regulate bcl-2 gene product in CD5+ leukaemic B-cells: in vitro/in vivo correlations. Br J Haematol 99:147–157, 1997.

152. M Aguilar-Santelises, ME Rottenberg, N Lewin, H Mellstedt, M Jondal. Bcl-2, Bax and p53 expression in B-CLL in relation to in vitro survival and clinical progression. Int J Cancer (Pred Oncol) 69:114–119, 1996.

153. C Pepper, P Bentley, T Hoy. Regulation of clinical chemoresistance by bcl-2 and bax onco-proteins in B-cell chronic lymphocytic leukaemia. Br J Haematol 95:513–517, 1996.

154. C Pepper, A Thomas, T Hoy, P Bentley. Chlorambucil resistance in B-cell chronic lympho-cytic leukaemia is mediated through failed bax induction and selection of high bcl-2-express-ing subclones. Br J Haematol 104:581–588, 1999.

155. S Kitada, J Andersen, S Akar, JM Zapata, S Takayama, S Krajewski, HG Wang, F Bullrich, CM Croce, KR Rai, J Hines, JC Reed. Expression of apoptosis-regulating proteins in chronic lymphocytic leukemia: Correlations with in vitro and in vivo chemoresponses. Blood 91: 3379–3389, 1998.

156. B Bellosillo, N Villamor, D Colomer, G Pons, E Montserrat, J Gil. In vitro evaluation of

fludarabine in combination with cyclophosphamide and/or mitoxantrone in B-cell chronic lymphocytic leukemia. Blood 94:2836–2843, 1999.

157. M Dancescu, M Rubio-Tujillo, G Biron, D Bron, G Delpesse, M Sarfati. Interleukin-4 protects chronic lymphocytic leukemia B cell from death by apoptosis and upregulates bcl-2 expression. J Exp Med 176:1319–1324, 1992.

158. P Francia Di Celle, A Carbone, D Marhis, D Zhou, S Sozzani, S Zupo, M Pini, A Mantovani, R Foa. Cytokine gene expression in B-cell chronic lymphocytic leukemia: Evidence of constitutive interleukin-8 (IL-8) mRNA expression and secretion of biologically active IL-8 protein. Blood 84:220–228, 1994.

159. P Francia Di Celle, S Mariani, L Riera, A Stacchini, G Reato, R Foa. Interleukin-8 induces the accumulation of B-cell chronic lymphocytic leukemia cells by prolonging survival in an autocrine fashion. Blood 87:4382–4389, 1996.

160. P Panayiotidis, K Ganeshaguru, SAB Jabbar, AV Hoffbrand. Interleukin-4 inhibits apoptotic cell death and loss of bcl-2 protein in B-cell chronic lymphocytic leukemia in vitro. Br J Haematol 83:439–446, 1993.

161. OS Frankfurt, JJ Byrnes, L Villa. Protection from apoptotic cell death by interleukin-4 is increased in previously treated chronic lymphocytic leukemia patients. Leuk Res 21:9–16, 1997.

162. S Molica, G Vitelli, D Levato, L Levato, A Dattilo, GM Gandolfo. Clinico-biological implications of increased serum levels of interleukin-8 in B-cell chronic lymphocytic leukemia. Haematologica 84:208–211, 1999.

163. Y Denizot, P Fixe, E Liozon, C Brigaudeau, V Praloran. Serum IL-6 concentrations in lymphomas. Br J Haematol 90:731–733, 1995.

164. J Hulkkonen, J Vilpo, L Vilpo, M Hurme. Diminished production of interleukin-6 in chronic lymphocytic leukaemia (B-CLL) cells from patients at advanced stages of disease. Br J Haematol 100:478–483, 1998.

165. J Jurlander, CF Lai, J Tan, CC Chou, CH Geisler, J Schriber, LE Blumenson, SK Narula, H Bauman, MA Caligiuri. Characterization of interleukin-10 receptor on B-cell chronic lymphocytic leukemia cells. Blood 89:4146–4152, 1997.

166. J Sjoberg, M Aguilar-Santelises, AM Sjogren, EK Pisa, A Ljungdahl, M Bjoorkholm, M Jondal, H Mellestedt, P Pisa. Interleukin-10 mRNA expression in B-cell chronic lymphocytic leukaemia inversely correlates with progression of disease. Br J Haematol 92:393–400, 1996.

167. L Fayad, MJ Keating, S O'Brien, M Talpaz, R Kurzrock. High serum interleukin-6 and serum interleukin-10 levels correlate with poor survival in chronic lymphocytic leukemia patients. J Clin Oncol 18(suppl 1):24a, 1999.

168. HJ Guss, SK Dower. Tumor necrosis factor ligand superfamily: Involvement in the pathology of malignant lymphomas. Blood 85:3378–3404, 1995.

169. R Foa, M Massaia, S Cardona, A Gillio Tos, A Bianchi, C Attisano, A Guarini, P Francia di Celle, MT Fierro. Production of tumor necrosis factor-alpha (TNF) by B-cell chronic lymphocytic leukemia cells: A possible regulatory role of TNF in the progression of the disease. Blood 76:393–400, 1990.

170. F Adami, A Guarini, M Pini, F Siviero, R Sancetta, M Massaia, L Trentin, R Foa, G Semenzato. Serum levels of tumour necrosis factor-alpha in patients with B-cell chronic lymphocytic leukaemia. Eur J Cancer 30A:1259–1263, 1994.

171. S Molica, G Vitelli, D Levato, G Crispino, M Dell'Olio, A Dattilo, R Matera, GM Gandolfo, P Musto. CD27 in B-cell chronic lymphocytic leukemia. Cellular expression, serum release and correlation with other soluble molecules belonging to nerve growth factor receptors (NGFr) superfamily. Haematologica 83:398–402, 1998.

172. MHJ van Oers, ST Pals, LM Evers, CE van der Schoot, G Koopman, JMG Bonfrer, RQ Hintzen, AEG Kr von dem Borne, RAW van Lier. Expression and release of CD27 in human B-cell malignancies. Blood 82:3430–3436, 1993.

173. S Molica, A Dattilo, G Crispino, D Levato, L Levato. Increased bcl-2/bax ratio in B-cell chronic lymphocytic leukemia is associated with a progressive pattern of disease. Haematologica 82:1122–1124, 1998.
174. TJ Kipps. Chronic lymphocytic leukemia. Curr Opin Hematol 5:244–253, 1998.
175. N Kalil, BD Cheson. Chronic lymphocytic leukemia. Oncologist 4:352–369, 1999.
176. D de Totero, G Reato, FR Mauro, A Cignetti, S Ferrini, A Guarini, M Gobbi, CE Grossi, R Foa. L-4 production and increased CD30 expression by unique CD8+ T-cell subset in B-cell chronic lymphocytic leukaemia. Br J Haematol 104:589–599, 1999.
177. S Molica, D Levato, A Dattilo. Natural history of early chronic lymphocytic leukemia. A single institution study with emphasis on the impact of disease progression on overall survival. Haematologica 84:1094–1099, 1999.
178. PM Carli, JW Coebergh, A Verdecchia. Variation in survival of adult patients with haematological malignancies in Europe since 1978. EUROCARE Working Group. Eur J Cancer 34 (14S):2253–2263, 1998.
179. DF Hayes. Designing tumor marker studies: will the results provide clinically useful information? Thirty-fifth Annual Meeting American Society of Clinical Oncology, May 15–18, 1999; Atlanta. Educational Book, pp 81–87.

13

Initial Approach to the Patient with Chronic Lymphocytic Leukemia

BRUCE D. CHESON

National Cancer Institute, National Institutes of Health, Bethesda, Maryland

Chronic lymphocytic leukemia (CLL) is characterized by a highly variable clinical course. Many patients may survive for decades without requiring treatment, whereas others die from disease-related complications within a few months of diagnosis, despite appropriate therapy. A number of prognostic factors are used to assign patients to a risk group that predicts outcome and, therefore, may be used to direct therapy (1–4). Patients with low-risk CLL (1) (Rai stage 0) often do not require therapy for many years after diagnosis and may eventually die of apparently unrelated causes. Many patients with intermediate-risk disease (Rai stages I and II) may also remain stable for years before requiring treatment. However, most patients with high-risk CLL (stages III and IV) need therapy at diagnosis. Therefore, the issues differ among these groups: when to initiate treatment is the most important consideration for patients with early-stage disease, whereas selecting the best therapy is more important for patients with advanced-stage CLL.

I. INITIAL APPROACH TO THE PATIENT WITH CLL

Currently available therapies do not cure patients with CLL, yet they may be associated with significant toxicities. As a result, the appropriate time to initiate therapy becomes an important decision, especially in patients with low-risk disease. Several studies have demonstrated that early intervention does not prolong the survival of patients with early stage CLL (5–9). The French Cooperative Group on CLL conducted two sequential studies, including 1535 previously untreated patients (5,8). In the first of these, patients were randomly assigned to treatment with daily oral chlorambucil (0.1 mg/kg/day) until disease progression or to observation. The response rate in the treated group was 86%, including

45% complete remissions (CRs). In the second trial, 926 patients received either intermittent chlorambucil (0.3 mg/kg/day for 5 days every month) plus prednisone (40 mg/m^2/day for 5 days every month) for 3 years or no initial treatment. The response to therapy in the treated group was 69% with 28% CRs.

Chlorambucil slowed progression to stages B and C in both trials, yet there was no survival advantage from early intervention in either study. In the first trial, after follow-up of more than 11 years, 49% of patients had still not progressed; however, 32% of the untreated patients and 27% of the initially treated patients (not including 22 patients with a fatal second malignancy) died of causes related to their disease. In the second study, 20% of the initially untreated patients died of causes assumed unrelated to CLL compared with 32% of the initially treated cases. Disease progression and infections, followed by second malignancies, mostly epithelial tumors, were the most frequent CLL-related causes of death in the treated group in both trials. Although there was an apparent increase in second malignancies in the treated group from the earlier trial, this finding was not apparent in the subsequent study. One possible explanation for this discrepancy is the difference in drug administration schedules (daily vs intermittent).

In a smaller study, Cancer and Leukemia Group B (CALGB), investigators (6) randomly assigned 51 patients to intermittent chlorambucil once a month or to no initial treatment. At 5 years from randomization, the proportion of patients exhibiting active disease was 70% in the untreated group and 55% in the treated group; however, there was no significant difference in survival between the two groups.

The CLL Trialists' Collaborative Group (9) attempted to conduct a meta-analysis of the results of all "properly randomized" trials beginning before the end of 1990. The database looking at the question of immediate versus deferred therapy included 2048 patients from six studies; all of the treatment arms contained chlorambucil (CLB) with or without steroids. The death rate was higher in those patients assigned to immediate therapy, but the difference was not significant. There was also a nonsignificant difference (3%) in survival at 10 years favoring deferred therapy. Because these were patients with early stage disease, more than half of the deaths were not clearly related to CLL.

On the basis of these observations, the general recommendation is that therapy should not be initiated in patients with early-stage CLL without specific indications, which include disease-related symptoms (e.g., fevers, chills, weight loss, pronounced fatigue), increasing bone marrow failure with anemia and/or thrombocytopenia, autoimmune anemia or thrombocytopenia, massive or progressive hepatosplenomegaly or lymphadenopathy, or recurrent infections (10). An elevated lymphocyte count alone is not sufficient to prompt therapy; however, a lymphocyte doubling time of <6 months may support the decision to treat (11,12).

II. SINGLE-AGENT CHEMOTHERAPY

Once the decision has been made that therapy is indicated, a limited number of effective treatment options are available. The most active classes of chemotherapy drugs include alkylating agents, such as CLB and cyclophosphamide, and the nucleoside analogs fludarabine, 2-chlorodeoxyadenosine (CdA) and 2′-deoxycoformycin (pentostatin; DCF) (13–15). CLB has been the traditional standard agent for several decades. It is available in tablet form, and its absorption by the gastrointestinal tract is almost complete. A more commonly used and less myelosuppressive schedule is 15 to 30 mg/m^2 every 2 weeks. Regimens of 20 to 40 mg/m^2 every 4 weeks or a daily schedule of 4 to 8 mg/m^2 for 4 to

8 weeks are also used. Responses are attained in approximately 30% to 70% of previously untreated patients, although few of these are complete using current response criteria (7,16,17). There is no demonstrated benefit from maintenance therapy after maximal response (18).

The activity of cyclophosphamide appears to be similar to CLB, but it is generally used only when CLB is poorly tolerated and in combination regimens.

Corticosteroids are less active than alkylating agents in CLL and should be reserved for patients with autoimmune complications because of the risks of bacterial, viral and fungal infections, diabetes, and osteoporosis.

III. PURINE ANALOGS

In the early 1980s, the purine analogs became available for clinical trials in CLL and related lymphoid malignancies. On the basis of their impressive activity, they have revolutionized our approach to the treatment of patients with CLL and other indolent lymphoid malignancies.

A large body of data now support fludarabine (2-fluoro-ara-AMP) as the most active agent for the treatment of CLL (Table 1).

The currently recommended schedule of administration of fludarabine is as an intravenous bolus of 25 mg/m^2 daily for 5 consecutive days once a month. Patients failing to respond to two to three courses should be considered for an alternate treatment. Patients who achieve a complete remission (CR) probably do not warrant additional courses of therapy. For those patients with a PR, therapy may be continued to best response plus two additional courses, not exceeding a year of therapy because of concerns of cumulative myelotoxicity. Other schedules have not been as active (25–27). The oral bioavailability of fludarabine is 50% to 60%, and an oral formulation is in clinical trials (28).

Fludarabine induces complete remissions in about 30% of previously untreated patients, with an overall response rate greater than 70% (Table 1) (17,20,21,29,30). Keating et al. (19) reported the results of long-term follow-up of 174 patients treated with fludara-

Table 1 Purine Analogs for Previously Untreated CLL

	Patients	Response rate (%)	
		CR	RR
Fludarabine			
Keating (19)	174	29	78
French Cooperative Group (20)	52	23	71
(21)	225	41	73
Rai (17)	170	20	63
CdA			
Delannoy (22)	19	47	74
Saven (23)	20	10	85
Robak (24)	194	45	83
DCF			
Dillman (15)	39 (26)[a]	3	26

[a] Number in parenthesis is previously untreated response rate for all patients
RR = Response rate.

bine alone ($n = 71$) or with prednisone ($n = 103$) as their initial therapy. The median age was 61 years, and 66 were in Rai stages III or IV. Only 9% had B symptoms, and most had good performance status: PS 0 in 93, PS 1 in 75, and PS 2 in 6. All patients were projected to receive six cycles of therapy, but the range of cycles administered ranged from 2 to 11. The overall response rate was 78%, including 29% CR, 32% nodular PR, and 17% PR, with a median survival of 63 months. The complete remission rate for fludarabine was 38% compared with 23% for fludarabine and prednisone, but the survival for the two regimens was the same. Additional patients experienced a tumor response, although not adequate to be classified as a PR. The median time to progression was 31 months, 37 months for the CRs, and 31 months for the nPRs. Factors predicting survival included patent age, Rai stage, beta$_2$-M, BUN, hemoglobin. Nine patients died during remission induction, six of infection, one of progressive CLL, one from cardiac failure, and one from a stroke. Five patients died while in remission of pulmonary infection (2), cardiac failure, stroke, liver cancer, and Hodgkin's disease. Those who achieve an immunophenotypic and molecular complete remission appear to experience a longer survival than those with only a clinical and hematological remission (32).

Fludarabine has been compared directly with alkylating agent-based regimens in several phase III trials (Table 2) (17,20,21).

In the North American Intergroup study conducted by CALGB, Southwest Oncology Group (SWOG), Eastern Cooperative Oncology Group (ECOG), and the National Cancer Institute of Canada Clinical Trials Group (NCIC-CTG) (17), 544 untreated patients with advanced stage and active disease were randomly assigned to either fludarabine using the standard schedule, chlorambucil (40 mg/m^2 single dose), or a combination of the two agents (fludarabine 20 mg/m^2 daily for 5 days; chlorambucil 20 mg/m^2 day 1). In each of the arms, chemotherapy was administered every 4 weeks for up to 12 months. Patients who had one of the single agents fail were crossed over to receive the alternate drug. The 166 patients in the fludarabine group had an overall response rate of 64%, including 20% complete remissions, which was significantly higher than with CLB (39% responses, 5% complete remissions; $P < 0.0001$). The differences in response rates were apparent for both the intermediate and high-risk groups. The duration of response with fludarabine was 28 months compared with 19 months with CLB ($P = 0.004$); the median progression-

Table 2 Randomized Trials of Fludarabine vs. Alkylating Agents in Untreated CLL

Investigator		Patients	CR	RR	RD	OS
Leporrier (33)	F	341	41	73	31 mo	74 mo
	CAP	240	14	60	28 mo	70 mo
	ChOP	357	30	73	28 mo	68 mo
Rai (34)	F	170	20	63	25 mo	66 mo
	Clb	181	4	37	14 mo	56 mo
	F/C	123	20	61	NR	55 mo
French (20)	F	52	23	71	NR	NR
	CAP	48	17	60	208 d	1580 d

F = fludarabine; Clb = chlorambucil; CAP = cyclophosphamide, doxorubicin, prednisone; ChOP = cyclophosphamide, doxorubicin, vincristine, prednisone; NR = not reported; RD = response duration; OS = overall survival; mo = months; d = days.

free survival was 20 months and 14 months for CLB ($P < 0.0003$), respectively. However, there was no apparent prolongation of survival (66 months for fludarabine vs 56 months for CLB), related in part to the crossover design of the study. The combination arm was prematurely closed, because it was more toxic than the single agents with no likelihood of being more effective than fludarabine alone.

A European collaborative group randomly assigned 196 patients with Binet stage A ($n = 2$), stage B ($n = 104$) or C ($n = 89$) to either fludarabine or one of two anthracycline-based regimens: cyclophosphamide doxorubicin, prednisone (CAP) or an attenuated cyclophosphamide, doxorubicin, vincristine, prednisone (CHOP) (20). A higher response rate (71% vs 60%) was attained with fludarabine in the untreated patients, although the difference was not significant. The advantage for fludarabine was significant for remission duration (median not reached for fludarabine vs 208 days with CAP), with a trend toward a survival advantage (median not reached vs 1580 days; $P = 0.087$).

In a subsequent trial by the International Working Group on CLL (IWCLL) (33), 651 stage B and 287 stage C patients were randomly assigned to fludarabine, CAP, or ChOP. The response rate with ChOP was 73%, 73% for fludarabine, and 59% for CAP, with clinical and hematological response rates of 30%, 41%, and 15%. Bone marrows were, unfortunately, not examined as part of the response definition. The median survival time was 81 months for stage B, 60 months for stage C, and 68 (ChOP), 70 (CAL), and 74 (fludarabine) Although fludarabine induced more myelosuppression, there was less nausea, vomiting, and hair loss. More patients on fludarabine became Coombs' positive, but the frequency of hemolysis was the same among the arms. The impression of the investigators was that fludarabine was the best tolerated of the regimens.

These results in aggregate establish fludarabine as the preferred initial treatment for most patients with CLL. The drug induces higher response rates with more CRs than alkylating agent or anthracycline-containing regimens, and the responses are more durable. However, CLB may be a reasonable first-line treatment option for patients who are elderly or those have a reduced performance status or an active infection. Another alternative is a 3-day schedule of fludarabine, which appears to be almost as active but with fewer associated toxicities (27).

The major toxicities associated with fludarabine at the currently used schedules are moderate myelosuppression and severe immunosuppression, with occasional neurotoxicity, particularly at higher than recommended doses (35–37). Lymphocyte counts decrease within weeks, particularly CD4 cells, which do not return to normal for a year or longer after treatment has been discontinued (30,36). Fludarabine is not significantly more myelotoxic than alkylating agent regimens but has been associated with increased opportunistic infections (17,20). Prophylactic antimicrobial therapy is not routinely recommended unless patients have had a history of infections (36,38). Similarly, the use of intravenous immunoglobulins should be reserved for patients with a documented history of recurrent bacterial infections because of the toxicity and expense of this treatment and lack of documented efficacy in the general CLL population (39).

Despite the prolonged immunosuppression, there is no apparent increase in the risk of secondary malignancies above what is expected in patients with CLL (40).

Tumor lysis syndrome is a rare complication of treatment of CLL with alkylating agents, radiation, combination chemotherapy, or fludarabine (41–46). Unfortunately, whereas prophylactic measures such as hydration or allopurinol are recommended, especially for patients with high lymphocyte counts or bulky disease, tumor lysis is not always preventable, and it may be fatal.

Table 3 Alkylator-based Combination Chemotherapy in Previously Untreated CLL

Regimen	Patients	CR(%)	PR(%)	Median survival (mo)
COP (57)	23	52	26	36
CVP (50)	27	6	27	22
COP (51)	62	23	59	47
COP (53)	34	6	32	22
M-2 (58)	37	30	51	47
CHOP (53)	36	19	64	62
CHOP (7)	14	14	36	60% 36 mo
CHOP (52)	77	56	16	64
POACH (55)	34	21	35	58
CMP (59)	48	13	42	33
CAP (56)	47	43	23	65
Epi/CLB (60)	7	14	57	NR
CAP (20)	48	17	43	17

CVP/COP = cyclophosphamide, vincristine, prednisone; M-2, melphalan; BCNU = cyclophosphamide, vincristine, prednisone; CHOP = CVP plus adriamycin; CAP = cyclophosphamide, doxorubicin, prednisone; POACH = prednisone, vincristine, cytarabine, cyclophosphamide, doxorubicin; CMP = cyclophosphamide, melphalan, prednisone.

Approximately 55% to 85% of patients who are treated with CdA as their initial therapy respond to this agent, but with only 10% to 15% complete remissions and with a duration of response that appears to be shorter than reported for fludarabine (Table 1) (23,24,47). Data with pentostatin as initial therapy are insufficient to assess its level of activity (Table 1) (15). Unfortunately, differences in response criteria make it difficult to compare these studies with each other and with the fludarabine trials.

The few other drugs studied as initial treatment have had too few patients evaluated for an adequate assessment or demonstrated limited activity (48,49).

IV. COMBINATION REGIMENS

Combination chemotherapy regimens based on alkylating agents are not clearly superior to single-agent therapy for CLL (Tables 2 and 3) (7,20,50–56). The most commonly used multiagent regimens include CLB plus prednisone or CVP. A wide range of responses have been reported with CP and CVP, varying with patient selection and definitions of response. Nevertheless, few of these responses are CRs, and the median survival is shorter than 2 years (Table 3) (7,16,50–52,57).

In the CLL Trialists' meta-analysis (9), the addition of steroids to CLB did not influence patient survival, but the number of patients was too small for an adequate analysis. The French Cooperative Group randomly assigned 151 patients with Binet stage B CLL to indefinite daily oral CLB and 140 to COP. There was no difference in response rate, reduction in clinical stage, or overall survival (61).

More aggressive regimens that include multiple alkylating agents or anthracyclines have also failed to show an advantage over less-intensive programs (55,56,58,59). One randomized trial suggested a survival advantage for an attenuated CHOP regimen (including doxorubicin at 25 mg/m^2 every 4 weeks) over COP in a small number of patients with stage C disease (53). Moreover, data from the same investigators suggest an advantage for CHOP over CAP (21). However, several other randomized trials and a meta-analysis have failed to confirm superiority for anthracycline-containing regimens (7,9,52,54). The CLL Trialists' meta-analysis included 10 trials, including 2035 (2022 evaluable) patients who were randomly assigned to either CLB or a combination regimen, 5 of which included CHOP. They were unable to detect a difference in 5-year survival.

In an attempt to improve on the activity of single-agent fludarabine, several investigators have combined the nucleoside with a variety of other agents. The addition of prednisone to fludarabine does not increase the response rate but is associated with more frequent opportunistic infections (30,38,62). Therefore, this combination should be reserved for patients who need steroids for other reasons, such as autoimmune phenomena, and concurrent trimethoprim-sulfamethoxazole or a suitable replacement for antimicrobial coverage, particularly for *Pneumocystis carinii*, should be delivered concurrently. Combinations of fludarabine with chlorambucil, anthracyclines, or related compounds, cytarabine, and alpha-interferon are not clearly better than fludarabine alone (17,63–70). O'Brien et al. have evaluated the combination of fludarabine cyclophosphamide in previously treated and untreated patients (71). Fludarabine was administered at a dose of 30 mg/m^2 daily for 3 days with cyclophosphamide at doses from 300 to 500 mg/m^2/day for 3 days. The activity was not clearly better than single-agent fludarabine when used as initial treatment. Flinn and coworkers (72) combined fludarabine at a dose of 20 mg/m^2 for 5 days, with cyclophosphamide at a dose of 600 mg/m^2 on day 1, with G-CSF support. The response rate in their 17 patients with CLL was 100%, including 47% complete remissions. Whether the differences in doses and schedules explain the different results is not clear. Nevertheless, these preliminary encouraging data have led to phase III studies.

Results of cladribine combined with prednisone or chlorambucil are not clearly better than cladribine alone but with significant myelosuppression (24,73). DCF has been combined with alkylating agents and steroids with high response rates but with considerable myelotoxicity and a high rate of opportunistic infections (74).

The limited experience with CAMPATH in untreated patients suggests a high level of activity, and this antibody may have a potential role as part of an initial approach (75). Rituximab has limited activity in relapsed and refractory CLL (76–78), but there are currently no data on the use of this antibody in previously untreated patients with this disease. Nevertheless, data suggest synergy between fludarabine and this antibody, and studies have been conducted to explore sequential and concurrent schedules of administration of the two agents (79). Moreover, a number of studies are underway to improve the activity of this antibody through modification of the dose or schedule or by attempting to enhance CD20 expression on the CLL cells (80–82).

V. SUMMARY

Over the past decade, there has been a change in our approach to the treatment of patients with CLL. Fludarabine has become the preferred initial therapy by many practicing hematologists and oncologists. Nevertheless, patients are still not cured, and it is not clear that survival has been improved by this agent. As a consequence, newer strategies need to be developed and rapidly made available for patients as part of their initial therapy. With newer and more active agents available, we need to revisit the question of early intervention and consider a fludarabine versus observation study for patients with indolent disease. For those patients who clearly require treatment, new approaches need to be actively

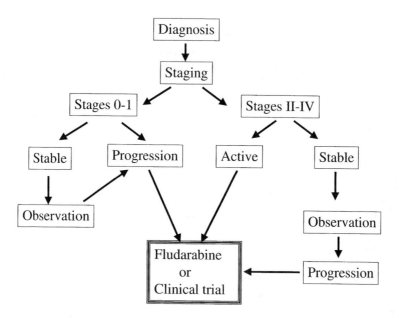

Figure 1 Recommended algorithm for the initial treatment of patients with CLL. Once the diagnosis has been confirmed and adequate staging conducted, therapy is initiated when indicated. For patients with limited, indolent disease, careful observation is usually recommended. For those with advanced stage, active disease, fludarabine is recommended as the initial therapeutic agent. Other options for these patients include high-quality clinical research studies.

developed, including combinations of fludarabine with other agents, such as rituximab or CAMPATH, new chemotherapy drugs, gene therapy, and other targeted therapies. It will become increasingly important to incorporate correlative laboratory studies into the design of the clinical trials to better understand how these approaches work or why they fail. By focusing our resources on high-quality clinical research, we may soon prolong the survival of these patients and eventually achieve the goal of curing CLL.

Suggested treatment algorithm for previously untreated patients with CLL (Fig. 1).

REFERENCES

1. KR Rai. A critical analysis of staging in CLL. In: RP Gale, KR Rai, eds. Chronic Lymphocytic Leukemia. Recent Progress and Future Direction. New York: Alan R. Liss, 1987, p 253.
2. J Zwiebel, BD Cheson. Prognostic factors in chronic lymphocytic leukemia. Semin Oncol 25: 42, 1998.
3. T Hamblin, Z Davis, A Gardiner, DG Oscier, FK Stevenson. Unmutated Ig Vh genes are associated with a more aggressive form of chronic lymphocytic leukemia. Blood 94:1848–1854, 1999.
4. RN Damle, T Wasil, F Fais, F Ghiotto, A Valetto, SL Allen, A Buchbinder, D Budman, K Dittmar, J Kolitz, SM Lichtman, P Schulman, VP Vinciguerra, KR Rai, M Ferrarini, N Chiorazzi. Ig V gene mutation status and CD38 expression as novel prognostic indicators in chronic lymphocytic leukemia. Blood 94:1840, 1999.
5. French Cooperative Group on Chronic Lymphocytic Leukemia F. Effects of chlorambucil and therapeutic decision in initial forms of chronic lymphocytic leukemia (stage A): results of a randomized trial on 612 patients. Blood 75:1414, 1990.

6. C Shustik, R Mick, R Silver, A Sawitsky, K Rai, L Shapiro. Treatment of early chronic lymphocytic leukemia: intermittent chlorambucil versus observation. Hematol Oncol 6:7, 1988.

7. Spanish Cooperative Group P. Treatment of chronic lymphocytic leukemia: a preliminary report of Spanish (PETHEMA) trials. Leuk Lymph 5:89, 1991.

8. G Dighiero, K Maloum, B Desablens, B Cazin, M Navarro, R Leblay, M Leporrier, J Jaubert, G Lepeu, B Dreyfus, JL Binet, P Travade. Chlorambucil in indolent chronic lymphocytic leukemia. French Cooperative Group on Chronic Lymphocytic Leukemia. New Engl J Med 338:1506, 1998.

9. CLL Trialists' Collaborative Group. Chemotherapeutic options in chronic lymphocytic leukemia: a meta-analysis of the randomized trials. CLL Trialists' Collaborative group. J Natl Cancer Inst 91:861, 1999.

10. BD Cheson, JM Bennett, M Grever, N Kay, MJ Keating, S O'Brien, KR Rai. National Cancer Institute-Sponsored Working Group guidelines for chronic lymphocytic leukemia: revised guidelines for diagnosis and treatment. Blood 87:4990, 1996.

11. E Montserrat, J Sanchez-Bisono, N Viñolas, C Rozman. Lymphocyte doubling time in chronic lymphocytic leukaemia: analysis of its prognostic significance. Br J Haematol 62:567, 1986.

12. E Montserrat, F Gomis, T Vallespí, A Rios, A Romero, J Soler, A Alcalá, M Morey, C Ferrán, J Díaz-Mediavilla, A Flores, S Woessner, J Batile, C González-Aza, M Rovira, J-C Reverter, C Rozman. Presenting features and prognosis of chronic lymphocytic leukemia in younger adults. Blood 78:1545, 1991.

13. MJ Keating. Chemotherapy of chronic lymphocytic leukemia. In: BD Cheson, eds. Chronic Lymphocytic Leukemia: Scientific Advances and Clinical Developments. New York: Marcel Dekker, Inc., 1993, p 297.

14. A Saven, CJ Carrera, DA Carson, E Beutler, LD Piro. 2-Chlorodeoxyadenosine treatment of refractory chronic lymphocytic leukemia. Leuk Lymph 5:133, 1991.

15. RO Dillman, R Mick, OR McIntyre. Pentostatin in chronic lymphocytic leukemia: a phase II trial of Cancer and Leukemia Group B. J Clin Oncol 7:433, 1989.

16. A Sawitsky, KR Rai, O Glidewell, RT Silver. Comparison of daily versus intermittent chlorambucil and prednisone therapy in the treatment of patients with chronic lymphocytic leukemia. Blood 50:1049, 1977.

17. KR Rai, B Peterson, L Elias, L Shepherd, J Hines, D Nelson, B Cheson, J Kolitz, CA Schiffer. A randomized comparison of fludarabine and chlorambucil for patients with previously untreated chronic lymphocytic leukemia. A CALGB, SWOG, CTC/NCI-C and ECOG intergroup study. Blood 88:141a(abstr 552), 1996.

18. JW Keller, WH Knospe, M Raney, CM Huguley, L Johnson, AA Bartolucci, GA Omura. Treatment of chronic lymphocytic leukemia using chlorambucil and prednisone with or without cycle-active consolidation therapy. A Southeastern Cancer Study Group trial. Cancer 58:1185, 1986.

19. MJ Keating, S O'Brien, S Lerner, C Koller, M Beran, LE Robertson, EJ Freireich, E Estey, H Kantarjian. Long-term follow-up of patients with chronic lymphocytic leukemia (CLL) receiving fludarabine regimens as initial therapy. Blood 92:1165, 1998.

20. French Cooperative Group on CLL, S Johnson, AG Smith, H Löffler, E Ösby, G Juliusson, B Emmerich, PJ Wyid, W Hiddemann. Multicentre prospective randomised trial of fludarabine versus cyclophosphamide, doxorubicin, and prednisone (CAP) for treatment of advanced-stage chronic lymphocytic leukemia. Lancet 347:1432, 1996.

21. S Leporrier, B Chevret, B Cazin, P Feugier, MJ Rapp, N Boudjerra, C Autrand, B Dreyfus, B Desablens, G Dighiero, P Travade, C Chastang, JL Binet. Randomized comparison of fludarabine, CAP and ChOP, in 695 previously untreated stage B and C chronic lymphocytic leukemia (CLL). Early stopping of the CAP accrual. Blood 90:529a(abstr 2357), 1997.

22. A Delannoy, P Martiat, JL Gala, V Deneys, A Ferrant, A Bosly, JM Schieff, JL Michaux.

2-Chlorodeoxyadenosine (CdA) for patients with previously untreated chronic lymphocytic leukemia (CLL). Leukemia 9:1130, 1995.

23. A Saven, RH Lemon, M Kosty, E Beutler, LD Piro. 2-Chlorodeoxyadenosine activity in patients with untreated chronic lymphocytic leukemia. J Clin Oncol 13:570, 1995.

24. T Robak, JZ Blonski, M Kasznicki, L Konopka, B Ceglarek, A Dmoszynska, M Soroka-Wojtaszko, AB Skotnicki, W Nowak, J Dwilewicz-Trojaczek, A Tomaszewska, A Hellmann, K Lewandowski, K Kuliczkowski, S Potoczek, B Zdziarska, J Hansz, R Kroll, M Komarnicki, J Holowiecki, P Grieb. Cladribine with or without prednisone in the treatment of previously treated or untreated B-cell chronic lymphocytic leukaemia—updated results of the multicentre study of 378 patients. Br J Haematol 108:357, 2000.

25. CA Puccio, A Mittelman, SM Lichtman, RT Silver, DR Budman, T Ahmed, EJ Feldman, M Coleman, PM Arnold, ZA Arlin, HG Chun. A loading dose/continuous infusion schedule of fludarabine phosphate in chronic lymphocytic leukemia. J Clin Oncol 9:1562, 1991.

26. A Kemena, S O'Brien, H Kantarjian, L Robertson, C Koller, M Beran, E Estey, W Plunkett, S Lerner, MJ Keating. A phase II clinical trial of fludarabine in chronic lymphocytic leukemia on a weekly low-dose schedule. Leuk Lymphoma 10:187, 1993.

27. LE Robertson, S O'Brien, H Kantarjian, C Koller, M Beran, M Andreef, S Lerner, W Plunkett, MJ Keating. A 3-day schedule of fludarabine in previously treated chronic lymphocytic leukemia. Leukemia 9:1444, 1995.

28. JM Foran, D Oscier, J Orchard, SA Johnson, M Tighe, M Cullen, PG de Takats, C Kraus, M Klein, TA Lister. Pharmacokinetic study of single doses of oral fludarabine phosphate. J Clin Oncol 17:1574, 1999.

29. MJ Keating, S O'Brien, H Kantarjian, W Plunkett, E Estey, C Koller, M Beran, EJ Freireich. Long-term follow-up of patients with chronic lymphocytic leukemia treated with fludarabine as a single agent. Blood 81:2878, 1993.

30. S O'Brien, H Kantarjian, M Beran, T Smith, C Koller, E Estey, LE Robertson, S Lerner, M Keating. Results of fludarabine and prednisone therapy in 264 patients with chronic lymphocytic leukemia with multivariate analysis-derived prognostic model for response to treatment. Blood 82:1695, 1993.

31. (Reference deleted in proof.)

32. LE Robertson, YO Huh, JJ Butler, WC Pugh, C Hirsch-Ginsberg, S Stass, H Kantarjian, MJ Keating. Response assessment in chronic lymphocytic leukemia after fludarabine plus prednisone: clinical, pathologic, immunophenotypic, and molecular analysis. Blood 80:29, 1992.

33. M Leporrier, S Chevret, B Cazin, N Boudjerra, P Feugier, B Desablens, M-J Rapp, J Jaubert, C Autrand, M Divine, B Dreyfus, JL Binet. Randomized comparison of fludarabine, CAP, and ChOP, in 938 previously treated stage B and C-chronic lymphocytic leukemia. In press.

34. KR Rai, BL Peterson, FR Appelbaum, J Kolitz, L Elias, L Shepherd, J Hines, G Threatte, RA Larson, BD Cheson, CA Schiffer. Fludarabine composed with chlorambucil as primary therapy for chronic lymphocytic leukemia. New Engl J Med 343:1750, 2000.

35. BD Cheson, D Vena, F Foss, JM Sorensen. Neurotoxicity of purine analogs: A review. J Clin Oncol 12:2216, 1994.

36. BD Cheson. Immunologic and immunosuppressive complications of purine analogue therapy. J Clin Oncol 13:2431, 1995.

37. BD Cheson. Toxicities associated with nucleoside analog therapy. In: BD Cheson, MJ Keating, W Plunkett, eds. Nucleoside Analogs in Cancer Therapy. New York: Marcel Dekker, Inc., 1997, p 451.

38. EJ Anaissie, DP Kontoyiannis, S O'Brien, H Kantarjian, L Robertson, S Lerner, MJ Keating. Infections in patients with chronic lymphocytic leukemia treated with fludarabine. Ann Intern Med 129:559, 1998.

39. S Molica, P Musto, F Chiurazzi, G Specchia, M Brugiatelli, L Cicoira, D Levato, F Nobile, M Carotenuto, V Liso, B Rotoli. Prophylaxis against infections with low-dose intravenous

immunoglobulins (IVIG) in chronic lymphocytic leukemia. Results of a crossover study. Haematologica 81:121, 1996.

40. BD Cheson, D Vena, J Barrett, B Freidlin. Second malignancies as a consequence of nucleoside analog therapy of chronic lymphoid leukemias. J Clin Oncol 17:2454, 1999.

41. BM Morse, SJ Shattil. Metabolic complications of aggressive therapy of chronic lymphocytic leukemia. Am J Med Sci 276:311, 1974.

42. R Kurlander, RS Stein, D Roth. Hyperkalemia complicating splenic irradiation of chronic lymphocytic leukemia. Cancer 36:926, 1975.

43. RD McCroskey, DF Mosher, CD Spencer, E Prendergast, WL Longo. Acute tumor lysis syndrome and treatment response in patients treated for refractory chronic lymphocytic leukemia with short-course, high-dose cytosine arabinoside, cisplatin, and etoposide. Cancer 66:246, 1990.

44. J Nomdedéu, R Martino, A Sureda, G Huidobro, R López, S Brunet, A Domingo-Albós. Acute tumor lysis syndrome complicating conditioning therapy for bone marrow transplantation in a patient with chronic lymphocytic leukemia. Bone Marrow Trans 13:659, 1994.

45. F Nakhoul, J Green, ZA Abassi, A Carter. Tumor lysis syndrome induced by fludarabine monophosphate: a case report. Eur J Haematol 56:254, 1996.

46. BD Cheson, JN Frame, D Vena, N Quashu, JM Sorensen. Tumor lysis syndrome: an uncommon complication of fludarabine therapy of chronic lymphocytic leukemia. J Clin Oncol 16: 2313, 1998.

47. G Juliusson, I Christiansen, MM Hansen, S Johnson, E Kimby, A Elmhorn-Rosenberhg, J Liliemark. Oral cladribine as primary therapy for patients with B-cell chronic lymphocytic leukemia. J Clin Oncol 14:2160, 1996.

48. S O'Brien, H Kantarjian, A Ellis, L Zwelling, E Estey, M Keating. Topotecan in chronic lymphocytic leukemia. Cancer 75:1104, 1995.

49. B Gahn, G Brittinger, G Dolken, H Döhner, B Emmerich, A Franke, M Freund, C Huber, R Kuse, T Scholten, W Hiddemann. Multicenter phase II study of oral idarubicin in treated and untreated patients with B-chronic lymphocytic leukemia. Leuk Lymph 37:169, 2000.

50. E Montserrat, A Alcala, R Parody, A Domingo, J Garcia-Conde, J Bueno, C Ferran, MA Sanz, M Giralt, D Rubio, I Anton, J Estape, C Rozman. Treatment of chronic lymphocytic leukemia in advanced stages. A randomized trial comparing chlorambucil plus prednisone versus cyclophosphamide, vincristine, and prednisone. Cancer 56:2369, 1985.

51. B Raphael, JW Andersen, R Silber, M Oken, D Moore, J Bennett, H Bonner, R Hahn, WH Knospe, J Mazza, J Glick. Comparison of chlorambucil and prednisone versus cyclophosphamide, vincristine, and prednisone as initial treatment for chronic lymphocytic leukemia: Long-term follow-up of an Eastern Cooperative Oncology Group randomized clinical trial. J Clin Oncol 9:770, 1991.

52. MM Hansen, E Andersen, H Birgens, BE Christensen, TG Christensen, C Geisler, K Meldgaard, D Pedersen. CHOP versus chlorambucil + prednisolone in chronic lymphocytic leukemia. Leuk Lymph 5:97, 1991.

53. French Cooperative Group on Chronic Lymphocytic Leukemia. Long-term results of the CHOP regimen in stage C chronic lymphocytic leukaemia. Br J Haematol 73:334, 1989.

54. E Kimby, H Millstedt. Chlorambucil/prednisone versus CHOP in symptomatic chronic lymphocytic leukemias of B-cell type. A randomized trial. Leuk Lymph 5:93, 1991.

55. MJ Keating, M Scouros, S Murphy, H Kantarjian, J Hester, KB McCredie, EM Hersh, EJ Freireich. Multiple agent chemotherapy (POACH) in previously treated and untreated patients with chronic lymphocytic leukemia. Leukemia 2:157, 1988.

56. MJ Keating, JP Hester, KB McCredie, et al. Long-term results of CAP therapy in chronic lymphocytic leukemia. Leuk Lymph 2:391, 1990.

57. M Liepman, ML Votaw. The treatment of chronic lymphocytic leukemia with COP chemotherapy. Cancer 41:1664, 1978.

58. S Kempin, BJ, III Lee, HT Thaler, B Koziner, S Hecht, T Gee, Z Arlin, C Little, D Straus, L Reich, E Phillips, H Al-Mondhiry, M Dowling, B Clarkson. Combination chemotherapy of advanced chronic lymphocytic leukemia: The M-2 protocol (vincristine, BCNU, cyclophosphamide, melphalan, and prednisone). Blood 60:1110, 1982.

59. E Montserrat, A Alcala, C Alonso, J Besalduch, JM Moraleda, J Garcia-Conde, M Gutierrez, F Gomis, J Garijo, MC Guzman, J Estape, C Rozman. A randomized trial comparing chlorambucil plus prednisone vs cyclophosphamide, melphalan, and prednisone in the treatment of chronic lymphocytic leukemia stages B and C. Nouv Rev Fr Hematol 30:429, 1988.

60. GM Smith, JA Child, DW Milligan, MA McEvoy, JA Murray. A pilot study of epirubicin and chlorambucil in the treatment of chronic lymphocytic leukemia (CLL). Hematol Oncol 9:315, 1991.

61. French Cooperative Group on Chronic Lymphocytic Leukemia. A randomized clinical trial of chlorambucil versus COP in stage B chronic lymphocytic leukemia. Blood 75:1422, 1990.

62. E Anaissie, DP Kontoyiannis, H Kantarjian, L Elting, LE Robertson, M Keating. Listeriosis in patients with chronic lymphocytic leukemia who were treated with fludarabine and prednisone. Ann Intern Med 117:466, 1992.

63. L Elias, D Stock-Novak, M Grever, J Weick, R Chapman, JE Godwin, S Balcerzak, F Appelbaum. A phase I trial of combination fludarabine and chlorambucil in chronic lymphocytic leukemia. Proc Am Soc Clin Oncol 10:221(abstr 745), 1991.

64. M Weiss, S Kempin, E Berman, A Eardley, T Gee. Results of a phase I study of fludarabine phosphate (FAMP) plus chlorambucil (CLB) in patients with chronic lymphocytic leukemia. Proc Am Soc Clin Oncol 11:276(abstr 914), 1992.

65. V Gandhi, B Nowak, MJ Keating, W Plunkett. Modulation of arabinosylcytosine metabolism by arabinosyl-2-fluoroadenine in lymphocytes from patients with chronic lymphocytic leukemia: Implications for combination therapy. Blood 74:2070, 1989.

66. V Gandhi, A Kemena, MJ Keating, W Plunkett. Fludarabine infusion potentiates arabinosylcytosine metabolism in lymphocytes of patients with chronic lymphocytic leukemia. Cancer Res 52:897, 1992.

67. S O'Brien, H Kantarjian, C Koller, L Robertson, M Beran, E Estey, S Lerner, M Keating. Fludarabine-prednisone: a highly effective regimen in chronic lymphocytic leukemia (CLL). Proc Am Soc Clin Oncol 11:260(abstr 850), 1992.

68. F Foss, D Ihde, R Phelps, A Fischmann, G Schechter, I Linniola, J Cotelingam, B Ghosh, J Phares, S Steinberg, J Stocker, A Bastian, E Sausville. Phase II study of fludarabine and interferon-alfa-2A in advanced mycosis fungoides/Sezary syndrome (MF/SS). Proc Am Soc Clin Oncol 11:315(abstr 1068), 1992.

69. MJ Rummel, G Käfer, M Pfreundschuh, E Jäger, U Reinhardt, PS Mitrou, D Hoelzer, L Bergmann. Fludarabine and epirubicin in the treatment of chronic lymphocytic leukaemia: a German multicenter phase II study. Ann Oncol 10:183, 1999.

70. F Bosch, M Perales, F Cobo, J Esteve, M Rafel, A López-Guillermo, JM Ribera, E Campo, E Montserrat. Fludarabine, cyclophosphamide and mitoxantrone (FCM) therapy in resistant or relapsed chronic lymphocytic leukemia (CLL) or follicular lymphoma (FL). Blood 90: 530a(abstr 2360), 1997.

71. S O'Brien, H Kantarjian, M Beran, S Lerner, J Gilbreath, MJ Keating. Fludarabine (FAMP) and cyclophosphamide (CTX) therapy in chronic lymphocytic leukemia (CLL). Int J Hematol 64:S56(abstr 214), 1996.

72. IW Flinn, JC Byrd, C Morrison, J Jamison, LF Diehl, T Murphy, S Piantadosi, E Seifter, RF Ambinder, G Vogelsang, MR Grever. Fludarabine and cyclophosphamide with filgrastim support in patients with previously untreated indolent lymphoid malignancies. Blood 96:71, 2000.

73. A Tefferi, R Levitt, CY Li, G Schroeder, LK Tschetter, JC Michalak, JE Krook, TE Witzig. Phase II study of 2-chlorodeoxyadenosine in combination with chlorambucil in previously untreated B-cell chronic lymphocytic leukemia. Ann Oncol 22:509, 1999.

74. MM Oken, S Lee, PA Cassileth, RL Krigel. Pentostatin, chlorambucil and prednisone for the treatment of chronic lymphocytic leukemia (CLL): Eastern Cooperative Oncology Group (ECOG) protocol E1488. Proc ASCO 17:6a(abstr 22), 1998.

75. H Mellstedt, Österborg, J Lundin, CF Björkholm, H Hagberg, R Hast, V Hjalmar, E Kimby, M Luthman, O Tullgren, B Werner. CAMPATH-1H therapy of patients with previously untreated chronic lymphocytic leukemia (CLL). Blood 92:490a(abstr 2019), 1998.

76. DG Maloney, AJ Grillo-López, CA White, D Bodkin, RJ Schilder, JA Neidhart, N Janakiraman, KA Foon, TM Liles, BK Dallaire, K Wey, I Royston, T Davis, R Levy. IDEC-C2B8 (Rituximab) anti-CD20-monoclonal antibody therapy in patients with relapsed low-grade non-Hodgkin's lymphoma. Blood 90:2188, 1997.

77. LD Piro, CA White, AJ Grillo-López, N Janakiraman, A Saven, TM Beck, C Varns, S Shuey, M Czuczman, JW Lynch, JE Kolitz, V Jain. Extended rituximab (anti-CD20 monoclonal antibody) therapy for relapsed or refractory low-grade or follicular non-Hodgkin's lymphoma. Ann Oncol 10:655, 1999.

78. U Winkler, M Jensen, O Manzke, H Schulz, V Diehl, A Engert. Cytokine-release syndrome in patients with B-cell chronic lymphocytic leukemia and high lymphocyte counts after treatment with an anti-CD20 monoclonal antibody (Rituximab, IDEC-C2B8). Blood 94:2217, 1999.

79. TA Johnson, OW Press. Synergistic cytotoxicity of iodine-131-anti-CD20 antibodies and chemotherapy for treatment of B-cell lymphomas. Int J Cancer 85:104, 2000.

80. JC Byrd, MR Grever, B Davis, MS Lucas, K Park, A Goodrich, C Morrison, T Murphy, L Kunkel, AJ Grillo-López, J Waselenko, IW Flinn. Phase I/II study of thrice weekly rituximab in chronic lymphocytic leukemia (CLL)/small lymphocytic lymphoma (SLL): a feasible and active regimen. Blood 94:704a (abstr 3114), 1999.

81. S O'Brien, DA Thomas, EJ Freireich, M Andreeff, FJ Giles, MJ Keating. Rituxan has significant activity in patients with CLL. Blood 94:603a (abstr 2684), 1999.

82. P Venugopal, S Sivaraman, X Huang, HK Chopra, T O'Brien, A Jajeh, HD Preisler. Upregulation of CD20 expression in chronic lymphocytic leukemia (CLL) cells by in vitro exposure to cytokines. Blood 92:247a (abstr 1009), 1998.

14

Management of the Patient with Relapsed or Refractory Chronic Lymphocytic Leukemia

**DEBORAH A. THOMAS, SUSAN M. O'BRIEN,
and MICHAEL J. KEATING**

The University of Texas M. D. Anderson Cancer Center, Houston, Texas

I. INTRODUCTION

Traditional first-line therapy for chronic lymphocytic leukemia (CLL) has been chlorambucil (CLB) with or without corticosteroids (1–15). Alternative alkylator-based regimens include cyclophosphamide (CTX) in combination with vincristine and prednisone (COP) (8,12,14,16–18); adriamycin and prednisone (CAP) (19–22); vincristine, adriamycin, and prednisone (CHOP) (13,20,23–24); CHOP with Ara-C (POACH) (25); melphalan and prednisone (CMP) (11), and others (26–28). In de novo CLL, alkylator regimens yield response rates of 60% to 80%, but with only a 10% to 25% rate of complete remission. Response rates in previously treated patients vary widely, ranging from 25% to 75%, but complete remissions were rarely achieved (Table 1). Recently, the nucleoside analogs fludarabine monophosphate (21,29–49), 2-chlorodeoxyadenosine (50–70), and deoxycoformycin (71–75), have demonstrated activity in previously treated patients with relapsed or alkylator-refractory disease (Tables 2–4). As observed with the alkylator regimens, response rates with nucleoside analogs are higher in previously untreated CLL than when administered in the salvage setting.

In randomized trials comparing fludarabine (Fludara; Berlex Laboratories, Inc., Richmond, VA) to akylator regimens (chlorambucil, CAP, CHOP), higher response rates and longer disease-free survival has been observed with the nucleoside analog for both untreated and previously treated patients (15,21,22). Although a survival advantage has not yet been demonstrated, fludarabine can be considered an attractive agent for front-line therapy (76). A recent publication by Keating and colleagues (77) detailed the encouraging

Table 1   Outcomes with Nonnucleoside or Alkylator Combination Regimens in CLL Patients

Author, year	Regimen	Status	No.	RR (%)	CR (%)	Response duration[a] (months)	Infection rate (%)[b] Any	No/Cycles	Fatal	Ref.
Sawitzky, 1977	CLB/P monthly	UT	29	55	10	16[c]	58	NA	NA	5
		PT	9	22	0					
	CLB/P daily	UT	29	40	17	7[c]	56			
		PT	12	33	0					
	P alone	UT	16	6	0	7[c]	53			
		PT	3	33	0					
Binet, 1977	MOPP	PT	23	30	17	NA	NA		NA	7
Liepman, 1978	COP	UT	23	78	52	NA	19	NA	8	16
		PT	13	62	31	NA				
Oken, 1979	COP	PT	18	44	11	13	17	NA	11	17
Kempin, 1982	M-2	UT	37	81	30	34	NA	NA	51	26
		PT	26	35	0	11				
Montserrat, 1985	CLB/P	UT	34	71	8[c]	NA	NA	NA	43	8
		PT	17	35						
	COP	UT	27	33	2[c]					
		PT	18	28						
Keating, 1988	POACH	UT	34	56	21	NA	NA	43/291 (15)	6	25
		PT	31	26	7	NA		36/137 (26)	16	
Ferrara, 1989	MiNa	UT	8	63	NA	NA	NA	NA	15	27
		PT	12	75						
Smith, 1991	CLB/epirubicin	UT	7	71	14	NA	20	NA	10	89
		PT	3	100	0					
Friedenberg, 1993	VAD	PT	31	21	0	6.5	61	NA	15	88
Molica, 1993	CLB/P + IFN	PT	8	37	0	4	100	NA	0	28
French Cooperative Group on CLL, 1996	CAP	UT	48	60	17	7	19	NA	9	21
		PT	48	27	6	6				
Itala, 1996	COP	PT	24	25	12	18	75	35/84 (42)	38	18

No., number of evaluable patients; RR, overall response rate (CR + partial response); CR, percentage with complete remission with or without lymphoid nodules in marrow; Ref, reference(s), UT, untreated; PT, previously treated; NA, not available; CLB/P, chlorambucil and prednisone; MOPP, nitrogen mustard, vincristine, procarbazine, and prednisone; COP, cyclophosphamide, vincristine, prednisone; M-2, vincristine, cyclophosphamide, BCNU, melphalan, and prednisone; POACH, cyclophosphamide, doxorubicin, vincristine, cytarabine, and prednisone; VAD, vincristine, doxorubicin, dexamethasone; MiNa, vincristine, cyclophosphamide, melphalan, peptichemio, and prednisone; IFN, interferon; CAP; cyclophosphamide, doxorubicin, prednisone.

[a] Median duration (months) of remission.

[b] Any; % patients experiencing either septicemia, pneumonia, minor infections, and/or fever unknown origin; No/cycles, number occurrences per number of cycles administered; Fatal, early infectious deaths.

[c] Represents overall CR rate or median duration of response for both untreated and previously treated patients.

Table 2 Responses to Fludarabine Monophosphate in Previously Treated CLL Patients

Author, year	Dose Schedule (mg/m²/day)	No.	RR (%)	CR (%)	Duration[a] (mo)	Reference
Grever, 1988	20 × 5	32	13	3	NA	29
Whelan, 1991	Standard	11	20	0	NA	33
Hiddeman, 1991	Standard	20	55	20	NA	34
Puccio, 1991	20 × 1, then 30 CI × 2	42	52	0	6	35
Keating, 1993	Standard or 30 × 5	78	59	15	21	36
O'Brien, 1993	30 × 5 (+prednisone)	169	52	37	22	37
Kemena, 1993	30 × 1 day weekly	46	24	15	NA	38
Zinzani, 1993	Standard	35	45	0	NA	39
Bergmann, 1993	Standard	18	67	NA	6	40
Spriano, 1994	Standard	21	48	5	NA	41
Fenchel, 1995	Standard	56	73	5	NA	42
Robertson, 1995	30 × 3	80	46	10	NA	43
Montserrat, 1996	Standard or 30 × 5	68	28	4	NA	44
French Cooperative Group on CLL, 1996	Standard	48	48	13	11	21
Gjedde, 1996	Standard	22	32	1	8	45
Angelopoulou, 1996	Standard	20	58	33	12	46
Sorensen, 1997	Standard ± prednisone	703	32	3	13	47
O'Brien, 1997	30 × 5 + G-CSF	25	32	20	25	48
Keating, 2000	Standard, + prednisone, or weekly	374	48	23	NA	49

No., number of evaluable patients; RR, overall response (CR + partial response); CR, percentage with complete remission with or without lymphoid nodules; NA, not available; Standard, fludarabine 25 mg/m²/day × 5 every 4 weeks; CI, continuous infusion.

[a] Median duration (months) of remission.

Table 3 Responses to 2-Chlorodeoxyadenosine in Previously Treated CLL Patients

Author, year	Dose schedule	Prior fludarabine? & sensitivity	No.	RR (%)	CR (%)	Duration[a] (mo)	Ref.
Piro, 1988	0.5–0.2 mg/kg/days CI × 7	NA	18	22	1	4.5	50
Saven, 1993	0.1 mg/kg/ days CI × 5–7 or	No	90	44	4	4	53
	0.028–0.14 mg/kg/days × 5	Refractory	14	0	0		
Juliusson, 1993	Standard	NA	18	67	39	9	54
O'Brien, 1994	4 mg/m²/days CI × 7	Refractory	28	7	0	4+, 14	58
Delannoy, 1994	4 mg/m²/days CI × 7 or 5.6 mg/m²/days × 5	All	22	32	1	2	59
		Refractory	6	0	0		
Tallman, 1995	0.1 mg/kg/days CI × 5–7	All	26	31	0	16[b]	30
		No	15	44	0		
		Yes	10	10	0		
Juliusson, 1996	Standard	All	52	58	31	20[b]	61
		Refractory	7	57	14		
Robak, 1996	Standard	All	92	36	5	NA	62
		Yes	1	0	0		
Brugiatelli, 1996	0.1 mg/kg/days × 5–7	No	16	62	31	8	63
Rondelli, 1997	6 mg/m²/days bolus × 5	All	19	68	11	NR (9)	65
		Sensitive	2	100	100		
		Refractory	3	66	0		
Betticher, 1998	0.7 mg/kg/cycle CI × 7 days	No	20	35	1	6	67
	0.5 mg/kg subq × 5 days	No	35	40	1	6	
Rai, 1998	Standard	No	8	63	13	NA	68
		Yes	6	17	0	NA	
Robak, 2000	Standard ± prednisone	No	184	48	12	13.5	70

No., number of evaluable patients; RR, overall response (CR + partial response); CR, percentage with complete remission with or without lymphoid nodules in marrow; Ref., Reference(s); CI, continuous infusion; Standard, 2-CdA 0.12 mg/kg/d bolus for 5 days; NA, not available; NR, not reached (time in parenthesis); subq, subcutaneous.
[a] Median duration (months) of remission.
[b] Actuarial estimate.

Table 4 Responses to Deoxycoformycin in Previously Treated CLL Patients

Author, year	Dose schedule	No. prior nucleoside	No.	RR (%)	CR (%)	Duration[a] (mo)	Ref.
Grever, 1985	4 mg/m² wkly or q. 2 wk	None	28	18	4	9	71
Dillman, 1989	4 mg/m² wkly × 3, then q. 2 wk	NA	26	15	4	NA	72
Ho, 1990	4 mg/m² wkly × 3, then q. 2 wk	NA	26	27	0	7	73
Dearden, 1990	4 mg/m² q. 1–2 wk	NA	17	35	0	6	74
Johnson, 1998	2 mg/m²/day × 5	17	24	29	8	7	75

No., number of evaluable patients; RR, overall response (CR + partial response); CR, percentage with complete remission with or without lymphoid nodules in marrow; Ref, reference; NA, not available; wkly, weekly; wk, weeks.
[a] Median duration (months) of remission.

experience and long-term follow-up of patients with de novo progressive or advanced CLL treated with single agent fludarabine as first-line therapy at the University of Texas M.D. Anderson Cancer Center (MDACC). The overall response rate was 78%, with a median survival of 63 months. Although durable remissions were observed, progression or disease recurrence was eventually seen in more than three-fourths of the patients. Forty-one of 63 patients (67%) who relapsed responded to retreatment with fludarabine; however, eventually some patients became refractory. No current standard of care exists for CLL patients who have been exposed to alkylators and have become fludarabine-refractory; reported salvage response rates with investigational agents range from 20% to 30%, with an expected median survival of less than 1 year (36,78). Clearly, new therapeutic strategies are needed to alter the natural history of the disease and prolong survival. Truly novel agents need to be identified that can effectively be combined in tolerable doses and schedules of administration, because complete remissions in a substantial number of patients are rarely achieved with monotherapy. Thus, chemotherapy agents with unique chemical structures directed at specific molecular targets or biological agents with selectivity toward leukemia cells need to be identified and explored.

Herein, we review the current literature regarding the (1) success of previously used salvage strategies, (2) preliminary results of ongoing clinical trials, and (3) role of autologous or allogeneic marrow transplantation in the management of the relapsed or refractory patient. The infectious complications of the disease and its therapy are discussed in addition to the known or postulated mechanisms of disease resistance and their relevance to novel agents currently in development. An algorithm is proposed to guide clinicians in their management of the relapsed or refractory CLL patient.

II. DEFINITION OF REFRACTORY CLL

Evaluation of prior treatment history in patients with CLL is often difficult, because the administration of CLB with or without corticosteroids is not standardized. Multiple alkylator regimens are often administered in succession such as chlorambucil with or without prednisone followed by COP. Currently, the definition of alkylator-refractory disease is arbitrary. A proposed definition applied to studies at the MDACC includes either failure

Table 5 Responses to Nucleoside Analogs in Previously Treated Patients by Alkylator Sensitivity

Author, year	Agent(s)	Response to prior alkylator therapy	No.	RR (%)	P value	Reference
O'Brien, 1993	Fludarabine +prednisone	All	169	52		
		sensitive	31	68	<0.001	37
		refractory	138	49		
Montserrat, 1996	Fludarabine	All	68	28		
		sensitive	18[a]	62	0.005	44
		refractory	57	20		
Keating, 2000	Fludarabine	All	374	48		
		sensitive	102	60	<0.01	49
		refractory	272	44		
Juliusson, 1996	2-CdA	All	52	58		
		sensitive	17	82	0.01	61
		refractory	35	46		
Betticher, 1998	2-CdA	All	55	38		
		sensitive	24	46	NS	67
		refractory	31	32		

[a] Seven patients active therapy, invaluable for response, distribution not specified.

to achieve a partial response or progression while on therapy (37,49). A generally accepted definition of fludarabine resistance includes (1) progression of disease during treatment, (2) failure to achieve partial response after at least two cycles, or (3) relapse within 6 months of treatment. Fludarabine-intolerance may be defined as (1) autoimmune hemolytic anemia (79–83) or idiopathic thrombocytopenia attributable to the agent during or within 1 month of therapy, or (2) greater than grade 2 pulmonary toxicity (84) or neurotoxicity (85–87) which would be prohibitive of further treatment. Similar definitions of failure are applied to the other nucleoside analogs 2-CdA and DCF, although the time required to achieve best clinical response reported in clinical trials differs from fludarabine.

Standard definitions are required for proper interpretation of clinical trials and development of new agents. For example, the determination of alkylator sensitivity is crucial to the interpretation of responses to subsequent treatments, because alkylator-refractory patients are less likely to respond to monotherapy with purine analogs than alkylator-sensitive or untreated patients (Table 5). An inherent mechanism of resistance, such as failure of apoptosis induction (rather than pharmacological cross-resistance) may account for such observations, and alternative treatment strategies could be used for patients demonstrating alkylator-resistant disease, such as administration of nucleoside analog combination therapy.

III. ALKYLATOR REGIMENS AS SALVAGE THERAPY

Traditional first-line therapy of CLL has been CLB with or without prednisone (1–15). Before the advent of the purine nucleoside analogs, treatment of relapsed or refractory patients included multiple aklylator-based regimens and anthracyline-based combinations.

A. Single-Agent Alkylator Trials

Single-agent CLB with or without prednisone was studied in three early trials. In the first study, Galton and colleagues (1) gave chlorambucil 4 to 8 mg/m^2 continuously for 4 to 8 weeks in 43 patients with de novo CLL. Responders included those with "relief of symptoms"; 77% of patients achieved an intitial response. Retreatment was administered in 33 patients; 70% responded to a second course, and 14 of 23 (61%) responded to a third course. The degree of benefit lessened with each retreatment, and the interval of response between courses became shorter. The subsequent addition of prednisone did not appear to improve either the quality or number of responses. Ezdinli and colleagues (2) treated 51 CLL patients with a daily dose of chlorambucil averaging 6 to 12 mg per day for 4 to 8 weeks. Reductions in lymphocyte count, adenopathy, and splenomegaly (in 75%, 33%, and 50% of the patients, respectively) occurred. Twenty to 30% of the patients exhibited improvements in anemia and thrombocytopenia. The retreatment response rate, however, was only 18%. The concept of intermittent therapy was introduced by Knospse and colleagues (3); a single dose of 0.4 mg/kg was given every 2 weeks with dose escalation by 0.1 mg/kg until either disease control or toxicity was observed. Seven of the 14 patients (50%) who were previously treated and were "sensitive" to alkylating agents responded, whereas only 2 of 9 patients (22%) who were resistant to continuous CLB responded to retreatment with intermittent chlorambucil. Further comparison to current salvage studies is not possible because of the lack of bone marrow response assessments in these studies.

B. Combination Alkylator Regimens

Han and colleagues (4) reported on the outcome of a double-blinded study in which 15 CLL patients who were treated with a combination of chlorambucil and prednisone were compared with 11 patients given chlorambucil alone. Chlorambucil was given at a dose of 6 mg/day continuously and prednisone at 30 mg/day for 6 weeks. Responding patients were maintained on chlorambucil, 2 to 4 mg/day, and prednisone, 15 to 20 mg/day. The overall response rate was 87% [20% complete response (CR) by marrow evaluation] for the combination versus 45% (9% CR) for single agent chlorambucil. The 2-year survival rates were 93% and 54%, respectively (P not significant).

Sawitsky et al. (5) from the Cancer and Leukemia Group B (CALGB) conducted a randomized trial comparing chlorambucil (0.4–0.8 mg/kg) and prednisone monthy, the combination daily (chlorambucil 0.08 mg/kg), and prednisone alone (0.8 mg/kg for 14 days, with 50% reduction days 15 and 29 for a 6-week course with maintenance 0.8 mg/kg daily for 7 days monthly) in both untreated and previously treated patients. The response rates in the latter group were 22%, 33%, and 33%, respectively; no CRs were observed (Table 1). Median survival in previously treated patients ranged from 8 to 15 months; responders fared as well as previously untreated responders. No significant difference in toxicity was observed between previously treated and untreated patients; however, chlorambucil doses were more often reduced in previously treated patients on the daily schedule because of myelosuppression.

The combination of cyclophosphamide, vincristine, and prednisone (COP) has been extensively studied in patients previously treated with CLB or without prednisone (Table 1). Leipman and Votaw (16) reported a response rate of 62% (31% CR rate) with the COP regimen (cyclophosphamide 400 mg/m^2 orally daily days 1–5, vincristine 1.4 mg/m^2 day 10, and prednisone 100 mg/m^2 daily days 1–5 every 3 weeks) in 13 previously treated patients (some with concurrent splenectomy). No significant differences in response, duration of response, or survival was noted between previously treated and untreated patients; specifics regarding prior therapy were not provided. Three fatal infections (8%) were observed during the induction phase of therapy. Oken and Kaplan (17) reported a response rate of 44% (11% clinical CR rate) in 18 patients with advanced alkylator-refractory CLL with a similar program (cyclophosphamide 800 mg/m^2 intravenously day 1 or 400 mg/m^2 orally days 1–5, vincristine 2 mg day 1, and prednisone 60 to 100 mg/m^2 orally days 1–5). Only one of five patients refractory to all prior therapy responded, whereas 54% of patients initially sensitive to prior therapy achieved either CR or partial response (PR). Median survival of responders was 37.5 months compared with 5 months for nonresponders; two (11%) treatment-related deaths were noted.

Montserrat et al. (8) randomly assigned 35 previously treated patients between CLB and prednisone versus COP (600 mg/m^2 IV day 6, vincristine 1 mg/m^2 day 6, and prednisone 60 mg/m^2 orally days 1–5). The overall response rate was 28% for 18 patients treated with COP and 35% for 17 patients administered chlorambucil and prednisone (Table 1). Median survival was 13.5 months for the previously treated group compared with 32 months for 61 untreated patients. In this study, 71% of the 58 deaths were related to infections, with 20 of those 41 patients (49%) succumbing to pneumonia. Details regarding differences in infection rates by treatment status (de novo or previously treated CLL) were not provided.

Other alkylator regimens studied include nitrogen mustard, vincristine, procarbazine, prednisone (MOPP). Binet et al. (7) reported the outcome of this regimen in 23 previously treated, advanced CLL patients. The overall response rate was 30% (13% CR rate). The Memorial Sloan-Kettering Cancer Center (MSKCC) reported a response rate of 35% (no complete remissions) with the M2 regimen (vincristine, cyclophosphamide, BCNU, melphalan, and prednisone) in 26 previously treated patients (26). A smaller study (MiNA) based on the M2 regimen but substituting an investigational drug (Peptochemio) for BCNU reported an overall response rate of 75% in 12 advanced CLL patients previously treated with chlorambucil and prednisone (27). Molica et al. (28) studied the addition of interferon-α to chlorambucil and prednisone in eight previously treated patients. The response rate was 37%; a high incidence of infections was observed (Table 1).

Thus, in previously treated patients (as in untreated patients), no alkylating agent combination regimen appeared superior to chlorambucil and prednisone on the basis of comparative trials, although sensitivity to prior alkylator therapy was not specified in most of these reports. However, small single-arm trials of multiple alkylating agent combinations suggest that increasing the dose intensity and/or heterogeneity of the agents may be associated with higher response rates than with conventional combinations (27).

C. Anthracycline-Containing (± Alkylators) Regimens

A randomized comparative trial reported by the French Cooperative Group (23) of COP (cyclosphosphamide 300 mg/m^2 orally days 1–5, vincristine 1 mg/m^2 intravenously day 1, and prednisone 40 mg/m^2 orally days 1–5) versus CHOP (the same three drugs with doxorubicin 25 mg/m^2 on day 1) was conducted in Binet stage C patients. Because of a significant improvement in survival observed for patients in the CHOP arm, the study was closed to accrual in 1986. A long-term follow-up of 70 patients confirmed the earlier report, with 36 and 34 patients treated with CHOP or COP, respectively (24). At the time of the analysis, 3-year survival rates were 71% for the group treated with CHOP versus

28% for those treated with COP ($P < 0.0001$), with corresponding median survivals of 62 and 22 months (24). Failures after COP (refractory or relapsed) received CHOP. Criticisms of the study included the small patient numbers and shorter median survival of the COP arm compared with other reported studies [<2 years as opposed to 4 years for Binet stage C patients treated with either chlorambucil or CAP (14)]. The activity of anthracyclines in CLL was evaluated further.

The multiagent chemotherapy regimen POACH (cyclophosphamide, doxorubicin, vincristine, cytarabine, and prednisone) was administered to both untreated and previously treated patients at the MDACC (25). Outcome was poorer in the previously treated patients, with an overall response rate of 26% compared with 56% (Table 1). A modified vincristine, doxorubicin, and dexamethasone (VAD) regimen was studied in 36 CLL patients with prior alkylator therapy but no more than two regimens (88). The response rate was 21% with no CRs observed. Response rate was greater (28% vs 16%) in those patients who had not received prior vincristine or doxorubicin. Mild to moderate neurotoxicity was observed in 36% of the patients, and 61% developed infections. Myelosuppression was severe in most patients. A pilot study of epirubicin and chlorambucil was conducted in 10 patients; the overall response rate was 80% (89). One complete and four partial responses were seen in seven untreated patients; all three previously treated patients achieved PRs. Further study is required to confirm this activity.

IV. NUCLEOSIDE ANALOGS AS SINGLE AGENTS

Until the late 1980s, the only agents with demonstrated activity in CLL were the alkylator compounds (especially chlorambucil and cyclophosphamide) and corticosteroids. No effective salvage strategy was available for patients who were refractory to these agents until the study of the nucleoside analogs fludarabine monophosphate, 2-chlorodeoxyadenosine (2-CdA), and deoxycoformycin (DCF). The literature describing the results of clinical trials of single-agent nucleoside therapy in previously treated CLL patients is summarized in Tables 2 through 4.

A. Fludarabine

Fludarabine (9-β-D-arabinofuranosyl-2-flouradenine-5′phosphate) is a water-soluble purine analog antimetabolite that is relatively resistant to adenosine deaminase. After administration, it is rapidly dephosphorylated to F-ara-A, concentrated intracellularly by a carrier-mediated transport system and then phosphorylated to its active metabolite, 2-fluoro-arabinofuranosyl-adenosine-triphosphate (F-ara-ATP) (90,91). The rate-limiting enzyme in the phosphorylation of F-ara-A is deoxycytidine kinase. Fludarabine inhibits both DNA and RNA synthesis by (1) termination of chain elongation after incorporation into DNA, (2) inhibition of DNA and RNA polymerases, and (3) inhibition of ribonucleotide reductase, which decreases intracellular deoxynucleotide levels. Huang et al. (92) recently demonstrated that fludarabine-mediated inhibition of mRNA and the consequent depletion of cell survival proteins may be instrumental for the cytotoxicity of relatively quiescent CLL cells.

Fludarabine was first studied in acute leukemias; severe and delayed neurotoxicity was observed when given in high doses by continuous infusion (125 to 150 mg/m²/d for 5–7 days) (85–87). Subsequent studies in chronic lymphoproliferative disorders at lower doses revealed significant activity, even in heavily pretreated patients. Response rates in refractory or relapsed low-grade B-cell Non-Hodgkin's lymphomas ranged from 31% to 61% (93–95). The activity of fludarabine in relapsed or alkylator-refractory CLL was first demonstrated by Grever and colleagues (29) in a Southwestern Oncology Group (SWOG) phase II protocol of 22 previously treated patients. One patient achieved CR, 3 had good PRs, and 15 (68%) had clinical improvement of their disease.

Subsequent clinical trials at the MDACC confirmed the highest therapeutic activity ever reported for a single agent in relapsed or refractory CLL (36–39,43,48,49). Keating and colleagues (36) gave fludarabine 25 to 30 mg/m^2/day for 5 days every 4 weeks to 78 previously treated patients, obtaining an overall response rate of 59% with a 15% CR rate. Survival correlated with response to therapy; those who failed fludarabine treatment had a median survival of 9 weeks. One of 17 patients (6%) responded to subsequent salvage therapy after failing fludarabine. The median time to progression in responders was 26 months. Relapse or progression was more likely to occur in patients with extensive prior therapy or fludarabine response other than CR. Of 32 patients who relapsed after fludarabine, 27 (84%) received salvage therapy. Retreatment with fludarabine generated a response in 27% of the patients; no patient responded to alternative salvage regimens. Toxicity observed with fludarabine included myelosuppression and infections, with complications more frequently observed among nonresponders and previously treated patients. Myelosuppression was associated with a nadir neutrophil count <500/µL and nadir platelet count of <50,000/µL in 56% and 25% of the courses, respectively. Of 337 courses of treatment evaluable for toxicity, 25 episodes (7%) of pneumonia and 28 episodes (8%) of fever of unknown origin (FUO) were noted. Septicemia (4 patients) and minor infections (16 patients) were less common. Other side effects such as nausea, vomiting, stomatitis, diarrhea, and neurotoxicity occured in less than 5% of the patients.

Although most studies have used a standard schedule of 25 mg/m^2/day for 5 days (total dose 125 mg/m^2), alternative schedules have been explored (Table 2). Puccio and colleagues (35) used a loading dose of 20 mg/m^2 followed by a 30 mg/m^2/day continuous infusion for 2 days (total dose 80 mg/m^2) every 4 weeks; response rate was 52% in 42 evaluable patients with no complete responses (defined by eradication of all CD5+ cells) achieved. Once weekly (38) and 3-day schedules (43) were explored at the MDACC; inferior response rates of 25% and 46% were observed, respectively (the latter with a lower CR rate and higher incidence of residual disease albeit with a lower infection rate compared with the 5-day schedule). Additional clinical trials of single-agent fludarabine in relapsed or refractory CLL are summarized in Table 2, with overall response rates ranging from 13% to 73% and CR rates from 0% to 37%. Response rates were higher in previously treated CLL patients with early-stage disease, minimal prior therapy, normal serum albumin, and age younger than 70 years (37,49). In addition, patients who were refractory to alkylator therapy had a lower response rate compared with those who were not (38% vs 93%) (36) (Table 5).

Seymour et al. (78) examined the survival of 91 patients aged 55 years or younger after relapse from (n = 49) or failure to (n = 42) fludarabine administered as either frontline or salvage therapy. The 49 fludarabine-responsive patients who relapsed had a median survival of 87 weeks from the time of relapse. Eighty-three percent of 14 patients who responded to fludarabine as first-line therapy achieved a second response with fludarabine retreatment; 60% of this latter group were alive at 4 years. Of 35 patients who relapsed after fludarabine as salvage therapy, only 7% responded to salvage treatments; however, median survival was 72 weeks from the time of relapse (4-year survival rate 16%). The median survival was 48 weeks in the 42 patients (46%) refractory to fludarabine, and the response rate to subsequent therapies was 11%. The authors concluded that investigation of innovative dose-intensive strategies such as allogeneic transplant were warranted in younger patients who failed or relapsed after fludarabine as salvage treatment because of the poor outcome with alternative modalities.

1.   Toxicities Related to Fludarabine Therapy

The major fludarabine-associated toxicities with currently recommended dosing schedules are myelosuppression and immunosuppression. Factors associated with a higher incidence of toxicity include older age, extensive prior therapy, and disease unresponsive to therapy. Fludarabine has been linked to the onset of autoimmune hemolytic anemia (79–83). The true incidence, causal relationship, and subsequent management of this complication (other than corticosteroid administration) remains controversial; however, it is generally recommended to avoid rechallenge. Nucleoside analog–induced CD4 lymphocytopenia may predispose to opportunistic infections; recovery may require a year or more after completion of therapy (37,77,96). Neurotoxicity is generally not observed unless administered at doses higher than recommended (85–87). Tumor lysis syndrome has been reported, although it is a rare (0.4%) complication that has occasionally been fatal (97). The incidence of secondary malignancies does not appear to be increased (98). Complications of immunosuppression are discussed further in the section entitled ''Infectious Complications of Salvage Therapy.''

2.   Prognostic Factors for Survival and Response to Fludarabine after Alkylator Therapy

The current management strategies for previously treated CLL are not well-defined, because the duration, intensity, and efficacy of previous therapy is not clearly specified in reported clinical trials of salvage therapy. Comparison of independently performed clinical trials is thus limited by the heterogeneity of the study population with regard to features that predict response, such as performance status, age, response to and extent of prior therapy, and stage of disease, among others. Therefore, the expected outcome with fludarabine salvage therapy in CLL patients previously treated with alkylators has not been clearly delineated.

Recently, the outcome of fludarabine salvage therapy in 724 patients (703 evaluable) with relapsed or alkylator-refractory CLL was reported by Sorensen and colleagues (46) of the National Cancer Institute. Thirty-two percent of evaluable patients responded, with 21 patients (3%) achieving CR. The median time to response was 4 months. In an assessment of baseline variables, only hemoglobin level predicted response. The median duration of response was 13.1 months. Overall survival for the group was 12.6 months and was influenced by pretreatment performance status, hemoglobin level, Rai stage, and age. Hematologic toxicity predominated, with grade 3 and 4 febrile neutropenia in 8.7% and 4.8% of the patients, respectively. The cause of death in 655 patients was disease in 74%, infection in 12%, cardiac events in 4%, other malignancies in 3%, and other causes in 8%. The prior treatment history and sensitivity were not provided, and outcome in the fludarabine-refractory group was not detailed.

A prognostic factor analysis for response and survival was conducted by Keating and colleagues (49) for 374 previously treated patients who received one of four single-agent fludarabine regimens as salvage therapy after resistance to or relapse from prior alkylator therapy. At least half of the patients were considered refractory to alkylator regimens as defined by failure to achieve at least a partial response or progression while on therapy. The fludarabine regimens were 25 to 30 mg/m²/day for 5 days every 4 weeks (36), 30 mg/m²/day for 5 days plus prednisone 30 mg/m²/day for 5 days every 4 weeks (37), 30 mg/m²/day once weekly (38), and 30 mg/m²/day for 3 days every 4 weeks (43). One-hundred and eighty-one patients (48%) responded to fludarabine salvage therapy, with 11%, 21%, and 16% meeting the criteria for the NCI response categories (99) of CR, nodular-PR, and PR, respectively. Most responders received treatment for six courses (range, 2–12 courses). The response rates ranged from 46% to 58%, except for the 43 patients treated with the weekly fludarabine schedule; only 23% achieved CR or PR. No differences in prognostic factors could be discerned among the four treatment groups, suggesting the dosing schedule was inferior.

When all 374 patients were analyzed, factors predicting any response included younger age, earlier Rai or Binet stage, preserved hemoglobin and/or platelet count, low white blood cell count, normal serum albumin and/or alkaline phosphatase, low LDH, normal serum creatinine, lower percentage of marrow lymphocytes, lower marrow cellularity, and minimal prior therapy (49). Patients refractory to alkylating agents had a lower response rate (44% vs 60%, $P < 0.01$). Multivariate analysis identified hemoglobin (<10 gm/dL, 10–11.9 gm/dL, or ≥ 12 gm/dL), albumin (<3.6 gm/dL, 3.6–4 gm/dL, or >4 gm/dL), and number of prior treatments (<4 or ≥ 4) as the three significant independent predictors of response. According to the model developed, the predicted response rate for patients in the worst or best subsets of all three categories was 13% versus 73%, respectively (Table 6).

A similar analysis was conducted for survival (49), which was similar among the three response categories of CR, nodular-PR, and PR. Univariate analysis of prognostic factors with a negative impact on survival included older age, advanced Rai or Binet stage, hepatomegaly, poor performance status, low hemoglobin level, low platelet count, high white blood cell count, low albumin, elevated alkaline phosphatase or LDH levels, high percentage of lymphocytes in the bone marrow, extensive prior therapy, and refractory CLL. Multivariate analysis revealed that seven factors predicted for survival: sex, age, number of prior treatments, performance status, hemoglobin, albumin, and alkaline phosphatase levels. Prognostic grouping allowed identification of a subset of patients with a particularly poor prognosis (death within 2 years of therapy). The models generated can

Table 6 Predictions of Probability of Response to Single-agent Fludarabine Salvage Therapy with Prior Alkylator Therapy

Hemoglobin (gm/dL)	No. prior therapies	Albumin (mg/dL)		
		<3.6	3.6–4	>4
<10	≥4	.13	.20	.31
	<4	.21	.31	.44
10–11.9	≥4	.21	.32	.45
	<4	.32	.46	.59
≥12	≥4	.33	.46	.60
	<4	.47	.61	.73

From Ref. 49 with permission.

be used to guide clinical decision making and assist in the design and analysis of clinical trials (Table 6).

B. 2-Chlorodeoxyadenosine

2-CdA (Leustatin; Ortho Biotech, Inc., Raritan, NJ) was first investigated by Piro and colleagues (50) of the Scripps Clinic in 18 previously treated patients with doses ranging from 0.5 to 0.2 mg/kg/day by continuous infusion for 7 days every 4 weeks; a partial response rate of 22% was achieved. Saven and colleages (53) reported a 44% response rate (4% CR rate by NCI criteria) in 90 patients with refractory or relapsed CLL treated with either bolus or continuous infusion 2-CdA. Although the CR rate was lower than observed with fludarabine in the salvage setting, more than 90% of the patients had advanced-stage disease, and all eight patients with Binet A or B stage CLL responded. The median duration of response was 4 months (range, 2–30 months). Infectious complications occurred in 18% of patients; three episodes of *Pneumocystis carinii* pneumonia (one with concurrent corticosteroids), and one episode of *Listeria* were documented. Thrombocytopenia (<50,000/μL) occurred in 25% of cases. Juliusson et al. (54) reported on the efficacy of a 2-hour bolus infusion (0.12 mg/kg daily for 5 days) in previously treated early-stage CLL. Overall response rate was 67%; 7 of 18 patients (39%) achieved CR. Other studies conducted with various bolus, continuous infusion, or subcutaneous schedules have reported response rates varying from 31% to 68% (Table 3).

2-CdA has a similar method of metabolism and activation within the cells to the triphosphate form as fludarabine and would be expected to exhibit clinical cross-resistance. Bromidge et al. (100) demonstrated in vitro cross-resistance between the two nucleoside analogs. However, Juliusson and colleagues (52) treated four consecutive patients who failed fludarabine with 2-CdA, and observed responses in all, including one CR. Other investigators have reported lack of efficacy of 2-CdA in similar patients (Table 3). O'Brien and colleagues (58) at the MDACC reported the largest experience with 2-CdA in fludarabine-refractory CLL patients. The overall response rate in 28 patients was 7% with no CRs observed. Sixty-five percent of courses were complicated by febrile episodes or infections, and 10 patients died within 60 days of starting therapy. Several investigators have corroborated the MDACC experience. No objective responses to 2-CdA therapy were observed either by Saven and colleagues (55) in 14 fludarabine-refractory patients or by Delannoy et al. (56) in 3 fludarabine-refractory patients, although reductions in lymphocyte counts were seen. Rai et al. (68) reported a 17% PR rate in six patients previously treated with fludarabine; responsiveness to the prior nucleoside analog therapy was not specified. Thus, 2-CdA does not appear to benefit fludarabine-refractory CLL patients, and alternative strategies should be pursued.

C. Deoxycoformycin

Several studies have been conducted with DCF (Nipent; Parke-Davis, Inc., Morris Plains, NJ) in various schedules; overall response rates range from 15% to 29% in previously treated patients (Table 4). Grever and colleagues (70) were the first to demonstrate the activity of DCF in CLL. Of 28 heavily pretreated patients with advanced refractory CLL or diffuse well-differentiated lymphocytic lymphoma (DWDLL) given DCF 4 mg/m² intravenously weekly or every other week, 16% achieved a response and 14% achieved clinical improvement. Eight episodes of pneumonia occurred, four of which were fatal.

Other infections observed included *Legionella* pneumonia, *Candida* sepsis, and disseminated herpes zoster. Dillman and colleagues (72) with the Cancer and Leukemia Group B (CALGB) administered DCF 4 mg/m^2 weekly for 3 weeks, then every 2 weeks in 26 previously treated patients. Response rates were similar to those of Grever et al. (71), although more patients (31%) exhibited a clinical improvement. In the previously untreated group, 46% of 13 patients achieved a PR; no complete responses were attained. Severe infections (including two septic deaths) were observed in 34% of patients. Nine cases of reactivated herpes virus, two cases of Candidiasis, and one case of *Pneumocystis carinii* pneumonia occurred, most within 6 weeks of initiating therapy. The European Organization for Research and Treatment of Cancer (EORTC) used a similar schedule to the CALGB in 26 patients with advanced CLL, most progressing on their previous regimen (73). Seven patients (27%) attained durable PRs (median 7 months, range 2 to 17), and all five patients who had only one prior therapy responded. Four patients (15%) had severe infections. Similar results were obtained by Johnson et al. (75) who administered DCF by daily bolus infusion for 5 days every 4 weeks to 24 heavily pretreated CLL patients, 17 of whom had received prior nucleoside analogs with either fludarabine ($n = 16$) or 2-CdA ($n = 1$). Complete responses were seen in two patients (8%) who had no prior nucleoside analog exposure. Five patients achieved a PR; two had prior nucleoside analogs with unknown responses.

Thus, it would appear that nucleoside analogs have significant activity in previously treated patients. The direct comparability of CR rates in these trials is somewhat limited by the recent revision of the response criteria by the NCI Working Group (99); a nodular CR (less than 30% lymphocytes but residual nodules in the bone marrow) was reclassified as a nodular PR. A survival analysis conducted by Keating and colleagues (101) failed to demonstrate a difference in survival by the NCI criteria of CR, nodular CR, or PR after salvage fludarabine treatment in contrast to alkylator regimens (8,16,17,25). However, a longer time to progression was observed for each more favorable response, including the absence of detectable CD5+CD19+ coexpressing lymphocytes by flow cytometry (101,102). Achieving a response to nucleoside analogs after alkylator therapy, however, does correlate with improved survival as demonstrated by several investigators (38,78). This suggests that the overall response rates are adequate measures to compare these agents. These, however, are heavily influenced by the heterogeneity of the patient populations treated and make direct comparisons of these independently conducted clinical trials of single agent nucleoside therapy difficult. With this caveat, and in the absence of randomized trials, fludarabine appears to have the greatest activity with the most favorable side effect profile among the nucleoside analogs tested to date.

V. COMBINATION CHEMOTHERAPY STRATEGIES WITH NUCLEOSIDE ANALOGS

Despite the significant response rates observed with single-agent purine analogs, the CR rate remains suboptimal (including elimination of minimal residual disease). Thus, combination chemotherapy strategies have been used to expound on the unique mechanisms of action of each agent in a synergistic fashion without augmenting toxicity. Corticosteroids have been reported to augment the activity of CLB (3). As discussed previously in the section entitled ''Anthracycline-Containing (±Alkylators) Regimens,'' members of the French Cooperative Group on CLL observed a survival benefit with the CHOP program compared with COP, suggesting a possible role for anthracyclines in improving outcome

(23,24). In vitro studies of the nonanthracycline DNA intercalator mitoxantrone suggested synergism with nucleoside analogs (103–105). The rationales for combining nucleoside analogs with aklyators agents include (1) individual activity of each class of chemotherapeutics; (2) lack of overlapping extramedullary toxicities; and (3) synergistic mechanisms of action, whereby inhibition of DNA repair by nucleoside analogs enhances retention of alkylating-agent–induced DNA cross-links (106–109). Combination regimens incorporating multimodality approaches such as biological agents or monoclonal antibodies are also being investigated.

A. Fludarabine and Corticosteroids

With the reported studies of chlorambucil and prednisone suggesting benefit of corticosteriods, a phase II clinical trial of prednisone 30 mg/m^2 for 5 days in combination with fludarabine, 30 mg/m^2 for 5 days, was conducted by O'Brien and colleagues (37) in 269 patients. The overall response rate was 52% (CR rate of 37%) in 169 previously treated alkylator-refractory CLL patients, similar to response rates reported with single-agent fludarabine. No difference in survival was observed with the combination compared with fludarabine alone. An increased incidence of opportunistic infections (14 episodes among 269 patients) with *Listeria monocytogenes* or *Pneumocystis carinii* occurred with the added immunosuppression favoring the investigation of other combinations (109,110).

An extensive evaluation of the quality of responses was conducted in 159 of these CLL patients (59%) by Robertson et al. (102). Most (77%) were previously treated. Residual disease was measured by flow cytometry for the expression of CD5 and monoclonal surface light chain and by polymerase chain reaction (PCR) for immunoglobulin gene rearrangement. Bone marrow evaluation for residual disease was performed after completion of six courses of fludarabine plus prednisone. There was no residual disease detectable by flow cytometry in 89% of CRs, 51% of nodular PRs, and 19% of PRs (the latter group had no identifiable morphological marrow involvement but had persistent lymphadenopathy). The overall survival was not different by marrow findings when comparing the CR or nodular PR groups. However, the 2-year progression-free survival rate was higher for CR patients without residual disease versus those with persistent marrow CLL identified by flow cytometry (84% vs 39%, $P < 0.001$). Posttreatment immunoglobulin gene rearrangement analysis using JH, Jκ, and Cλ probes demonstrated germline configuration in five of seven CRs and two of eight nodular PRs assayed. Thus, the absence of detectable minimal residual disease was predictive of a longer time to progression and was remarkably attained, in some patients, with fludarabine and prednisone as salvage therapy. Other investigators have confirmed the correlation of longer time to progression with absence of residual disease (112–115). Recent reports of minimal residual disease studies after autologous or allogeneic bone marrow transplant (BMT) have also demonstrated a higher probability of relapse after failure to eradicate clonal disease as measured by PCR amplification of immunoglobulin genes (116–119).

B. Fludarabine and Anthracyclines or Mitoxantrone

The combination of fludarabine and doxorubicin was investigated in a phase I to II study performed at the MDACC by Robertson and colleagues (120). Thirty patients with previously treated CLL (including 25 who had received prior fludarabine) were given fludarabine (intravenously either at 30 mg/m^2 days 1–3 or days 1–4, or 25 mg/m^2 days 1–4) and doxorubicin 50 mg/m^2 day 1. Prednisone was administered to the first 17 patients but subsequently discontinued on recognition of the (1) failure to improve response rate with the addition of prednisone to fludarabine (37), and (2) increased incidence of opportunistic infections with the combination (37,110,111). Although the overall response rate was 55%, the CR rate was only 3%. The combination was not pursued further.

Mitoxantrone induces apoptosis of CLL cells in vitro, and synergism with fludarabine has been demonstrated by several investigators (103–105). McLaughlin and colleagues (121) at the MDACC reported significant activity of the fludarabine/mitoxantrone/dexamethasone (FND) regimen for 51 patients with recurrent or refractory indolent non-Hodgkin's lymphoma. The overall response rate was 94%, with 47% of patients achieving CR. Most toxicities were related to myelosuppression or opportunistic infections. This combination was thus pursued in CLL but without corticosteroids, because of the previous negative experience with the fludarabine and prednisone combination (37).

The regimen containing fludarabine 30 mg/m^2 days 1 to 3 and mitoxantrone 10 mg/m^2 day 1 was administered to 53 previously treated patients and reported by O'Brien et al. (122). As illustrated in Table 7, response differed by prior treatment status and sensitivity to prior fludarabine. In the 15 patients who had only prior alkylator exposure, the overall response rate was 60% (7% CR, 20% nodular PR, 33% PR). In the patients previously treated with both alkylators and fludarabine, the overall response rate was 42% for fludarabine-sensitive patients versus 17% for those resistant to fludarabine. Overall, the combination of fludarabine and mitoxantrone did not appear significantly more efficacious than fludarabine alone (Table 8).

C. Fludarabine and Alkylators

The combination of fludarabine with alkylators is particularly attractive because of the strong rationale for synergistic cytotoxicity. The inhibitory effect of fludarabine on DNA repair was demonstrated in vitro when human colon carcinoma cell lines were exposed to cisplatin with or without fludarabine (106). The cells were then analyzed for repair of interstrand cross-links induced by cisplatin. At 10 hours after exposure, 40% of the cross-links had been removed by repair mechanisms in those treated with cisplatin alone, but only 5% had been removed in cells exposed to the combination. Koehl et al. (109) reported similar findings in human leukemia cell lines and in leukemia cells from five patients with CLL. In this study, all DNA cross-links had been removed within 6 to 8 hours after exposure to cyclophosphamide alone, whereas less than 20% had been removed after treatment in conjunction with fludarabine. These findings provide scientific rationale for studying nucleoside analog combinations with chlorambucil or cyclophosphamide.

The Southwest Oncology Group (SWOG) conducted a phase I study of fludarabine and chlorambucil in 21 patients with heavily pretreated CLL (123). Chlorambucil, 15 or 20 mg/m^2, was given orally on day 1 and fludarabine, 10 to 20 mg/m^2 days 1–5 every 28 days. The maximally tolerated dose was chlorambucil, 15 mg/m^2, with fludarabine, 20 mg/m^2. Dose-limiting toxicity was thrombocytopenia, and multiple course administrations were limited in dose by myelosuppression. The overall response rate was 53% (one CR) in 17 evaluable patients treated at various dose levels. Prior treatment history was not provided. Another combination study was conducted by Weiss and colleagues (124) at the Memorial Sloan-Kettering Cancer Center in 15 heavily pretreated CLL patients. The trial was designed to escalate fludarabine from 10 to 20 mg/m^2 days 1–5 with a fixed dose of chlorambucil of 20 mg/m^2 days 1 and 15. After unacceptable myelosuppression

Table 7 Nucleoside Combination Strategies for Salvage Therapy in Previously Treated CLL

Author, year	Regimen	Treatment status & sensitivity	No.	RR (%)	CR (%)	nPR (%)	PR (%)	Ref.
Robertson, 1995	F + doxorubicin (FA)	All	29	55	5	17	35	120
		Only ALK	5	60	—	20	40	
		N ± ALK, responsive to N	19	59	—	NA	NA	
		N ± ALK, resistant to N	5	40	—	NA	NA	
O'Brien, 1998	F + mitoxantrone (FM)	UT	35	77	20	46	11	122
		Only ALK	15	60	7	20	33	
		N ± ALK, responsive to N	26	42	11	7	24	
		N ± ALK, resistant to N	12	17	—	—	17	
Giles, 1999	F + cisplatin (PF) ± ara-C (PFA)	All	41	19	—	—	19	125
		Responsive to N	11	27	—	—	27	
		Resistant to N	30	16	—	—	16	
Frewin, 1999	F + CTX (FC1)	UT (1) or N-responsive (4), N-refractory (1 PR)	6	71	28	NA	NA	126
O'Brien, 1998	F + CTX (FC2)	UT	20	80	35	30	15	122
		Only ALK	14	79	21	21	37	
		N ± ALK, responsive to N	35	80	23	23	48	
		N ± ALK, resistant to both	24	38	16	16	18	
Van De Neste, 2000	2-CdA + CTX	All	13	62	8	8	46	132
		Only ALK	2	100	50	—	50	
		N ± ALK, responsive to N	6	50	—	17	33	
		N ± ALK, resistant to N	5	60	—	—	60	

No., number of evaluable patients; RR, overall response (CR + nPR + PR); CR, percentage with complete remission; nPR, nodular PR; PR, partial response; F, fludarabine; CTX, cyclophosphamide; ALK, alkylator; N, nucleotide analog; UT, untreated; FC1, fludarabine 25 mg/m² days 1–3, CTX 250 mg/m² days 1–3; FC2, fludarabine 30 mg/m² days 1–3, CTX 300 mg/m² days 1–3; NA, not available.

Table 8 Single-agent Fludarabine Versus Fludarabine Combinations

Prior treatment	RR			% of Assessable patients	CR[a]		
	F	FM	FC	P value	F	FM	FC
Untreated	79	77	94	NS	30	20	44
Only aklyator	56	60	79	0.09	13	7	21
F ± alkylator (responsive to F)	37	42	80	<0.001	9	11	9

RR, overall response rate (CR + PR); CR, complete response; F, fludarabine; M, mitoxantrone; C, cyclophosphamide; NS, not significant.
[a] Not significantly different compared to fludarabine alone.
From Ref. 122 with permission.

was observed at the first dose level, the protocol was modified to administer only one dose of chlorambucil on day 1. The maximally tolerated dose was fludarabine 15 mg/m² days 1–5 with chlorambucil. The predominant toxicity was again thrombocytopenia (grade 3 or 4 in 73%), and the dose-limiting toxicity was infection. The overall response rate was 26%; one patient achieved CR for 28 months. Sensitivity to prior therapy was not specified.

Giles et al. (125) at the MDACC reported an early study in advanced heavily pre-treated patients receiving salvage therapy with continuous infusion cisplatin 100 mg/m² days 1–4 and fludarabine 30 mg/m² days 3–4 ($n = 13$). In 26 patients, continuous infusion ara-C, 500 mg/m² day 4, was added. Seventy-three percent of the patients were previously nucleoside analog refractory. The response rate overall was 19% in 41 treated patients (Table 7). No difference in response was observed with or without ara-C. Toxicities in-cluded (1) tumor lysis syndrome in three patients, (2) dialysis-dependent renal failure in one patient, and (3) infections, with 10 episodes of pneumonia (*Aspergillus* in one patient) and 14 episodes of fever of unknown origin. One patient had cryptococcal meningitis. Significant myelosuppression was observed in more than half of the patients.

A small phase II trial of fludarabine, 25 mg/m² days 1 to 3, combined with cyclo-phosphamide, 250 mg/m² days 1–3, demonstrated activity in five of seven patients with CLL (126). A larger phase II trial of fludarabine, 30 mg/m² days 1–3, and cyclophospha-mide in 73 previously treated (and 20 untreated) patients was then conducted at the MDACC (122). The cyclophosphamide was initially given 500 mg/m² days 1–3 in the first 12 patients; however, significant myelosuppression led to dose reductions. The dose of cyclophosphamide was 350 mg/m²/day in the subsequent 27 patients, then 300 mg/m²/day for the remainder of the trial. The overall response rates were 80% for patients with either (1) prior alkylator therapy only or (2) prior fludarabine and alkylator therapy who were considered nucleoside analog sensitive (Table 7). More than one-third of pa-tients who had failed sequential treatments of single-agent fludarabine and alkylator(s) responded to the combination; the overall response rate in this subgroup was 38% (4% CR, 16% nodular PR, and 18% PR).

Comparison of the fludarabine/cyclophosphamide regimen with single-agent flu-darabine in previously treated patients demonstrated a significant increase in response rate with the combination from 37% to 80% ($P < 0.001$) for patients who had prior exposure to alkylators and were considered sensitive to their prior nucleoside analog regimen (Ta-ble 8). A similar trend favoring the combination was observed in those patients who had only received prior alkylator therapy (56% vs 79%, $P = 0.09$), although statistical signifi-cance was not achieved. A trend to higher CR rates was also appreciated, especially in the previously untreated group.

Other investigators have confirmed the activity and tolerance of the fludarabine and cyclophosphamide combination in CLL and low-grade lymphomas (127–129). Compari-son with dose-intensified chlorambucil suggests better tolerance and higher response rates with the combination regimen (129).

D. Fludarabine Combinations in Alkylator-Refractory Patients

In previously untreated patients, there is no apparent difference in response rates with fludarabine as a single agent or in combination with either mitoxantrone or cyclophospha-mide (Table 8). However, an increase in response rate is observed in patients who were resistant to prior alkylating agents with the fludarabine/cyclophosphamide or fludarabine/

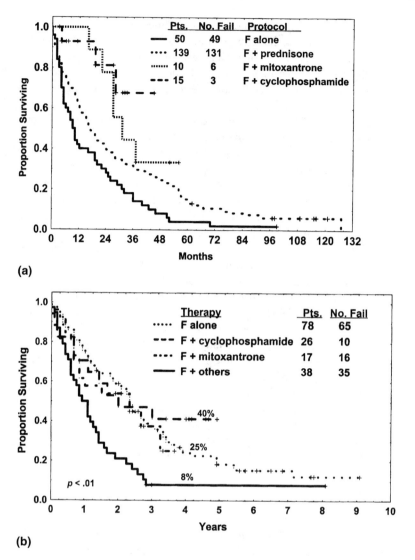

Figure 1 (a) Survival of alkylator-refractory fludarabine-naive CLL patients treated with various fludarabine regimens. (b) Survival of fludarabine retreated CLL patients by fludarabine regimen.

mitoxantrone regimens compared with single agent fludarabine (69% or 60% vs 38%, respectively) (130). The duration of response was also longer for patients treated with fludarabine/cyclophosphamide compared with fludarabine/mitoxantrone or single-agent fludarabine. An early analysis revealed a significant survival advantage for the combination with 2-year survival rates of 80% for fludarabine/cyclophosphamide versus 35% for fludarabine alone (Fig. 1) (130).

E. 2-Chlorodeoxyadenosine Combinations

A phase I study of 2-CdA and chlorambucil in previously treated CLL or low-grade lymphoma was conducted by Tefferi and colleagues (131) at the Mayo Clinic; the maximum tolerated dose of 2-CdA combined with chlorambucil given 30 mg/m^2 orally every 2 weeks was 2 mg/m^2/day for 7 days by continuous infusion. Severe and protracted cytopenias were seen with higher doses of 2-CdA, associated with life-threatening infections in some instances. Extramedullary toxicities included nausea, vomiting, anorexia, and fatigue. Cumulative myelosuppression was observed after administration of two courses. Only partial responses of short duration (less than 6 months) were observed.

Van Den Neste and colleagues (132) performed a phase I to II study of 2-CdA 5.6 mg/m^2 days 1–3 with escalating doses of cyclophosphamide ranging from 200 to 300 mg/m^2 days 1–3 in previously treated patients. Although acute neutropenia was the dose-limiting toxicity, prolonged thrombocytopenia prohibited further treatment delivery in 31% of patients. Eight of 13 patients (62%) responded. One patient refractory to chlorambucil without prior nucleoside therapy achieved CR. Three of five patients (60%) considered resistant to nucleoside analogs responded to the combination. Response outcome by prior treatment status is detailed in Table 7.

A phase II trial conducted at the MDACC of 2-CdA 4 mg/m^2 days 1–3 and cyclophosphamide 350 mg/m^2 days 1–3 was conducted in 30 previously treated CLL patients; 24 had received prior nucleoside analogs (all but one fludarabine; one had prior 2-CdA) (133). Eleven patients (37%) were considered refractory to their previous regimen. The median number of prior therapies was 2 (range, 1–5). The response rate was 33% with a 15% CR rate. Six patients (60%) maintained their response with a median follow-up of 8 months (range, 2–14). Toxicities included grade 4 neutropenia in 22%, febrile neutropenia in 11%, and grade 3–4 infections in 4% of patients.

F. Deoxycoformycin Combinations

Trials incorporating DCF into combination programs are underway. A phase I to II study of untreated or minimally treated CLL patients was conducted by the Eastern Cooperative Oncology Group (ECOG) with DCF 2 mg/m^2 day 1, prednisone 80 mg orally days 1 to 5, and chlorambucil 30 mg/m^2 orally day 1 every 2 weeks for 9 to 18 months (134). Preliminary results showed a CR rate of 44%, with an overall response rate of 87%. Disease-free survival was greater than 32 months. Thirty-three percent of patients had infections, and dose reductions were required in most on subsequent courses. Twenty-five percent of patients developed herpes zoster infection (no prophylaxis was administered), and one case of *Pneumocystis carinii* pneumonia occurred. A phase II study using DCF 2 mg/m^2 day 1 and chlorambucil 30 mg/m^2 orally day 1 every 3 weeks for 8 cycles with GM-CSF support is planned (135).

A phase II study of theophylline, DCF, and CLB was conducted by Byrd and colleagues (136,137). The rationale for incorporation of the methylxanthine compound is the proposed potentiation of cytotoxicity with chemotherapy in p53-deficient cells through the abrogation of the G_2/M cell-cycle checkpoint. Theophylline administration results in accumulation of cyclic adenosine monophosphate (cAMP), thereby inducing apoptosis by way of a pathway unique to both fludarabine and chlorambucil. Down-regulation of *bcl-2* (antiapoptotic protein) mRNA is observed after in vitro exposure to theophylline. A pilot study demonstrated clinical responses in 11 of 12 refractory CLL patients treated with theophylline and an alkylator (either cyclophosphamide or chlorambucil); no activity was observed with single-agent theophylline (137). The current regimen included theophylline dosed to serum levels of 10 to 20 µg/mL days 1 to 9, chlorambucil either 20 mg/m^2 or 30 mg/m^2 day 8, and DCF 2 mg/m^2 day 8 every 3 weeks. Five of seven (71%)

evaluable previously treated CLL patients achieved partial responses; accrual was ongoing. Reductions in bcl-2 and p27 protein expression correlated with responses (136).

Weiss and colleagues (138,139) at the MSKCC initiated a phase I to II clinical trial of DCF in combination with cyclophosphamide in previously treated patients. DCF was administered at a fixed dose of 4 mg/m^2 day 1 with escalating cyclophosphamide doses ranging from 600 to 2000 mg/m^2 day 1 every 21 days for six cycles. G-CSF was administered in addition to prophylaxis for *P. carinii* pneumonia and herpes virus. Preliminary results indicated activity. Several episodes of tumor lysis syndrome were observed.

In summary, the MDACC combination trials of fludarabine with prednisone (37), doxorubicin, (120), mitoxantrone (122), and cisplatin with or without ara-C (125) were disappointing in that none of these combinations increased the response rate compared with fludarabine alone and in some cases may have increased the incidence of toxic side effects. However, the preliminary results of the nucleoside analog and alkylator combinations, particularly fludarabine and cyclophosphamide, are encouraging. Higher response rates were observed in CLL patients treated with the latter combination compared with single-agent fludarabine in the salvage setting. Those who derived the most benefit from the combination had received (1) only prior alkylator treatment (e.g., were nucleoside analog naive) or (2) prior fludarabine and alkylator therapy and were nucleoside-analog sensitive. An early analysis also demonstrated a survival benefit for the combination compared with the fludarabine or fludarabine plus prednisone regimens (130). The fludarabine and cyclophosphamide combination appears to be well tolerated with significant outcome improvements in previously treated patients, and phase II trials incorporating anti-CD20 monoclonal antibodies are underway at the MDACC. Preliminary findings suggest that molecular remissions are attainable with such "triple therapy" (140). Although activity is evident, the alkylator regimens with either 2-CdA or DCF require further study to determine the optimal schedules, because severe myelosuppression appears to be more frequent with these combinations.

VI. RETREATMENT WITH NUCLEOSIDE ANALOGS

The literature is sparse regarding expectation of outcome in patients receiving retreatment with nucleoside analog therapy on relapse of their CLL. As described earlier, the experience with 2-CdA salvage therapy in patients refractory to prior fludarabine suggests that such sequential treatments should not be administered (55,56,58). Sorenson et al. (47) noted that 27 of 212 patients (13%) relapsing after single-agent fludarabine as salvage therapy (prior alkylator regimens) were retreated with fludarabine on relapse; the reported response rate was 25%, and the median survival after retreatment was 14 months. Specifics regarding prior fludarabine and alkylator sensitivity were not provided in this subgroup. Reported response rates in patients resistant to single-agent fludarabine retreated with fludarabine in combination regimens (e.g., doxorubicin, mitoxantrone, cyclophosphamide, or cisplatin ± ara-C) range from 16% to 40% compared with 28% to 80% for those responsive to prior fludarabine (Table 7).

Keating and colleagues (77) reported the long-term outcome of fludarabine therapy in de novo CLL; more than 67% of patients responded to fludarabine retreatment with subsequent relapse, usually administered in the form of combination therapy. Recently, a retrospective analysis was performed evaluating the outcome of 203 relapsed or refractory CLL patients previously treated with fludarabine who received subsequent salvage therapy at the MDACC (141). Prior fludarabine therapy had been given either as a single agent (46%), in combination with prednisone (48%), or with other agents such as cisplatin, doxorubicin, or mitoxantrone (6%). One-third of patients were refractory to alkylators, 30% were refractory to fludarabine, and 17% were refractory to both. More than 60% of patients had received more than one prior therapy (range, 1–7), and 54% were advanced Rai stage III to IV. One hundred fifty-nine of these patients (78%) were retreated with fludarabine alone (or in combination with other agents) on relapse after or failure of the previous regimen. Salvage programs included (1) fludarabine alone or in combination with mitoxantrone (122), cyclophosphamide (122), or other agents (125); (2) 2-CdA; (3) phase I to II chemotherapeutic agents such as topotecan (142), paclitaxel, and others; and (4) bone marrow transplant (BMT). The response rates for the fludarabine combinations ranged from 21% to 65%, favoring the fludarabine/cyclophosphamide regimen (Table 9). The response rates for 2-CdA and investigational agents were poor: 7% each with no complete responses observed; more than 60% of these patients were deemed fludarabine-refractory. The 2-year survival rate for these groups was 15%. Only three patients received allogeneic BMT; one achieved a durable CR.

The multivariate analysis determined the following pretreatment features to be favorable for response: prior fludarabine-sensitivity, preserved hemoglobin level (greater than 13 g/dL), preserved platelet count (greater than 100,000/μL), minimal prior therapy, and fludarabine-based salvage treatment. The quality and duration of prior fludarabine response was also indicative of response to retreatment with fludarabine (Table 9). For example, the response rate to fludarabine retreatment in the fludarabine-sensitive group with only one prior therapy (either alone or with prednisone) was 85%; the CR rate was 22%. As observed with previous studies, responders has a significantly longer survival than nonresponders (Fig. 2). Survival was influenced by a number of prior therapies, prior treatment sensitivity, and salvage regimen administered (fludarabine-based versus nonfludarabine-containing). The incidence of infection for the entire group (203 patients) administered 590 courses of therapy included 34 episodes (6%) of pneumonia, 15 episodes (3%) of sepsis, 53 episodes (9%) of fever of unknown origin, 45 episodes (8%) of minor infections, and 22 episodes of herpes reactivation (4%). Most serious infections were related to gram-negative rods such as *Psuedomonas aerugionosa* or fungal infections such as *Aspergillus* spp. No episodes of *Pneumocystis carinii* pneumonia or *Listeria* were documented.

Therefore, the relapsed or refractory CLL patients who may benefit from retreatment with fludarabine-based regimens include those with (1) previous durable response to fludarabine, (2) minimal prior therapy, and (3) favorable disease characteristics such as preserved hematopoiesis, low β_2-microglobulin, and earlier stage disease. Salvage therapy strategies must incorporate prior treatment sensitivity into expectation for response; patients who have an expected response rate of 20% or less should be encouraged to participate in clinical trials (Fig. 3).

VII. BONE MARROW OR STEM CELL TRANSPLANT

High-dose chemotherapy is limited by the associated toxicities of myelosuppression requiring stem cell rescue. High-dose alkylating agents appeared to be beneficial in a study conducted by Jaksic and collaborators (10) from the International Society for Chemo- and Immunotherapy (IGCS, Vienna) CLL Group, which compared a high-dose continuous chlorambucil regimen with an intermittent chlorambucil and prednisone combination. A 2-to-1 randomization between (1) single-agent chlorambucil, 15 mg daily, until CR or toxicity (prednisone was added if organomegaly persisted despite peripheral lymphocyte

Table 9 Response to Retreatment with Fludarabine or Fludarabine Combinations by Prior Therapy and Sensitivity

Parameter	Category	No. (%)	RR (%)	CR (%)	P value
Any	All	159	43	10	—
Regimen	Fludarabine alone	78 (49)	47	12	0.05
	+ cyclophosphamide	26 (16)	65	15	
	+ mitoxantrone	17 (11)	47	12	
	+ others	38 (24)	21	3	
No. prior therapies	1	70 (44)	64	17	<0.01
	2–3	47 (29)	32	4	
	>3	42 (26)	19	5	
Prior fludarabine	Sensitive	126 (79)	51	13	<0.01
	Refractory	33 (21)	12	—	
	Sensitive (No prior alkylators)	64 (40)	72	19	—
	Sensitive—only 1 prior therapy (No prior alkylators)	24 (15)	85	22	—
Prior akylators	Sensitive or naive	111 (70)	52	14	<0.01
	Refractory	48 (30)	23	2	
Fludarabine sensitive					
Prior response	CR	34 (27)	71	35	<0.01
	Nodular PR	61 (48)	46	5	
	PR	31 (25)	35	3	
Prior time to progression (mo)	≤18	48 (34)	39	10	0.02
	>18–26	47 (33)	41	13	
	>26	47 (33)	62	13	
No. prior fludarabine treatments	1	63 (50)	71	19	<0.0001
	2	16 (13)	38	13	
	≥3	47 (37)	32	7	

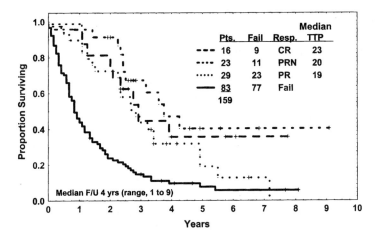

Figure 2 Survival of 159 relapsed or refractory fludarabine-exposed CLL patients retreated with fludarabine-based regimens by response; median time to progression (TTP) was similar for the three response groups.

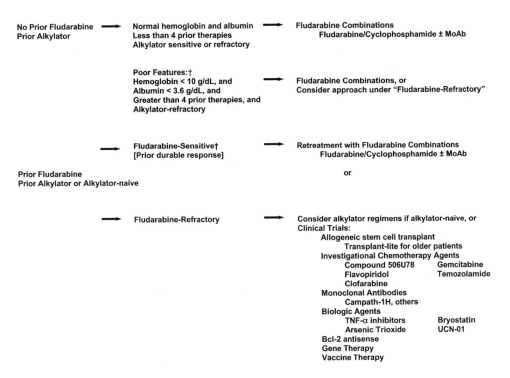

Figure 3 Algorithm for the management of the relapsed or refractory CLL patient. Refer to text and Table 6 for details.

response), or (2) chlorambucil, 75 mg every 4 weeks for 6 doses, with prednisone, 50 mg daily for 2 weeks reduced to 25 mg then 15 mg at 2 week intervals for 6 weeks during the first course with resumption to 30 mg daily for 1 week every 4 weeks. After CR, patients received 15 mg CLB twice weekly for at least 3 years. The patients in the high-dose arm ($n = 129$) had an overall response rate of 89% with a 70% clinical CR rate compared with the second schedule ($n = 52$) with rates of 50% and 31%, respectively (bone marrows were not used to evaluate response). Survival was longer (6 years vs 3 years, $P < 0.01$) in the high-dose single-agent arm. The total alkylator dose delivered was six times higher than the combination regimen, suggesting a dose-response relationship.

Autologous BMT has not been widely applied because of the persistence of residual disease at the time of marrow harvest and ineffective marrow purging techniques (Table 10). Investigators from the Dana Farber Cancer Institute have reported results of autologous intensifications with purged marrow in patients achieving remissions with front-line induction regimens (143). Twelve patients were treated with cyclophosphamide plus total body irradiation (TBI) with infusion of monoclonal antibody-purged marrow; the CR rate was 91%. Several patients treated in this manner became negative for immunoglobulin gene rearrangements by PCR assessments of marrow. Ten patients had maintained their response with a median follow-up of 6 months. The experience with autologous intensifications at other centers, including MDACC, has been less promising with reported relapse rates of 50% to 56% (144,145). The treatment-related mortality ranged from 8% to 19%. Longer follow-up of the MDACC study demonstrated a relapse rate of 71% within 18 months of autologous transplant (146). The use of more effective purging techniques (147), purging agents, and stem cell mobilizations (148,149) may improve outcome with autologous intensifications in future clinical trials.

Allogeneic BMT, however, has demonstrated efficacy (Table 10). The European Bone Marrow Transplant Registry (EBMTR) and the International Bone Marrow Transplant Registry (IBMTR) have demonstrated response rates of 70% to 94% (150,151). Michallet at al. (151) recently reported the European Group results in HLA-identical sibling BMT in patients younger than 60 years. Most patients received conditioning with high-dose cyclophosphamide plus TBI and cyclosporine and/or methotrexate for graft-versus-host disease (GVHD) prophylaxis. The 3-year probability of survival was 46% (95% confidence interval, 32%–60%). Acute GVHD grade II to IV occurred in 37% of the patients at risk. Five patients (9%) died of progressive CLL, and 25 (46%) died of treatment-related complications. Data from the Dana Farber Cancer Institute included eight patients treated with T-cell–depleted allogeneic BMT with cyclophophosphamide plus TBI administered as the preparative regimen (143). Only one case of acute GVHD was observed; six of which had received prior fludarabine. The response rate was 88% with six CRs and one CR with minimal residual disease; event-free survival was 75% with a median follow-up of 1 year.

Khouri and colleagues at the MDACC (144) reported similar results with a lower incidence of GVHD, perhaps related to prior immunosuppressive therapy with purine analogs as noted in the Dana Farber report. Using the same preparative regimen and T-cell depletion, 11 patients received allogeneic or syngeneic (one patient) BMT. All patients had refractory or relapsed disease, and most were heavily pretreated. The response rate was 82%, with most (64%) complete responses. No instance of acute GVHD higher than grade 2 occurred, and only one patient developed chronic GVHD. Ninety percent of the patients remained alive with a median follow-up of 1 year. An update of the early results at the MDACC included 15 patients, 10 of whom had been reported in the previous study

Table 10   Bone Marrow Transplant in Relapsed or Refractory CLL

Investigator (yr) comment	No.	Median age (yr)	No. prior therapies	Interval from Diagnosis[a]	Response (%)	TRM (%)	BMT-related or infectious deaths	Relapse (%)	% EFS[b] (follow-up)	% Survival[b] (X yr)
Allogeneic										
Michallet, 1991 No prior fludarabine	17	40 (32–49)	2 (0–3)	44 (5–96)	94, CR 6, NR	24	1 ED; 1 graft failure 2 GVHD	12	NA (26, 4–48)	53 (2)
Rabinowe, 1993 Six prior fludarabine	8	40 (31–54)	2.6 (1–6)	41 (17–85)	88, CR 12, PD	12	1 PCP pneumonia	12	75 (12,6–18)	NA
Khouri, 1994 All prior fludarabine	11	42 (25–55)	3 (1–4)	40 (15–98)	64, CR 9, nPR 9, PR	9	1 Aspergillus	—	91 (11, 2–36)	90 (1)
Michallet, 1996 No prior fludarabine	54	41 (21–58)	NA	37 (5–130)	70, HR	46	10 GVHD; 4 VOD 2 Graft failures; 2 ARDS 2 Pneumonitis; 4 other 1 Hemorrhage	NA	43 (27, 5–80)	46 (3)
Khouri, 1997 All prior fludarabine	15	43 (25–55)	3 (1–6)	40 (13–119)	73, CR 20, PR	27	1 Aspergillus; 2 cGVHD 1 Adenovirus	20	53 (35, 3–60)	57 (4)
Khouri, 1998 "Transplant-lite" All prior fludarabine	6	60 (51–71)	3 (1–6)	NA	33, CR 33, PR 33, NR	33	1 cGVHD 1 PCP pneumonia	NA	NA	NA
Toze, 2000 3 prior fludarabine	7	44 (32–53)	3 (1–4)	NA	83, CR 17, NR 1, NE	14	1 Aspergillus	—	57 (24, 11–72)	57 (2)
Pavletic, 2000 15 prior fludarabine	23	46 (29–60)	2 (1–6)	19 (4–160)	87, CR 9, PD 1, NE	35	1 ED; 1 Adenovirus 1 MOF; 2 GVHD 2 Aspergillus	5	65 (26, 9–115)	62 (5)
Autologous										
Rabinowe, 1993 Minimal disease state	12[c]	45 (27–54)	3 (1–4)	25 (12–115)	91, CR 9, PD 1, NE	8	1 Alveolar hemorrhage	—	83 (6, 2–31)	NA
Khouri, 1994	11[c]	59 (37–66)	3 (2–5)	49.5 (15–147)	55, CR 36, nPR	9	1 CMV pneumonia	56	27 (4–29)	40 (1)
Pavletic, 1998 Minimal disease state	16	49 (44–60)	2 (1–3)	11 (5–58)	100, CR	19	1 Early death 1 Cerebral bleed	50	37 (41, 22–125)	68 (3)

HR, hematologic remission; CR, complete remission; nPR, nodular PR; PR, partial remission; PD, progressive disease; NE, not evaluable; NA, not available; ED, early death; GVHD, graft-versus-host-disease, cGVHD, chronic GVHD; TRM, treatment-related mortality; VOD, veno-occlusive disease; MOF, multiorgan failure.

[a] Months.

[b] Event-free and overall survival percentage with median follow-up and range in months.

[c] Purged.

(146). Event-free survival was 53% with a median follow-up of 3 years, and the relapse rate was 20%. The absence of severe acute GVHD was again noted; however, two patients died of complications related to chronic GVHD. Similar outcomes have been observed by other investigators (152,153) and are summarized in Table 10.

Achievement of molecular CR (defined by absence of clonal lymphocytes in the marrow by flow cytometry and PCR for immunoglobulin gene rearrangements) with autologous or allogeneic BMT has been demonstrated (166–119,154,155). Disease-free survival appears to be superior in patients without minimal residual disease after transplantation, and the detection of clonal disease predicts a high probability of relapse (116–119).

Because of the advanced age of most patients with CLL, BMT currently has a limited role in the management of refractory or relapsed disease. Nonmyeloablative or "minitransplant" strategies have been investigated by Khouri and colleagues (156) at the MDACC. Six older patients (median age, 60 years; range, 51–71) with advanced, heavily pretreated relapsed or refractory CLL received cyclophosphamide, 300 mg/m^2, and fludarabine, 30 mg/m^2 days-5, -4, and -3 with infusion of stem cells day 0 and short-term GVHD prophylaxis. In the three CLL patients who engrafted, two achieved CR and one had a PR. Autologous reconstitution occurred within 2 to 3 weeks without sequelae in the three who failed to engraft. One of three patients who failed to engraft had a partial response. The other two failures received subsequent therapy, including a second allogeneic BMT or donor lymphocyte infusion (DLI). Death from liver failure ensued in the first patient. The DLI induced a dramatic regression of bulky lymphadenopathy, but the patient later succumbed to *Pneumocystis carinii* pneumonia. An apparent graft-versus-leukemia affect has been reported by other investigators coinciding with the onset of GVHD or DLI infusions (157–160). With these encouraging preliminary results, the potential roles of nonmyeloablative transplants and donor lymphocyte infusions in the management of relapsed or refractory CLL need to be explored further in the context of clinical trials.

Thus, studies with allogeneic BMT (with minimum follow-up of 2 years) report long-term survival rates of 46% to 62% with apparent plateaus on the survival curve. Khouri et al. (161) demonstrated a survival benefit for allogeneic BMT compared with matched controls (by Rai stage, number of prior therapies, and status of disease) in younger patients previously treated with fludarabine (3-year survival rate 58% in 24 patients vs 25% in 48 patients, respectively, $P = 0.004$). Reduction in morbidity and mortality are paramount for future trials; the newer conditioning regimens incorporating monoclonal antibodies such as Campath-1H (see "Investigational Agents and Innovative Strategies") offer promise in addition to the nonmyeloablative approaches (162). Therefore, allogeneic BMT should be considered in any young patient with relapsed or refractory CLL for whom an HLA-identical donor has been identified. The potential benefits (e.g., cure) should be balanced by the attendant risks of morbidity and mortality (e.g., GVHD or infection). Patients with poor prognostic features are reasonable candidates; younger patients who are fludarabine refractory have an expected median survival of 11 months and a less than 20% probability of responding to subsequent therapies (78,163). Several factors appear to influence outcome with allogeneic BMT in the salvage setting, including (1) purine nucleoside analog sensitivity and extent of prior therapy, (2) age, (3) tumor burden before transplant, and (4) donor source.

Although promising, bone marrow or stem cell transplant should not be performed outside the context of clinical trials (161,164–168). It is imperative that future trials refine and address the transplant-related issues of the (1) best candidates, (2) optimal timing, (3) best method such as autologous versus allogeneic versus nonmyeloablative allogeneic, (4) best conditioning regimen, (5) impact of prior therapy, including nucleoside analogs, (6) purging techniques for autologous transplants and their effect on outcome, (7) clinical significance of minimal residual disease or molecular remission after BMT, and (8) role of posttransplant or maintenance therapy.

VIII. SPLENECTOMY

Indications for splenectomy in patients with CLL generally include hypersplenism, symptomatic splenomegaly, or autoimmune hemolytic anemia/thrombopenia unresponsive to standard interventions such as corticosteroids, intravenous gammaglobulin, and/or cyclosporin (169,170). The therapeutic benefit of splenectomy in CLL has been demonstrated in several early studies (171–175). The more recent literature is reviewed herein. In a retrospective analysis, Neal et al. (176) reviewed 57 patients who underwent splenectomy for cytopenia(s) or symptomatic splenomegaly at the Mayo Clinic between 1975 and 1991. Durable recovery of hemoglobin to ≥ 11 g/dL or platelet count to $\geq 100,000/\mu L$ was seen in 77% of patients with anemia, 70% with thrombopenia, and 64% with both cytopenias. The response was sustained for at least 1 year in more than 85% of patients, and transfusion-requirements were significantly decreased. The preoperative mortality was 4% with a morbidity of 26%. The median duration of hospital stay was 9 days (range, 5–24 days). Median survival postoperatively was 41 months in responders compared with 14 months in nonresponders. No preoperative parameters predicted response outcome.

Seymour et al. (177) conducted a retrospective case-controlled study of 55 previously treated patients (aklylators, fludarabine, or both) who underwent splenectomy at the MDACC from 1971 to 1993 and compared their outcome with that of 55 patients treated with fludarabine alone. The two groups were matched for various prognostic factors such as sex, age, hemoglobin level, serum albumin level, Rai stage, number of prior therapies, and time from diagnosis. Most patients benefitted from splenectomy, with improvements in neutrophil count and hemoglobin level. Larger spleen weight correlated with response ($P = 0.05$). The perioperative mortality (within 30 days of procedure) was 9% and was related to septic complications in all cases. Preoperative Zubrod performance status 2 or greater was the most significant predictor of perioperative mortality ($P = 0.05$). Morbidities included pneumonia/atelectasis in 25% of the patients and minor infections in 18%. No difference in overall survival was detected between splenectomized patients and matched controls; however, a trend toward improved survival with splenectomy in Rai stage IV patients (51% $\pm$ 9 vs 28% $\pm$ 9, $P = 0.15$) was observed. The study was then expanded to 77 patients (51 previously treated, 66%) who were splenectomized from 1970 to 1994 (178). Hematological responses were seen in 20 of 29 patients (69%) whose preoperative hemoglobin was ≤ 10 g/dL and in 11 of 18 patients (61%) whose preoperative platelet count was less than 50,000/μL. Fifty-five percent of patients with both cytopenias preoperatively had a hematological response. Postoperative infections occurred in 25 patients (32%), with pneumonia in 11 cases (44%). The perioperative mortality rate was 7.8% and was not significantly different than the mortality rate of 11.7% seen in 18 patients treated with three courses of fludarabine ($P = 0.418$). Median survival of all patients who underwent splenectomy was 34 months compared with 25 months for matched case-control patients treated with fludarabine ($P = 0.266$). In a subset analysis, splenectomized Rai stage IV patients had a longer median survival compared with case-matched controls (19 vs 10 months for hemoglobin $\leq$10 g/dL, and 17 vs 4 months for platelet count $\leq$50,000/ μL, both P = 0.025).

Although these retrospective studies are subject to selection bias and other factors, it seems that good performance status patients with Rai stage III to IV CLL and clinically significant cytopenias may benefit from splenectomy in selected cases. In fact, hematological improvements derived from the procedure may allow subsequent administration of adequate doses of myelosuppressive chemotherapy. Thus, the role of splenectomy should be studied further in a prospective fashion.

IX. RADIOTHERAPY

Radiation therapy was one of the first measures used in the treatment of CLL. Total body irradiation (179–182), [32]P (183), thymic/mediastinal irradiation (184–186), extracorporeal irradiation of blood (183), and phototherapy (187) have all been used. Total body irradiation was not found to be superior to conventional chemotherapy in randomized trials (179,180,188). In a randomized ECOG study, either high-dose (150 rad, n = 26) or low-dose (50 rad, n = 15) irradiation was administered to forty-one CLL patients (188). The response rate was 73%; no complete responses were achieved. Nearly three-fourths of patients experienced severe thrombocytopenia and/or neutropenia with the high-dose TBI. Chemotherapy with chlorambucil/prednisone was administered to 26 patients with an overall response rate of 77% (23% CR rate). No difference in overall survival was observed between the two arms, although the median duration of response was longer with chemotherapy compared with irradiation. Thus, radiation therapy essentially has a pallia tive role in the management of relapsed or refractory CLL for treatment of bulky lymph nodes or splenomegaly which is not amenable to chemotherapy or alternative strategies (189). In patients who are not surgical candidates, low-dose splenic irradiation may be an alternative to splenectomy (189–191).

X. INFECTIOUS COMPLICATIONS OF SALVAGE THERAPY

A high risk of infectious complications occurs in CLL (192), related both to immunosuppression from the underlying disease [hypogammaglobulinemia with humoral dysfunction (192,193), defective cell-mediated immunity (110,111), neutrophil phagocytic dysfunction (194,195)], and the attendant complications of prolonged myelosuppression and lymphocytopenia that may be observed with alkylator (Table 1) or nucleoside analog (Table 11) therapy. In 1973, Twomey et al. (197) reported a higher incidence of infections in CLL patients compared with age-matched controls. The incidence and severity of infections were noted to be increased in patients with advanced stage disease or lack of response to alkylator therapy. In a retrospective analysis of 125 patients followed over a 10-year period, 199 infections were recorded during 447 person-years (196). Forty-seven were severe (9.8 per 100 person-years), and 72 were moderate (16 per 100 person-years). The 5-year risk for a severe infection was 26%, with hazard analysis demonstrating a constant pattern of risk over time. Twenty-one of 71 deaths (29.5%) were attributed to infectious causes in this study. Although most early studies reporting outcome with alkylator-based regimens in previously treated CLL focused on response rather than infectious complications, the incidence of early death (first 3 months of therapy) resulting from infections ranged from 6% to 51% with salvage alkylator-based regimens (Table 1).

Table 11 Infection Rates Observed with Single-agent Nucleoside Analogs in CLL

Author, year	Regimen	No.	Status	Episodes				Incidence[a]
				Any	Minor/FUO	Major	Fatal	No./Cycles (%)
Puccio, 1991	Fludarabine	51	PT	53	25	18	10	53/236 (22)
		22	Responders	40	21	16	3	40/149 (27)
		29	Nonresponders	13	4	2	7	13/87 (15)
Zinzani, 1993	Fludarabine	41	PT	21	6	14	3	NA
Keating, 1993	Fludarabine	78	PT	109	60	49	NA	109/437 (25)
O'Brien, 1993	F + prednisone	169	PT	254	113	112	4	254/886 (29)
Kemena, 1993	F weekly	46	PT	37	19	17	NA	37/211 (17)
Robertson, 1995	F × 3 days	80	PT	63	32	26	NA	63/451 (14)
O'Brien, 1997	F + G-CSF	25	PT	60	36	24	3	24/83 (29)
Sorensen, 1997	Fludarabine	724	PT	48%	26%	22%	0.3%	NA
O'Brien, 1994	2-CdA	28	PT	41	19	12	NA	41/48 (85)
Tallman, 1995	2-CdA	26	PT	19	12	7	3	NA
Robak, 1996	2-CdA	18	UT	4	4	—	—	NA
		92	PT	55	33	14	8	NA
Betticher, 1998	2-CdA	20	PT-IV	14	7	6	1	14/41 (34)
		35	PT-SQ	7	6	1	—	7/89 (8)
Ho, 1990	DCF	26	PT	15	11	4	—	NA
Johnson, 1998	DCF	29	PT	9	7	NA	2	20/88 (23)

No., number of patients or episodes; PT, previously treated; UT, untreated; IV, intravenous; SQ, subcutaneous; F, fludarabine; NA, not available; (—), none.
[a] Any infection.

In a randomized trial of single-agent fludarabine versus CAP in untreated and previously treated CLL, the incidence of early death from infection (4% vs 3%, respectively) or overall incidence of infection (23% vs 19%, respectively) did not appear different between the two arms (21). Direct comparison by prior treatment status was not reported. However, the incidence of infectious complications with fludarabine in the salvage setting ranged from 14% to 29% and appeared to be higher in nonresponders than responders (Table 11). Anaissie and colleagues (111) examined the risk factors for infection in 402 patients who received fludarabine with or without prednisone at the MDACC. Two-thirds of patients were previously treated with alkylator regimens (some with anthracyclines), and 50% had advanced Rai stage III or IV disease. One-third of patients were hypogammaglobulinemic. The number of patients with infections was higher in previously treated patients [144 of 248 (58%)] compared with untreated patients [53 of 154 (34%)] ($P <$ 0.001). *Listeria monocytognes* or *Pneumocystis carinii* pneumonia occurred in 12 of 170 previously treated patients (7%) versus 2 of 119 untreated patients (2%) who received fludarabine plus prednisone ($P =$ 0.036). Risk factors for major infections included advanced Rai stage, previous alkylator therapy, fludarabine-refractory status, low serum albumin level, increased creatinine or β_2-microglobulin level, poor performance status, and poor response to therapy. A baseline absolute granulocyte count $>1000/\mu L$ before therapy was protective. Treatment with 2-CdA has been associated with severe serious infectious complications (Table 11). Previous chemotherapy, advanced age, lymphopenia, and prior infection within 6 months of commencing 2-CdA were risk factors for the development of a serious infection in one study (58). The infection rate appeared higher in patients who were fludarabine-refractory.

Use of G-CSF in conjunction with fludarabine in previously treated CLL patients has been shown to reduce the incidence of granulocytopenia $<1000/\mu L$ (45% vs 79%, $P =$ 0.002) and pneumonia (8% vs 37%, $P =$ 0.004) compared with controls treated with fludarabine alone (48). The incidence of other infections; however, was not affected, perhaps because of other factors such as humoral or cellular-mediated immunity. The induction of CD4 lymphopenia by nucleoside analogs may predispose to opportunistic infections, particularly when combined with corticosteroids (37,110,111). The CD4 count typically falls to 150 to 200/μL after three courses of standard dose fludarabine therapy (43). Five of 19 patients (26%) with absolute CD4 counts $<50/\mu L$ had zoster infections compared with 9 of 139 patients (6%) with CD4 counts above that level as measured after the third treatment cycle (111). Reactivation of herpes simplex virus (199) and *Listeriosis* was also observed with the lower CD4 count. Three different single-agent fludarabine schedules in previously treated CLL patients [5 days (36), 5 days with prednisone (37), and 3 days (43)] were compared with respect to development of CD4 lymphopenia (43). The 3-day schedule had a more gradual rate of decline after three courses (CD4 counts 500–600/μL). The incidence of myelosuppression, major infections, and minor bacterial infections was substantially less with the 3-day schedule compared with the 5-day regimen (43).

A changing spectrum of pathogens has been observed. Fungal infections with endemic mycosis were typically associated with akylating agent regimens; however, an increasing incidence of opportunistic mycotic infections with *Candida* spp and *Aspergillus* spp has been observed with prolonged and profound neutropenia, broad-spectrum antibiotic use, and prior history of corticosteroid exposure (198). The major cause of early death in 147 patients with fludarabine-refractory CLL treated at the MDACC was associated with various pathogens: gram-negative rods, opportunistic fungi, *P. carinii, Legionella* spp, mycobacteria, and reactivated disseminated herpes viruses (198). A similar pattern of infections has been reported with DCF; infections were usually seen within the first few weeks of therapy and were significantly more common in pretreated patients with advanced stage CLL (72,200). The spectrum of pathogens included *S. pneumoniae, Pseudomonas* bacteremia, herpes simplex virus, varicella zoster, disseminated candidiasis, and *P. carinii.* In earlier studies, prophylaxis for *P. carinii* and herpes virus was not routinely administered. Although most herpes virus infections are localized, occasional dissemination may be observed in particularly susceptible CLL patients [e.g., IgG3 deficiency (20) or CD4 count <50/μL (111)].

Newer agents such as biological response modifiers and monoclonal antibodies appear to have a lower incidence of infectious complications. However, exceptions include the monoclonal antibody Campath-1H (see "Investigational Agents and Innovative Strategies"), which appears to cause a high frequency of opportunistic infections (herpes virus, varicella zoster virus, *P. carinii, Cryptococcus, Listeria,* and opportunistic fungi) in the absence of anti-infective prophylaxis (198,199). Cytomegalovirus (CMV) infection appears to be increased in fludarabine-refractory patients treated with Campath-1H. In addition, bone marrow transplant recipients appear to be at increased risk for atypical infection (Table 10); delayed or defective reconstitution of their immune system may account for these observations (202).

Prophylactic strategies and improved supportive care measures to reduce the incidence of infection are needed to prolong the survival of the relapsed or refractory CLL patient. Interventions such as the use of prophylactic anti-infective agents (203–205), growth factors (48,206), intravenous gammaglobulins (192), vaccination, stimulation of cellular immunity, and alternative methods of drug administration [e.g., subcutaneous 2-CdA (67), or the 3-day schedule of fludarabine in older patients (43)] need to be studied. Supportive care strategies are discussed in detail by Ravandi and colleagues in Chapter 22.

XI. ALGORITHM FOR THE MANAGEMENT OF REFRACTORY OR RELAPSED CLL

A proposed management strategy for the relapsed or refractory CLL patient is outlined in Figure 3. Nucleoside analog naïve patients with prior alkylator exposure who have indications for therapy according to the NCI criteria (99) should receive a nucleoside analog–based alkyator combination. Fludarabine combinations with cyclophosphamide have been well studied, and early analysis suggested increased response rates and prolongation of survival compared with single-agent fludarabine in the salvage setting. This regimen is being studied with the incorporation of the monoclonal antibody rituximab at the MDACC, with encouraging preliminary results (140). Those patients who relapse after a prior durable meaningful response to fludarabine (or other nucleoeoside analog) have minimal prior therapy, and favorable disease features are likely to respond to retreatment. Supportive care measures to reduce the incidence of infection in this setting are paramount. Younger patients who have received prior fludarabine as salvage therapy should be considered for allogeneic bone marrow transplant strategies in the context of a clinical trial. Patients who are refractory to single-agent fludarabine (or other nucleoside analogs) or nucleoside analog combination regimens are unlikely to benefit from retreatment with nucleoside analogs with expected response rates less than 20% to 30%. Previously treated patients with poor risk features and/or nucleoside-refractory disease should be encouraged to participate in clinical trials of novel therapeutic strategies or investigational agents.

XII. MECHANISMS OF DISEASE RESISTANCE

Approximately 99% of the neoplastic B cells are in the G_0/G_1 phase of the cell cycle, resulting in accumulation caused by dysregulation of apoptosis or programmed cell death (207). Most antitumor agents exert their cytotoxic effect through induction of apoptosis. This process is mediated by means of an increased expression of the tumor suppressor protein p53, resulting in an increase in *bax* (proapoptotic protein) and decrease in *bcl-2* (antiapoptotic protein), resulting in a favorable *bcl-2/bax* ratio promoting programmed cell death (207,208–210). p53 also increases MDM-2 (resistance protein) expression, which results in binding and inactivation of p53, acting as a homeostatic negative regulator (211). Increased expression of multidrug resistance (MDR1) P_{170} glycoproteins in CLL has been correlated with adverse clinical features and poor outcome (212–219). Elevated *bcl-2* levels enhance resistance to cytotoxic effects of various agents in vitro, including cyclophosphamide, cisplatin, mitoxantrone, doxorubicin, cytarabine, dexamethasone, nitrosureas, vincristine, fludarabine, and 2-CdA (208–210,220,221). Clinically, higher levels of *bcl-2/bax* have been correlated with disease progression (by mRNA analysis) and refractoriness to chemotherapy (by protein assays) (208–210,222). Robertson et al. (223) reported a shorter survival in CLL patients with higher levels of *bcl-2* protein.

Because of the role of p53 in apoptosis, Newcomb et al. (224) studied the spectrum of p53 mutations in CLL and identified mutations at codon 209 and transversions at codon 273 of the p53 gene. DNA strand bias was also observed, as seen in carcinogen-induced carcinomas of the lung, esophagus, and head and neck. Dohner et al. (225) studied the significance of p53 deletions by FISH with a genomic p53 DNA probe in 90 patients with CLL. Seventeen percent of the patients exhibited a monoallelic p53 gene deletion by FISH with loss of band 17p13 by G-banding analysis. None of 12 patients with a p53 deletion responded to nucleoside analogs compared with 20 responders in 36 patients (56%) without a deletion ($P < 0.001$). Other investigators have also detected p53 derangements in CLL (226–228). Identification of frequently associated chromosomal aberrations such as deletion of band 14 on the long arm of chromosome 13 and trisomy 12 suggest that other tumor-suppressor genes and/or proto-oncogenes may be responsible for disease progression (207). Cytokine-mediated biological effects are also paramount in the regulation of apoptosis (222,229–234).

Messenger RNA has been detected in CLL cells for IL-1β, transforming growth factor-β (TGF-β), tumor necrosis factor-alpha (TNF-α), IL-6, IL-7, and IL-8. Foa and colleagues (235) detected circulating levels of TNF-α in 20 of 24 CLL patients (83%) assayed. The proliferative effect of TNF-α has been demonstrated and appears to be enhanced by activation of CLL cells. Correction of abnormal in vitro hematopoiesis was observed in cultures of CLL cells from 11 of 15 patients (73%) after use of specific TNF-α neutralizing monoclonal antibodies (236). In vitro, interleukin-4 has been shown to inhibit apoptosis in CLL cells of previously treated patients (237), and antisense oligodeoxynucleotides to IL-4 have abrogated this effect (238). Transduction of cell-survival and cell-death signals occurs by means of CD40 and Fas receptors present on the surface of CLL cells (239). The mean soluble CD40 ligand (CD40L) appears to be higher in CLL patients than controls (240). In vitro, CD40L appeared to prolong survival of CLL cells by mediating resistance to Fas ligand and fludarabine in a dose-dependent manner, and this effect could be reversed with CD40L antibodies. Angiogenesis (241,242) and alteration of adhesion molecules (243,244) are also postulated to play a role in the progression of CLL.

Several mechanisms of resistance common to both nucleoside analogs and alkylating agents have been proposed and include (1) alteration in DNA repair-synthesis activity, (2) increased glutathione sulfhydryl groups, and (3) failed *bax* induction. MDR1 gene expression may account for resistance to vinca alkaloids and anthracyclines. The role of *bcl-2/bax* in mediating fludarabine resistance remains controversial. Thomas et al. (228) reported a correlation between induction of apoptosis by fludarabine and the ratio of *bcl-2* to *bax*; fludarabine-sensitive cells had low or undetectable *bcl-2/bax* ratios. Both elevated *bcl-2* expression and lack of endonuclease enzymatic activity has been reported in fludarabine-resistant cells, resulting in resistance to apoptosis (245).

In vitro studies have been performed attempting to correlate drug sensitivities using (MTT) assays with in vivo clinical resistance. Johnston et al. (211) studied cells from 31 patients with CLL in vitro with 2-CdA, fludarabine, and chlorambucil. Protein levels of *bax* and *bcl-2* were measured in CLL cells from 25 patients and found to be higher in leukemic cells than normal B cells. However, no correlation between drug sensitivity or cellular levels of MDM-2 mRNA could be ascertained. Treatment of CLL cells with wild-type p53 resulted in both increased p53 and MDM-2 mRNA; however, no changes in *bax* or *bcl-2* were detected. CLL cells with p53 mutations were highly resistant to both chlorambucil and the nucleoside analogs.

Continued scientific research to discover means to restore sensitivity of the malignant cells to nucleoside analogs and to develop drugs with novel mechanisms of action is needed to improve the outcome of patients with relapsed or refractory CLL (246).

XIII. INVESTIGATIONAL AGENTS AND INNOVATIVE STRATEGIES

Several clinical trials of single-agent therapy have reported suboptimal responses in treatment of the relapsed or refractory CLL patient, including intravenous topotecan (142), mitoguanzone (247), and cyclosporin (169,170). However, several agents studied in recently completed or current clinical trials appear promising.

A. Monoclonal Antibodies

1. Campath-1H

Campath-1H (Leukosite, Inc., Cambridge, MA) is a monoclonal humanized form of a rat antibody active against CD52, an antigen present on nearly all normal B and T lymphocytes. The function of this 21 to 28 kDa phosphatidylinositolglycan(PIG)-anchored glycoprotein is not known but is found at a density of up to 5×10^5 receptors/cell on more than 95% of normal and malignant B and T lymphocytes (248). CD52-positive lymphocytes are depleted with sparing of normal hematopoietic stem cells, because the antigen is not present on granulocytes, platelets, or progenitor cells (249). Complement-mediated lysis is induced because of the close proximity of the epitope to the cell surface membrane, whereas antibody-dependent cellular cytotoxicity (ADCC) is elicited only by certain isotypes (250,251).

In early studies, Campath-1H was given to heavily pretreated CLL and non-Hodgkin's lymphoma (NHL) patients intravenously three times weekly for 4 to 16 weeks (252–254). Infusional events included shaking chills, fever, transient hypotension, and/or rash responsive to prophylactic interventions, and tolerance occurred with continued use. More than three-fourths of patients responded, with 47% achieving CR. Campath-1H, however, was not effective in reducing bulky lymphadenopathy (255). Significant responses were also seen in patients with T cell prolymphocytic transformations, because CD52 is strongly expressed on these malignant lymphocytes (256). The predominant morbidity was opportunistic infections such as *P. carinii* and *Cytomegalovirus*. Transient myelosuppression was also observed.

A pivotal trial was subsequently conducted from April to July 1998 with use of prophylactic trimethoprim-sulfamethoxazole and antiviral agents to reduce the incidence of infectious complications (257). Ninety-two patients with fludarabine-resistant, advanced-stage B-cell CLL were given Campath-1H with gradual dose escalation from 5 mg, 10 mg, to 30 mg intravenously days 1 to 3 followed by 30 mg three times weekly for 4 to 12 weeks. The median age was 66 years (range, 32–86). Seventy-six percent had advanced Rai stage III to IV disease, and most were heavily pretreated (median number prior regimens 3; range, 2–7). More than one-third of patients had a β_2-microglobulin level greater than 5 mg/dL. Patients who had received prior bone marrow transplant were ineligible. The overall response rate was 33% with a 2% CR rate; 60% of patients had stable disease. Factors predicting response included lower β_2-microglobulin level (18% vs 42%, $P < 0.05$), platelet count >50,000/μL (40% vs 12%, $P < 0.05$), and nodal size less than 3 cm (44% vs 13% with >5 cm nodes, $P < 0.05$). Median time to relapse and median overall survival were 5+ and 12+ months, respectively (257). Toxicities included grade 3 to 4 infusion-related events such as fever (19%), rigors (13%), and dyspnea (12%) despite premedication. Tolerance developed as treatment continued. Approximately 50% of patients exhibited neutropenia and thrombocytopenia, with recovery seen 1 to 2 months after completion of therapy. Grade 3 to 4 infections included pneumonia (9%), bacteremia (8%), and sepsis (6%). The overall incidence of infection was 19%, with five deaths (5%) related to infectious complications.

The role of Campath-1H is being explored further in several therapeutic strategies: (1) eradication of minimal residual disease after fludarabine treatment, (2) combination programs with fludarabine or other monoclonal antibodies, (3) purging bone marrow for autologous intensifications, and (4) incorporation into bone marrow transplant conditioning regimens and/or GVHD prophylaxis. A subcutaneous formulation has been developed and is currently in clinical trials (258).

2. Rituximab

The CD20 antigen is a 32-kDa hydrophobic transmembrane protein expressed on pre-B and mature B lymphocytes (259–261). Rituximab (IDEC Pharmaceuticals, San Diego, CA; Genentech, Inc., San Francisco, CA) is a chimeric humanized mouse antibody against CD20, which has been extensively explored in lymphoproliferative disorders (262–266). It induces apoptosis (267) in addition to both complement- and antibody-mediated cellular cytotoxicity (268). In the pivotal trial, four weekly doses of 375 mg/m^2 resulted in an overall response rate of 48% in relapsed or refractory low-grade or follicular non-Hodgkin's lymphoma (NHL) (263). Infusion-related events were manageable and included fever, nausea, chills, asthenia, and headache. Marrow *bcl-2* negativity by PCR could be achieved by responders at 3 months after the completion of treatment. Those patients with the International Working Formulation (IWF) subtypes B, C, and D responded better than those with IWF subtype A (tissue equivalent of CLL) (58% vs 12%, $P < 0.05$). Response rate was higher in patients with less bulky (< 5 cm) adenopathy (55% vs 38%, $P < 0.05$), and chemosensitive relapse (53% vs 36%, $P < 0.05$). Long-term follow-up revealed a mean duration of response of 11.6 months, with nearly 30% of patients in remission for more than 20 months (265). Responses have been achieved with retreatment. Because of its activity, it was the first monoclonal antibody therapy approved by the Food and Drug Administration for the treatment of relapsed or refractory low-grade or follicular CD20-positive NHL. A higher response rate (63% overall) was reported in a subsequent phase II trial of eight weekly standard doses of rituximab in relapsed or refractory NHL, suggesting a dose-response relationship (266).

Several recent trials have been conducted with rituximab in relapsed or refractory CLL. Because of the low response rates observed in IWF A NHL patients (269), a dose escalation study (initial dose of 375 mg/m^2 followed by three weekly fixed doses ranging from 500–2250 mg/m^2) was conducted by O'Brien and colleagues in 40 patients with refractory or relapsed CLL (270). Although the response rate was 40%, no complete responses were seen. The response rate was higher in patients treated at higher dose levels (1500–2250 mg/m^2) and in chemosensitive patients. No significant toxicities were observed. An dose intensity regimen of thrice weekly rituximab was investigated in 27 patients with refractory/relapsed CLL ($n = 21$) or small lymphocytic lymphoma (SLL) by Byrd and colleagues (271). The response rate was 46% in 13 evaluable CLL patients and 60% in 5 evaluable SLL patients.

Although tumor lysis syndrome and severe infusion-related toxicity has been reported in patients with high lymphocyte counts, rituximab is otherwise well tolerated without appreciable immunosuppression (272,273). In combination trials with CHOP therapy in NHL, 95% of 40 de novo or previously treated patients treated thus far have responded [(55% CR, 40% PR) (274)]. Clinical trials of rituximab in CLL include combinations with cytotoxic chemotherapy or other agents: (1) either concurrently or sequentially with fludarabine by the CALGB in chemotherapy-naïve patients, (2) concurrently with fludarabine and cyclophosphamide at MDACC in both untreated and previously treated patients (140), and (3) in combination with other monoclonal antibodies such as Campath-1H in relapsed or refractory disease. Up-regulation of CD20 surface antigen by concomitant administration of cytokines such as GM-CSF or TNF-α may increase the number of available CD20 binding sites and thereby augment cytotoxic response; such studies are underway (275).

B. Other Monoclonal Antibodies, Radioimmunoconjugates, and Immunotoxins

Future progress with monoclonal antibodies will depend on (1) engineered monoclonal antibodies with enhanced antigen binding and ability to activate natural effector mechanisms, (2) up-regulation of the target antigens with cytokines, and (3) identification of synergistic combinations of cell surface epitopes that trigger apoptosis. In addition to CD52 and CD20, antibody targets such as Hu-1D10, Lym-1, and CD19 (with ricin) have been identified. Anti-B1, a murine anti-CD20 monoclonal antibody, has been linked to iodine-131 (276,277,278) or yttrium-90 (279,280) in an effort to increase efficacy with selective radiation targeting. Radioimmunoconjugate therapy strategies are being explored in minimal residual disease states in CLL; concomitant myelosuppression prohibits exploration in relapsed or refractory disease outside the setting of stem cell rescue (281,282). Immunotoxins are targeted therapies that are delivered by their selectivity for the desired antigen; DAB486IL-2 replaces the native receptor binding domain of diphtheria toxin with IL-2 (283,284) and recombinant anti-TAC(FV)-PE38 fuses anti-CD25 antibody to a truncated *Pseudomonas* exotoxin (285). Clinical trials with these agents are ongoing for previously treated lymphoproliferative disorders.

C. Oral Agents

Oral chemotherapy is attractive with regard to both quality of life issues and costs. An oral formulation of fludarabine has been developed with 10-mg immediate-release tablets. A pharmacokinetic study was performed in 27 previously treated patients with B-cell CLL or low-grade NHL. Oral fludarabine (Schering Health Care Limited, Burgess Hill, West Sussex, United Kingdom) was administered at a random dose of 50 mg, 70 mg, or 90 mg on day 1 followed by intravenous fludarabine 25 mg/m^2 days 2 to 5 for at least three cycles every 28 days (286). Most patients had received chlorambucil; five patients (18%) had prior fludarabine and 2 (7%) had previous 2-CdA. Measurements of the plasma metabolite, 2-fluoro-arabinsofuranosyl-adenine (2F-ara-A) were performed. Pharmacokinetic studies after single-dose administration revealed a dose-independent bioavailability of approximately 55% (range, 30%–80%) with low intraindividual variation. Systemic exposure after oral administration, however, was dose-dependent and comparable to intravenous dosing. Interindividual variation was observed with the oral formulation as seen with the intravenous form because of differences in metabolism rather than absorption. Major toxicity was related to myelosuppression or infection; other toxicities included nausea/vomiting and alopecia. Response rate in 18 assessable patients with low-grade NHL was 50% with a CR rate of 28%. Response rate in seven assessable B-cell CLL patients was 71%; however, no CRs were observed.

Recently, a phase II study was conducted with oral fludarabine in CLL; 78 patients with prior alkylator therapy but näive to purine analogs were treated (287). Most patients were in the intermediate or high-risk Rai stage categories. With the noted bioavailability of approximately 50%, the drug was administered 40 mg/m^2 days 1 to 5 every 28 days for 6 to 8 courses. Thirty-five of 78 (45%) withdrew early because of adverse events ($n = 25$), disease progression ($n = 8$), or withdrawal of consent ($n = 2$). An intention-to-treat analysis revealed an overall response rate of 41% with a CR rate of 18% according to the NCI criteria. Thirty-two percent of patients required dose reduction, most for myelosuppression. Hematological toxicities included grade 3 to 4 granulocytopenia in 54%, thrombocytopenia in 36%, and anemia in 24%. Autoimmune hemolytic anemia occurred in 5% of cases. The incidences of nausea/vomiting and diarrhea were higher than those observed with intravenous fludarabine; however, few were severe (grade 3–4).

Oral anthracycline administration was recently investigated in a phase II study of idarubicin (4-demethoxydaunorubicin) in both untreated ($n = 7$) and previously treated ($n = 12$) patients with CLL (288). The dose-limiting toxicity of phase I clinical trials was myelosuppression; a total dose of 40 to 50 mg/m^2 orally was recommended for phase II trials. Idarubicin was administered orally 15 mg/m^2 daily for 3 consecutive days every 4 weeks with antiemetic prophylaxis. Overall response rate was 26%, with no CRs observed. Toxicities included nausea, vomiting, and diarrhea. Combination studies were recommended.

D. Nelarabine

Nelarabine (Compound 506U78) was developed after an observation that deficiency of the enzyme purine nucleoside phosphorylase (PNP) induced severed T-cell lymphopenia. The accumulated deoxyguanosine derivative, ara-G, was toxic to T lymphoblastoid cells. Nelarabine is a methoxy derivative of ara-G, which is more soluble. After intravenous infusion, nelarabine is converted to ara-G by adenosine deaminase. After intracellular uptake, ara-G is converted to ara-GTP and inserted into DNA. Nelarabine undergoes rapid deamination, resulting in a half-life of only 16 minutes. However, the ara-G half-life in the plasma is 3 to 4 hours (289,290). Pharmacokinetics reveal a strong correlation between the dose of nelarabine and the plasma ara-G levels achieved (289).

The MDACC participated in three multi-institutional clinical trials with this agent (289–291). Phase I dose escalation studies were conducted in refractory leukemias, with doses ranging from 20 to 60 mg/kg over 1 hour daily for 5 days. Activity was observed, with the highest response rates in T-cell acute lymphoblastic leukemia (ALL) or lymphoblastic lymphoma (LL). Higher intracellular ara-GTP levels were achieved in patients with T-ALL/LL and lower levels in T-CLL. Cellular pharmacokinetic studies demonstrated a strong correlation between clinical response and intracellular ara-GTP levels ($P < 0.01$). Dose-limiting toxicity was neurotoxicity; cumulative peripheral neuropathy was noted at all dose levels. The latter was more common in patients who had received prior vincristine.

A subsequent phase I study was performed with an alternate-day schedule 1, 3, and 5, with doses ranging from 1.2 g/m^2 to 2.9 g/m^2/day. The maximum tolerated dose was determined to be 2.9 g/m^2 with dose-limiting neurotoxicity, including somnolence. A combination study of fludarabine (30 mg/m^2 days 3 and 5) and nelarabine (1.2 g/m^2 days 1, 3, 5) was also conducted. Overall, 37 patients with CLL ($n = 16$), CLL with transformation to PLL or large cell lymphoma (LCL) ($n = 9$), or T-cell CLL/PLL ($n = 12$) were treated at the MDACC (291). Most patients were older than 60 years of age (59%), had received at least two prior regimens (73%), and had alkylator- and fludarabine-refractory disease (68%) with advanced Rai II to IV stage (84%).

The response rate was 31% in B-CLL (one CR) and 25% in T-CLL, with 2 CRs seen. None of the patients with transformation to PLL or LCL responded. Response appeared to be independent of response to prior therapy, immunophenotype (T versus B), or dose. The major toxicities observed included somnolence, fatigue, weakness, tremor, ataxia, myalgia, and peripheral neuropathy. Grade 3 toxicity was observed in 10% to 15% of the patients. Myelosuppression was modest, with acute neurotoxicity observed usually mild and reversible. Peripheral neuropathy occurred predominantly after three or more courses of therapy. A multi-institutional phase II trial is ongoing with nelarabine administered 1.5 g/m^2 days 1, 3, and 5 in B-cell CLL. In addition, the response rate with the combination of fludarabine and nelarabine appeared promising and warrants further study.

E. New Nucleoside Analogs and Chemotherapeutic Agents

Several new agents are currently in clinical trials (Table 12). Clofarabine (2-chloro-9[2′-deoxy-2′fluro-β-D-arabinofuranosyl]9H-purine-6-amine, Cl-F-ara-A) is a unique nucleoside analog being studied at the MDACC (292). Its mechanisms of action include both inhibition of ribonucleotide reductase and inhibition of DNA polymerase; the two mechanisms shared by both fludarabine (F-ara-A) and 2-CdA. Troxacitabine [(−)-2′-deoxy-3′-oxacytidine] is an L-enantiomer form of a nucleoside analog that undergoes phosphorylation to its mono-, di-, and triphosphate forms and is incorporated into DNA (but not RNA) (293,294). The triphospate form inhibits the replicative and repair DNA polymerases in addition to inducing DNA chain termination. However, unlike the other nucleoside analogs, troxacitabine is unable to inhibit ribonucleotide reductase. Flavopiridol (Aventa Pharmaceuticals, Inc., Canada) is a novel synthetic flavone that inhibits intracellular protein kinases CDK1, CDK2, CDK4, leading to an arrest in cell cycle progression at G_1 and G_2M (295). Other proposed mechanisms of action include induction of apoptosis independent of p53, and caspase 3 cleavage (296).

Table 12 Investigational Agents in Clinical Trials for Relapsed or Refractory CLL

Agent	Description	Mechanism(s) of action
Clofarabine	2-Chloro-2'-fluoro-deoxy-9-β-D-arabinofuranosyladenine	Inhibition RNR Inhibition DNA polymerase
Troxacitabine	L-nucleoside analog	Inhibition DNA polymerase DNA chain termination
Compound 506U78	Methoxy-derivative of ara-G	Inhibition purine nucleoside phosphorylase
FMdC	2'-deoxy-2'-(fluormethylene) cytidine Resistant to deactivation by cytidine deaminase	Inhibition RNR DNA chain termination Induction of apoptosis Inhibition angiogenisis
Flavopiridol	Synthetic flavone	Inhibition cyclin-dependent kinase Induction of rapid apoptosis
Bryostatin	Natural from marine bryozoan *Bugula neritina*	Induction of terminal differentiation Induction of cytokines
UCN-01	Hydroxylated derivative of staurosporine	Inhibition PKC Activation of CDC2 kinase Induction of apoptosis
Arsenic trioxide	Organic arsenical	Induction of apoptosis Induction of terminal differentiation
PS-341	Proteasome inhibitor	Inhibitor proteasomes Induction of apoptosis
Bcl-2 antisense	Oligonucleotides (short, single-stranded DNA molecule)	Heteroduplexes to target messenger RNA Induction of apoptosis
TNFR:Fc	Neutralizes TNF-α receptor	Modulation nuclear transcription factors
9-Aminocampothecin	Topoisomerase I inhibitor	Stabilization DNA topoisomerase I complex

PKC, protein kinase C; RNR, ribonucleotide reductase.

F. Biological Agents

Resistance to apoptosis frequently develops in the setting of refractory or multiply relapsed CLL. The 26S proteasome degrades regulatory proteins involved in transcription factor activation and apoptosis, as well as the proteolytic degradation of damaged, oxidized, or misfolded proteins. Blocking proteasome function can lead to an inhibition of cell growth and/or programmed cell death, thereby arresting or blunting disease progression (297). PS-341 is a proteasome inhibitor currently in clinical trials for relapsed or refractory CLL.

As described earlier, most B-CLL cells contain high levels of the antiapoptotic protein *bcl-2* and high *bcl-2/bax* ratios have been associated with in vitro resistance to cytotoxic agents. Down-regulation of *bcl-2* results in a lower *bcl-2/bax* ratio favoring cell death. Antisense olgionucleotides are short (15–25 bases) synthetic single-stranded DNA molecules that form heteroduplexes with the target messenger RNA, ultimately decreasing *bcl-2* protein expression (298). Phase I clinical trials in lymphomas have demonstrated a favorable toxicity profile with preliminary activity (299). Arsenic trioxide is an organic arsenical that down-regulates the *bcl-2* protein expression in B-cell leukemia cell lines and induces apoptosis and terminal differentiation (300).

Basic fibroblast growth factor (bFGF) (an angiogenesis mediator) up-regulates the expression of *bcl-2* in B-CLL cell lines. In a recent study at the MDACC with assays of plasma bFGF among leukemia subtypes, CLL exhibited the highest levels of bFGF (compared with normals, chronic myelogenous leukemia, chronic myelomonocytic leukemia, AML, and myelodysplastic syndromes, AML, and ALL) (242). Thus, clinical study of antiangiogenesis agents is warranted. Bryostatin 1 is a natural compound isolated from the marine bryozoan *Bugula neritina*. Its actions include stimulation of hematopoietic and immune systems and terminal differentiation of CLL to hairy cell leukemia by morphology and immunophenotype (by means of induction of CD11c, tartrate-resistant acid phosphatase, and CD22) (301,302). Preliminary activity has been reported (303,304). Inhibition of TNF-α has been shown to restore hematopoiesis in vitro (236); high levels of this cytokine have been detected in CLL patients (235). Inhibitors of TNF-α include recombinant human soluble tumor necrosis factor receptor (p75), fusion protein (TNFR:Fc), thalidomide, and other agents.

G.   Gene Therapy and Vaccine Strategies

Abnormalities in T-cell function and acquired immune deficiency have been noted in CLL. Increased susceptibility to infection results from defects in both antibody- and cellular-mediated immune function. Anergy to vaccines and/or skin test antigens is frequently observed. The suppressive effects appear to be mediated by TGF-β or soluble CD27 factors produced by the leukemia cells. Although large quantities of class II major histocompatibility antigens are expressed on the surface of the CLL cells, T cell reactivity does not occur (even after neutralizing TGF-β). Thus, the surface immunophenotype appears favorable for tolerance of the T cell. However, exposure to a large number of activated T cells expressing CD154 (CD40 ligand) results in the appearance of several costimulatory surface acessory molecules on the leukemia cell, including ICAM-1 (CD54), B7-1 (CD80), and B7-2 (CD86) (305,306). These are crucial to the proliferative T-cell response to presented antigens. In vitro, insertion of a gene encoding the recombinant form of the CD40 ligand by means of a crippled adenovirus vector (Ad-CD154) successfully resulted in such a phenomenon. These findings are currently being explored further in phase I to II clinical trials (307).

XIV.   FUTURE DIRECTIONS

Prospects for long-term, disease-free survival continue to improve with the discovery and application of new therapeutic strategies aimed at eradication of CLL at the molecular level, including elimination of minimal residual disease as detected by PCR immunoglobulin gene rearrangements. The combined modality approach to CLL may result in an increased proportion of complete remissions, and ultimately true eradication of disease. A palliative approach to the management of multiply relapsed or fludarabine-refractory CLL should be supplanted by enrollment into clinic trials to promote drug discovery (307–310). Improvements in supportive care strategies are paramount to reduce the fatal infectious complications of salvage therapy in refractory or relapsed CLL. Continued intensive research to further understand the biology of CLL and its heterogeneity is required, and novel therapeutic agents are needed to counter mechanisms of drug resistance. The incorporation of potentially curative strategies earlier in the disease course is paramount to alter the natural history of CLL.

REFERENCES

1. DAG Galton, E Wiltshaw, L Szur, JV Dacie. The use of chlorambucil and steroids in the treatment of chronic lymphocytic leukemia. Br J Haematol 7:73, 1961.
2. EZ Ezdinli, L Stutzman, C William August, D Firat. Corticosteroid therapy for lymphomas and chronic lymphocytic leukemia. Cancer 23:900, 1969.
3. WH Knospe, V Loeb Jr, CM Huguley Jr. Biweekly chlorambucil treatment of chronic lymphocytic leukemia. Cancer 33:555, 1974.
4. T Han, EZ Ezdinli, K Shimaoka, DV Desai. Chlorambucil vs. combined chlorambucil-corticosteroid therapy in chronic lymphocytic leukemia. Cancer 31:502, 1973.
5. A Sawitsky, KR Rai, O Glidewell, RT Silver. Comparison of daily versus intermittent chlorambucil and prednisone therapy in the treatment of patients with chronic lymphocytic leukemia. Blood 50:1049, 1977.
6. KR Rai, A Sawitsky, EP Cronkit, AD Chanana, RN Levy, BS Paternack. Clinical staging of chronic lymphocytic leukemia. Blood 46:219, 1975.
7. JL Binet, M Leporrier, G Dighiero. A clinical staging system for chronic lymphocytic leukemia. Cancer 40:855, 1977.
8. E Montserrat, A Alcala, R Parody, A Domingo, J Garcia-Conde, J Bueno, C Ferran, MA Sanz, M Giralt, D Rubio, I Anton, J Estape, C Rozman, and participating members of Pethema, Spanish Cooperative Group for Hematological Malignancies Treatment, Spanish Society of Hematology. Treatment of chronic lymphocytic leukemia in advanced stages. A randomized trial comparing chlorambucil plus prednisone versus cyclophosphamide, vincristine, and prednisone. Cancer 56:2369, 1985.
9. JW Keller, WH Knospe, M Raney, CM Huguley Jr, L Johnson, AA Bartolucci, GA Omura. Treatment of chronic lymphocytic leukemia using chlorambucil and prednisone with or without cycle-active consolidation chemotherapy. A Southeastern Cancer Study Group Trial. Cancer 58:1185, 1986.
10. B Jaksic, M Brugiatelli. High dose continuous chlorambucil vs intermittent chlorambucil plus prednisone for treatment of B-CLL-IGCI CLL-01 trial. Nouv Rev Fr Hematol 30:437, 1988.
11. E Montserrat, A Alcala, C Alonso, J Besalduch, JM Moraleda, J Garcia-Conde, M Gutierrez, F Gomis, J Garijo, MC Guzman, J Estape, C Rozman, and participating members of Pethema, Spanish Society of Hematology. A randomized trial comparing chlorambucil plus prednisone vs cyclophosphamide, melphalan, and prednisone in the treatment of chronic lymphocytic leukemia stages B and C. Nouv Rev Fr Hematol 30:429, 1988.
12. The French Cooperative Group on Chronic Lymphocytic Leukemia. A randomized clinical trial of chlorambucil versus COP in stage B chronic lymphocytic leukemia. Blood 75:1422, 1990.
13. MM Hansen, E Andersen, H Birgens, BE Christensen, TG Christensen, C Geisler, K Meldgaard, D Pedersen. CHOP versus chlorambucil + prednisolone in chronic lymphocytic leukemia. Leuk Lymphoma 5:97, 1991.
14. B Raphael, JW Anderson, R Silber, M Oken, D Moore, J Bennett, H Bonner, R Hahn, WH Knospe, J Mazza, J Glick. Comparison of chlorambucil and prednisone versus cyclophosphamide, vincristine, and prednisone as intitial treatment for chronic lymphocytic leukemia: Long-term follow-up of an Eastern Cooperative Oncology Group Randomized Clinical Trial. J Clin Oncol 9:770, 1991.
15. KR Rai, B Peterson, L Elias, L Shepherd, J Hines, D Nelson, B Cheson, J Kolitz, CA Schiffer. Cancer and Leukemia Group B. A randomized comparison of fludarabine and chlorambucil

for patients with previously untreated chronic lymphocytic leukemia. A CALGB, SWOG, CTG/NCI-C and ECOG Inter-Group Study. Blood 88(suppl 1):141a (abstr. 552), 1996.

16. M Liepman, ML Votaw. The treatment of chronic lymphocytic leukemia with COP chemotherapy. Cancer 41:1664, 1978.

17. MM Oken, ME Kaplan. Combination chemotherapy with cyclophosphamide, vincristine, and prednisone in the treatment of refractory chronic lymphocytic leukemia. Cancer Treat Rep 63:441, 1979.

18. M Itala, K Remes. The COP regimen is not a feasible treatment for advanced, refractory chronic lymphocytic leukemia. Leuk Lymph 23:137, 1996.

19. MJ Keating, JP Hester, KB McCredie, MA Burgess, WK Murphy, EJ Freireich. Long-term results of CAP therapy in chronic lymphocytic leukemia. Leuk Lymph 2:391, 1990.

20. The French Cooperative Group on Chronic Lymphocytic Leukemia. Comparison of fludarabine, cyclophosphamide/doxorubicin/prednisone, and cyclophosphamide, doxorubicin/vincristine/prednisone in advanced forms of chronic lymphocytic leukemia: Preliminary results of a controlled clinical trial. Semin Oncol 20:21, 1993.

21. S Johnson, AG Smith, H Loffler, E Osby, G Juliusson, B Emmerich, PJ Wyld, W Hiddemann. Multicentre prospective randomised trial of fludarabine versus cyclophosphamide, doxorubicin, and prednisone (CAP) for treatment of advanced-stage chronic lymphocytic leukaemia. The French Cooperative Group on CLL. Lancet 347:1432, 1996.

22. M Leporrier, S Chevret, B Cazin, P Feugier, MJ Rapp, N Boudjerra, C Autrand, B Dreyfus, B Desablens, G Dighiero, Ph Trarade, Cl Clastang, JL Binet. French Cooperative Group in CLL. Randomized comparison of fludarabine, CAP, and CHOP, in 695 previously untreated stage B and C chronic lymphocytic leukemia (CLL). Early stopping of the CAP accrual. Blood 90(suppl 1):529a (abstr. 2357), 1997.

23. The French Cooperative Group on Chronic Lymphocytic Leukemia. Effectiveness of "CHOP" regimen in advanced untreated chronic lymphocytic leukaemia. Lancet 14:1346, 1986.

24. The French Cooperative Group on Chronic Lymphocytic Leukemia. Long-term results of the CHOP regimen in stage C chronic lymphocytic leukemia. Br J Haematol 73:334, 1989.

25. MJ Keating, M Scouros, S Murphy, H Kantarjian, J Hester, KB McCredie, EM Hersh, EJ Freireich. Multiple agent chemotherapy (POACH) in previously treated and untreated patients with chronic lymphocytic leukemia. Leukemia, 2:157, 1988.

26. S Kempin, BH Lee III, HT Thaler, B Koziner, S Hecht, T Gee, Z Arlin, C Little, D Straus, L Reich, E Phillips, H Al-Mondhiry, M Dowling, K Mayer, B Clarkson. Combination chemotherapy of advanced chronic lymphocytic leukemia: The M-2 protocol (vincristine, BCNU, cyclophosphamide, melphalan, and prednisone). Blood 60:1110, 1982.

27. F Ferrara, L Del Vecchio, G Mele, V Rametta, F Ronconi, R Montouri. A new combination chemotherapy for advanced chronic lymphocytic leukemia (vincristine, cyclophosphamide, melphalan, peptichemio, and prednisone protocol). Cancer 64:789, 1989.

28. S Molica. Combined use of alpha 2B-interferon, chlorambucil, and prednisone in the treatment of previously treated B-chronic lymphocytic leukemia. Am J Hematol 42:334, 1993.

29. MR Grever, KJ Kopecky, CA Coltman, JC Files, BR Greenberg, JJ Hutton, R Talley, DD Von Hoff, SP Balcerzak. Fludarabine monophosphate: A potentially useful agent in chronic lymphocytic leukemia. Nouv Rev Fr Hematol 30:457, 1988.

30. MJ Keating, H Kantarjian, M Talpaz, J Redman, C Koller, B Barlogie, W Velasquez, W Plunkett, EJ Freireich, KB McCredie. Fludarabine: A new agent with major activity against chronic lymphocytic leukemia. Blood 74:19, 1989.

31. M Grever, J Leiby, E Kraut, E Metz, J Neidhart, S Balcerak, L Malspeis. A comprehensive phase I and II clinical investigation of fludarabine phosphate. Semin Oncol 17:39, 1990.

32. MJ Keating, H Kantarjian, S O'Brien, C Koller, M Talpaz, J Schachner, CC Childs. Fludarabine: A new agent with marked cytoreductive activity in untreated chronic lymphocytic leukemia. J Clin Oncol 9:44, 1991.

33. JS Whelan, CL Davis, S Rule, M Ranson, OP Smith, AB Mehta, D Catovsky, AZ Rohatiner, TA Lister. Fludarabine phosphate for the treatment of low grade malignancy. Br J Cancer 64:120, 1991.

34. W Hiddemann, R Rottmann, B Wormann, A Thiel, M Essink, C Ottensmeier, M Freund, T Buchner, J van de Loo. Treatment of advanced chronic lymphocytic leukemia by fludarabine. Results of a clinical phase-II study. Ann Hematol 63:1, 1991.

35. CA Puccio, A Mittelman, SM Lichtman, RT Silver, DR Budman, T Ahmed, EJ Feldman, M Coleman, PM Arnold, ZA Arlin, et al. A loading dose/continuous infusion schedule of fludarabine phosphate in chronic lymphocytic leukemia. J Clin Oncol 9:1562, 1991.

36. MJ Keating, S O'Brien, H Kantarjian, W Plunkett, E Estey, C Koller, M Beran, EJ Freireich. Long-term follow-up of patients with chronic lymphocytic leukemia treated with fludarabine as a single agent. Blood 81:2878, 1993.

37. S O'Brien, H Kantarjian, M Beran, T Smith, C Koller, E Estey, LE Robertson, S Lerner, M Keating. Results of fludarabine and prednisone therapy in 264 patients with chronic lymphocytic leukemia with multivariate analysis-derived prognostic model for response to treatment. Blood 82:1695, 1993.

38. A Kemena, S O'Brien, H Kantarjian, L Robertson, C Koller, M Beran, E Estey, W Plunkett, S Lerner, MJ Keating. Phase II clinical trial of fludarabine in chronic lymphocytic leukemia on a weekly low-dose schedule. Leuk Lymphoma 10:187, 1993.

39. PL Zinzani, F Lauria, D Rondelli, D Benfenati, D Raspadori, M Bocchia, A Gozzetti, M Cavo, TM Cirio, F Zaja, et al. Fludarabine in patients with advanced and/or resistant B-chronic lymphocytic leukemia. Eur J Haematol 51:93, 1993.

40. L Bergmann, K Fenchel, B Jahn, PS Mitrou, D Hoelzer. Immunosuppressive effects and clinical response of fludarabine in refractory chronic lymphocytic leukemia. Ann Oncol 4: 371, 1993.

41. M Spriano, M Clavio, P Carrara, L Canepa, M Miglino, I Pierri, L Celesti, E Rossi, R Vimercati, R Bruni, et al. Fludarabine in untreated and previously treated B-CLL patients: A report on efficacy and toxicity. Haematologica 79:218, 1994.

42. K Fenchel, L Bergmann, P Wijermans, A Engert, H Pralle, PS Mitrou, V Diehl, D Hoelzer. Clinical experience with fludarabine and its immunosuppressive effects in pretreated chronic lymphocytic leukemias and low-grade lymphomas. Leuk Lymphoma 18:485, 1995.

43. LE Robertson, S O'Brien, H Kantarjian, C Koller, M Beran, M Andreeff, S Lerner, W Plunkett, MJ Keating. A 3-day schedule of fludarabine in previously treated chronic lymphocytic leukemia. Leukemia 9:1444, 1995.

44. E Montserrat, JL Lopez-Lorenzo, F Manso, A Martin, E Prieto, J Arias-Sampedro, MN Fernandez, FJ Oyarzabal, J Odriozola, A Alcala, J Garcia-Conde, R Guardia, F Bosch. Fludarabine in resistant or relapsing B-cell chronic lymphocytic leukemia: The Spanish Group experience. Leuk Lymphoma 21:467, 1996.

45. SB Gjedde, MM Hansen. Salvage therapy with fludarabine in patients with progressive B-chronic lymphocytic leukemia. Leuk Lymphoma 21:317, 1996.

46. MA Angelopoulou, C Poziopoulos, VA Boussiotis, F Kontopidou, GA Pangalis. Fludarabine monophosphate in refractory B-chronic lymphocytic leukemia: Maintenance may be significant to sustain response. Leuk Lymphoma 21:321, 1996.

47. JM Sorensen, DA Vena, A Fallavollita, HG Chun, BD Cheson. Treatment of refractory chronic lymphocytic leukemia with fludarabine phosphate via the group C protocol mechanism of the National Cancer Institute: Five-year follow-up report. J Clin Oncol 15:458, 1997.

48. S O'Brien, H Kantarjian, M Beran, C Koller, M Talpaz, S Lerner, MJ Keating. Fludarabine and granulocyte colony-stimulating factor (G-CSF) in patients with chronic lymphocytic leukemia. Leukemia 11:1631, 1997.

49. MJ Keating, TL Smith, S Lerner, S O'Brien, LE Robertson, H Kantarjian, EJ Freireich. Prediction of prognosis following fludarabine used as secondary therapy for chronic lymphocytic leukemia. Leuk Lymphoma 37:71, 2000.

50. LD Piro, CJ Carrera, E Beutler, DA Carson. 2-Chlorodeoxyadenosine: An effective new agent for the treatment of chronic lymphocytic leukemia. Blood 72:1069, 1988.

51. E Beutler, LD Piro, A Saven, AC Kay, R McMillan, R Longmire, CJ Carrera, P Morin, DA Carson. 2-Chlorodeoxyadenosine (2-CdA): A potent chemotherapeutic and immunosuppressive nucleoside. Leuk Lymphoma 5:1, 1991.

52. G Juliusson, A Elmhorn-Rosenborg, J Liliemark. Response to 2-chlorodeoxyadenosine in patients with B-cell chronic lymphocytic leukemia resistant to fludarabine. N Engl J Med 327:1056, 1992.

53. A Saven, LD Piro. 2-Chlorodeoxyadenosine in the treatment of hairy cell leukemia and chronic lymphocytic leukemia. Leuk Lymphoma 11 (suppl 2):109, 1993.

54. G Juliusson, J Liliemark. High complete remission rate from 2-chloro-2'-deoxyadenosine in previously treated patients with B-cell chronic lymphocytic leukemia: Response predicted by rapid decrease of blood lymphocyte count. J Clin Oncol 11:679, 1993.

55. A Saven, RH Lemon, LD Piro. 2-Chlorodeoxyadenosine for patients with B-cell chronic lymphocytic leukemia resistant to fludarabine. N Engl J Med 328:812, 1993.

56. A Delannoy, G Hanique, A Ferrant. 2-Chlorodeoxyadenosine for patients with B-cell chronic lymphocytic leukemia resistant to fludarabine. N Engl J Med 328:812, 1993.

57. G Juliusson, J Liliemark. Retreatment of chronic lymphocytic leukemia with 2-chlorodeoxyadenosine (CdA) at relapse following CdA-induced remission: No acquired resistance. Leuk Lymphoma 13:75, 1994.

58. S O'Brien, H Kantarjian, E Estey, C Koller, B Robertson, M Beran, M Andreeff, S Pierce, M Keating. Lack of effect of 2-chlorodeoxyadenosine therapy in patients with chronic lymphocytic leukemia refractory to fludarabine therapy. N Engl J Med 330:319, 1994.

59. A Delannoy, A Ferrant, P Martiat, L Montfort, C Doyen, G Sokal, JL Michaux. 2-Chlorodeoxyadenosine therapy in advanced chronic lymphocytic leukaemia. Nouv Rev Fr Hematol 36:311, 1994.

60. MS Tallman, D Hakimian, C Zanzig, DK Hogan, A Rademaker, E Rose, D Variakojis. Cladribine in the treatment of relapsed or refractory chronic lymphocytic leukemia. J Clin Oncol 13:983, 1995.

61. G Juliusson, J Liliemark. Long-term survival following cladribine (2-chlorodeoxyadenosine) therapy in previously treated patients with chronic lymphocytic leukemia. Ann Oncol 7:373, 1996.

62. T Robak, M Blasinka-Morawiec, E Krykowski, M Kasznicki, A Pluzanska, P Potemski, A Hellmann, JM Zaucha, K Lewandowski, A Dmoszynska, J Hansz, M Komarnicki, L Konopka, T Durzynski, B Ceglarek, A Sikorska, S Kotlarek-Haus, G Mazur, I Urasinski, B Zdziarska, S Maj, I Kopec, AB Skotnicki, J Dwilewicz-Trojaczek, P Grieb, et al. Intermittent 2-hour intravenous infusions of 2-chlorodeoxyadenosine in the treatment of 110 patients with refractory or previously untreated B-cell chronic lymphocytic leukemia. Leuk Lymphoma 22:509, 1996.

63. M Brugiatelli, B Holowiecka, A Dmoszynska, O Krieger, A Planinc-Peraica, B Labar, V Callea, F Morabito, B Jaksic, J Holowiecki, D Lutz. 2-Chlorodeoxyadenosine treatment in non-Hodgkin's lymphoma and B-cell chronic lymphocytic leukemia resistant to conventional chemotherapy: Results of a multicentric experience, International Society for Chemo-Immunotherapy. Ann Hematol 73:79, 1996.

64. A Saven. The Scripps Clinic experience with cladribine (2-CdA) in the treatment of chronic lymphocytic leukemia. Semin Hematol 33 (1 suppl 1):28, 1996.

65. D Rondelli, F Lauria, PL Zinzani, D Raspadori, MA Ventura, P Galieni, S Birtolo, F Forconi, R Algeri, S Tura. 2-Chlorodeoxyadenosine in the treatment of relapsed/refractory chronic lymphoproliferative disorders. Eur J Haematol 58:46, 1997.

66. M Mitterbauer, E Hilgenfeld, A Wilfing, U Jager, WU Knauf. Is there a place for 2-CDA in the treatment of B-CLL? Leukemia 11 (suppl 2):S35, 1997.

67. DC Betticher, D Ratschiller, SF Hsu Schmitz, A von Rohr, U Hess, G Zulian, M Wernli,

A Tichelli, A Tobler, MF Fey, T Cerny. Reduced dose of subcutaneous cladribine induces identical response rates but decreased toxicity in pretreated chronic lymphocytic leukaemia. Swiss Group for Clinical Cancer Research (SAKK). Ann Oncol 9:721, 1998.

68. KR Rai. Cladribine for the treatment of hairy cell leukemia and chronic lymphocytic leukemia. Semin Oncol 25(3 suppl 7):19, 1998.

69. T Robak, JZ Blonski, H Urbanska-Rys, M Blasinska-Morawiec, AB Skotnicki. 2-Chlorodeoxyadenosine (Cladribine) in the treatment of patients with chronic lymphocytic leukemia 55 years old and younger. Leukemia 13:518, 1999.

70. T Robak, JZ Blonski, M Kasznicki, L Konopka, B Ceglarek, A Dmoszynska, M Soroka-Wojtaszko, AB Skotnicki, W Nowak, J Dwilewicz-Trojaczek, A Tomaszewska, A Hellmann, K Lewandowski, K Kuliczkowski, S Potoczek, B Zdziarska, J Hansz, R Kroll, M Komarnicki, J Holowiecki, P Grieb. Cladribine with or without prednisone in the treatment of previously treated and untreated B-cell chronic lymphocytic leukaemia—Updated results of the multicentre study of 378 patients. Br J Haematol 108:357, 2000.

71. MR Grever, JM Leiby, EH Kraut, HE Wilson, JA Neidhart, RL Wall, SP Balcerzak. Low-dose deoxycoformycin in lymphoid malignancy. J Clin Oncol 3:1196, 1985.

72. RO Dillman, R Mick, OR McIntyre. Pentostatin in chronic lymphocytic leukemia: A phase II trial of Cancer and Leukemia group B. J Clin Oncol 7:433, 1989.

73. AD Ho, J Thaler, P Styckmans, B Coiffier, M Luciani, P Sonneveld, K Lechner, S Rodenhuis, ME Peetermans, F de Cataldo, et al. Pentostatin in refractory chronic lymphocytic leukemia: A phase II trial of the European Organization for Research and Treatment of Cancer. J Natl Cancer Inst 82:1416, 1990.

74. C Dearden, D Catovsky. Deoxycoformycin in the treatment of mature B-cell malignancies. Br J Cancer 62:4, 1990.

75. SA Johnson, D Catovsky, JA Child, AC Newland, DW Milligan, R Janmohamed. Phase I/II evaluation of pentostatin (2'-deoxycoformycin) in a five day schedule for the treatment of relapsed/refractory B-cell chronic lymphocytic leukaemia. Invest New Drugs 16:155, 1998.

76. BD Cheson. Therapy for previously untreated chronic lymphocytic leukemia: A reevaluation. Semin Hematol 35(3 suppl 3):14, 1998.

77. MJ Keating, S O'Brien, S Lerner, C Koller, M Beran, LE Robertson, EJ Freireich, E Estey, H Kantarjian. Long-term follow-up of patients with chronic lymphocytic leukemia (CLL) receiving fludarabine regimens as initial therapy. Blood 92:1165, 1998.

78. JF Seymour, LE Robertson, S O'Brien, S Lerner, MJ Keating. Survival of young patients with chronic lymphocytic leukemia failing fludarabine therapy: A basis for the use of myeloablative therapies. Leuk Lymphoma 18:493, 1995.

79. Y Bastion, B Coiffier, C Dumontet, ED Spinouse, PA Bryon. Severe autoimmune hemolytic anemia in two patients treated with fludarabine for chronic lymphocytic leukemia. Ann Oncol 3:171, 1992.

80. H Myint, JA Copplestone, J Orchard, V Craig, D Curtis, AG Prentice, MD Hamon, DG Oscier, TJ Hamblin. Fludarabine-related autoimmune haemolytic anaemia in patients with chronic lymphocytic leukaemia. Br J Haematol 91:341, 1995.

81. G Tertian, J Cartron, C Bayle, A Rudent, T Lambert, G Tchernia. Fatal intravascular autoimmune hemolytic anemia after fludarabine treatment for chronic lymphocytic leukemia. Hematol Cell Ther 38:359, 1996.

82. H Gonzalez, V Leblond, N Azar, L Sutton, J Gabarre, JL Binet, JP Vernant, G Dighiero. Severe autoimmune hemolytic anemia in eight patients treated with fludarabine. Hematol Cell Ther 40:113, 1998.

83. RB Weiss, J Freiman, SL Kweder, LF Diehl, JC Byrd. Hemolytic anemia after fludarabine therapy for chronic lymphocytic leukemia. J Clin Oncol 16:1885, 1998.

84. PG Hurst, MP Habib, H Garewal, M Bluestein, M Paquin, BR Greenberg. Pulmonary toxicity associated with fludarabine monophosphate. Invest New Drugs 5:207, 1987.

85. RP Warrell, E Berman. Phase I and II study of fludarabine phosphate in leukemia: Therapeutic efficacy with delayed central nervous system toxicity. J Clin Oncol 4:74, 1986.

86. HG Chun, B Leyland-Jones, SM Caryk, DF Hoth. Central nervous system toxicity of fludarabine phosphate. Cancer Treatment Rep 70:1225, 1986.

87. BD Cheson, DA Vena, FM Foss, JM Sorensen. Neurotoxicity of purine analogs: A review. J Clin Oncol 12:2216, 1994.

88. WR Friedenberg, J Anderson, BC Wolf, PA Cassileth, MM Oken. Modified vincristine, doxorubicin, and dexamethasone regimen in the treatment of resistant or relapsed chronic lymphocytic leukemia. An Eastern Cooperative Oncology Group Study. Cancer 15:2983, 1993.

89. GM Smith, JA Child, DW Milligan, MA Mcevoy, JA Murray. A pilot study of epirubicin and chlorambucil in the treatment of chronic lymphocytic leukemia (CLL). Hematol Oncol 6:315, 1991.

90. W Plunkett, V Gandhi, P Huang, LE Robertson, LY Yang, V Gregoire, E Estey, MJ Keating. Fludarabine: Pharmacokinetics, mechanisms of action, and rationales for combination therapies. Semin Oncol 20(suppl 7):2, 1993.

91. JC Adkins, DH Peters, A Markham. Fludarabine: An update of its pharmacology and use in the treatment of hematological malignancies. Drugs 53:1005, 1997.

92. P Huang, A Sandoval, E Van Den Neste, MJ Keating, W Plunkett. Inhibition of RNA transcription: a biochemical mechanism of action against chronic lymphocytic leukemia cells by fludarabine. Leukemia 14:1405, 2000.

93. HS Hochster, K Kim, MD Green, RB Mann, RS Neiman, MM Oken, PA Cassileth, P Stott, P Ritch, MJ O'Connell. Activity of fludarabine in previously-treated non-Hodgkin's low-grade lymphoma: Results of an Eastern Cooperative Oncology Group study. J Clin Oncol 10:28, 1992.

94. W Hiddemann, M Unterhalt, C Pott, B Wormann, D Sandford, M Freund, A Engert, W Gassmann, W Holtkamp, J Seufert, et al. Fludarabine single-agent therapy for relapsed low-grade non-Hodgkin's lymphoma: A phase II study of the German low-grade non-Hodgkin's lymphoma study group. Semin Oncol 20:28, 1993.

95. PL Zinzani, F Lauria, D Rondelli, D Benfenati, D Raspadori, M Bocchia, M Bendandi, A Gozzetti, F Zaja, R Fanin, et al. Fludarabine: An active agent in the treatment of previously-treated and untreated low-grade non-Hodgkin's lymphoma. Ann Oncol 4:575, 1993.

96. BD Cheson. Immunologic and immunosuppressive complications of purine analogue therapy. J Clin Oncol 13:2431, 1995.

97. BD Cheson, JN Frame, D Vena, N Quashu, JM Sorensen. Tumor lysis syndrome: An uncommon complication of fludarabine therapy of chronic lymphocytic leukemia. J Clin Oncol 16: 2313, 1998.

98. BD Cheson, DA Vena, J Barrett, B Freidlin. Second malignancies as a consequence of nucleoside analog therapy for chronic lymphoid leukemias. J Clin Oncol 17:2454, 1999.

99. BD Cheson, JM Bennett, M Grever, N Kay, MJ Keating, S O'Brien, KR Rai. National Cancer Institute-sponsored Working Group guidelines for chronic lymphocytic leukemia: Revised guidelines for diagnosis and treatment. Blood 87:4990, 1996.

100. TJ Bromidge, DL Turner, DJ Howe, SA Johnson, SA Rule. In vitro chemosensitivity of chronic lymphocytic leukemia to purine analogues-correlation with clinical course. Leukemia 12:1230, 1998.

101. MJ Keating, S O'Brien, L Robertson, Y Huh, H Kantarjian, W Plunkett. Chronic lymphocytic leukemia—Correlation of response and survival. Leuk Lymphoma 11 (suppl 2):167, 1993.

102. LE Robertson, YO Huh, JJ Butler, WC Pugh, C Hirsch-Ginsberg, S Stass, H Kantarjian, MJ Keating. Response assessment in chronic lymphocytic leukemia after fludarabine plus prednisone: Clinical, pathologic, immunophenotypic, and molecular analysis. Blood 80:29, 1992.

103. F Morabito, I Callea, G Console, C Stelitano, G Sculli, M Filangeri, B Oliva, C Musolino,

P Iacopino, M Brugiatelli. The in vitro cytotoxic effect of mitoxantrone in combination with fludarabine or pentostatin in B-cell chronic lymphocytic leukemia. Haematologica 82:560, 1997.

104. B Bellosillo, D Colomer, G Pons, J Gil. Mitoxantrone, a topoisomerase II inhibitor, induces apoptosis of B-chronic lymphocytic leukaemia cells. Br J Haematol 100:142, 1998.

105. B Bellosillo, N Villamor, D Colomer, G Pons, E Montserrat, and J Gil. In vitro evaluation of fludarabine in combination with cyclophosphamide and/or mitoxantrone in B-cell chronic lymphocytic leukemia. Blood 94:2836, 1999.

106. LY Yang, L Li, MJ Keating, W Plunkett. Arabinosyl-2-fluoroadenine augments cisplatin cytotoxicity and inhibits cisplatin-DNA cross-link repair. Mol Pharmacol 47:1072, 1995.

107. A Sandoval, U Consoli, W Plunkett. Fludarabine-mediated inhibition of nucleotide excision repair induces apoptosis in quiescent human lymphocytes. Clin Cancer Res 2:1731, 1996.

108. L Li, X Liu, AB Glassman, MJ Keating, M Stros, W Plunkett, LY Yang. Fludarabine triphosphate inhibits nucleotide excision repair of cisplatin-induced DNA adducts in vitro. Cancer Res 57:1487, 1997.

109. U Koehl, L Li, B Nowak, V Ruiz van Haperen, B Kornhuber, D Schwabe, S O'Brien, M Keating, W Plunkett, LY Yang. Fludarabine and cyclophosphamide: Synergistic cytotoxicity associated with inhibition of interstrand cross-link removal. Proc Am Assoc Cancer Res 38: 2 (abstr. 10), 1997.

110. E Anaissie, DP Kontoyiannis, H Kantarjian, L Elting, LE Robertson, M Keating. Listeriosis in patients with chronic lymphocytic leukemia who were treated with fludarabine and prednisone. Ann Intern Med 117:466, 1992.

111. EJ Anaissie, DP Kontoyiannis, S O'Brien, H Kantarjian, L Robertson, S Lerner, MJ Keating. Infections in patients with chronic lymphocytic leukemia treated with fludarabine. Ann Intern Med 129:559, 1998.

112. L Soper, B Bernhardt, A Eisenberg, B Cacciapaglia, L Bennett, A Sanda, M Baird, R Silver, P Benn. Clonal immunoglobulin gene rearrangements in chronic lymphocytic leukemia: A correlative study. Am J Hematol 27:257, 1988.

113. M Brugiatelli, V Callea, F Morabito, B Oliva, P Francia Di Celle, MT Fierro, A Neri, R Foa. Immunologic and molecular evaluation of residual disease in B-cell chronic lymphocytic leukemia patients in clinical remission phase. Cancer 63:1979, 1989.

114. F Vuillier, JF Claisse, C Vandenvelde, P Travade, C Magnac, S Chevret, B Desablens, JL Binet, G Dighiero. Evaluation of residual disease in B-cell chronic lymphocytic leukemia patients in clinical and bone-marrows remission using CD5-CD19 markers and PCR study of gene rearrangements. Leuk Lymphoma 7:195, 1992.

115. E Cabezudo, E Matutes, M Ramrattan, R Morilla, D Catovsky. Analysis of residual disease in chronic lymphocytic leukemia by flow cytometry. Leukemia 11:1909, 1997.

116. D Provan, L Bartlett-Pandite, C Zwicky, D Neuberg, A Maddocks, P Corradini, R Soiffer, J Ritz, LM Nadler, JG Gribben. Eradication of polymerase chain reaction-detectable chronic lymphocytic leukemia cells is associated with improved outcome after bone marrow transplantation. Blood 88:2228, 1996.

117. JL Schultze, JW Donovan, JG Gribben. Minimal residual disease detection after myeloablative chemotherapy in chronic lymphatic leukemia. J Mol Med 77:259, 1999.

118. S Schey, G Ahsan, R Jones. Dose intensification and molecular responses in patients with chronic lymphocytic leukaemia: A phase II single centre study. Bone Marrow Transplant 24:989, 1999.

119. J Mattsson, M Uzunel, M Remberger, P Ljungman, E Kimby, O Ringden, H Zetterquist. Minimal residual disease is common after allogeneic stem cell transplantation in patients with B cell chronic lymphocytic leukemia and may be controlled by graft-versus-host disease. Leukemia 14:247, 2000.

120. LE Robertson, S O'Brien, H Kantarjian, C Koller, M Beran, M Andreeff, S Lerner, MJ Keating. Fludarabine plus doxorubicin in previously treated chronic lymphocytic leukemia. Leukemia 9:943, 1995.

121. P McLaughlin, FB Hagemeister, JE Romaguera, AH Sarris, O Pate, A Younes, F Swan, M Keating, F Cabanillas. Fludarabine, mitoxantrone, and dexamethasone: an effective new regimen for indolent lymphoma. J Clin Oncol 14:1262, 1996.

122. S O'Brien. Clinical challenges in chronic lymphocytic leukemia. Semin Hematol 35:22, 1998.

123. L Elias, D Stock-Novack, DR Head, MR Grever, JK Weick, RA Chapman, JE Godwin, EN Metz, FR Appelbaum. A phase I trial of combination fludarabine monophosphate and chlorambucil in chronic lymphocytic leukemia: A Southwest Oncology Group study. Leukemia 7:361, 1993.

124. M Weiss, T Spiess, E Berman, S Kempin. Concomitant administration of chlorambucil limits dose intensity of fludarabine in previously treated patients with chronic lymphocytic leukemia. Leukemia 8:1290, 1994.

125. FJ Giles, SM O'Brien, V Santini, V Gandhi, W Plunkett, JF Seymour, LE Robertson, HM Kantarjian, MJ Keating. Sequential cis-platinum and fludarabine with or without arabinosyl cytosine in patients failing prior fludarabine therapy for chronic lymphocytic leukemia: A phase II study. Leuk Lymphoma 36:57, 1999.

126. R Frewin, D Turner, M Tighe, S Davies, S Rule, S Johnson. Combination therapy with fludarabine and cyclophosphamide as salvage treatment in lymphoproliferative disorders. Br J Haematol 104:612, 1999.

127. M Lazzarino, E Orlandi, M Montillo, A Tedeschi, G Pagnucco, C Astori, A Corso, E Brusamolino, L Simoncini, E Morra, C Bernasconi. Fludarabine, cyclophosphamide, and dexamethasone (FluCyD) combination is effective in pretreated low-grade non-Hodgkin's lymphoma. Ann Oncol 10:59, 1999.

128. IS Lossos, O Paltiel, A Polliack. Salvage chemotherapy using a combination of fludarabine and cyclophosphamide for refractory or relapsing indolent and aggressive non-Hodgkin's lymphomas. Leuk Lymphoma 33:155, 1999.

129. M Hallek, M Wilhelm, B Emmerich, H Dohner, HP Fostitsch, O Sezer, M Herold, W Knauf, R Busch, B Schmitt, CM Wendtner, R Kuse, M Freund, A Franke, F Schriever, C Nerl, E Thiel, W Hiddemann, G Brittinger, and the GCLLSG. Fludarabine plus cyclophosphamide (FC) and dose-intensified chlorambucil (DIC) for the treatment of chronic lymphocytic leukemia: Results of two phase II studies (CLL-2 protocol) of the German CLL Study Group (GCLLSG). Blood 94(suppl 1):313a (abstr. 1402), 1999.

130. MJ Keating. Chronic lymphocytic leukemia. Semin Oncol 26 (5 suppl 14):107, 1999.

131. A Tefferi, TE Witzig, JM Reid, CY Li, MM Ames. Phase I study of combined 2-chlorodeoxyadenosine and chlorambucil in chronic lymphoid leukemia and low-grade lymphoma. J Clin Oncol 12:569, 1994.

132. E Van Den Neste, I Louviaux, JL Michaux, A Delannoy, L Michaux, A Sonet, A Bosly, C Doyen, P Mineur, M Andre, N Straetman, E Coche, C Venet, T Duprez, A Ferrant. Phase I/II study of 2-chloro-2'-deoxyadenosine with cyclophosphamide in patients with pretreated B cell chronic lymphocytic leukemia and indolent non-Hodgkin's lymphoma. Leukemia 14:1136, 2000.

133. M Montillo, A Tedeschi, F DiRaimondo, S O'Brien, S Lerner, E Morra, MJ Keating. Phase II study of 2-chlorodeoxyadenosine (2-CdA) and cyclophosphamide (CP) in patients with chronic lymphocytic leukemia. Blood 94(suppl 1):127a (abstr. 559), 1999.

134. MM Oken, S Lee, PA Cassileth, RL Krigel. Pentostatin, chlorambucil, and prednisone for the treatment of chronic lymphocytic leukemia: Eastern Cooperative Oncology Group Protocol E1488. Proc Am Soc Clin Oncol 17:6a (abstr. 22), 1998.

135. JK Waselenko, MR Grever, M Beer, MA Lucas, JC Byrd. Pentostatin (Nipent) and chloram-

bucil with granulocyte-macrophage colony-stimulating factor support for patients with previously untreated, treated, and fludarabine-refractory B-cell chronic lymphocytic leukemia. Semin Oncol 27(2 suppl 5):44, 2000.

136. JC Byrd, CR Willis, JK Waselenko, K Park, A Goodrich, C Morrison, MA Lucas, C Shinn, LF Diehl, MR Grever, IW Flinn. Theophylline, pentostatin, and chlorambucil; A dose escalation study to modulate intrinsic biologic resistance mechanisms in patients with relapsed lymphoproliferative disorders. Blood 94(suppl 1):308b (abstr. 4602), 1999.

137. JC Byrd, MR Grever, JK Waselenko, CR Willis, K Park, A Goodrich, MA Lucas, C Shinn, IW Flinn. Theophylline, pentostatin (Nipent), and chlorambucil: a dose-escalation study targeting intrinsic biologic resistance mechanisms in patients with relapsed lymphoproliferative disorders. Semin Oncol 27(2 suppl 5):37, 2000.

138. M Weiss, P Maslak, D Scheinberg, S Kossman. A phase I study of pentostatin and cyclophosphamide (CTX) for previously treated patients with CLL. Blood 94(suppl 1):316b (abstr. 4637), 1999.

139. MA Weiss. A phase I and II study of pentostatin (Nipent) with cyclophosphamide for previously treated patients with chronic lymphocytic leukemia. Semin Oncol 27(2 suppl. 5):41, 2000.

140. MJ Keating, S O'Brien, J Cortes, F Giles, H Kantarjian. Fludarabine and cyclophosphamide combined with Rituxan (FCR) is a potent cytoreductive regimen as initial therapy of chronic lymphocytic leukemia. Proc Am Soc Clin Oncol 19:8a (abstr. 21), 2000.

141. D Thomas, S O'Brien, H Kantarjian, FJ Giles, S Lerner, and MJ Keating. Outcome in 203 patients (pts) with relapsed or refractory B-cell chronic lymphocytic leukemia (CLL) with salvage therapy (Rx): Retreatment with fludarabine (FLU). Blood 92 (suppl 1):102a (abstr. 419), 1998.

142. S O'Brien, H Kantarjian, A Ellis, L Zwelling, E Estey, M Keating. Topotecan in chronic lymphocytic leukemia. Cancer 75:1104, 1995.

143. SN Rabinowe, RJ Soiffer, JG Gribben, H Daley, AS Freedman, J Daley, K Pesek, D Neuberg, G Pinkus, PR Leavitt, et al. Autologous and allogeneic bone marrow transplantation for poor prognosis patients with B-cell chronic lymphocytic leukemia. Blood 82:1366, 1993.

144. IF Khouri, MJ Keating, HM Vriesendorp, CL Reading, D Przepiorka, YO Huh, BS Andersson, KW van Besien, RC Mehra, SA Giralt, et al. Autologous and allogeneic bone marrow transplant for chronic lymphocytic leukemia: Preliminary results. J Clin Oncol 12:748, 1994.

145. ZS Pavletic, PJ Bierman, JM Vose, MR Bishop, CD Wu, JL Pierson, JP Kollath, DD Weisenburger, A Kessinger, JO Armitage. High incidence of relapse after autologous stem-cell transplantation for B-cell chronic lymphocytic leukemia or small lymphocytic lymphoma. Ann Oncol 9:1023, 1998.

146. IF Khouri, D Przepiorka, K van Besien, S O'Brien, JL Palmer, S Lerner, RC Mehra, HM Vriesendorp, BS Andersson, S Giralt, M Korbling, MJ Keating, RE Champlin. Allogeneic blood or marrow transplantation for chronic lymphocytic leukaemia: Timing of transplantation and potential effect of fludarabine on acute graft-versus-host disease. Br J Haematol 97:466, 1997.

147. U Paulus, N Schmitz, K Viehmann, N von Neuhoff, P Dreger. Combined positive/negative selection for highly effective purging of PBPC grafts: Towards clinical application in patients with B-CLL. Bone Marrow Transplant 20:415, 1997.

148. M Michallet, A Thiebaut, P Dreger, K Remes, N Milpied, G Santini, M Hamon, B Bjorkstrand, E Kimby, A Belhabri, ML Tanguy, JF Apperley. Peripheral blood stem cell (PBSC) mobilization and transplantation after fludarabine therapy in chronic lymphocytic leukaemia (CLL): A report of the European Blood and Marrow Transplantation (EBMT) CLL subcommittee on behalf of the EBMT Chronic Leukaemias Working Party (CLWP). Br J Haematol 108:595, 2000.

149. M Itala, TT Pelliniemi, A Rajamaki, K Remes. Autologous blood cell transplantation in B-

CLL: Response to chemotherapy prior to mobilization predicts the stem cell yield. Bone Marrow Transplant 19:647, 1997.

150. M Michallet, B Corront, D Hollard, A Gratwohl, N Milpied, C Dauriac, S Brunet, J Soler, JP Jouet, H Esperou Bourdeau, W Arcese, F Witz, A Moine, FE Zwaan. Allogenic bone marrow transplantation in chronic lymphocytic leukemia: 17 cases. Report from the EBMTG. Bone Marrow Transplant 7:275, 1991.

151. M Michallet, E Archimbaud, G Bandini, PA Rowlings, HJ Deeg, G Gahrton, E Montserrat, C Rozman, A Gratwohl, RP Gale. HLA-identical sibling bone marrow transplantation in younger patients with chronic lymphocytic leukemia. European Group for Blood and Marrow Transplantation and the International Bone Marrow Transplant Registry. Ann Intern Med 124:311, 1996.

152. ZS Pavletic, ER Arrowsmith, PJ Bierman, SA Goodman, JM Vose, SR Tarantolo, RS Stein, G Bociek, JP Greer, CD Wu, JP Kollath, DD Weisenburger, A Kessinger, SN Wolff, JO Armitage, MR Bishop. Outcome of allogeneic stem cell transplantation for B cell chronic lymphocytic leukemia. Bone Marrow Transplant 25:717, 2000.

153. CL Toze, JD Shepherd, JM Connors, NJ Voss, RD Gascoyne, DE Hogge, HG Klingemann, SH Nantel, TJ Nevill, GL Phillips, DE Reece, HJ Sutherland, MJ Barnett. Allogeneic bone marrow transplantation for low-grade lymphoma and chronic lymphocytic leukemia. Bone Marrow Transplant 25:605, 2000.

154. A Sadoun, S Patri, V Delwail, JC Chomel, M Cogne, A Brizard, A Kitzis, F Guilhot. Molecular remission after allogeneic bone marrow transplantation for chronic lymphocytic leukemia. Bone Marrow Transplant 13:217, 1994.

155. C Martinez, R Martino, S Brunet, A Sureda, J Nomdedeu, A Garcia, J Soler, A Domingo-Albos. Allogeneic stem cell transplantation for advanced low-grade lymphoproliferative disorders: Report of six cases. Haematologica 81:330, 1996.

156. IF Khouri, M Keating, M Korbling, D Przepiorka, P Anderlini, S O'Brien, S Giralt, C Ippoliti, B von Wolff, J Gajewski, M Donato, D Claxton, N Ueno, B Andersson, A Gee, R Champlin. Transplant-lite: Induction of graft-versus-malignancy using fludarabine-based nonablative chemotherapy and allogeneic blood progenitor-cell transplantation as treatment for lymphoid malignancies. J Clin Oncol 16:2817, 1998.

157. G Rondon, S Giralt, Y Huh, I Khouri, B Andersson, M Andreeff, R Champlin. Graft-versus-leukemia effect after allogeneic bone marrow transplantation for chronic lymphocytic leukemia. Bone Marrow Transplant 18:669, 1996.

158. J Mehta, R Powles, S Singhal, T Iveson, J Treleaven, D Catovsky. Clinical and hematologic response of chronic lymphocytic and prolymphocytic leukemia persisting after allogeneic bone marrow transplantation with the onset of acute graft-versus-host disease: Possible role of graft-versus-leukemia. Bone Marrow Transplant 17:371, 1996.

159. M deMagalhaes-Silverman, A Donnenberg, L Hammert, J Lister, D Myers, J Simpson, E Ball. Induction of graft-versus-leukemia effect in a patient with chronic lymphocytic leukemia. Bone Marrow Transplant 20:175, 1997.

160. J Mehta, R Powles, S Kulkarni, J Treleaven, S Singhal. Induction of graft-versus-host disease as immunotherapy of leukemia relapsing after allogeneic transplantation: Single-center experience of 32 adult patients. Bone Marrow Transplant 20:129, 1997.

161. IF Khouri, MJ Keating, R Champlin. Hematopoietic stem cell transplantation for chronic lymphocytic leukemia. Curr Opin Hematol 5:454, 1998.

162. GM Cull, AP Haynes, JL Byrne, GI Carter, G Miflin, P Rebello, G Hale, H Waldmann, NH Russell. Preliminary experience of allogeneic stem cell transplantation for lymphoproliferative disorders using BEAM-CAMPATH conditioning: An effective regimen with low procedure-related toxicity. Br J Haematol 108:754, 2000.

163. M de Lima, S O'Brien, S Lerner, MJ Keating. Chronic lymphocytic leukemia in the young patient. Semin Oncol 25:107, 1998.

164. P Dreger, N von Neuhoff, R Kuse, R Sonnen, B Glass, L Uharek, R Schoch, H Loffler, N

Schmitz. Early stem cell transplantation for chronic lymphocytic leukaemia: A chance for cure? Br J Cancer 77:2291, 1998.

165. IW Flinn, G Vogelsang. Bone marrow transplantation for chronic lymphocytic leukemia. Semin Oncol 25:60, 1998.

166. IF Khouri, MJ Keating. High-dose chemotherapy for chronic lymphocytic leukemia: Eligibility, timing, and benefit? Ann Oncol 9:131, 1998.

167. JK Waselenko, JM Flynn, JC Byrd. Stem-cell transplantation in chronic lymphocytic leukemia: The time for designing randomized studies has arrived. Semin Oncol 26:48, 1999.

168. P Dreger, M Michallet, N Schmitz. Stem-cell transplantation for chronic lymphocytic leukemia: The 1999 perspective. Ann Oncol 11 (suppl 1):49, 2000.

169. E Van Den Neste, M Maerevoet, P Martiat, A Ferrant, A Delannoy, JL Michaux. Cyclosporin A in the treatment of refractory B chronic lymphocytic leukemia (B-CLL). Leukemia 9:1102, 1995.

170. K Nishii, N Katayama, H Mitani, T Matsumoto, H Miwa, K Kita, H Shiku. Effects of cyclosporin A on refractory B-cell chronic lymphocytic leukemia. Int J Hematol 71:59, 2000.

171. A Ferrant, JL Michaux, G Sokal. Splenectomy in advanced chronic lymphocytic leukemia. Cancer 58:2130, 1986.

172. JR Delpero, JA Gastaut, YP Letreut, A Caamano, N Mathieu-Tubiana, D Maraninchi, C Simon-Lejeune, B Mascret, AP Blanc, G Sebahoun, et al. The value of splenectomy in chronic lymphocytic leukemia. Cancer 59:340, 1987.

173. RS Stein, D Weikert, V Reynolds, JP Greer, JM Flexner. Splenectomy for end-stage chronic lymphocytic leukemia. Cancer 59:1815, 1987.

174. G Majumdar, AK Singh. Role of splenectomy in chronic lymphocytic leukaemia with massive splenomegaly and cytopenia. Leuk Lymphoma 7:131, 1992.

175. R Thiruvengadam, M Piedmonte, M Barcos, T Han, ES Henderson. Splenectomy in advanced chronic lymphocytic leukemia. Leukemia 4:758, 1990.

176. TF Neal Jr, A Tefferi, TE Witzig, J Su, RL Phyliky, DM Nagorney. Splenectomy in advanced chronic lymphocytic leukemia: A single institution experience with 50 patients. Am J Med 93:435, 1992.

177. JF Seymour, JD Cusack, SA Lerner, RE Pollock, MJ Keating. Case/control study of the role of splenectomy in chronic lymphocytic leukemia. J Clin Oncol 15:52, 1997.

178. JC Cusack Jr, JF Seymour, S Lerner, MJ Keating, RE Pollock. Role of splenectomy in chronic lymphocytic leukemia. J Am Coll Surg 185:237, 1997.

179. RE Johnson. Total body irradiation of chronic lymphocytic leukemia. Relationship between therapeutic response and prognosis. Cancer 37:2691, 1976.

180. RE Johnson, U Ruhl. Treatment of chronic lymphocytic leukemia with emphasis on total body irradiation. Int J Radiat Oncol Biol Phys 1:387, 1976.

181. P Jacobs, HS King. A randomized prospective comparison of chemotherapy to total body irradiation as initial treatment for the indolent lymphoproliferative diseases. Blood 69:1642, 1987.

182. P Rubin, JM Bennett, C Begg, MJ Bozdech, R Silber. The comparison of total body irradiation vs chlorambucil and prednisone for remission induction of active chronic lymphocytic leukemia: an ECOG study. Part I: total body irradiation-response and toxicity. Int J Radiat Oncol Biol Phys 7:1623, 1981.

183. Editorial. Radiotherapy for chronic lymphocytic leukemia. Lancet 1:82, 1979.

184. AD Novetsky, LB Garner, SM Lichter. Multiple remissions induced by mediastinal irradiation in a patient with chronic lymphocytic leukemia. Radiology 143:549, 1982.

185. F Richards Jr, CL Spurr, C Ferree, DD Blake, M Raben. The control of chronic lymphocytic leukemia with mediastinal irradiation. Am J Med 64:947, 1978.

186. F Richards Jr, CL Spurr, TF Pajak, DD Blake, M Raben. Thymic irradiation. An approach to chronic lymphocytic leukemia. Am J Med 57:862, 1974.

187. JS Wieselthier, TL Rothstein, TL Yu, T Anderson, MC Japowicz, HK Koh. Inefficacy of

extracorporeal photochemotherapy in the treatment of B-cell chronic lymphocytic leukemia: Preliminary results. Am J Hematol 41:123, 1992.

188. JM Bennett, B Raphael, D Moore, R Silber, MM Oken, P Rubin. Comparison of chlorambucil and prednisone vs. total body irradiation and chlorambucil/prednisone vs. cytoxan, vincristine, prednisone for the therapy of active chronic lymphocytic leukemia: A long term follow-up of two ECOG studies. In: RP Gale, KR Rai, eds. Chronic Lymphocytic Leukemia: Recent Progress and Future Direction UCLA Symposium on Molecular and Cellular Biology. New series. Vol. 59. New York: Alan Liss, 1987, p 317.

189. K Aabo, S Walbom-Jorgensen. Spleen irradiation in chronic lymphocytic leukemia (CLL): Palliation in patients unfit for splenectomy. Am J Hematol 19:177, 1985.

190. G De Rossi, C Biagini, M Lopez, V Tombolini, F Mandelli. Treatment by splenic irradiation in 22 chronic lymphocytic leukemia patients. Tumori 68:511, 1982.

191. D Catovsky, S Richards, J Fooks, TJ Hamblin. (MRC Working Party on Leukaemia in Adults). CLL trials in the United Kingdom. Leuk Lymph 5 (suppl):105, 1991.

192. VA Morrison. The infectious complications of chronic lymphocytic leukemia. Semin Oncol 25:98, 1998.

193. M Itala, H Helenius, J Nikoskelainen, K Remes. Infections and serum IgG levels in patients with chronic lymphocytic leukemia. Eur J Haematol 48:266, 1992.

194. HI Zeya, E Keku, F Richards 2d, CL Spurr. Monocyte and granulocyte defect in chronic lymphocytic leukemia. Am J Pathol 95:43, 1979.

195. M Itala, O Vainio, K Remes. Functional abnormalities in granulocytes predict susceptibility to bacterial infections in chronic lymphocytic leukaemia. Eur J Haematol 57:46, 1996.

196. S Molica, D Levato, L Levato. Infections in chronic lymphocytic leukemia. Analysis of incidence as a function of length of follow-up. Haematologica 78:374, 1993.

197. JJ Twomey. Infections complicating multiple myeloma and chronic lymphocytic leukemia. Arch Intern Med 132:562, 1973.

198. S Tsiodras, G Samonis, MJ Keating, DP Kontoyiannis. Infection and immunity in chronic lymphocytic leukemia. Mayo Clin Proc 75:1039, 2000.

199. JC Byrd, LH McGrail, DR Hospenthal, RS Howard, NA Dow, LF Diehl. Herpes virus infections occur frequently following treatment with fludarabine: Results of a prospective natural history study. Br J Haematol 105:445, 1999.

200. PJ O'Dwyer, AS Spiers, S Marsoni. Association of severe and fatal infections and treatment with pentostatin. Cancer Treat Rep 70:1117, 1986.

201. HM Chapel, C Bunch. Mechanisms of infection in chronic lymphocytic leukemia. Semin Hematol 24:291, 1987.

202. A Zomas, J Mehta, R Powles, J Treleaven, T Iveson, S Singhal, B Jameson, B Paul, S Brincat, D Catovsky. Unusual infections following allogeneic bone marrow transplantation for chronic lymphocytic leukemia. Bone Marrow Transplant 14:799, 1994.

203. JC Byrd, JB Hargis, KE Kester, DR Hospenthal, SW Knutson, LF Diehl. Opportunistic pulmonary infections with fludarabine in previously treated patients with low-grade lymphoid malignancies: A role for *Pneumocystis carinii* pneumonia prophylaxis. Am J Hematol 49: 135, 1995.

204. J Mehta, R Powles, S Singhal, U Riley, J Treleaven, D Catovsky. Antimicrobial prophylaxis to prevent opportunistic infections in patients with chronic lymphocytic leukemia after allogeneic blood or marrow transplantation. Leuk Lymphoma 26:83, 1997.

205. T Sudhoff, M Arning, W Schneider. Prophylactic strategies to meet infectious complications in fludarabine-treated CLL. Leukemia 11 (suppl 2):S38, 1997.

206. M Itala, TT Pelliniemi, K Remes, S Vanhatalo, O Vainio. Long-term treatment with GM-CSF in patients with chronic lymphocytic leukemia and recurrent neutropenic infections. Leuk Lymphoma 32:165, 1998.

207. JC Reed. Molecular biology of chronic lymphocytic leukemia: Implications for therapy. Semin Hematol 35(3 suppl 3):3, 1998.

208. C Pepper, P Bentley, T Hoy. Regulation of clinical chemoresistance by bcl-2 and bax onco-proteins in B-cell chronic lymphocytic leukaemia. Br J Haematol 95:513, 1996.

209. C Pepper, T Hoy, DP Bentley. Bcl-2/Bax ratios in chronic lymphocytic leukaemia and their correlation with in vitro apoptosis and clinical resistance. Br J Cancer 76:935, 1997.

210. C Pepper, A Thomas, T Hoy, P Bentley. Chlorambucil resistance in B-cell chronic lympho-cytic leukaemia is mediated through failed Bax induction and selection of high Bcl-2-express-ing subclones. Br J Haematol 104:581, 1999.

211. JB Johnston, P Daeninck, L Verburg, K Lee, G Williams, LG Israels, MR Mowat, A Beg-leiter. p53, MDM-2, BAX and BCL-2 and drug resistance in chronic lymphocytic leukemia. Leuk Lymphoma 26:435, 1997.

212. C Shustik, N Groulx, P Gros. Analysis of multidrug resistance (MDR-1) gene expression in chronic lymphocytic leukemia (CLL). Br J Haematol 79:50, 1991.

213. G Majumdar, AK Singh. P-glycoprotein expression in drug-resistant chronic lymphoprolifer-ative disorder. Leuk Lymphoma 5:387, 1991.

214. P Sonneveld, K Nooter, JTM Burghouts, H Herwiejer, HJ Adriaansen, JJM van Dongen. High expression of the MDR-3 multidrug resistance gene in advanced-stage chronic lymphocytic leukemia. Blood 79:1496, 1992.

215. RL Sparrow, FJ Hall, H Siregard, MB van der Weyden. Common expression of the multidrug resistance marker P-glycoprotein in B-cell chronic lymphocytic leukemia and correlation with in vitro drug resistance. Leuk Res 17:941, 1993.

216. J Wallner, H Gisslinger, B Gisslinger, A Gsur, M Goltz, S Zochbauer, R Pirker. MDR1 gene expression in chronic lymphocytic leukemia. Leuk Lymphoma 13:333, 1994.

217. G Wulf, H Kluding, AD Ho, M Doerner, H Doehner, C Manegold, W Hunstein. Multidrug resistance phenotype in patients with chronic lymphocytic leukemia as detected by immuno-fluorescence (FACS) and Northern blot analysis. Leukemia Res 18:475, 1994.

218. V Ribrag, L Massade, AM Faussat, F Dreyfus, C Bayle, A Gouyette, JP Marie. Drug resis-tance mechanisms in chronic lymphocytic leukemia. Leukemia 10:1944, 1996.

219. WR Friedenberg, SK Spencer, C Musser, TF Hogan, KA Rodvold, DA Rushing, JJ Mazza, DA Tewksbury, JJ Marx. Multi-drug resistance in chronic lymphocytic leukemia. Leuk Lymphoma 34:171, 1999.

220. F Morabito, C Stelitano, I Callea, M Filangeri, B Oliva, G Sculli, V Callea, F Nobile, M Brugiatelli. In vitro sensitivity of chronic lymphocytic leukemia B-cells to fludarabine, 2-chlorodeoxyadenosine and chlorambucil: Correlation with clinico-hematological and immu-nophenotypic features. Haematologica 81:224, 1996.

221. F Morabito, M Filangeri, I Callea, G Sculli, V Callea, NS Fracchiolla, A Neri, M Brugiatelli. Bcl-2 protein expression and p53 gene mutation in chronic lymphocytic leukemia: Correla-tion with in vitro sensitivity to chlorambucil and purine analogs. Haematologica 82:16, 1997.

222. M Aguilar-Santelises, R Magnusson, SB Svenson, A Loftenius, B Andersson, H Mellstedt, M Jondal. Expression of interleukin-1 alpha, interleukin-1 beta and interleukin-6 in chronic B lymphocytic leukaemia (B-CLL) cells from patients at different stages of disease progres-sion. Clin Exp Immunol 84:422, 1991.

223. LE Robertson, W Plunkett, K McConnell, MJ Keating, TJ McDonnell. Bcl-2 expression in chronic lymphocytic leukemia and its correlation with the induction of apoptosis and clinical outcome. Leukemia 10:456, 1996.

224. EW Newcomb, S el Rouby, A Thomas. A unique spectrum of p53 mutations in B-cell chronic lymphocytic leukemia distinct from that of other lymphoid malignancies. Mol Carcinog 14:227, 1995.

225. H Dohner, K Fischer, M Bentz, K Hansen, A Benner, G Cabot, D Diehl, R Schlenk, J Coy, S Stilgenbauer, et al. p53 gene deletion predicts for poor survival and non-response to therapy with purine analogs in chronic B-cell leukemias. Blood 85:1580, 1995.

226. G Gaidano, P Ballerini, JZ Gong, G Inghirami, A Neri, EW Newcomb, IT Magrath, DM Knowles, R Dalla-Favera. p53 mutations in human lymphoid malignancies: Association with

Burkitt lymphoma and chronic lymphocytic leukemia. Proc Natl Acad Sci USA 88:5413, 1991.

227. S El Rouby, A Thomas, D Costin, CR Rosenberg, M Potmesil, R Silber, EW Newcomb. p53 gene mutation in B-cell chronic lymphocytic leukemia is associated with drug resistance and is independent of MDR1/MDR3 gene expression. Blood 82:3452, 1993.

228. A Thomas, S El Rouby, JC Reed, S Krajewski, R Silber, M Potmesil, EW Newcomb. Drug-induced apoptosis in B-cell chronic lymphocytic leukemia: Relationship between p53 gene mutation and bcl-2/bax proteins in drug resistance. Oncogene 12:1055, 1996.

229. M Schena, G Gaidano, D Gottardi, F Malavasi, LG Larsson, K Nilsson, F Caligaris-Cappio. Molecular investigation of the cytokines produced by normal and malignant B lymphocytes. Leukemia 6:120, 1992.

230. A Biondi, V Rossi, R Bassan, T Barbui, S Bettoni, M Sironi, A Mantovani, A Rambaldi. Constitutive expression of the interleukin-6 gene in chronic lymphocytic leukemia. Blood 73:1279, 1989.

231. PF di Celle, A Carbone, D Marchis, D Zhou, S Sozzani, S Zupo, M Pini, A Mantovani, R Foa. Cytokine gene expression in B-cell chronic lymphocytic leukemia: Evidence of constitutive interleukin-8 (IL-8) mRNA expression and secretion of biologically active IL-8 protein. Blood 84:220, 1994.

232. JE Reitte, KL Yong, P Panayiotidis, AV Hoffbrand. Interleukin-6 inhibits apoptosis and tumour necrosis factor induced proliferation of B-chronic lymphocytic leukaemia. Leuk Lymphoma 22:83, 1996.

233. OS Frankfurt, JJ Byrnes, L Villa. Protection from apoptotic cell death by interleukin-4 is increased in previously treated chronic lymphocytic leukemia patients. Leuk Res 21:9, 1997.

234. WR Friedenberg, SA Salzman, SM Phan, JK Burmester. Transforming growth factor-β and multidrug resistance in chronic lymphocytic leukemia. Med Oncol 16:110, 1999.

235. R Foa, M Massaia, S Cardona, AG Tos, A Bianchi, C Attisano, A Guarini, PF di Celle, MT Fierro. Production of tumor necrosis factor-alpha by B-cell chronic lymphocytic leukemia cells: A possible regulatory role of TNF in the progression of the disease. Blood 76:393, 1990.

236. R Michalevicz. Restoration of in vitro hematopoiesis in B-chronic lymphocytic leukemia by antibodies to tumor necrosis factor. Leuk Res 15:111, 1991.

237. LA Iciek, SA Delphin, J Stavnezer. CD40 cross-linking induces Ig epsilon germline transcripts in B cells via activation of NF-kappaB: Synergy with IL-4 induction. J Immunol 158: 4769, 1997.

238. K Ikizawa, K Kajiwara, T Koshio, N Matsuura, Y Yanagihara. Inhibition of IL-4 receptor upregulation on B cells by antisense oligodeoxynucleotide suppresses IL-4 induced human IgE production. Clin Exp Immunol 100:383, 1995.

239. D Wang, GJ Freeman, H Levine, J Ritz, MJ Robertson. Role of the CD40 and CD95 (APO-1/Fas) antigens in the apoptosis of human B-cell malignancies. Br J Haematol 97:409, 1997.

240. A Younes, V Snell, U Consoli, K Clodi, S Zhao, JL Palmer, EK Thomas, RJ Armitage, M Andreeff. Elevated levels of biologically active soluble CD40 ligand in the serum of patients with chronic lymphocytic leukemia. Br J Haematol 100:135, 1998.

241. A Konig, T Menzel, S Lynen, L Wrazel, A Rosen, A Al-Katib, E Raveche, JL Gabrilove. Basic fibroblast growth factor (bFGF) upregulates the expression of bcl-2 in B cell chronic lymphocytic leukemia cell lines resulting in delaying apoptosis. Leukemia 11:258, 1997.

242. A Aguayo, S O'Brien, M Keating, T Manshouri, C Gidel, B Barlogie, M Beran, C Koller, H Kantarjian, M Albitar. Clinical relevance of intracellular vascular endothelial growth factor levels in B-cell chronic lymphocytic leukemia. Blood 96:768, 2000.

243. AP Jewell, KL Yong, CP Worman, FJ Giles, AH Goldstone, PM Lydyard. Cytokine induction of leucocyte adhesion molecule-1 (LAM-1) expression on chronic lymphocytic leukaemia cells. Leukemia 6:400, 1992.

244. AP Jewell, KL Yong. Regulation and function of adhesion molecules in B-cell chronic lymphocytic leukaemia. Acta Haematol 97:67, 1997.

245. DJ McConkey, J Chandra, S Wright, W Plunkett, TJ McDonnell, JC Reed, M Keating. Apoptosis sensitivity in chronic lymphocytic leukemia is determined by endogenous endonuclease content and relative expression of BCL-2 and BAX. J Immunol 156:2624, 1996.

246. S O'Brien, A del Giglio, M Keating. Advances in the biology and treatment of B-cell chronic lymphocytic leukemia. Blood 85:307, 1995.

247. PH Wiernik, LI Gordon, MM Oken, JE Harris, MJ O'Connell. Evaluation of mitoguazone in patients with refractory chronic lymphocytic leukemia: A phase II study (P-H482) of the Eastern Cooperative Oncology Group. Leuk Lymphoma 35:375, 1999.

248. G Hale. Synthetic peptide mimotope of the CAMPATH-1 (CD52) antigen, a small glycosyl-phosphatidylinositol-anchored glycoprotein. Immunotechnology, 1:175, 1995.

249. B Hertenstein, B Wagner, D Bunjes, C Duncker, A Raghavachar, R Arnold, H Heimpel, H Schrezenmeier. Emergence of CD52-, phosphatidylinositolglycan-anchor-deficient T lymphocytes after in vivo application of Campth-1H for refractory B-cell non-Hodgkin lymphoma. Blood 86:1487, 1995.

250. WC Rowan, G Hale, JP Tite, SJ Brett. Cross-linking of the CAMPATH-1H antigen (CD52) triggers activation of normal human T lymphocytes. Int Immunol 7:69, 1995.

251. G Hale, M Clark, H Waldmann. Therapeutic potential of rat monoclonal antibodies: isotype specificity of antibody-dependent cell-mediated cytotoxicity with human lymphocytes. J Immunol 134:3056, 1985.

252. G Hale, MJ Dyer, MR Clark, JM Phillips, R Marcus, L Riechmann, G Winter, H Waldmann. Remission induction in non-Hodgkin lymphoma with reshaped human monoclonal antibody CAMPATH-1H. Lancet 2:1394, 1988.

253. SH Lim, G Davey, R Marcus. Differential response in a patient treated with Campath-1H monoclonal antibody for refractory non-Hodgkin lymphoma. Lancet 341:432, 1993.

254. A Osterborg, MJ Dyer, D Bunjes, GA Pangalis, Y Bastion, D Catovsky, H Mellstedt. Phase II multi-center study of human CD52 antibody in previously treated chronic lymphocytic leukemia, European Study Group of CAMPATH-1H Treatment in Chronic Lymphocytic Leukemia. J Clin Oncol 15:1567, 1997.

255. MJ Dyer, SM Kelsey, HJ Mackay, E Emmett, P Thornton, G Hale, H Waldmann, AC Newland, D Catovsky. In vivo 'purging' of residual disease in CLL with Campath-1H. Br J Haematol 97:669, 1997.

256. R Pawson, MJ Dyer, R Barge, E Matutes, PD Thornton, E Emmett, JC Kluin-Nelemans, WE Fibbe, R Willemze, D Catovsky. Treatment of T-cell prolymphocytic leukemia with human CD52 antibody. J Clin Oncol 15:2667, 1997.

257. MJ Keating, J Byrd, K Rai, I Flinn, V Jain, JL Binet, R Bolin, P Hillmen, M Hutchinson. Campath-1H Collaborative Study Group. Blood 94(suppl 1):705a (abstr. 3118), 1999.

258. AL Bowen, A Zomas, E Emmett, E Matutes, MJ Dyer, D Catovsky. Subcutaneous Campath-1H in fludarabine-resistant/relapsed chronic lymphocytic and B-prolymphocytic leukemia. Br J Haematol 96:617, 1997.

259. DA Einfeld, JP Brown, MA Valentine, EA Clark, JA Ledbetter. Molecular cloning of the human B cell CD20 receptor predicts a hydrophobic protein with multiple transmembrane domains. EMBOJ 7:711, 1988.

260. NM Almasri, RE Duque, J Iturrapse, E Everett, RC Braylan. Reduced expression of CD20 antigen as a characteristic marker for chronic lymphocytic leukemia. Am J Hematol 40:259, 1992.

261. L Ginaldi, M De Martinis, E Matutes, N Farahat, R Morilla, D Catovsky. Levels of expression of CD19 and CD20 in chronic B cell leukaemias. J Clin Pathol 51:364, 1998.

262. DG Maloney, AJ Grillo-Lopez, CA White, D Bodkin, RJ Schilder, JA Neidhart, N Janakiraman, KA Foon, TM Liles, BK Dallaire, K Wey, I Royston, T Davis, R Levy. IDEC-C2B8 (Rituximab) anti-CD20 monoclonal antibody therapy in patients with relapsed low-grade non-Hodgkin's lymphoma. Blood 90:2188, 1997.

263. P McLaughlin, A Grillo-Lopez, BK Link, R Levy, MS Czuczman, ME Williams, MR Heyman, I Bence-Bruckler, CA White, F Cabanillas, V Jain, AD Ho, J Lister, K Wey, D Shen, BK

Dallaire. Rituximab chimeric anti-CD20 monoclonal antibody therapy for relapsed indolent lymphoma: Half of patients respond to a four-dose treatment program. J Clin Oncol 16:2825, 1998.

264. B Coiffier, C Haioun, N Ketterer, A Engert, H Tilly, D Ma, P Johnson, A Lister, M Feuring-Buske, JA Radford, R Capdeville, V Diehl, F Reyes. Rituximab (anti-CD20 monoclonal antibody) for the treatment of patients with relapsing or refractory aggressive lymphoma: A multicenter phase II study. Blood 92:1927, 1998.

265. P McLaughlin, AJ Grillo-Lopez, DG Maloney, BK Link, R Ley, MS Czuczman, F Cabanillas, BK Daliare, CA White. Efficacy controls and long-term follow-up of patients treated with rituximab for relapsed or refractory low-grade or follicular NHL. Blood 92(suppl 1): 414a (abstr. 1712), 1998.

266. L Piro, CA White, AJ Grillo-Lopez, N Janakiraman, TM Beck, K Selander, S Dowden, M Czuczman, JW Lynch, JE Kolitz, V Jain. Rituxan: Interim analysis of a phase II study of once weekly times eight dosing in patients with relapsed low-grade or follicular non-Hodgkin's lymphoma. Blood 90(suppl 1):510a (abstr. 2272), 1997.

267. TF Tedder, AW Boyd, AS Freedman, LM Nadler, SF Schlossman. The B cell surface molecule B1 is functionally linked with B cell activation and differentiation. J Immunol 135:973, 1985.

268. ME Reff, C Carner, KS Chambers, PC Chinn, JE Leonard, R Raab, RA Newman, N Hanna, DR Anderson. Depletion of B cells in vivo by a chimeric mouse human monoclonal antibody to CD20. Blood 83:435, 1994.

269. JM Foran, AZ Rohatiner, D Cunningham, RA Popescu, P Solal-Celigny, M Ghielmini, B Coiffier, PW Johnson, C Gisselbrecht, F Reyes, JA Radford, EM Bessell, B Souleau, A Benzohra, TA Lister. European phase II study of rituximab (chimeric anti-CD20 monoclonal antibody) for patients with newly diagnosed mantle-cell lymphoma and previously treated mantle-cell lymphoma, immunocytoma, and small B-cell lymphocytic lymphoma. J Clin Oncol 18:317, 2000.

270. S O'Brien, D Thomas, EJ Freireich, M Andreeff, FJ Giles, MJ Keating. Rituxan has significant activity in patients with CLL. Blood 94(suppl 1):603a (abstr. 2684), 1999.

271. JC Byrd, MR Grever, B Davis, MS Lucas, K Park, A Goodrich, C Morrison, T Murphy, L Kunkel, A Grillo-Lopez, JK Waselenko, IW Flinn. Phase I/II study of thrice weekly Rituximab in chronic lymphocytic leukemmia (CLL)/small lymphocytic lymphoma (SLL): A feasible and active regimen. Blood 94(suppl 1):704a (abstr. 3114), 1999.

272. M Jensen, U Winkler, O Manzke, V Diehl, A Engert. Rapid tumor lysis in a patient with B-cell chronic lymphocytic leukemia and lymphocytosis treated with an anti-CD20 monoclonal antibody (IDEC-C2B8, rituximab). Ann Hematol 77:89, 1998.

273. JC Byrd, JK Waselenko, TJ Maneatis, T Murphy, FT Ward, BP Monahan, MA Sipe, S Donegan, CA White. Rituximab therapy in hematologic malignancy patients with circulating blood tumor cells: Association with increased infusion-related side effects and rapid blood tumor clearance. J Clin Oncol 17:791, 1999.

274. MS Czuczman, AJ Grillo-Lopez, CA White, M Saleh, L Gordon, AF LoBuglio, C Jonas, D Klippenstein, B Dallaire, C Varns. Treatment of patients with low-grade B-cell lymphoma with the combination of chimeric anti-CD20 monoclonal antibody and CHOP chemotherapy. J Clin Oncol 17:268, 1999.

275. P Venugopal, S Sivaraman, XK Huang, J Nayini, SA Gregory, HD Preisler. Effects of cytokines on CD20 antigen expression on tumor cells from patients with chronic lymphocytic leukemia. Leuk Res 24:411, 2000.

276. C Klingbeil, DH Hsu. Pharmacology and safety assessment of humanized monoclonal antibodies for therapeutic use. Toxicol Pathol 27:1, 1999.

277. MS Kaminski, KR Zasadny, IR Francis, MC Fenner, CW Ross, AW Milik, J Estes, M Tuck, D Regan, S Fisher, SD Glenn, RL Wahl. Iodine-131-anti-B1 radioimmunotherapy for B-cell lymphoma. J Clin Oncol 14:1974, 1996.

278. KR Rai. Future strategies toward the cure of indolent B-cell malignancies. New biologic therapies. Semin Hematol 36(4 suppl 5):12, 1999.

279. GA Wiseman, CA White, TE Witzig, LI Gordon, C Emmanouilides, A Raubitschek, N Janakiraman, J Gutheil, RJ Schilder, S Spies, DH Silverman, AJ Grillo-Lopez. Radioimmunotherapy of relapsed non-Hodgkin's lymphoma with zevalin, a 90Y-labeled anti-CD20 monoclonal antibody. Clin Cancer Res 5:3281s, 1999.

280. TE Witzig, BR Leigh, LI Gordon, JL Murray, GA Wiseman, MS Czuczman, BL Pohlman, AJ Grillo-Lopez, CA White. Interim results from a prospective randomized controlled trial comparing Zevalin radioimmunotherapy to rituximab immunotherapy for B-cell non-Hodgkin's lymphoma (NHL): Resistance to prior chemotherapy vs. response rate. Proc Am Soc Clin Oncol 19:29a (abstr. 105), 2000.

281. OW Press, JF Eary, FR Appelbaum, PJ Martin, CC Badger, WB Nelp, S Glenn, G Butchko, D Fisher, B Porter, et al. Radiolabeled-antibody therapy of B-cell lymphoma with autologous bone marrow support. N Engl J Med 329:1219, 1993.

282. OW Press, JF Eary, FR Appelbaum, PJ Martin, WB Nelp, S Glenn, DR Fisher, B Porter, DC Matthews, T Gooley, et al. Phase II trial of ^{131}I-anti-B1 (anti-CD20) antibody therapy with autologous stem cell transplantation in relapsed B cell lymphomas. Lancet 346:336, 1995.

283. CF LeMaistre, FE Craig, C Meneghetti, B McMullin, K Parker, J Reuben, DH Boldt, M Rosenblum, T Woodworth. Phase I trial of a 90-minute infusion of the fusion toxin DAB 486IL-2 in hematological cancers. Cancer Res 53:3930, 1993.

284. CF LeMaistre, MN Saleh, TM Kuze, F Foss, LC Platanias, G Schwartz, M Ratain, A Rook, CO Freytes, F Craig, J Reuben, JC Nichols. Phase I trial of a ligand fusion-protein (DAB 389IL-2) in lymphomas expressing the receptor for interleukin-2. Blood 91:399, 1998.

285. RJ Kreitman, WH Wilson, JD White, M Stetler-Stevenson, ES Jaffe, S Giardina, TA Waldmann, I Pastan. Phase I trial of recombinant immunotoxin anti-Tac(Fv)-PE38 (LMB-2) in patients with hematologic malignancies. J Clin Oncol 18:1622, 2000.

286. JM Foran, D Oscier, J Orchard, SA Johnson, M Tighe, MH Cullen, PG de Takats, C Kraus, M Klein, TA Lister. Pharmacokinetic study of single doses of oral fludarabine phosphate in patients with ''low-grade'' non-Hodgkin's lymphoma and B-cell chronic lymphocytic leukemia. J Clin Oncol 17:1574, 1999.

287. MA Boogaerts, A Van Hoof, D Catovsky, M Kovacs, M Montillo, S Tura, JL Binet, W Feremans, R Marcus, E Montserrat, G Verhoef, M Klein. Treatment of alkylator resistant chronic lymphocytic leukemia with oral fludarabine phosphate. Blood 94(suppl 1):704a (abstr. 3113), 1999.

288. B Gahn, G Brittinger, G Dolken, H Dohner, B Emmerich, A Franke, M Freund, C Huber, R Kuse, T Scholten, W Hiddemann. Multicenter phase II study of oral idarubicin in treated and untreated patients with B-chronic lymphocytic leukemia. Leuk Lymphoma 37:169, 2000.

289. V Gandhi, W Plunkett, CO Rodriguez Jr, BJ Nowak, M Du, M Ayres, DF Kisor, BS Mitchell, J Kurtzberg, MJ Keating. Compound GW506U78 in refractory hematologic malignancies: Relationship between cellular pharmacokinetics and clinical response. J Clin Oncol 16:3607, 1998.

290. DF Kisor, W Plunkett, J Kurtzberg, B Mitchell, JP Hodge, T Ernst, MJ Keating, V Gandhi. Pharmacokinetics of nelarabine and 9-beta-D-arabinofuranosyl guanine in pediatric and adult patients during a phase I study of nelarabine for the treatment of refractory hematologic malignancies. J Clin Oncol 18:995, 2000.

291. S O'Brien, D Thomas, H Kantarjian, E Freireich, C Koller, J Cortes, F Giles, C Bivens, S Lerner, J Hodge, N Spector, M Keating. Compound 506 has activity in mature lymphoid leukemia. Blood 92(suppl 1):490a (abstr. 2022), 1998.

292. P Kozuch, N Ibrahim, F Khuri, P Hoff, E Estey, V Gandhi, M Du, MB Rios, W Plunkett, MJ Keating, H Kantarjian. Phase I clinical and pharmacologic study of clofarabine. Blood 94(suppl 1):127a (abstr 558), 1999.

293. KL Grove, X Guo, SH Liu, Z Gao, CK Chu, YC Cheng. Anticancer activity of beta-L-dioxolane-cytidine, a novel nucleoside analogue with the unnatural L configuration. Cancer Res 55:3008, 1995.

294. SH Liu, KL Grove, YC Cheng. Unique metabolism of a novel antiviral L-nucleoside analog, 2′-fluoro-5-methyl-beta-L-arabinofuranosyluracil: A substrate for both thymidine kinase and deoxycytidine kinase. Antimicrob Agents Chemother 42:833, 1998.

295. MD Losiewicz, BA Carlson, G Kaur, EA Sausville, PJ Worland. Potent inhibition of CDC2 kinase activity by the flavenoid L86-8275. Biochem Biophys Res Com 210:589, 1995.

296. JC Byrd, C Shinn, JK Waselenko, EJ Fuchs, TA Lehman, PL Nguyen, IW Flinn, LF Diehl, E Sausville, MR Grever. Flavopiridol induces apoptosis in chronic lymphocytic leukemia cells via activation of caspase-3 without evidence of bcl-2 modulation or dependence on functional p53. Blood 92:3804, 1998.

297. J Chandra, I Niemer, J Gilbreath, KO Kliche, M Andreeff, EJ Freireich, M Keating, DJ McConkey. Proteasome inhibitors induce apoptosis in glucocorticoid-resistant chronic lymphocytic leukemic lymphocytes. Blood 92:4220, 1998.

298. C Pepper, A Thomas, T Hoy, F Cotter, P Bentley. Antisense-mediated suppression of Bcl-2 highlights its pivotal role in failed apoptosis in B-cell chronic lymphocytic leukaemia. Br J Haematol 107:611, 1999.

299. A Webb, D Cunningham, F Cotter, PA Clarke, F di Stefano, P Ross, M Corbo, Z Dziewanowska. BCL-2 antisense therapy in patients with non-Hodgkin lymphoma. Lancet 349:1137, 1997.

300. W Zhang, K Ohnishi, K Shigeno, S Fujisawa, K Naito, S Nakamura, K Takeshita, A Takeshita, R Ohno. The induction of apoptosis and cell cycle arrest by arsenic trioxide in lymphoid neoplasms. Leukemia 12:138, 1998.

301. NR Wall, RM Mohammad, KB Reddy, AM Al-Katib. Bryostatin 1 induces ubiquitination and proteasome degradation of Bcl-2 in the human acute lymphoblastic leukemia cell line, Reh. Int J Mol Med 5:165, 2000.

302. A Al-Katib, RM Mohammad, M Dan, ME Hussein, A Akhtar, GR Pettit, LL Sensenbrenner. Bryostatin 1-induced hairy cell features on chronic lymphocytic leukemia cells in vitro. Exp Hematol 21:61, 1993.

303. ML Varterasian, RM Mohammad, DS Eilender, K Hulburd, DH Rodriguez, PA Pemberton, JM Pluda, MD Dan, GR Pettit, BD Chen, AM Al-Katib. Phase I study of bryostatin 1 in patients with relapsed non-Hodgkin's lymphoma and chronic lymphocytic leukemia. J Clin Oncol 16:56, 1998.

304. ML Varterasian, RM Mohammad, MS Shurafa, K Hulburd, PA Pemberton, DH Rodriguez, V Spadoni, DS Eilender, A Murgo, N Wall, M Dan, AM Al-Katib. Phase II trial of bryostatin 1 in patients with relapsed low-grade non-Hodgkin's lymphoma and chronic lymphocytic leukemia. Clin Cancer Res 6:825, 2000.

305. K Kato, MJ Cantwell, S Sharma, TJ Kipps. Gene transfer of CD40-ligand induces autologous immune recognition of chronic lymphocytic leukemia B cells. J Clin Invest 101:1133, 1998.

306. R Buhmann, A Nolte, D Westhaus, B Emmerich, M Hallek. CD40-activated B-cell chronic lymphocytic leukemia cells for tumor immunotherapy: stimulation of allogeneic versus autologous T cells generates different types of effector cells. Blood 93:1992, 1999.

307. WG Wierda, MJ Cantwell, LZ Rassenti, E Avery, JA Johnson, TJ Kipps. CD154 (CD40-ligand) gene immunization of chronic lymphocytic leukemia: A phase I study. Blood 92(suppl 1):489a (abstr. 2018), 1998.

308. E Montserrat. New therapeutic issues in CLL. Hematol Cell Ther 39(suppl 1):S45, 1997.

309. JC Byrd, KR Rai, EA Sausville, MR Grever. Old and new therapies in chronic lymphocytic leukemia: Now is the time for a reassessment of therapeutic goals. Semin Oncol 25:65, 1998.

310. MJ Keating. Chronic lymphocytic leukemia in the next decade: Where do we go from here? Sem Hematol 35(suppl 3):27, 1998.

15

The Use of Therapeutic Monoclonal Antibodies in Chronic Lymphocytic Leukemia

MARTIN J. S. DYER*

Royal Marsden Hospital, London, England

ANDERS ÖSTERBORG

Karolinska Hospital, Stockholm, Sweden

I. INTRODUCTION

That antibodies have the specificity to deliver targeted therapy for human disease was realized soon after their description in the 1890s (1). The first therapeutic attempts in malignancy were reported in France by Hericourt and Richet as early as 1895 (2). Their conclusion, based on observations made on the effects of crude antisera raised in donkeys and other animals and in patients with advanced disease, was that antibody therapy should be combined with radical surgery, which sounds remarkably modern. Since then, however, therapeutic antibodies have had a long and largely undistinguished history in oncology (3).

The introduction of monoclonal antibodies (MAbs) in the 1980s allowed some of the barriers to effective antibody therapy of malignancy to be recognized (4). Furthermore, the advances of genetic engineering and cell culture methods have allowed the almost routine production of large quantities of humanized antibodies (5). Several antibodies have shown considerable potential in a variety of clinical settings, and some of them have now found a routine therapeutic role in oncological practice. Some of the conditions necessary for effective MAb action in vivo and some recent data on the use of CD52 (CAMPATH-1) and CD20 (Rituximab) MAbs in the treatment of lymphoid malignancies and specifically chronic lymphocytic leukemia (CLL), are reviewed here.

---

* *Current affiliation*: University of Leicester, Leicester, England.

II. GENERAL CONSIDERATIONS

CLL and related leukemias are ideal diseases for experimental therapy with MAbs. First, the disease is usually only slowly progressive, allowing sequential observations to be made in the one patient—this is of importance when comparing related reagents as shown later. Second, the presence of tumor cells in the blood allows quantitative assessment of the effects of each MAb—if there are no effects on cells in the blood, that are accessible to MAb, there are not likely to be effects on infiltrated lymph nodes or on extranodal masses. Third, CLL patients are immunocompromised, limiting the potential for neutralizing anti-globulin responses.

MAb therapy should ideally be directed against tumor-specific antigens. In the case of lymphoid malignancies, this is feasible because of the expression of immunoglobulin or T-cell receptor molecules specific for the leukemic clone. MAbs raised to the idiotypic determinants of tumor immunoglobulin have been used with some success in the treatment of low-grade B-cell lymphomas (6). These reagents may function by the activation of an idiotype immune network cascade as much as by direct action of the MAb itself. However, this approach suffers from the necessity of producing reagents for each individual patient. Moreover, antigen (idiotype)-negative tumor cells may appear as a result of the anti-idiotypic antibody therapy, thereby limiting their potential for repeated administration to the patient (7).

Another approach is to use passive serotherapy with MAbs directed against cell-surface differentiation antigens expressed on both normal and malignant cells. This is not strictly tumor-specific therapy but rather the ablation of a specific lineage of malignant (and corresponding normal) cells, with the anticipation that normal cells will ultimately be regenerated from normal stem cells. The advantage of this approach is that the one MAb may be used for a variety of different malignancies, with the disadvantage being the transient reduction or loss of normal cells.

Many MAbs of this kind of different specificities have been used in the lymphoid malignancies. Two divergent strategies have emerged. Use of MAbs on their own as unconjugated reagents depends either on the ability of the MAb itself either to kill cells directly (e.g., to deliver an apoptotic signal) or to activate effector mechanisms such as complement, T cells, neutrophils and so forth, to recreate and target the anti-inflammatory response, which the tumor has somehow managed to avoid. Most unconjugated MAbs are not effective in vivo for reasons discussed later, and therefore many groups have focused on the use of MAbs conjugated to some form of toxic reagent (such as radioisotopes, cytotoxic drugs/prodrugs, toxins). These reagents rely solely on the toxic moiety to destroy the malignant cell, with the MAb relegated to the role of a passive vector.

Both approaches have their own problems. For conjugated MAbs, the major problem is that only a fraction (<0.1% of the injected dose) of intact MAb will actually localize within the tumor, the bulk being taken up by Fc and other receptors expressed in organs such as liver, spleen, and lung; nonspecific uptake in these sites may result in significant side effects. Nevertheless, because lymphoid malignancies are mostly radiosensitive, radiolabeled MAbs including CD20 MAbs have been used principally in relapsed low-grade B-non-Hodgkin's lymphoma (NHL) and shown considerable activity in a variety of settings, although this approach has not yet been tested in CLL (8,9). MAbs conjugated with toxins have shown incredible potency both in vitro and in animal models, but side effects such as capillary-leak syndrome and the inherent immunogenicity of the toxins themselves

Table 1 Barriers to Effective Therapy with Unmodified MAbs

A. Properties of antigen	Secretion/shedding of antigen
	Low level expression
	Modulation
	"Permissive" for lysis/apoptosis
B. Properties of target cell	"Cellular defense mechanisms"
C. Properties of MAb	Immunogenicity
	Correct isotype
	Ability to trigger apoptosis
	Accessibility to tumor masses
D. Effector mechanisms	Quantity (previous chemotherapy)
	Activation
	Recruitment to tumor sites

have limited their usefulness in patients (10). The effects of conjugated MAbs will not be discussed further in this review.

The major barriers to effective therapy with unconjugated MAbs are summarized in Table 1 and discussed following with particular reference to CD20 and CD52.

A. Properties of the Target Antigen

From the outset, it has been clear that the nature of the target antigen has an important role in determining the likelihood of therapeutic success. First, it seems likely that the target antigen must be sufficiently abundant to allow the Mab molecules to activate effector mechanisms. Second, cross-linking by bivalent MAb may result in very rapid internalization (antigenic modulation), which in vivo can occur in minutes and renders a cell effectively antigen negative for prolonged periods thereafter. Nonmodulating, abundant antigens such as CD20 and CD52 are therefore favored, although modulation and therapeutic efficacy can be overcome by the use of monovalent MAbs (11).

However, for reasons that are not clear, only some antigens "permit" cell lysis with human complement and antibody-dependent cellular cytotoxicity (ADCC) effectors. A comparison of rat MAbs against CD45, CD52, and major histocompatibility (MHC) class I antigens (all of which are abundantly expressed and nonmodulating) showed that only the CD52 and the MHC class I MAbs were lytic with human complement (12). Significant lysis with CD45 MAbs was only seen with the use of synergistic pairs of MAbs. Other antigens that are potential targets for therapy have also been defined (13). Despite these antigens being permissive for both complement and cell-mediated lysis in vitro, only some of these antigens allow effective in vivo therapy in animal models and then only in some, and not all, antigen-bearing cell lines. The biological and biochemical reasons underlying these discrepancies between in vitro and in vivo antibody activities remain unknown.

B. Properties of the Target Cell

Antigen expression on the target cell may not be sufficient to allow lysis, and the nature of the target cell is also of profound importance. Among lymphoid malignancies, sensitivity to complement-mediated lysis in vitro by CD52 MAbs varied over a 200-fold range.

T-cell prolymphocytic leukemia (T-PLL) is inherently sensitive to CD52 MAbs both in vitro and in vivo. This, in part, may reflect the high CD52 antigen density on this cell type (14). In contrast, monocytes and monocytic leukemias were completely resistant to CAMPATH-1 MAbs in vivo despite expressing comparable amounts of antigen (15). The cause of this variability is unknown but may reflect the action of membrane proteins that protect cells against attack by homologous complement or the presence of specific genetic defects that underly the pathogenesis of the disease, resulting in inactivation of specific pathways (16).

C. Properties of the MAb Molecule

The properties of the MAb molecule are of crucial importance for effective MAb action. First, as described later, only some immunoglobulin heavy-chain isotypes will successfully interact with both human complement and Fc receptors to permit cell lysis; the latter function appears to be essential for in vivo lymphocyte depletion in man. Only those immunoglobulin isotypes capable of interacting with human Fc receptors to elicit ADCC appear to be able to deplete in vivo. Second, MAb produced in either mice or rats will be immunogenic even in immunocompromised recipients. However, genetic engineering methods can now be used to generate either partially or wholly humanized MAbs or MAb fragments, which should preclude most neutralizing antiglobulin responses, although anti-idiotypic and antiallotype responses may still occur. Despite their large size intact, MAbs remain the preferred constructs at present because of the rapid clearance of MAb fragments.

CAMPATH-1H is a fully humanized MAb and contains the six complementarity determining regions of the rat IgG2a MAb "grafted" onto the backbone of human IgG1 and κ genes (17). IgG1 is the preferred human isotype for both ADCC and complement-mediated lysis (18). The CD20 rituximab is not fully humanized and contains the entire variable region segments along with the human IgG1/κ constant region gene segments; this is therefore a "chimeric" MAb. Although this in theory should make the CD20 MAb more immunogenic than a fully reshaped version, it does not seem to be an important issue, because CLL patients are immunosuppressed as a result of their disease and the immunosuppressive nature of the MAb. Both CAMPATH-1H and rituximab can therefore be used repeatedly for a given patient with little danger of a neutralizing antiglobulin arising.

Regarding humanized antibodies, the cells in which the antibody is produced and the conditions under which they are grown may influence the antibody glycosylation patterns (19,20). These changes may profoundly influence both biodistribution and effector functions.

Finally, intact Mabs are large molecules and access to bulky lymph nodes or extra-nodal masses may be limited. Animal experiments (21) and imaging studies with radiolabeled MAbs indicate that MAb will penetrate into lymph nodes but only at lower concentrations than achieved in the peripheral blood; this and the lack of suitable effector cells may seriously compromise MAb action at such sites. These data suggest that the optimal timing of MAb therapy may be once bulk disease has been eradicated by conventional therapy. Furthermore, it is likely that previous chemotherapy will also deplete and impair effector cell functions; this is an argument for the use of MAb early in the course of the disease.

III. THE CD52 ANTIGEN AND THE CAMPATH-1 MAbs

The CD52 antigen is composed of only 12 amino acids attached indirectly to the cell membrane through a GPI anchor. Despite the short length of the peptide, there are two allelic forms; the possible biological significance of these alleles is not known (22). The peptide is heavily glycosylated and the complete structure of the antigen has been established (23). The function(s) of the antigen, however, remains unknown. Whether CD52, like other GPI-linked proteins, is a component of glycolipid ''rafts'' or ''microdomains'' and therefore implicated in signal transduction is also not known (24).

CD52 is expressed at high levels (approximately 500,000 molecules/cell) on most normal and malignant mature lymphocytes of both T- and B-cell lineages and therefore potentially comprises about 5% of the total cell surface; it is not expressed on hemopoietic stem cells (25–27). Therapeutically, the broad lymphoid expression of CD52 suggests that all malignant lymphopoietic progenitor cells may express the target antigen; all normal lymphoid progenitor cells would, however, also be similarly targeted with resulting profound lymphopenia. Patients with rheumatoid arthritis treated with CAMPATH-1H rapidly regenerate normal numbers of B cells and CD8 T cells but do not recover normal numbers of CD4 T cells in the peripheral blood (28). CAMPATH-1H–induced lymphopenia is associated with increased opportunistic infections for up to 8 to 12 weeks after MAb infusion, particularly in heavily pretreated patients (29). Long-term follow-up has shown that this deficiency in blood CD4+ve-T cells does not appear to be associated with any long-term clinical sequelae.

CD52 does not modulate either in vitro or in vivo in the presence of bivalent MAb. This, and the close proximity of the antigenic epitope to the membrane, may be important in allowing cell lysis. Cross-linking CD52 MAbs may induce apoptosis under some in vitro conditions (30). However, the possible clinical significance of this is difficult to assess, because most cell lines lose expression of CD52. We have not observed CAMPATH-1H–induced apoptosis in vivo as adjudged by Annexin V staining and DNA laddering in patients with a high peripheral blood lymphocyte count (M. Dyer, unpublished observations, 1999). Furthermore, the MAb appears to have no apoptotic effect on cells within the CNS; MAb administered intrathecally remained bound to infiltrating B-PLL cells 24 hours later (31). Appearance of CD52-negative tumor cells after CAMPATH-1H treatment is extremely rare (compare the appearance of CD20-negative tumors after rituximab), and it has been possible to treat some patients successfully with multiple courses of MAb. In contrast, appearance of CD52 negative, normal T cells is not uncommon either after or indeed during the course of CAMPATH-1H (32,33).

A series of rat and human CD52 MAbs has been generated, which has allowed some of the conditions for effective MAb action in vivo to be determined. The original rat IgM Mab (CAMPATH-1M) was selected in a screen for MAbs that would lyse lymphocytes with human complement (34). Initial therapeutic attempts were made with the rat IgM MAb (31,35). Subsequently, a rat IgG2a CD52 MAb was produced; this MAb elicited complement-mediated lysis but not ADCC, with human complement and effector cells. A rat IgG2b class-switch variant (CAMPATH-1G) was derived from this (i.e., the IgG2a and IgG2b MAb have identical variable region genes and differ only in their constant region gene segments) (36). CAMPATH-1G is able to interact effectively with human Fc receptors and thus elicits ADCC.

Clinical experience with the series of rat MAbs showed the importance of immunoglobulin heavy chain isotype (15,31). All CD52 MAbs are highly effective at eliciting cell lysis with human complement in vitro, but only those MAbs that elicit ADCC with human effector cells seem to be effective in vivo. This point was shown in two patients with CLL, who had progressed to B-cell prolymphocytic leukemia, who consecutively received rat IgM, IgG2a, and IgG2b CAMPATH MAbs. The rat IgM MAb (CAMPATH-1M), despite depleting serum complement did not result in lymphocyte depletion, whereas the rat IgG2b resulted in lymphocyte depletion with no effect on serum complement, (Fig. 1 and 2). Similarly, the human IgG1 MAb CAMPATH-1H depletes cells without any detectable changes in complement levels, indicating that complement binding is necessary but not sufficient. An exception to these "rules" is the human IgG4 variant of CAMPATH-1H, which from in vitro testing should not elicit ADCC and yet is capable of depleting cells in patients (37).

Further experience with CAMPATH-1G, in a series of patients with a variety of lymphoproliferative diseases, showed that small (nonsaturating) doses of this MAb could readily deplete lymphocytes from peripheral blood, bone marrow, and spleen, whereas lymph nodes and extranodal masses were largely unaffected (15,31). Similar small doses (approximately 100 mg) of the genetically reshaped human IgG1 CD52 Mab, CAMPATH-1H, produced in a rat myeloma cell line Y0, also induced remission in the first two patients with advanced B-NHL (38); both patients were in leukemic phase with predominantly hematological disease. More recent clinical experience with commercial CAMPATH-1H produced in Chinese hamster ovary (CHO) cells is reviewed later, but the preferential

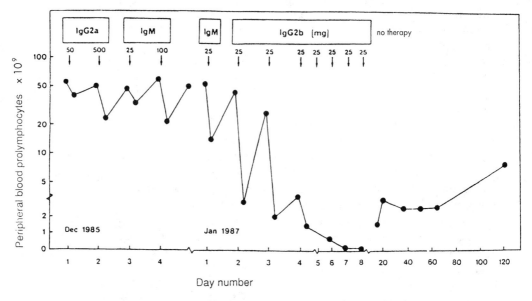

Figure 1   Comparison of rat CD52 MABs of differing isotype in a patient with B-CLL–PLL. This patient with B-CLL was treated in December 1985 with rat IgM and IgG2a MAbs. By January 1987, the disease had progressed to B-PLL, and further attempts were made with both rat IgM and IgG2b (CAMPATH-1G) MAbs. MAbs were infused at the doses shown, and the peripheral blood lymphocyte count monitored. With the IgG2b but not the IgM or the IgG2a CD52 MAbs, there was rapid clearance of lymphocytes from the blood, confirming the importance of immunoglobulin isotype. (From Ref. 15 with permission.)

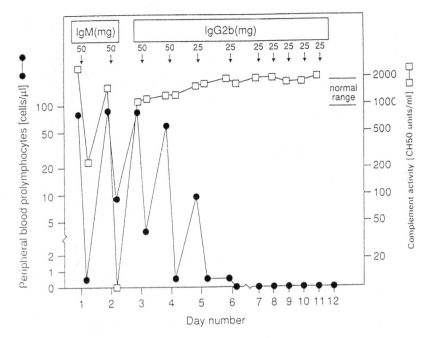

Figure 2   Activation of complement by rat IgM but not IgG2b CD52 MAbs. A patient with B-PLL refractory to CHOP chemotherapy received IgM and IgG2b MAbs at the doses indicated. Infusions of the IgM MAb resulted in only very temporary falls in the blood lymphocyte count with cells returning into the blood within 5 minutes of stopping the MAb infusion (closed circles); similar results had been seen in other studies (35). Nevertheless, each IgM infusion was associated with massive decreases in CH50, C3, and C4 levels (open squares). In contrast, the IgG2b MAb resulted in clearance of blood and in this case bone marrow also with no change in serum complement levels. (From Ref. 15 with permission.)

effect of CAMPATH-1 MAbs for tumor cells in peripheral blood and bone marrow with relatively little effect in lymph nodes was confirmed. These data suggested that CAMPATH-1H might be useful primarily for patients with hematological disease.

IV.   THE CD20 ANTIGEN AND THE CD20 MAbs

The CD20 antigen shows little physical similarity to CD52. CD20 is a transmembrane, unglycosylated phosphoprotein of 33 to 37 kDa that is expressed in hemopoietic tissues exclusively on cells of the B-cell lineage (39). CD20 protein is nonmodulating and is thought to cross the extracellular membrane four times with a single short extracellular domain of about 50 amino acids. MAbs have been generated against different epitopes within this loop, and only some of these have biological activity. The proximity of the antigen to the cell surface may, as with CD52, explain some aspects of the efficacy of the MAb in eliciting lysis.

Like CD52, the precise functions of CD20 are not yet known. However, overall the structure of the molecule is similar to that of proteins forming channels, and it is possible that the protein is involved in regulation of calcium flux (39,40). CD20 appears to be involved in cell signaling and in the modulation of B-cell growth and differentiation, although the CD20 mutant mouse in which the gene has been inactivated shows no major defect within the B-cell lineage (41). Some MAbs (including 1F5—see later) induce both activation and proliferation of resting normal tonsillar B cells and apoptosis in a range of malignant B-cell lines (42–44). Apoptosis of malignant B cells was dependent on cross-linking and associated with increased calcium flux (43,44). The mechanisms by which these effects are mediated remain obscure. Cross-linking of CD20 by MAb activates non-receptor tyrosine kinases, resulting in phosphorylation of phospholipase C-gamma and also causes redistribution of CD20 to an insoluble membrane compartment "microdomains," which interestingly contain high concentrations of GPI-linked molecules such as CD52 (45). Explanation of the mechanisms by which CD20 MAbs activate malignant B-cell apoptosis (such as activation of Src tyrosine kinases) may open new therapeutic strategies. Although a direct comparison with CD52 MAbs has not been made, the rate of apoptosis induction with CD20 MAbs is much faster and more pronounced than that seen with CD52 MAbs in vitro.

Comparison of the in vivo effects of CD20 and CD52 MAbs sheds light on their probable modes of action. Like CD52, CD20 is expressed at high density (100,000 molecules/cell) on most malignant mature B cells, although antigen density is lower on B-CLL. Similarly, CD20 MAbs of the appropriate isotype will elicit both complement lysis and ADCC, although not to the same extent as with CD52 MAbs. Preliminary therapeutic efforts with CD20 MAbs were made with a mouse IgG2a, 1F5 (46). Four patients with relapsed B-cell lymphoma received incremental doses of MAb, with one patient receiving 2380 mg. As with CAMPATH MAbs, cells were cleared rapidly from the peripheral blood. However, even in these initial experiments, at the higher doses, major effects were also seen on lymph nodes. These preliminary results were confirmed in cynomolgus monkeys with a chimeric human CD20 using the human IgG1 constant region genes and the variable region genes of the mouse MAb 2B8 (47); again, lymph node depletion of B cells was observed. Initial and subsequent studies have confirmed the clinical value of the chimeric C2B8 CD20 MAb in a variety of B-cell malignancies, but principally in low-grade B-cell follicular lymphomas (48,49). A striking feature of these studies is the lymph nodal regression, although "bulky" disease tends to be more resistant.

Although equivalent doses of either rat or human CD52 MAbs have not been used, CD52 MAbs have failed to show major, consistent effects against lymph nodes, suggesting that CD52 and CD20 MAbs deplete cells by fundamentally different mechanisms. It is likely that the success of the CD20 MAbs in this compartment is due to their ability to elicit apoptosis, circumventing the need for the activated effector cells necessary for CD52 MAbs. The rapid and direct induction of cell death by CD20 MAbs may also explain the tumor lysis syndrome that is occasionally seen in patients with a high blood lymphocyte count treated with this MAb. In contrast, this phenomenon has not been seen in patients treated with CD52 MAbs, despite many of these being leukemic.

V. CLINICAL EXPERIENCE WITH MAbs IN CLL

Many patients with CLL can be managed with conventional therapies for a long time. Although the initial response to standard therapy with chlorambucil or other alkylating agents is good, progression of the disease ultimately occurs as resistance to alkylating agents develops (50). Major responses have been reported with the purine analogs fludarabine and cladribine, either at diagnosis (51,52) or at relapse (53,54). Nevertheless, the disease remains incurable, and the outlook is poor for those who fail to respond or relapse (55,56). Thus, there is a need for new therapeutic approaches for patients with CLL using agents with different mechanisms of action. To date, most experience with MAb therapy in patients with CLL relates to the use of CD52 (CAMPATH-1H) and anti-CD20 (rituximab) MAb.

A. CAMPATH-1H in CLL

CAMPATH-1H was originally used in patients with NHL. As noted earlier, Hale et al. (38) noted substantial tumor regression in two patients with advanced NHL. However, observations in additional patients revealed that the response rate in patients with NHL was no higher than 20% (57,58). The modest overall response rate was due primarily to a poor efficacy in bulky lymph nodes, whereas a high frequency of tumor regression was observed in the blood and bone marrow (58). Lymphocytic leukemias and, in particular, CLL might therefore be the preferred disorder for therapy with CAMPATH-1H. The results from the published trials on CAMPATH-1H in CLL are summarized in Table 2.

In a phase II trial, 29 CLL patients with heavily pretreated alkylating agent-refractory or -relapsing disease were treated with CAMPATH-1H (59). The dose of CAMPATH-1H was 30 mg delivered intravenously three times per week for up to 12 weeks. The overall response rate was 42% (11 partial and 1 complete remission). CLL cells were rapidly eliminated from blood in 28 of 29 patients (97%). Complete remission in the bone marrow was obtained in 36%, whereas enlarged lymph nodes were normalized in only two patients, confirming the preferential effect of CAMPATH-1H on tumor cells in blood and bone marrow. The median response duration was 12 months. Fever and rigor related to CAMPATH-1H infusions were seen predominantly during the first infusions but disappeared in most patients on repeated administrations. Apart from long-lasting lymphocytopenia, which occurred in all patients, the hematological toxicity was moderate. Twenty percent of the patients had WHO grade IV neutropenia develop (59). This study indicated that CAMPATH-1H appeared to be a drug with major activity in CLL. The long-lasting lymphocytopenia induced by CAMPATH-1H may result in an increased risk of opportunistic and other serious infections (58,59). Prophylactic treatment with acyclovir and cotrimoxazole has been successfully used in more recent trials (see later) and is therefore now generally recommended.

As discussed previously, the reason for a differential response at various tumor sites is not clear but may be related to a poor bioavailability of CAMPATH-1H in bulky lymph nodes and thus a low MAb concentration on the tumor-cell surface (60). In addition, lack of effector cells in bulky lymph nodes may result in less activity of Mabs at such locations (61).

In another study, CAMPATH-1H was administered as subcutaneous injections to seven patients with fludarabine-resistant/relapsed CLL and B-cell prolymphocytic leukaemia (62). Four of the seven patients responded. A local injection-site reaction was observed after the first doses but disappeared during subsequent injections. Notably, three of the patients had reactivation of cytomeagalovirus (CMV) develop; two of these patients required therapy with ganciclovir. The beneficial effect of CAMPATH-1H in fludarabine-refractory CLL patients has been confirmed in two recently completed multicenter trials. A high frequency of complete remission (34%) was reported among 29 patients with fludarabine nonresponsive CLL (63). In the pivotal trial, which was recently presented

Table 2 Summary of Clinical Trials on CAMPATH-1H (anti-CD52) in Patients with CLL

No. of patients	Previous therapy	Response rate[a] (%)			Response duration (mo)	Remarks	Reference
		CR	PR	OR			
29	Alkylating agents[a]	4	38	42	12	36% achieved a CR in the bone marrow	(59)
7	Fludarabine	14	43	57	11	Subcutaneous administration	(62)
29	Fludarabine	34	25	59	17	Lymphadenopathy predicted for a worse response	(63)
92	Fludarabine	2	31	33	9+	Responses were least common with bulky disease	(64)
6	Fludarabine	83	17	100	—	Patients with minimal residual disease	(69)
15	Purine analogs	60	13	73	—	T-PLL patients	(72)
9	None	33	56	89	12+	78% achieved a CR in the bone marrow	(67)
11	None	27	46	73	—	Early interim analysis. Subcutaneous administration	(68)

[a] CR, complete remission; PR, partial remission, OR, overall response rate.

by Keating et al. (64), 92 patients with advanced fludarabine-refractory B-CLL received CAMPATH-1H three times weekly for up to 12 weeks. The overall response rate was 33% with an acceptable overall toxicity profile.

In conclusion, CAMPATH-1H appears to be an effective treatment for patients with advanced CLL.

As indicated earlier, previous chemotherapy and advanced disease/high tumor burden may impair the effector functions and hinder MAb actions, which supports the use of MAb early in the course of the disease or in patients with minimal residual disease (65,66). To address this question, CAMPATH-1H was given to a small cohort of patients with symptomatic but previously untreated CLL; eight of nine patients responded with durable remissions, one of whom persisted in an unmaintained CR 7 years after end of CAMPATH-1H therapy (67). Preliminary data from an ongoing phase II trial on the use of subcutaneous CAMPATH-1H as first-line therapy in CLL patients indicate that the overall response ratio in this cohort may be around 80%. Around two-thirds of the patients may obtain a complete remission in the bone marrow, which, however, may require long-term administration (up to 18 weeks) of CAMPATH-1H (68). This is in contrast to the peripheral blood, from which the CLL cells were cleared within 2 to 3 weeks (59). Thus, long-term treatment with CAMPATH-1H might be important to achieve a remission of high quality. The optimal length of CAMPATH-1H therapy thus still remains to be finally determined, as well as the clinical value of CAMPATH-1H in the upfront setting.

Intravenous administration of CAMPATH-1H is almost invariably associated with first-dose reactions such as fever, rigor, and nausea (58,59). These side effects appear to be either absent or milder after subcutaneous administration without negatively affecting the rate of or time to clearance of CLL cells from the blood (62,67,68). Taking into consideration the practical aspects (self-administration at home), the subcutaneous route may therefore be the preferred route of CAMPATH-1H (and other MAbs) in the future. The bioavailability and pharmacokinetics after subcutaneous administration and the possible immunogenic concerns (subcutaneous MAb may result in more anti-idiotypic and other antiglobulin responses) however, need, to be studied in detail. Furthermore, it needs to be clarified whether subcutaneous MAb is equally effective as intravenously administered MAb, particularly in the presence of bulk disease. Further studies are underway to compare the intravenous and subcutaneous routes with regard to toxicity and efficacy.

CAMPATH-1H may be used also for in vivo purging or to eradicate minimal residual disease. Dyer et al. (69) reported six patients with CLL who had been treated to maximal response with fludarabine. Five of these patients achieved a complete remission in blood and bone marrow (analyzed by flow-cytometry) after CAMPATH-1H therapy, and two of the patients underwent a subsequent autologous transplantation without complications (69). Achieving polymerase chain reaction–negativity in the blood seems to be a realistic goal after CAMPATH-1H treatment (70). This effect may be achievable without negatively influencing the human hematopoetic progenitor cells (26). Further studies are currently underway to explore the role of CAMPATH-1H for in vivo purging and eradication of minimal residual disease.

T-cell prolymphocytic leukemia (T-PLL) is a rare and chemotherapy-resistant disease with a median survival of 6 months (71), which is particularly sensitive to CAMPATH-1H therapy. A response rate of 73% (11 of 15 patients) with nine complete remissions was seen in chemotherapy-refractory patients after CAMPATH-1H treatment (72). Retreatment with the MAb resulted in second complete remissions in some of the patients. These results were recently confirmed by others (73). The response was, however, of short duration in most patients, indicating that CAMPATH-1H should be combined with other treatment modalities when used in patients with T-PLL. Use of CAMPATH-1H has allowed the harvesting of uncontaminated stem cells in some T-PLL patients as assessed by both dual color flow cytometry and by nested polymerase chain reaction of clonal T cell receptor gene rearrangements (74). Three of these patients have undergone autologous transplantation, one in first complete remission, but all three have relapsed and died of progressive disease in less than 2 years after transplantation (M. Dyer, et al., submitted). It seems likely that the cause of relapse in these patients is from MAb "sanctuary sites." Whether this disappointing situation can be improved with the use of radiolabeled CAMPATH-1H as additional "consolidation" will be determined.

Finally, two patients with T-PLL in this series (72) had profound bone marrow aplasia develop after successful remission induction with CAMPATH-1H. The reasons for this are not clear; comparable bone marrow aplasia has not been observed in any other patient groups treated with CAMPATH Mabs.

B. Rituximab Therapy in CLL

Rituximab (chimeric anti-CD20 MAb) has rapidly become part of the routine management of patients with low-grade follicular lymphomas. Intravenous doses of 375 mg/m^2 given once weekly for 4 weeks induced a response rate of 48% in patients with relapsed low-grade NHL (75). Toxicity was usually limited to mild to moderate flulike symptoms predominantly during the first infusion.

However, the response rate among patients with a small lymphocyte lymphoma (SLL) phenotype treated in that study was only 12% (75). Similar results on SLL have recently been reported by others (76,77). A rituximab study on patients with CLL revealed that only 1 of 15 treated achieved a partial remission after standard doses of rituximab (78). Notably, the responding patient had high levels of CD20 staining, which is not the case in most patients with CLL. Therefore, the weak expression of CD20 on CLL cells (79) may be a mechanism for the lack of response to rituximab in CLL. Notably, the nonresponse to rituximab was obvious despite a dramatic reaction of the peripheral blood lymphocytosis observed in many of the patients, which was in contrast to the no change observed in the posttreatment bone marrow examination (78). In addition, the reduction of the leukemic CLL cells was transient, because the number of CLL cells in blood had started to increase 1 to 2 months after the last rituximab infusion (80). This effect is thus in marked contrast to what has been observed in CLL after treatment with CAMPATH-1H.

Importantly, the rapid reduction of CLL cells from the blood after rituximab administration may be associated with a risk of tumor lysis syndrome or severe cytokine-release syndrome developing (81–83). The risk of severe first-dose effects developing seemed to correlate with the lymphocyte count at baseline (82,83). Moreover, severe symptoms occurred at the time of peak serum levels of interleukin-6 and tumor necrosis factor-alpha (83). It is important to note that such dramatic effects have usually not been observed after treatment with CAMPATH-1H, indicating that a different dosing schedule with prolonged application of small doses of MAb may improve the safety of rituximab in CLL.

To try to improve the efficacy of rituximab in CLL, a dose-escalation study of rituximab has been initiated. Preliminary data indicate that a response rate of at least 40% may be achieved in CLL using high doses of rituximab (84). Pharmacokinetic data have shown that higher serum rituximab concentrations correlated with response to therapy in NHL patients and that SLL/CLL patients usually had low levels (75). Therefore, a phase I/II trial of high doses of rituximab, administered thrice weekly, has been initiated. An interim analysis revealed a response rate of 50% in 18 evaluable patients, with a correlation between the intensity of CD20 expression on the tumor cells and the clinical effect (85). Thus, the dose, schedule of administration, and the density of CD20 expression may be of importance for the clinical effects of rituximab in CLL/SLL patients.

VI. CONCLUSIONS

MAbs, and in particular CAMPATH-1H, will become integrated as part of the standard therapy in CLL. Major clinical responses are achieved in 30% to 40% of patients with advanced, chemotherapy-refractory disease. The safety and toxicity profile is acceptable. Promising effects have been reported when used as first-line treatment and for eradication of minimal residual disease. Subcutaneous administration may be the preferred route, although much work needs to be done to confirm this point. The effect of other MAbs, including rituximab, still need to be confirmed in CLL. Further improvement can be envisaged. Radiolabeled MAbs have not yet been tested in CLL. Combining MAb therapy with recombinant cytokines may be beneficial, as well as the combination of MAbs and chemotherapeutic agents. The clinical possibilities of synergistic interactions between CAMPATH-1H and rituximab (as well as other MAbs) remain to be explored. An important issue will be the financial cost for the health care system for regular clinical use.

ACKNOWLEDGMENTS

We gratefully acknowledge the continued support and enthusiasm of Dr. Geoff Hale and Professor Hermann Waldmann at the Therapeutic Antibody Centre in Oxford, UK, whose production of the CAMPATH-1 MAbs has allowed these studies to progress.

REFERENCES

1. P Ehrlich. On Immunity with special reference to the cell of life. Proc Roy Soc London 66: 424–448, 1890.
2. J Hericourt, C Richet. "Physiologie pathologique": de la serotherapie dans le traitment du cancer. C R Hebd Seanc Acad Sci Paris 121:567–569, 1895.
3. GA Currie. Eighty years of immunotherapy: a review of immunological methods used for the treatment of human cancer. Br J Cancer 26:141–153, 1972.
4. J Ritz, SF Schlossman. Utilization of monoclonal antibodies in the treatment of leukemia and lymphoma. Blood 59:1–11, 1982.
5. G Winter, C Milstein. Man-made antibodies. Nature 349:293–299, 1991.
6. TA Davis, DG Maloney, DK Czerwinski, TM Liles, R Levy. Anti-idiotype antibodies can induce long-term complete remissions in non-Hodgkin's lymphoma, without eradicating the malignant clone. Blood 92:1184–1190, 1998.
7. DG Maloney, S Brown, DK Czewinski, TM Liles, SM Hart, RA Miller, R Levy. Monoclonal anti-idiotype antibody therapy of B-cell lymphomas: The addition of a short course of chemotherapy does not interfere with the antitumor effect nor prevent the emergence of idiotype-negative variant cells. Blood 80:1502–1510, 1992.
8. RL Wahl, KR Zasadny, D MacFarlane, IR Francis, CW Ross, J Estes, S Fisher, D Regan, S Kroll, MS Kaminski. Iodine-131 anti-B1 antibody for B-cell lymphoma: an update on the Michigan Phase I experience. J Nucl Med, 39 (8 suppl):21S–27S, 1998.

9.   OW Press. Radiolabeled antibody therapy of B-cell lymphomas. Semin Oncol 26(5 suppl 14): 58–65, 1999.

10. JE O'Toole, D Esseltine, TJ Lynch, JM Lambert, ML Grossbard. Clinical trials with blocked ricin immunotoxins. Curr Top Microbiol Immunol 234:35–56, 1998.

11. M Clark, C Bindon, M Dyer, P Friend, G Hale, S Cobbold, R Calne, H Waldmann. The improved lytic function and in vivo efficacy of monovalent monoclonal CD3 antibodies. Eur J Immunol 19:381–388, 1989.

12. CI Bindon, G Hale, H Waldmann. Importance of antibody specificity for complement mediated lysis by monoclonal antibodies. Eur J Immunol 18:1507–1514, 1988.

13. AL Tutt, RR French, TM Illidge, J Honeychurch, HM McBride, CA Penfold, DT Fearon, RM Parkhouse, GG Klaus, MJ Glennie. Monoclonal antibody therapy of B-cell lymphoma: signaling activity on tumor cells appears to be more important than recruitment of effectors. J Immunol 169:3176–3185, 1998.

14. L Ginaldi, M De Martinis, E Matutes, N Farahat, R Morilla, MJS Dyer, D Catovsky. Levels of expression of CD52 in normal and leukemic B and T cells: correlation with in vivo therapeutic responses to Campath-1H. Leuk Res 22:185–191, 1998.

15. MJS Dyer, G Hale, RE Marcus, H Waldmann. Remission induction in patients with lymphoid malignancies using unconjugated CAMPATH-1 monoclonal antibodies. Leukemia Lymphoma 2:179–190, 1990.

16. I Vorechovsky, L Luo, MJ Dyer, D Catovsky, PL Amlot, JC Yaxley, L Foroni, L Hammarström, AD Webster, MA Yuille. Clustering of missense mutations in the ataxia-telangiectasia gene in a sporadic T-cell leukaemia. Nat Genet 17:96–9, 1997.

17. L Riechmann, M Clark, H Waldmann, G Winter. Reshaping human antibodies for therapy. Nature 332:323–327, 1998.

18. M Bruggemann, GT Williams, CI Bindon, MR Clark, MR Walker, R Jefferis, H Waldmann, MS Neuberger. Comparison of the effector functions of human immunoglobulins using a matched set of chimeric antibodies. J Exp Med 166:1351–1361, 1987.

19. MR Lifely, C Hale, S Boyce, MJ Keen, J Phillips. Glycosylation and biological activity of CAMPATH-1H expressed in different cell lines and grown under different culture conditions. Glycobiology 5:813–822, 1995.

20. P Umana, J Jean-Mairet, R Moudry, H Amstutz, JE Bailey. Engineered glycoforms of an antineuroblastoma IgG1 with optimized antibody-dependent cellular cytotoxic activity. Nat Biotechnol 17:176–180, 1999.

21. JF de Kroon, RA de Paus, HC Kluin-Nelemans, PM Kluin, CA van Bergen, AJ Munro, G Hale, R Willemze, JH Falkenburg. Anti-CD45 and anti-CD52 (CAMPATH) monoclonal antibodies effectively eliminate systemically disseminated human non-Hodgkin's lymphoma B-cells in SCID mice. Exp Hematol 24:919–926, 1996.

22. A Treumann, MR Lifely, P Schneider, MA Ferguson. Primary structure of CD52. J Biol Chem 270:6088–6099, 1995.

23. C Hale, M Bartholomew, V Taylor, J Stables, P Topley, J Tite. Recognition of CD52 allelic gene products by CAMPATH-1H antibodies. Immunology 88:183–190, 1996.

24. K Simons, E Ikonen. Functional rafts in cell membranes. Nature 387:569–572, 1997.

25. G Hale, MQ Xia, HP Tighe, MJ Dyer, H Waldmann. The CAMPATH-1 antigen (CDw52). Tissue Antigens 35:118–127, 1990.

26. MH Gilleece, TM Dexter. Effect of Campath-1H antibody on human hematopoietic progenitors in vitro. Blood 82:807–812, 1993.

27. JR Salisbury, NT Rapson, JD Codd, MV Rogers, AB Nethersell. Immunohistochemical analysis of CDw52 antigen expression in non-Hodgkin's lymphomas. J Clin Pathol 47:313–317, 1994.

28. S Brett, G Baxter, H Cooper, JM Johnston, J Tite, N Rapson. Re-population of blood lymphocyte sub-populations in rheumatoid arthritis patients treated with the depleting humanized monoclonal antibody, CAMPATH-1H. Immunology 88:13–19, 1996.

29. SC Tang, K Hewitt, MD Reis, NL Berinstein. Immunosuppressive toxicity of CAMPATH-1H monoclonal antibody in the treatment of recurrent low-grade lymphoma. Leukemia Lymphoma 24:93–101, 1996.

30. W Rowan, J Tite, P Topley, SJ Brett. Cross-linking of the CAMPATH-1 antigen (CD52) mediates growth inhibition in human B- and T-lymphoma cell lines, and subsequent emergence of CD52-deficient cells. Immunology 95:427–436, 1998.

31. MJS Dyer, G Hale, FGJ Hayhoe, H Waldmann. Effects of CAMPATH-1 antibodies in vivo in patients with lymphoid malignancies: influence of antibody isotype. Blood 73:1431–1439, 1989.

32. B Hertenstein, B Wagner, D Bunjes, C Duncker, A Raghavachar, R Arnold, H Heimpel, H Schrezenmeier. Emergence of CD52-, phosphatidylinositolglycan-anchor-deficient T lymphocytes after in vivo application of Campath-1H for refractory B-cell non-Hodgkin lymphoma. Blood 86:1487–1492, 1995.

33. A Österborg, A Werner, E Halapi, J Lundin, U Harmenberg, H Wigzell, H Mellstedt. Clonal CD8+ and CD52− T cells are induced in responding B cell lymphoma patients treated with Campath-1H (anti-CD52). Eur J Haematol 58:5–13, 1997.

34. G Hale, S Bright, G Chumbley, T Hoang, D Metcalf, AJ Munro, H Waldmann. Removal of T cells from bone marrow for transplantation: a monoclonal antilymphocyte antibody fixes human complement. Blood 62:873–882, 1983.

35. G Hale, DM Swirsky, FGJ Hayhoe, H Waldmann. Effects of monoclonal anti-lymphocyte antibodies in vivo in monkeys and humans. Mol Biol Med 1:321–334, 1983.

36. G Hale, SP Cobbold, H Waldmann, G Easter, P Matejtschuk, RR Coombs. Isolation of low-frequency class-switch variants from rat hybrid myelomas. J Immunol Methods 103:59–67, 1987.

37. JD Isaacs, MG Wing, JD Greenwood, BL Hazleman, G Hale, H Waldmann. A therapeutic human IgG4 monoclonal antibody that depletes target cells in humans. Clin Exp Immunol 106:427–433, 1996.

38. G Hale, MJ Dyer, MR Clark, JM Phillips, R Marcus, L Riechmann, G Winter, H Waldmann. Remission induction in non-Hodgkin lymphoma with reshaped human monoclonal antibody CAMPATH-1H. Lancet 2:1394–1399, 1988.

39. TF Tedder, P Engel. CD20: a regulator of cell-cycle progression of B lymphocytes. Immunol Today 15:450–454, 1994.

40. TF Tedder, M Streuli, SF Schlossman, H Saito. Isolation and structure of a cDNA encoding the B1 (CD20) cell-surface antigen of human B lymphocytes. Proc Natl Acad Sci USA 85:208–212, 1988.

41. TL O'Keefe, GT Williams, SL Davies, MS Neuberger. Mice carrying a CD20 gene disruption. Immunogenetics 48:125–132, 1998.

42. EA Clark, G Shu, JA Ledbetter. Role of the Bp35 cell surface polypeptide in human B-cell activation. Proc Natl Acad Sci USA 82:1766–1770, 1985.

43. D Shan, JA Ledbetter, OW Press. Apoptosis of malignant human B Cells by ligation of CD20 with monoclonal antibodies. Blood 91:1644–1652, 1998.

44. H Taji, Y Kagami, Y Okada, M Andou, Y Nishi, H Saito, M Seto, Y Morishima. Growth inhibition of CD20-positive B lymphoma cell lines by IDEC-C2B8 anti-CD20 monoclonal antibody. Jpn J Cancer Res 89:748–756, 1998.

45. MJ Polyak, SH Tailor, JP Deans. Identification of a cytoplasmic region of CD20 required for its redistribution to a detergent-insoluble membrane compartment. J Immunol 161:3242–3248, 1998.

46. OW Press, F Appelbaum, JA Ledbetter, PJ Martin, J Zarling, P Kidd, ED Thomas. Monoclonal antibody 1F5 (anti-CD20) serotherapy of human B cell lymphomas. Blood 69:584–591, 1987.

47. ME Reff, K Carner, KS Chambers, PC Chinn, JE Leonard, R Raab, RA Newman, N Hanna, DR Anderson. Depletion of B cells in vivo by a chimeric mouse human monoclonal antibody to CD20. Blood 83:435–445, 1994.

48. DG Maloney, TM Liles, DK Czerwinski, C Waldichuk, J Rosenberg, A Grillo-Lopez, R Levy. Phase I clinical trial using escalating single-dose infusion of chimeric anti-CD20 monoclonal antibody (IDEC-C2B8) in patients with recurrent B-cell lymphoma. Blood 84:2457–2466, 1994.

49. DG Maloney. Preclinical and phase I and II trials of rituximab. Semin Oncol 26(5 suppl 14): 74–78, 1999.

50. D Catovsky, S Richards, J Fooks, et al. CLL trials in the United Kingdom. The Medical Research Council CLL trials 1, 2 and 3. Leuk Lymph 6:105–112, 1991.

51. MJ Keating, H Kantarjian, S O'Brien, C Koller, M Talpaz, J Schachner, CC Childs, EJ Freireich, KB McCredie. Fludarabine: a new agent with marked cytoreductive activity in untreated chronic lymphocytic leukemia. J Clin Oncol 9:44–49, 1991.

52. A Saven, RH Lemon, M Kosty, E Beutler, LD Piro. 2-Chlorodeoxyadenosine activity in patients with untreated chronic lymphocytic leukemia. J Clin Oncol 13:570–574, 1995.

53. MJ Keating, H Kantarjian, M Talpaz, J Redman, C Koller, B Barlogie, W Velasquez, W Plunkett, EJ Freireich, KB McCredie. Fludarabine: a new agent with major activity against chronic lymphocytic leukemia. Blood 74:19–25, 1989.

54. G Juliusson, J Liliemark. High complete remission rate from 2-chloro-2'-deoxyadenosine in previously treated patients with B-cell chronic lymphocytic leukemia: response predicted by rapid decrease of blood lymphocyte count. J Clin Oncol 11:679–689, 1993.

55. MJ Keating, S O'Brien, H Kantarjian, W Plunkett, E Estey, C Koller, M Beran, EJ Freireich. Long-term follow-up of patients with chronic lymphocytic leukemia treated with fludarabine as a single agent. Blood 81:2878–2884, 1993.

56. G Juliusson, J Liliemark. Retreatment of chronic lymphocytic leukemia with 2-chlorodeoxyadenosine (CdA) at relapse following CdA-induced remission: No aquired resistance. Leuk Lymph 13:75–80, 1994.

57. SH Lim, G Davey, R Marcus. Differential response in a patient treated with Campath-1H monoclonal antibody for refractory non-Hodgkin lymphoma. Lancet 341:432–433, 1993.

58. J Lundin, A Österborg, G Brittinger, D Crowther, H Dombret, A Engert, A Epenetos, C Gisselbrecht, D Huhn, U Jaeger, J Thomas, R Marcus, N Nissen, C Poynton, E Rankin, R Stahel, M Uppenkamp, R Willemze, H Mellstedt. CAMPATH-1H monoclonal antibody in therapy for previously treated low-grade non-Hodgkin's lymphomas: a phase II multicenter study. European Study Group of CAMPATH-1H Treatment in Low-Grade Non-Hodgkin's Lymphoma. J Clin Oncol 16:3257–3263, 1998.

59. A Österborg, M Dyer, D Bunjes, GA Pangalis, Y Bastion, D Catovsky, H Mellstedt. Phase II multicenter study of human CD52 antibody in previously treated chronic lymphocytic leukemia. J Clin Oncol 15:1567–1574, 1997.

60. J Shetye, J Frödin, B Christensson, C Grant, B Jacobsson, S Sundelius, M Sylven, P Biberfeld, H Mellstedt. Immunohistochemical monitoring of metastatic colorectal carcinoma in patients treated with monoclonal antibodies (MAb17-1A). Cancer Immunol Immunother 27:154–162, 1988.

61. M Dyer. The role of CAMPATH-1 antibodies in the treatment of lymphoid maligancies. Semin Oncol 26(suppl 14):52–57, 1999.

62. AL Bowen, A Zomas, E Emmett, E Matutes, M Dyer, D Catovsky. Subcutaneous CAMPATH-1H in fludarabine-resistant/relapsed chronic lymphocytic and B-prolymphocytic leukaemia. Br J Haematol 96:617–619, 1997.

63. B Kennedy, A Rawstron, P Evans, A English, A Haynes, N Russel, J Byrne, G Hale, G Morgan, P Hillman. Campath-1H therapy in 29 patients with refractory CLL: "True" complete remission is an attainable goal. Blood 94(suppl 1):603a, 1999.

64. M Keating, J Byrd, K Rai, I Flinn, V Jain, J Binet, R Bolin, P Hillman, M Hutchinson. Multicenter study of Campath-1H in patients with chronic lympocytic leukemia (B-CLL) refractory to fludarabine. Blood 94(suppl 1):705a, 1999.

65. G Riethmuller, E Schneider-Gadicke, G Schlimok, W Schmiegel, R Raab, K Hoffken, R

Gruber, H Pichlmaier, H Hirche, R Pichlmayr, et al. Randomised trial of monoclonal antibody for adjuvant therapy of resected Dukes' C colorectal carcinoma. German Cancer Aid 17-1A Study Group. Lancet 343:1177–1183, 1994.

66. G Riethmuller, E Holz, G Schlimok, W Schmiegel, R Raab, K Hoffken, R Gruber, I Funke, H Pichlmaier, H Hirche, P Buggisch, J Witte, R Pichlmayr. Monoclonal antibody therapy for resected Dukes' C colorectal cancer: seven-year outcome of a multicenter randomized trial. J Clin Oncol 16:1788–1794, 1998.

67. A Österborg, A Fassas, A Anagnostopoulos, M Dyer, D Catovsky, H Mellstedt. Humanized CD52 monoclonal antibody CAMPATH-1H as first-line treatment in chronic lymphocytic leukaemia. Br J Haematol 93:151–153, 1996.

68. H Mellstedt, A Österborg, J Lundin, M Björkholm, F Celsing, H Hagberg, R Hast, V Hjalmar, E Kimby, M Luthman, O Tullgren, B Werner. CAMPATH-1H therapy of patients with previously untreated chronic lymphocytic leukemia (CLL). Abstract. Blood 92(suppl. 1):490a, 1998.

69. M Dyer, S Kelsey, H Mackay, E Emmett, P Thornton, G Hale, H Waldmann, A Newland, D Catovsky. In vivo "purging" of residual disease in CLL with Campath-1H. Br J Haematol 97:669–672, 1997.

70. G DelleKarth, K Laczika, C Scholten, K Lechner, U Jaeger, I Schwarzinger, I Simonitsch. Clearance of PCR-detectable lymphoma cells from the peripheral blood, but not bone marrow after therapy with campath-1H. Am J Hematol 50:146–152, 1995.

71. E Matutes, V Brito-Babapulle, J Swansbury, J Ellis, R Morilla, C Dearden, A Sempere, D Catovsky. Clinical and laboratory features of 78 cases of T-prolymphocytic leukemia. Blood 78:3269–3274, 1991.

72. R Pawson, M Dyer, R Barge, E Matutes, PD Thornton, E Emmett, JC Kluin-Nelemans, WE Fibbe, R Willemze, D Catovsky. Treatment of T-cell prolymphocytic leukemia with human CD52 antibody. J Clin Oncol 15:2667–2672, 1997.

73. B Cazin, M Wetterwald, M Ojeda, B Mahé, F Bauters. Campath-1H in the treatment of T-prolymphocytic leukemia (T-PLL). Blood 94(suppl 1):125a, 1999.

74. PJJS De Schouwer. Gene rearrangements in T-cell prolymphocytic leukaemia. PhD thesis, University of London, 1999.

75. P McLaughlin, AJ Grillo-Lopez, BK Link, R Levy, MS Czuczman, ME Williams, MR Heyman, I Bence-Bruckler, CA White, F Cabanillas, V Jain, AD Ho, J Lister, K Wey, D Shen, BK Dallaire. Rituximab chimeric anti-CD20 monoclonal antibody therapy for relapsed indolent lymphoma: half of patients respond to a four-dose treatment program. J Clin Oncol 16:2825–2833, 1998.

76. J Foran, A Rohatiner, D Cunningham, R Popescu, P Solal-Celigny, M Ghielmini, B Coiffier, P Johnson, C Gisselbrecht, F Reyes, J Radford, E Bessell, B Souleau, A Benzohra, T Lister. European Phase II study of rituximab (chimeric anti-CD20 monoclonal antibody) for patients with newly diagnosed mantle-cell lymphoma and previously treated mantle-cell lymphoma, immunocytoma, and small B-cell lymphocytic lymphoma. J Clin Oncol 18:317–324, 2000.

77. LD Piro, CA White, AJ Grillo-López, N Janakiraman, A Saven, TM Beck, C Varns, S Shuey, M Czuczman, JW Lynch, JE Kolitz, V Jain. Extended rituximab (anti-CD20 monoclonal antibody) therapy for relapsed or refractory low-grade or follicular non-Hodgkin's lymphoma. Annals of Oncology 10:655–661, 1999.

78. DT Nguyen, JA Amess, H Doughty, L Hendry, LW Diamond. IDEC-C2B8 anti-CD20 (rituximab) immunotherapy in patients with low-grade non-Hodgkin's lymphoma and lymphoproliferative disorders: evaluation of response on 48 patients. Eur J Haematol 62:76–82, 1999.

79. NM Almasri, RE Duque, J Iturraspe, E Everett, RC Braylan. Reduced expression of CD20 antigen as a characteristic marker for chronic lymphocytic leukemia. Am J Hematol 40:259, 1992.

80. M Ladetto, L Bergui, I Ricca, S Campana, A Pileri, C Tarella. Rituximab anti-CD20 mono-

clonal antibody induced marked but transient reductions of peripheral blood lymphocytes in chronic lymphocytic leukemia patients. Med Oncol 17:203–210, 2000.

81. M Jensen, U Winkler, O Manzke, V Diehl, A Engert. Rapid tumor lysis in a patient with B-cell chronic lymphocytic leukemia and lymphocytosis treated with an anti-CD20 monoclonal antibody (IDEC-C2B8, rituximab). Ann Hematol 77:89–91, 1998.

82. U Winkler, M Jensen, O Manzke, H Schulz, V Diehl, A Engert. Cytokine-release syndrome in patients with B-cell chronic lymphocytic leukemia and high lymphocyte counts after treatment with an anti-CD20 monoclonal antibody (rituximab, IDEC-C2B8). Blood 94:2217–2224, 1999.

83. JC Byrd, JK Waselenko, TJ Maneatis, T Murphy, FT Ward, BP Monahan, MA Sipe, S Donegan, CA White. Rituximab therapy in hematologic malignancy patients with circulating blood tumor cells: association with increased infusion-related side effects and rapid blood tumor clearance. J Clin Oncol 17:791–795, 1999.

84. S O'Brien, D Thomas, E Freireich, M Andreef, F Giles, M Keating. Rituxan has significant activity in patients with CLL. Blood 94(suppl 1):603a, 1999.

85. JC Byrd, MR Grever, B Davis, MS Lucas, K Park, A Goodrich, C Morrison, T Murphy, L Kunkel, A Grillo-Lopez, JK Waselenko, IW Flinn. Phase I/II study of thrice weekly rituximab in chronic lymphocytic lymphoma (SLL): A feasible and active regimen. Blood 94(suppl 1): 704a, 1999.

16

Genomic Aberrations in B-Cell Chronic Lymphocytic Leukemia

STEPHAN STILGENBAUER and HARTMUT DÖHNER

University of Ulm, Ulm, Germany

PETER LICHTER

Deutsches Krebsforschungszentrum, Heidelberg, Germany

I. INTRODUCTION

B-cell chronic lymphocytic leukemia (B-CLL) is the most common leukemia in adults. Despite the high incidence, the knowledge on the genomic aberrations underlying B-CLL pathogenesis is still limited. This is mainly related to the low in-vitro mitotic activity of the tumor cells, which has made conventional cytogenetic studies by chromosome banding difficult. On the other hand, analyses based on molecular genetic techniques such as Southern blot analysis or polymerase chain reaction (PCR) have been limited by the fact that candidate genes are known only for few chromosome regions affected in B-CLL. By fluorescence in-situ hybridization (FISH) genomic abnormalities can be detected on the single cell level in nondividing cells, circumventing the need to obtain metaphase chromosomes from B-CLL cells. The genomic regions can be detected with DNA probes available from genome-wide libraries without the need of prior candidate gene identification. By FISH with a disease-specific probe set aberrations can now be detected in more than 80% of B-CLL cases. In contrast to other types of low-grade lymphoma the by far most frequent type of genomic aberration in B-CLL are deletions. The most frequent deletion cluster regions involve band 13q14, followed by 11q22–q23, 17p13, and 6q21. Common gains of chromosomal material are trisomies 12q, 8q, and 3q. Translocations involving the immunoglobulin heavy chain gene locus (*IgH*) at 14q32, which are frequently observed in other types of lymphoma, are rare events in B-CLL. Genes targeted by the aberrations in B-CLL appear to be *p53* in band 17p13 and *ATM* in a subset of cases with 11q22–q23 deletions. However, for most of the frequently affected genomic regions in B-CLL, the search for candidate genes is ongoing. In addition to the delineation of critical regions, FISH allowed the accurate evaluation of the incidence of genomic aberrations in B-CLL. This provided the valid basis for a correlation of the abnormalities with clinical phenotype and survival. Deletions 17p13 (*p53*) and 11q22–q23 have proven to be among the most important independent prognostic factors identifying subgroups of patients with rapidly progressive disease and inferior survival. In addition, deletion 17p13 (*p53*) has been shown to predict for nonresponse to therapy with purine analogs. The study of genomic aberrations may lead to a better understanding of the molecular pathogenesis of the disease. Furthermore, the prognostic significance of these aberrations may have implications for a better risk-adapted management of B-CLL patients in the near future.

II. TECHNICAL APPROACHES FOR THE GENETIC ANALYSIS OF B-CLL

A. Conventional Chromosome Banding Analysis

Chromosome abnormalities in B-CLL were initially studied by conventional metaphase chromosome analysis of short-term in-vitro cultures. A key problem in these early studies was the very low metaphase yield and until the late 1970s no chromosome abnormality characteristic for B-CLL was identified (1). In the 1980s the application of B-cell mitogens such as TPA, lipopolysaccharide, pokeweed mitogen, anti-human IgM, B-cell growth factor, and anti-CD40 antibody allowed the stimulation of B cells to divide in vitro and led to the identification of recurrent chromosome aberrations (2–9). However, even then, frequently only metaphase spreads without clonal abnormalities were obtained. In a study combining immunophenotyping and karyotyping, it was demonstrated that despite the use of B-cell mitogens, the normal metaphase spreads obtained from B-CLL samples frequently originated from nonleukemic T-cells (10). Despite improved cell culture techniques, in the early 1990s clonal chromosome abnormalities were detectable in only 40% to 50% of B-CLL cases. Furthermore, the identification and characterization of the aberrations were often hampered by poor chromosomes quality (11–13).

B. Fluorescence In-Situ Hybridization

Over recent years, the development of molecular cytogenetic techniques such as FISH has greatly improved the diagnostic accuracy for the detection of genomic aberrations in tumor cells (14,15). Specific DNA sequences in interphase cells or metaphase spreads are delineated by FISH with cloned DNA fragments, which are visualized by fluorescence microscopy. This allows the detection of numerical and structural aberrations because copy number changes in the tumor cell genome are identified by aberrant signal numbers per cell, whereas translocation breakpoints can be identified by the aberrant spatial distribution pattern of the fluorescence signals (see color plate for Fig. 1 [noted as Figure 16.1]). The spatial resolution for the detection of aberrations by FISH is superior to that of conventional chromosome banding. Whereas by chromosome banding analysis only large abnormalities are detected [i.e., rearranged or deleted chromosome bands corresponding to several megabasepairs (Mb) of DNA] FISH allows the identification of genomic aberrations in the range of several kilobase pairs (kb). Ideal FISH probes are fragments of 40- to 150-kb size, [i.e., DNA fragments cloned into cosmid, P1-derived artificial chromosome [PAC], or bacterial artificial chromosome [BAC] vectors] (14,15). Moreover, for the detection of genomic aberrations the region involved does not need to be well characterized at the molecular level. In contrast to analyses by PCR-based approaches, no sequence information of the region under investigation needs to be available. Probes can be selected from the continuously growing number of physically mapped fragments cloned in yeast artificial chromosomes (YACs), PACs, BACs, or cosmids that are available as genome-wide libraries.

The diagnostic potential of FISH is not restricted to the study of metaphase chromosomes. By selection of adequate probes numerical and structural aberrations can also be detected in interphase nuclei, an approach referred to as "interphase cytogenetics" (see color plate for Fig. 1 [noted as Figure 16.1]) (16,17). The metaphase cells obtained from B-CLL specimens are often not representative for the leukemic clone. This, together with its better spatial resolution, results in the much higher sensitivity of the interphase cytogenetic approach to detect genomic aberrations in B-CLL (Fig. 2). However, because of the restricted number of fluorochromes available, only a limited number of probes can be combined in a single hybridization experiment. Therefore, to analyze multiple regions of interest several experiments are necessary, and a comprehensive screening is labor intensive.

C. Comparative Genomic Hybridization

By comparative genomic hybridization (CGH) a genome-wide screening for chromosome imbalances in a tumor genome can be performed without the knowledge of candidate regions involved in the respective tumor type (18–20). Differently labeled total genomic DNA samples, one derived from the tumor cells and the other derived from normal tissue, are hybridized simultaneously as probes to normal metaphase spreads. Chromosome regions overrepresented in the tumor such as trisomies, polysomies, or DNA amplifications

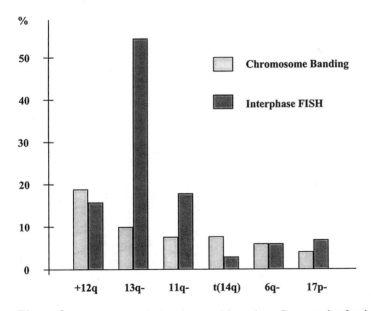

Figure 2 Comparison of Metaphase and Interphase Cytogenetics for the Detection of Chromosome Aberrations in B-CLL. The incidence of trisomy 12 (+12q) deletions affecting 13q (13q−), 11q (11q−), 6q (6q−), and 17p (17p−), as well as translocations of band 14q32, t(14q), are compared as observed by chromosome banding (11,12) and by interphase FISH (142).

can be detected by a stronger hybridization signal in the respective regions of the metaphase chromosomes compared with a homogenous staining of the differently labeled control DNA. Correspondingly, regions underrepresented in the tumor genome such as monosomies or deletions can be detected by a weaker staining of the respective target regions in the metaphase chromosomes compared with the staining by the control DNA. In a study directly comparing CGH data with banding results in B-CLL, a high proportion of cases with aberrations only detectable by CGH was found (21). This observation was frequently due to the failure of B-CLL cells to divide and sometimes due to complex karyotypes. Therefore, CGH provides a valuable additional technology for a genome-wide screening for chromosome imbalances in B-CLL. The delineation of critical regions by CGH has been instrumental for the selection of DNA probes that can be used for a rapid screening of large numbers of B-CLL cases by interphase cytogenetics.

D. Molecular Genetic Techniques

In B-CLL the analysis of genomic aberrations at the molecular genetic level has been limited by the lack of candidate genes in almost all recurrently involved genomic segments. In addition, the contamination of B-CLL specimens with nonclonal cells can influence the sensitivity of molecular approaches such as quantitative Southern blot or microsatellite analyses. Deletion screening detecting loss of heterozygosity (LOH) by quantitative Southern blot or microsatellite analyses and in particular mutation analyses of candidate genes by single-strand conformational polymorphism (SSCP) or DNA sequence analysis have been limited to a few regions. Only recently, a pathogenic role was identified for specific genes such as *p53* and *ATM* in subsets of B-CLL patients (see later), allowing molecular genetic screening in patient samples.

III. INCIDENCE OF CHROMOSOME ABNORMALITIES IN B-CLL

A. Chromosome Banding Studies

Initial reports on recurrent chromosome abnormalities in B-CLL as detected by chromosome banding were published in the late 70s and early 80s. Various abnormalities were reported, but the first aberration described as a recurrent aberration was trisomy 12 (2–6,22). Trisomy 12 was subsequently confirmed as a frequent aberration in B-CLL in several studies (23–31). In the late 80s another recurrent aberration was described involving the long arm of chromosome 13 (13q). Structural abnormalities, mostly deletions and less frequently translocations, involving band 13q14 were found by several groups (28,32–34). In several smaller series, this abnormality was observed at the same frequency or even more frequently than trisomy 12. Other chromosome aberrations identified at varying frequencies by chromosome banding were deletions of 6q (6,25,26,30,31), 11q (25,26,28, 33,35) and 17p (30), partial or total trisomy 3 (23,25,28), and translocations involving band 14q32 (3,6,23,25,27,30,31,36–38). Frequently, the 14q32 abnormality was the result of a t(11;14)(q13;q32), which today is considered the genetic hallmark of mantle cell lymphoma (MCL) (39). Therefore, many of the tumors reported as B-CLL exhibiting the t(11;14(q13;q32) in early chromosome banding reports may have been leukemic MCL cases.

Among the largest compilations of chromosome banding data in B-CLL were the reports of the *First* and *Second International Working Party on Chromosomes in CLL* (IWCCLL) (11,12). In the Second IWCCLL, 662 B-CLL patients from 11 institutions were studied, and chromosomes were successfully obtained in 604 cases. Clonal chromosome aberrations were identified in 311 of the 662 cases (47%), and the single most common aberration was trisomy 12 (19% of the evaluable cases), followed by structural aberrations of chromosomes 13 (10%), 14 (8%), 11 (8%), 6 (6%), and 17 (4%) (12). However, in more than half of the cases studied either no metaphase spreads were obtained or no clonal abnormality was found.

B. Interphase Cytogenetic Studies

The identification of chromosome regions recurrently involved in aberrations by chromosome banding studies and CGH provided the basis for the development of DNA probe sets allowing a comprehensive assessment of genomic aberrations in B-CLL. Our probe set is designed for the identification of the most important numerical and structural abnormalities, including trisomy 12 and deletions in several chromosome regions, such as 13q14, 11q22.3–q23.1, 6q21, 6q27, and 17p13, as well as of other less frequently occurring aberrations. With the application of these probes on large series of B-CLL patients it became apparent that the prevalence of specific aberrations is higher than assumed on the basis of the data from chromosome banding studies. As detected by interphase cytogenetics, the most common aberration in B-CLL is 13q14 deletion, which is found in approximately 50% of cases. The next most common aberrations are 11q22–q23 deletion (approximately 20%), trisomy 12 (15%–20%), 6q21 deletion (5%–10%), and 17p13 deletion (5%–10%). The discrepancy of the incidence of individual aberrations as detected by chromosome banding analysis and interphase cytogenetics may to some degree reflect differences in patient selection but is to a larger extent likely related to the different sensitivity of the techniques.

The sensitive detection of genomic aberrations in B-CLL by interphase FISH provided the basis for a more accurate correlation of the abnormalities with clinical parameters such as disease progression, response to therapy, and survival. These studies have indicated that the genomic aberrations are among the most important independent risk factors in B-CLL. This has led to the evaluation of the prognostic significance of genomic aberrations in large prospective multicenter treatment trials. Furthermore, while recurrently involved regions were identified by chromosome banding, interphase analyses and molecular techniques have allowed the narrowing of the critical genomic regions and the identification of candidate genes involved in the pathogenesis or progression of B-CLL.

IV. CHARACTERIZATION OF GENOMIC ABERRATIONS IN B-CLL

A. Deletions in Band 13q14 and Identification of Candidate Genes

Chromosome banding series in the late 1980s initially pointed to the recurrent involvement of the long arm of chromosome 13 in B-CLL (28,31–34). At the resolution power of metaphase chromosome analysis, most cases with 13q14 aberrations are deletions, whereas some appear as balanced translocations. However, it was later demonstrated by molecular genetic techniques that the translocation breakpoints in 13q14 are accompanied by submicroscopic deletions.

Genomic regions frequently involved in deletions are assumed to harbor tumor suppressor genes, which by deletion of one allele and mutation of the remaining copy are inactivated. A prominent tumor suppressor gene located in band 13q14 is the retinoblastoma gene (*RB1*) (40). In addition to hereditary and sporadic retinoblastoma, a variety of other tumors are thought to be related to loss of function resulting from inactivation of both alleles by mutation and/or deletion. *RB1* encodes a nuclear phosphoprotein involved in cell cycle control and transcriptional regulation (40). By molecular techniques, monoallelic deletions of *RB1* were frequently found in B-CLL, but abnormalities disrupting both alleles of *RB1*, in line with the two-hit model for tumor suppressor gene inactivation, were rarely observed (41–44).

Therefore, a search for other tumor suppressor genes in this region was initiated. Because translocation breakpoints involving 13q14 were found to leave *RB1* intact while they were associated with loss of a more telomeric genomic region in vicinity of the marker *D13S25*, a novel tumor suppressor gene was postulated to be located approximately 1.6 cM telomeric of *RB1* (44,45). Subsequent molecular genetic studies aimed at localizing the critical region more precisely (44–50). Devilder et al. (47) initially located the critical region between *D13S25* and the more distal marker *D13S294*. However, a comparison of *RB1* and *D13S25* deletions in 85 B-CLL tumors led us to hypothesize that the critical region was located centromeric of *D13S25*. Our finding was supported by Liu et al., who found a critical region involving the marker *D13S319* located between *RB1* and *D13S25* (48,49). Bullrich et al., (50) identified a minimal deletion region between *D13S25* and the marker *206XF12* located less than 550 kb proximal of *D13S25*.

To localize the critical genomic region and to identify candidate genes from this segment, several groups have constructed high-resolution physical maps spanning several hundred kilobases at the *RB1–D13S25* interval (51–55). Kalachikov et al. (51) identified a critical deletion region of approximately 300 kb around the *D13S272* marker. Deletions of this segment were observed in 54% B-CLLs tested and were frequently homozygous. Furthermore, a large number of novel expressed sequences were identified from this critical region. Liu et al. (52) found a 10-kb minimal deletion interval immediately centromeric to *D13S272* and identified two candidate genes, *Leu1* and *Leu2*, located in this region. However, no mutational inactivation of these genes was found. Bouyge-Moreau et al. (53) identified a 550-kb critical region but also found no mutational inactivation of *Leu1* and *Leu2* (56).

We constructed a 1.4-Mb sized contig of DNA fragments at the critical *D13S273– D13S25* interval and used these clones to study a series of 322 B-CLL cases. Included in this analysis were 30 MCLs, because a similar deletion cluster region at 13q14 was observed in this disease (55,57). The frequency of 13q14 deletion was 51% in B-CLL and even 70% in MCL. A commonly deleted segment involving marker *D13S272* was identified, and several cDNA fragments were isolated from this region (55). Two of them, *ep272-3-t5* and *ep272-3-t4*, corresponded to the *Leu1* and *Leu2* genes, respectively, which were described in the study by Liu et al. (52). However, also in our experiments no evidence for mutational disruption of these genes was observed, and therefore the search for the tumor suppressor gene involved in B-CLL in band 13q14 is currently ongoing. Interestingly, a similar 13q14 deletion region as in B-CLL was recently described in multiple myeloma. This raises the question whether the same putative tumor suppressor gene is involved in both diseases (58).

An independent deletion region affecting the *BRCA2* gene in band 13q12 was postulated in one study (59). However, in several subsequent reports no recurrent deletion of *BRCA2* was observed. Panayiotidis et al. found no case of *BRCA2* loss among 24 B-CLL, and in our study only a single case with *BRCA2* deletion without 13q14 loss was observed among 105 B-CLL (55,60).

B. Deletions of Chromosome Bands 11q22–q23 and *ATM* as Candidate Gene

In a compilation of data from the *Catalog of Chromosome Aberrations in Cancer*, one of the most common structural aberrations resulting in loss of chromosomal material in the categories "lymphoproliferative disorders" and "NHLs" were aberrations affecting the region 11q21–q25 (61). However, abnormalities involving 11q were only observed in 49 of 604 (8%) cytogenetically evaluable cases in the Second IWCCLL study (12). Most of these aberrations resulted from the translocation t(11;14)(q13;q32), which today is considered the cytogenetic hallmark of MCL. By molecular studies, the rearrangement of the *CCND1* (*BCL1*) gene with the *IgH* locus, the molecular counterpart of the t(11; 14)(q13;q32), is very infrequently found in B-CLL (see section on 14q32 aberrations).

11q Aberrations other than translocations at 11q13 were observed in less than 5% of B-CLL cases in the Second IWCCLL (12). Also, in three recently published large series, each on several hundred B-CLL cases, 11q deletions did not occur as a frequent aberration (62–64). However, the frequency of 11q deletions has probably been underestimated in many chromosome banding studies in B-CLL. Evidence for the significance of chromosomal loss in 11q came from several smaller studies, and in a recent report 11q deletions were the second most common chromosome aberration after 13q deletion and were of prognostic significance (25,26,28,33,35,65,66). Regarding the characterization of the critical 11q region in B-CLL, until recently only scarce data have been available. In one FISH study of 15 hematological neoplasms with 11q deletions, a commonly deleted segment at 11q23.1 containing the neural cell adhesion molecule (NCAM) gene was found, whereas the *BCL1* locus at 11q13 and the *MLL* gene at 11q23.3 were located outside the critical region (67).

To refine the critical region affected by the 11q deletions in B-CLL, we performed a molecular cytogenetic study applying interphase FISH in 40 B-CLL, showing 11q deletion (68) with probes from a YAC contig spanning bands 11q14.3–q23.3 (69). All 11q deletions were found to affect a single minimal deletion region of 2 to 3 Mb in bands 11q22.3–q23.1 in which were also two translocation breakpoints located. A similar deletion segment was confirmed by another group (70). Among the genes located in this region, *RDX* (radixin) and *ATM* (ataxia telangiectasia mutated) appeared as candidate tumor suppressor genes because of their function. *RDX* has homology to the neurofibromatosis-type 2 gene (*NF2*) (71), whereas evidence for a growth suppressor function of *ATM* came from murine knockout models and from its involvement in cell cycle checkpoint control and DNA maintenance (72). Furthermore, deletions and missense mutations leading to disruption of both *ATM* alleles have been reported in T prolymphocytic leukemia, indicating a tumor suppressor function of *ATM* (73,74). It was postulated that *ATM* may also be affected in B-CLL on the basis of the observation of absent *ATM* protein expression in subsets of B-CLL, and indeed a mutational disruption of *ATM* was demonstrated in B-CLL (75–78). Although in the study by Bullrich et al. *ATM* mutations found in B-CLL cells were also observed in the germ line, suggesting a predisposition of heterozygous *ATM* mutation carriers to develop B-CLL (76), this was not observed in our series (78). Furthermore, in our series *ATM* mutations were only observed in 5 of 22 B-CLL cases with 11q22–q23 deletions. Therefore, the possibility that additional genes in 11q22–q23 may be altered in B-CLL has to be considered. This is in marked contrast to the situation in MCL in which deletion 11q22–q23 has recently been identified as frequent alteration (79,80). In MCL, all cases with loss of 11q material showed mutational disruption of the remaining *ATM* allele, strongly arguing for a tumor suppressor function of *ATM* in MCL (81).

C. Trisomy 12 as a Recurrent Aberration in B-CLL

In the early 80s, trisomy 12 was reported as the first recurrent chromosome aberration of B-CLL and in subsequent reports was almost invariably found as the most frequent chromosome aberration occurring at a frequency of less than 10% to more than 25% of cases (6,23–31). The identification of a critical region has been difficult by chromosome banding analyses, because only few B-CLL cases were reported exhibiting a partial trisomy 12 (8,30,82). The segment recurrently found duplicated included bands 12q13–q21.2, indicating that this region may contain an oncogene likely involved in the pathogenesis of B-CLL. As shown by restriction fragment length polymorphism (RFLP) analyses, trisomy 12 in B-CLL results from duplication of one homolog rather than from loss of one homolog and triplication of the remaining one (83).

The molecular cytogenetic approach by interphase FISH has been widely used to study trisomy 12 in B-CLL (8,62,84–90) (Table 1). The frequencies of trisomy 12 in the FISH studies ranged from 10% to 20% in European series to more than 30% in two studies from the United States (85,87). These differences may be related to patient selection but may also be due to different geographical distribution of this chromosome aberration. However, in all studies the frequency of trisomy 12 was greater when assessed by interphase FISH using DNA probes recognizing the repetitive sequences of the centromeric and pericentromeric region than when conventional chromosome banding techniques were used. For example, in our initial series of 42 patients, trisomy 12 was observed in 4 cases (10%) by banding and in 6 cases (14%) by interphase FISH (8). In the extended analysis of 245 B-CLL cases by interphase FISH, 36 (15%) exhibited trisomy 12, which was only the third most common chromosome aberration after deletion 13q14 and deletion 11q22–q23 (91). Toward the identification of a minimal duplication segment of chromosome 12, we identified a B-CLL tumor with isolated overrepresentation of a fragment in 12q13–q14 (21). Merup et al. analyzed a complex chromosome 12 rearrangement found in a lymphoproliferative tumor by FISH and found bands 12q13–q15 amplified at the highest

Table 1 Correlation of Specific Chromosome Aberrations with the Clinical Characteristics and Outcome in Patients with B-CLL

	Chromosome banding	Interphase cytogenetics
Trisomy 12	Atypical morphology	Atypical morphology
	Stronger SmIg + FMC7 expression	Stronger SmIg + FMC7 expression
	Advanced stages	
	Shorter survival times (controversial)	Shorter survival times
13q Aberrations	Favorable prognosis	No data
11q Aberrations	Rapid disease progression	Extensive lymphadenopathy
		Advanced stages
		Shorter treatment-free interval
		Shorter survival times
17p Aberrations	Shorter survival times	Shorter treatment-free interval
		Shorter survival times
		Resistance to treatment

frequency (92). Dierlamm et al. observed partial trisomy 12 in 11 of more than 1000 cases of B-NHL by FISH, and bands 12q13–q22 were identified as the minimally duplicated region (93). An alternative approach to identify and localize amplification segments in the genome is comparative genomic hybridization (CGH) (21). Particularly useful to this end could be the recently developed DNA-chip technology allowing a high-resolution mapping of copy number aberrations by hybridization to cloned DNA fragments instead of entire chromosomes (94,95).

D. Deletion 6q in Lymphoid Neoplasms

Deletions involving the long arm of chromosome 6 are observed as recurrent aberration in the entire spectrum of lymphoid neoplasms (61). In B-CLL, 6q deletions were found in 6% of evaluable cases by chromosome banding in the Second IWCCLL study (12). The aberrations were diverse, but bands 6q15 and 6q23 were most frequently affected. In a comprehensive molecular genetic analysis of several subtypes of malignant lympho- mas, at least two independent deletion cluster regions were identified, one at 6q21–q23 and another at 6q25–q27 (96). The deletion region in 6q21–q23 was linked to small lymphocytic lymphoma (SLL), which is considered the lymphomatous counterpart of B-CLL (97). A proximal location of the minimal deletion region in 6q was also found in several recent studies. Merup et al. observed 6q deletions in 6% of B-CLL with a critical deletion region spanning markers D6S283 through D6S270 in 6q21 (98). Gaidano et al. found 6q deletions in only 4 of 100 B-CLL tumors by Southern blot analysis (99). How- ever, the probes used in this study were located in band 6q27, which may not be the critical segment of chromosome 6 most frequently lost in B-CLL. In our interphase FISH study of 285 B-CLL patients, probes for 6q21 and 6q27 were used (100). The incidence of 6q deletion was 7%, and all deletions were found with the probe mapping to 6q21, whereas the 6q27 region was deleted in one-third of these cases only. No case of 6q27 deletion without 6q21 deletion was observed. Similarly, Zhang et al. determined a 4–5 Mb minimal deletion region in band 6q21 in a variety of lymphomas and lymphoid leuke- mias (101). A number of genes are known to be located in the critical 6q21 region, but at present none of these has been shown to be involved in lymphoma or leukemia develop- ment.

E. Deletion 17p13 and Mutation of *p53* in B-CLL

Evidence for an involvement of the *p53* gene and its chromosomal site in band 17p13 in B-CLL initially came from molecular genetic studies. On the basis of its prominent role in the pathogenesis of other types of cancer, *p53* was studied as a candidate gene despite the fact that 17p abnormalities were only very infrequently observed in B-CLL by chromo- some banding (12). By SSCP analysis and by sequencing of the PCR amplified gene fragments, Gaidano et al. found *p53* mutations in 6 of 40 (15%) B-CLL tumors (102). Subsequently, several groups found *p53* mutations at a frequency ranging from 10% to 15% (99,103,104). Until the recently observed disruption of *ATM* by mutations in B-CLL, *p53* was the only gene shown to be involved in the pathogenesis of B-CLL. The disruption of one allele by point mutation together with deletion of the second allele is the hallmark of the inactivation of a recessively acting tumor suppressor gene such as *p53*. However, structural aberrations of chromosome 17 were only observed in 4% of cytogenetically evaluable B-CLL in the IWCCLL studies (11,12). Recently, Geisler and coworkers found chromosome 17 aberrations at a frequency of 4% among 480 B-CLL patients using chromosome banding analysis (63). Evidence for a more frequent disruption of chromosome 17 in B-CLL came from smaller chromosome banding series. Bird et al. (30) observed abnormalities leading to deletion of 17p in 5 of 31 (16%) of evaluable cases. Although the involvement of *p53* in B-CLL was largely based on molecular genetic studies demonstrating intragenic mutations, we applied FISH using a *p53* genomic probe to screen for deletions in a large series of patients with chronic B-cell leukemias (105). In our initial series of 100 cases of chronic B-cell leukemias, we identified 17 (17%) tumors that exhibited a *p53* gene deletion, whereas in an extended series of 214 B-CLL patients, the frequency of *p53* loss was 9% (91). The difference in incidence between the two studies is most likely due to patient selection, because in the extended series only leukemias with the morphological and immunophenotypical characteristics of classical B-CLL were included, and in the initial study a high frequency of deletions was found among prolymphocytic variants. Thus, in classical B-CLL *p53* appears to be disrupted by deletion or mutation in approximately 9% to 15% of cases as detected by interphase FISH and DNA sequence analyses.

F. Rearrangement and Mutation at the *IgH* locus at 14q32

Translocations involving chromosome 14, mostly at band 14q32 where the immunoglobulin heavy chain gene locus (*IgH*) resides, were frequently reported in chromosome banding studies of B-CLL (3,6,11,23,25,27,30,31,36,37,38). In the Second IWCCLL, aberrations involving chromosome 14 were reported in 8% of evaluable cases (12). The 14q32 abnormalities were frequently the result of the translocation t(11;14)(q13;q32). However, this aberration, leading to the fusion of the *BCL1* locus at 11q13 to *IgH* at 14q32 with subsequent overexpression of cyclin D1 (*CCND1*), is today considered the hallmark of MCL and may also occur at a low frequency in lymphoproliferative disorders distinct from classical B-CLL (39,106–108). Early molecular studies also suggested a role for *CCND1* in the pathogenesis of B-CLL, because the breakpoints of the translocation were cloned from two tumors initially diagnosed as B-CLL (109–111). However, on re-evaluation these cases were later classified as MCL (39). A consistent feature of recent analyses is that no evidence for a frequent occurrence of the t(11;14) or involvement of *CCND1* in B-CLL was found (99,112–115). Accordingly, in a series of 100 B-CLL cases diagnosed based on the criteria of the International Workshop on Chronic Lymphocytic Leukemia (116) and the National Cancer Institute–sponsored Working Group (117), no rearrangements of *CCND1* were detected (99). Therefore, the differential diagnosis of MCL should strongly be considered in leukemic lymphoproliferative disorders resembling B-CLL but exhibiting the t(11;14) or *CCND1* expression.

A pathogenic role was also proposed for *BCL2* on the basis of rearrangements at 18q21 (118,119). The translocation t(14;18) is considered to be characteristic of follicular NHL, but overexpression of *BCL2* without the t(14;18) is also consistently observed in other lymphoid neoplasms such as B-CLL. Whereas the breakpoints of the t(14;18)(q32; q21) in follicular NHL are located in the major breakpoint region (mbr) or the minor cluster region (mcr) at the 3′ portion of *BCL2*, the breakpoints in B-CLL tumors were localized 5′ of *BCL2*, with preferential juxtaposition of *BCL2* to the immunoglobulin light chains. However, when tested in large series of classical B-CLL, *BCL2* rearrangements were only rare events in almost all subsequent molecular genetic studies (99,114,120–122).

Another rearrangement involving the *IgH* locus at 14q32, the t(14;19)(q32;q13) (37,38), was observed in 6 cases among 4487 lymphoproliferative disorders (123). Five of these six tumors were classified as B-CLL. From the 19q13 breakpoint region, the *BCL3* gene encoding an I-kB-like protein, which functions as a transcriptional coactivator, was cloned (123–127). The low incidence of t(14;19)(q32;q13) rearrangements in lymphoproliferative disorders was confirmed by Southern blot analysis of 1150 tumors (123).

Thus, rearrangements of the *IgH* locus at 14q32 with *BCL*-type proto-oncogenes appear to be rare events in B-CLL, and their observation in a lymphoid neoplasm should lead to a careful evaluation for features of low-grade NHL other than B-CLL. Considering molecular genetic data, the "14q+" marker observed as a recurrent aberration in early chromosome banding studies of B-CLL appears not to be a frequent aberration in this disease.

Another genetic parameter of the immunoglobulin genes, the mutation status of their variable portion (*IgV*), has recently gained attention in B-CLL (128,129). In these studies approximately half of the B-CLL cases showed mutated *IgV*, a feature physiologically observed in postgerminal center B-cells. Therefore, two types of B-CLL were proposed, one with a pregerminal center cell of origin and another derived from postgerminal center B cells. Furthermore, the mutational status of *IgV* correlated with the expression level of CD38 in one study but not in the other (130,131). To resolve these discrepancies and to correlate the *IgV* mutation status with other biological features of potential pathogenic significance in B-CLL, further studies are necessary.

G. Infrequent Genetic Abnormalities of B-CLL

Knowledge on other genomic aberrations of B-CLL came either from genome-wide screening analyses, such as chromosome banding and CGH, or from candidate gene approaches focused on genes involved in other malignancies. The latter approach led us to study 50 cases of chronic B-cell leukemias by FISH for deletion of the *CDKN2A* (*p16*) gene in band 9p21, which is disrupted in a wide variety of malignancies (132). In agreement with data from chromosome banding studies and Southern blot analyses, we did not detect deletions of *CDKN2* in B-CLL (132–135).

Several genomic regions infrequently but recurrently involved in aberrations in B-CLL were detected by chromosome banding and CGH. These aberrations are commonly gains of chromosomal regions, such as trisomy 3, which has been reported at low frequency in B-CLL (23,25,28). Chromosome banding and CGH data suggested that the minimally duplicated segment comprised the distal region of the long arm, which may therefore contain an oncogene of pathogenic significance in B-CLL (21). In addition, although trisomy 3 was known to occur in B-CLL on the basis of banding data, gains of genetic material on chromosome arm 8q were identified as novel aberrations by CGH (21). For the infrequently involved chromosome regions candidate genes remain to be identified.

V. CLINICAL SIGNIFICANCE OF GENOMIC ABERRATIONS IN B-CLL

A. Correlation of Chromosome Banding Karyotype with Outcome in B-CLL

In the multicenter studies of the First and Second IWCCLL, the relation between chromosome aberrations as detected by conventional cytogenetic techniques and clinical parameters was evaluated in a large number of B-CLL patients (11,12). In these studies, a normal karyotype was associated with a better survival (median, 15 years) compared with the group of B-CLL with clonal aberrations (median, 7.7 years). Among the patients with clonal abnormalities, those with complex aberrations had an inferior survival compared with the patients with single aberrations. On the evaluation of subgroups defined by single aberrations, trisomy 12 was associated with a poor survival. In contrast, patients with structural aberrations of chromosome 13 seemed to have a more favorable outcome, with survival probabilities similar to those with a normal karyotype (11,12). However, neither the presence of clonal aberrations nor the number of clonal aberrations were independent prognostic parameters in multivariate analysis.

A novel basis for a correlation of specific genomic aberrations with clinical characteristics and outcome was provided by the interphase cytogenetic approach. However, until recently, only a limited number of reports on the basis of interphase analyses have been published, and only single aberrations have been studied, not taking into account the potential impact of various aberrations within a single B-CLL case.

B. Clinical Significance of 11q22–q23 Deletion in B-CLL

Evidence for a prognostic role of 11q loss came from two recent reports (66,91). B-CLL cases with 11q loss had more rapid disease progression and shorter survival times. By interphase FISH the 11q22–q23 deletion was the second most common abnormality observed in 43 of 214 (20%) tumors of our series. It was associated with a characteristic clinical presentation (91). Patients with B-CLL and 11q deletion had more advanced disease stages, and they exhibited extensive lymphadenopathy as assessed by the extent of peripheral lymph node involvement and the frequency of mediastinal or abdominal lymphadenopathy. Furthermore, these patients had a more rapid disease progression as shown by a shorter treatment-free period (9 months vs 43 months; $P < 0.001$). In survival analysis, the prognostic impact of the 11q deletion was age-dependent; in patients younger than 55 years, the median survival time was significantly shorter in the 11q deletion group (64 months vs 209 months; $P < 0.001$), whereas in patients 55 years of age and older there was no significant difference (94 months vs 111 months; $P = 0.82$). Multivariate analysis with survival as a dependent variable revealed deletion 11q as independent risk factor (91). A similar prognostic impact also depending on the age of the patients was described for B-CLL with loss of *ATM* protein (75). Thus, 11q deletions identify a new clinical subset of B-CLL characterized by extensive lymph node involvement, rapid disease progression, and inferior survival (see also Fig. 3 and Fig. 4). The prognostic impact of the 11q deletion appears to be more prominent among young (≤55 years) patients. Therefore, this aberration could serve as a parameter to identify B-CLL patients who may benefit from intensified treatment protocols such as high-dose therapy with autologous or allogeneic stem cell transplantation.

C. Clinical Significance of Trisomy 12

In the chromosome banding analyses of the First and Second IWCCLL, patients with trisomy 12 had the shortest survival probability among patients with single chromosome abnormalities (11,12). Also, in single center studies trisomy 12 was the first chromosome aberration associated with shorter treatment-free intervals (136) and shorter overall survival (26). However, this adverse prognostic effect was only shown in univariate analysis, and it could not be confirmed by other single center studies (24,25,30,31).

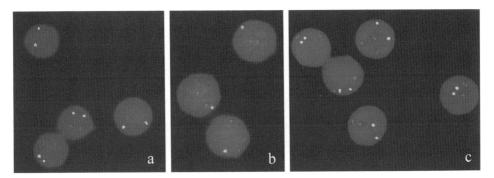

Figure 16.1 Examples of FISH images demonstrating genomic aberrations in B-CLL. (a) B-CLL with biallelic 13q14 deletion. Three of the four nuclei show no red hybridization signal of a DNA probe containing marker *D13S272* demonstrating biallelic loss of this genomic region. The single cell with two red and two green signals probably represents a nonleukemic T- or B-cell from the specimen. (b) B-CLL with monoallelic 11q22–q23 deletion as demonstrated by the single green signal of a probe recognizing the *ATM* gene. Two red signals of a control probe indicate a high hybridization efficiency. (c) B-CLL with trisomy 12q. Three red hybridization signals are present in three of the five nuclei. In the cell to the upper left, the left signal is composed of a doublet representing two signals in different focal planes.

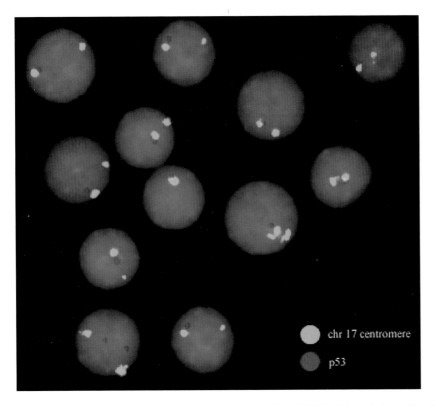

chr 17 centromere

p53

Figure 24.3 FISH analysis shows monoallelic p53 deletion in a B-PLL. The red signal identifies the p53 gene and the green signal the chromosome 17 centromere.

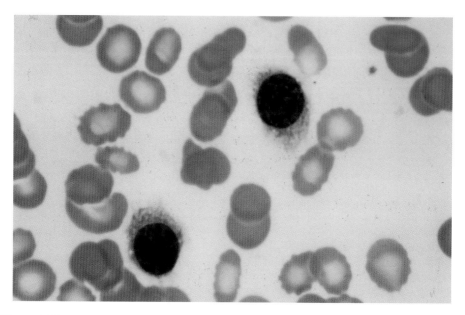

Figure 26.1 Peripheral blood smear from a patient with hairy cell leukemia shows circulating hairy cells with slightly eccentric nuclei, loosely condensed chromatin, and "hairy" cytoplasmic borders. Wright's stain.

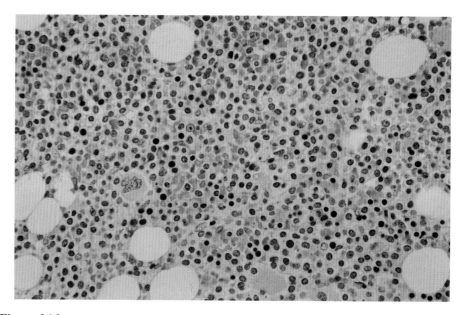

Figure 26.2 Bone marrow trephine biopsy with extensive infiltration by hairy cells characterized by round to oval nuclei and abundant cytoplasm. Hematoxylin and eosin stain.

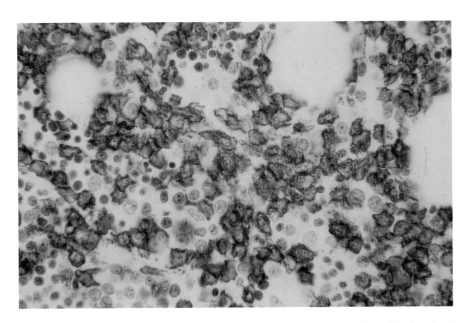

Figure 26.3 Bone marrow trephine biopsy with extensive involvement by hairy cell leukemia. The malignant cells are highlighted by immunostains for CD20, a B-cell marker. Immunostain (CD20).

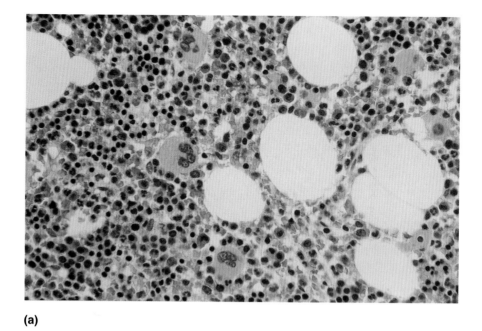

(a)

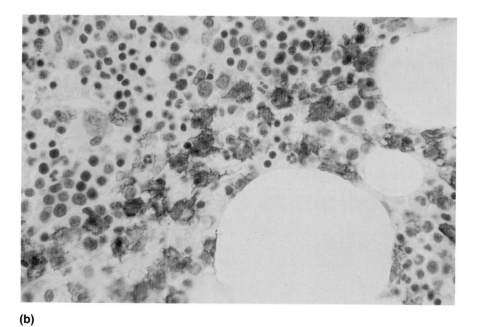

(b)

Figure 26.6 (a) Bone marrow trephine biopsy from a patient with hairy cell leukemia 3 months after therapy with 2-CdA. No evidence of disease is apparent by routine staining. Hematoxylin and eosin stain. (b) Bone marrow trephine biopsy after immunostain for CD20. Minimal residual disease characterized by scattered clusters of hairy cells is highlighted by positivity for CD20. Immunohistochemistry (CD20).

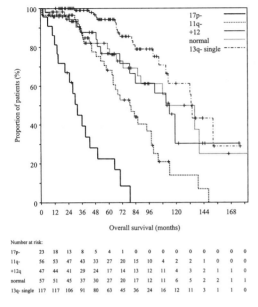

Number at risk:															
17p-	23	18	13	8	5	4	1	0	0	0	0	0	0	0	0
11q-	56	53	47	43	33	27	20	15	10	4	2	2	1	0	0
+12q	47	44	41	29	24	17	14	13	12	11	4	3	2	1	1
normal	57	51	45	37	30	27	20	17	12	11	6	5	2	2	1
13q- single	117	117	106	91	80	63	45	36	24	16	12	11	3	1	1

Figure 3 Estimated survival probabilities from the date of diagnosis in 325 CLL patients. The median survival times for the 17p deletion (17p−) (n = 23), 11q deletion (11q−) (n = 56), 12q trisomy (+12) (n = 47), normal karyotype (normal) (n = 57), and 13q deletion as single abnormality (13q− single) (N = 117) groups were 32, 79, 114, 111, and 133 months, respectively.

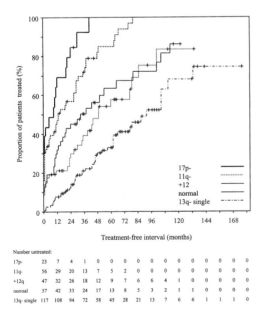

Number untreated:															
17p-	23	7	4	1	0	0	0	0	0	0	0	0	0	0	0
11q-	56	29	20	13	7	5	2	0	0	0	0	0	0	0	0
+12q	47	32	26	18	12	9	7	6	6	4	1	0	0	0	0
normal	57	42	33	24	17	13	8	5	3	2	1	1	0	0	0
13q- single	117	108	94	72	58	45	28	21	13	7	6	6	1	1	1

Figure 4 Probabilities of disease progression as assessed by the treatment free interval in 325 CLL patients. The median treatment free intervals for 17p deletion (17p−) (n = 23), 11q deletion (11q−) (n = 56), 12q trisomy (+12) (n = 47), normal karyotype (normal) (n = 57), and 13q deletion as single abnormality (13q− single) (N = 117) groups were 9, 13, 33, 49, and 92 months respectively. The differences between the curves were statistically highly significant (P < 0.001).

In our interphase cytogenetic study, trisomy 12 was observed in 36 of 245 (15%) B-CLL and represented only the third most common abnormality after deletions of 13q14 and 11q22–q23 (8,91). As assessed by interphase cytogenetics, trisomy 12 is significantly associated with an increased number of atypical lymphocytes or prolymphocytes among the leukemic cells and also frequently with an atypical immunophenotype (62,88,89). The effect of trisomy 12 on survival was studied by Escudier et al., who assessed 83 B-CLL tumors for the presence of trisomy 12 by FISH and by chromosome banding (87). The group of patients with trisomy 12 was found to have an inferior outcome compared with the group with diploid karyotypes (7.8 years vs 14.4 years) but not compared with the overall group without trisomy 12. Furthermore, patients with trisomy 12 were more heavily pretreated and had advanced Binet stages. The response to therapy with fludarabine was similar for the groups with or without trisomy 12, but the trisomy 12 group showed a tendency toward earlier disease progression after treatment.

D. Clinical Significance of 6q Deletion

In a single center chromosome banding study by Oscier et al., shorter treatment-free intervals were observed for the group of B-CLL patients with 6q deletions (31). Accordingly, in follicular NHL, deletion 6q has been defined as a negative prognostic factor (137). In contrast, in the multicenter IWCCLL studies, no adverse prognostic effect of 6q deletions was found (11,12). In our interphase cytogenetic study of 285 B-CLL cases, 6q deletion was significantly associated with a higher tumor mass as measured by higher white blood cell counts (median 49.3×10^9/L vs 31.7×10^9/L; $P = 0.036$) and more lymphadenopathy (100). The sum of the products of the diameters of the largest cervical, axillar, and inguinal lymph nodes (median 7.3 cm^2 vs 3.0 cm^2; $P = 0.029$) and the largest lymph node diameters (median, 4.0 cm vs 2.0 cm; $P = 0.008$) were higher in the group of patients with 6q deletion. However, overall survival (131 vs 132 months) and treatment-free intervals were similar in the groups with and without 6q deletion (100). Therefore, B-CLL with 6q deletion appeared to be associated with a high tumor mass but not with inferior outcome.

E. Clinical Significance of 17p Deletion or *p53* Mutation

Evidence for the involvement of *p53* in a subset of B-CLL cases came from a study by El-Rouby et al., who identified *p53* mutations by SSCP analyses (104). Abnormalities of *p53* had a strong prognostic impact and were also predicting for treatment failure. Furthermore, aberrations involving 17p13, the genetic locus of *p53*, were observed as the only aberration of prognostic significance in a recent trial of 480 untreated B-CLL patients (63). In our initial FISH study, 17 of 100 chronic B-cell leukemias exhibited a monoallelic *p53* deletion and the presence of such deletions had clinical implications (105). Patients with a *p53* deletion had significantly shorter survival times than patients without a deletion. In addition, a correlation between 17p13 deletion and treatment failure was identified; whereas 56% of patients without *p53* deletion showed a response to treatment with purine analogs, none of the patients with a *p53* deletion did (105). Multivariate analysis revealed *p53* deletion as the strongest prognostic factor for survival, followed by established clinical prognostic parameters such as age, stage, and hemoglobin level. In an extended analysis including B-CLL cases only, *p53* deletion was observed in 25 of 189 (13%) tumors. The survival probability from the time of diagnosis was significantly shorter for patients with *p53* deletion (see also Figs. 3 and 4). Therefore, with *p53* alteration by deletion or mutation, a biological parameter became available that predicts treatment response and survival of B-CLL patients.

F.   Clinical Impact of *IgH* Translocations and *IgV* Mutations

Among the aberrations associated with inferior survival in early cytogenetic studies on B-CLL were translocations involving chromosome band 14q32, leading to the formation of a "14q+" chromosome (11,25). In the First IWCCLL, patients with a 14q+ had shorter survival times than those with trisomy 12 (11). However, the 14q+ abnormality was frequently the result of the reciprocal translocation t(11;14)(q13;q32), which is strongly associated with MCL (39). Considering the dismal prognosis of MCL, the inferior outcome of such patients is not surprising. In some studies, the occurrence of the t(11;14) was associated with "atypical" B-CLL, which has been described as a disorder with inferior survival compared with "typical" B-CLL (138–140) However, the distinction of these cases from leukemic MCL remains controversial, and the similar clinical course of "atypical" B-CLL with *CCND1* overexpression and MCL suggests that these two disorders may belong to the same disease category (140). In a B-cell lymphoid leukemia with cytogenetic or molecular evidence of the t(11;14)(q13;q32) or *CCND1* overexpression, a pathological diagnosis of MCL should therefore be considered.

Recently, the mutation status of the immunoglobulin genes' variable region (*IgV*) was used to divide B-CLL into two groups: one with a proposed pregerminal center (*IgV*unmutated) cell of origin and one of postgerminal center (*IgV*mutated) origin (128,129). These two groups have been associated with distinct clinical characteristics. Whereas the group of B-CLL cases with unmutated *IgV* genes showed rapid disease progression, the group with mutated *IgV* genes followed an indolent clinical course with long survival probabilities. Although *IgV* mutational status and clinical outcome correlated with expression levels of CD38 in one study (129,131), this was not found in another analysis (130). Therefore, it is still a matter of debate whether CD38 expression can serve as a surrogate marker for *IgV* mutation status and prognosis. Also, it will be interesting to correlate the *IgV* mutation status with clinical parameters in subgroups defined by genomic aberrations as described earlier.

VI.   PERSPECTIVE

The knowledge on genomic aberrations in B-CLL has been rapidly expanding over recent years and has led to the identification of genes involved in disease progression and clinical risk groups. However, for most of the frequently involved genomic regions candidate genes remain to be identified. The isolation of such genes may give insight into the molecular pathogenesis of B-CLL and may provide parameters of diagnostic and prognostic significance. Genomic aberrations such as *p53* alterations and 11q22–q23 deletions have already been shown to be among the strongest independent factors for survival. However, to draw a comprehensive portrait of genomic lesions of a B-CLL tumor, techniques that allow a rapid and accurate genome wide screening are mandatory. To achieve this, disease-specific sets of DNA probes are necessary that can be applied for interphase cytogenetics or for the recently developed approach of matrix-CGH on the basis of DNA chip technology (94,95). If genomic aberrations predict the outcome independently of established clinical parameters such as stage, they may become helpful in the diagnostic workup of a B-CLL patient (see also Figs. 3 and 4) (141,142). Biological risk parameters may allow the identification of early stage B-CLL patients who are at high risk for rapid disease progression or resistance to therapy. The prognostic impact of genomic aberrations may be particularly helpful in B-CLL patients of young age who are candidates for experimental treatment approaches with curative potential such as high-dose chemotherapy followed by autologous or allogeneic hematopoietic stem cell transplantation. To address this issue molecular cytogenetic studies are under way in large prospective clinical treatment trials.

REFERENCES

1. F Mitelman, G Levan. Clustering of aberrations to specific chromosomes in human neoplasms. Hereditas 89:207–232, 1978.
2. KH Robèrt, E Möller, G Gahrton, H Eriksson, B Nilsson. B-cell activation of peripheral blood lymphocytes from patients with chronic lymphocytic leukaemia. Clin Exp Immunol 33:302–308, 1978.
3. K Autio, O Turunen, O Penttilä, E Erämaa, A de la Chapelle, J Schröder. Human chronic lymphocytic leukemia: Karyotypes in different lymphocyte populations. Cancer Genet Cytogenet 1:147–155, 1979.
4. JN Hurley, SM Fu, HG Kunkel, RSK Chaganti, J German. Chromosome abnormalities of leukaemic B lymphocytes in chronic lymphocytic leukaemia. Nature 283:76–78, 1980.
5. G Gahrton, KH Robèrt, K Friberg, L Zech, AG Bird. Extra chromosome 12 in chronic lymphocytic leukaemia (letter) Lancet 1:146–147, 1980.
6. G Gahrton, KH Robèrt, K Friberg, L Zech, AG Bird. Nonrandom chromosomal aberrations in chronic lymphocytic leukemia revealed by polyclonal B-cell-mitogen stimulation. Blood 56:640–647, 1980.
7. DG Oscier. Cytogenetic and molecular abnormalities in chronic lymphocytic leukaemia. Blood Reviews 8:88–97, 1994.
8. H Döhner, S Pohl, M Bulgay-Mörschel, S Stilgenbauer, M Bentz, P Lichter. Detection of trisomy 12 in chronic lymphoid leukemias using fluorescence in situ hybridization. Leukemia 7:516–520, 1993.
9. DH Crawford, D Catovsky. In vitro activation of leukaemia B cells by interleukin-4 and antibodies to CD40. Immunology 80:40–44, 1993.
10. K Autio, E Elonen, L Teerenhovi, S Knuutila. Cytogenetic and immunologic characterization of mitotic cells in chronic lymphocytic leukemia. Eur J Haematol 39:289–298, 1986.
11. G Juliusson, DG Oscier, M Fitchett, FM Ross, G Stockdill, MJ Mackie, AC Parker, GL Castoldi, A Cuneo, S Knuutila, E Elonen, G Gahrton. Prognostic subgroups in B-cell chronic lymphocytic leukemia defined by specific chromosomal abnormalities. N Engl J Med 323:720–724, 1990.
12. G Juliusson, D Oscier, G Gahrton, for the International Working Party on Chromosomes in CLL (IWCCLL). Cytogenetic findings and survival in B-cell chronic lymphocytic leukemia. Second IWCCLL compilation of data on 662 patients. Leuk Lymphoma 5:21–25, 1991.
13. G Juliusson, G Gahrton. Chromosome aberrations in B-cell chronic lymphocytic leukemia. Pathogenetic and clinical implications. Cancer Genet Cytogenet 45:143–160, 1990.
14. P Lichter, DC Ward. Is non-isotopic in situ hybridization finally coming of age? Nature 345:93–95, 1990.
15. P Lichter, M Bentz, S Joos. Detection of chromosomal aberrations by means of molecular cytogenetics: Painting of chromosomes and chromosomal subregions and comparative genomic hybridization. Methods Enzym 254:334–359, 1995.
16. AM Joseph, JR Gosden, AC Chandley. Estimation of aneuploidy levels in human spermatozoa using chromosome specific probes and in situ hybridization. Hum Genet 66:234–238, 1984.
17. T Cremer, J Landegent, A Brückner, HP Scholl, M Schardin, HD Hager, P Devilee, PP Pearson, M van der Ploeg. Detection of chromosome aberrations in the human interphase nucleus by visualization of specific target DNAs with radioactive and non-radioactive in situ hybridization techniques: diagnosis of trisomy 18 with probe L1.84. Hum Genet 74:346–352, 1986.

18. A Kallioniemi, O-P Kallioniemi, D Sudar, D Rutovitz, JW Gray, F Waldman, D Pinkel. Comparative genomic hybridization for molecular cytogenetic analysis of solid tumors. Science 258:818–821, 1992.

19. S Du Manoir, MR Speicher, S Joos, E Schröck, S Popp, H Döhner, G Kovacs, M Robert-Nicoud, P Lichter, T Cremer. Detection of complete and partial chromosome gains and losses by comparative genomic in situ hybridization. Hum Genet 90:590–610, 1993.

20. S Joos, H Scherthan, MR Speicher, J Schlegel, T Cremer, P Lichter. Detection of amplified genomic sequences by reverse chromosome painting using genomic tumor DNA as probe. Hum Genet 90:584–589, 1993.

21. M Bentz, K Huck, S du Manoir, S Joos, CA Werner, K Fischer, H Döhner, P Lichter. Comparative genomic hybridization in chronic B-cell leukemias reveals a high incidence of chromosomal gains and losses. Blood 85:3610–3618, 1995.

22. EW Fleischman, EL Prigogina. Karyotype pecularities of malignant lymphomas. Hum Genet 35:269–279, 1977.

23. M Morita, J Minowada, AA Sandberg. Chromosomes and causation of human cancer and leukemia. XLV. Chromosome patterns in stimulated lymphocytes of chronic lymphocytic leukemia. Cancer Genet Cytogenet 3:293–306, 1981.

24. T Han, H Ozer, N Sadamori, L Emrich, GA Gomez, ES Henderson, JL Bloom, AA Sandberg. Prognostic importance of cytogenetic abnormalities in patients with chronic lymphocytic leukemia. N Engl J Med 310:288–292, 1984.

25. S Pittman, D Catovsky. Prognostic significance of chromosome abnormalities in chronic lymphocytic leukaemia Br J Haematol 58:649–660, 1984.

26. G Juliusson, KH Robèrt, A Öst, K Friberg, P Biberfeld, B Nilsson, L Zech, G Gahrton. Prognostic information from cytogenetic analysis in chronic B-lymphocytic leukemia and leukemic immunocytoma. Blood 65:134–141, 1985.

27. PC Nowell, EC Vonderheid, E Besa, JA Hoxie, L Moreau, JB Finan. The most common chromosome change in 86 chronic B cell or T cell tumors: A 14q32 translocation. Cancer Genet Cytogenet 19:219–227, 1986.

28. FM Ross, G Stockdill. Clonal chromosome abnormalities in chronic lymphocytic leukemia patients revealed by TPA stimulation of whole blood cultures. Cancer Genet Cytogenet 25:109–121, 1987.

29. T Han, N Sadamori, AMW Block, H Xiao, ES Henderson, L Emrich, AA Sandberg. Cytogenetic studies in chronic lymphocytic leukemia, prolymphocytic leukemia and hairy cell leukemia: A progress report. Nouv Rev Fr Hematol 30:393–395, 1988.

30. ML Bird, Y Ueshima, JD Rowley, JM Haren, JW Vardiman. Chromosome abnormalities in B cell chronic lymphocytic leukemia and their clinical correlations. Leukemia 3:182–191, 1989.

31. DG Oscier, J Stevens, TJ Hamblin, RM Pickering, R Lambert, M Fitchett. Correlation of chromosome abnormalities with laboratory features and clinical course in B-cell chronic lymphocytic leukaemia. Brit J Haematol 76:352–358, 1990.

32. M Fitchett, MJ Griffiths, DG Oscier, S Johnson, M Seabright. Chromosome abnormalities involving band 13q14 in hematologic malignancies. Cancer Genet Cytogenet 24:143–150, 1987.

33. L Zech, H Mellstedt. Chromosome 13— A new marker for B-cell chronic lymphocytic leukemia. Hereditas 108:77–84, 1988.

34. LC Peterson, LL Lindquist, S Church, NE Kay. Frequent clonal abnormalities of chromosome band 13q14 in B-cell chronic lymphocytic leukemia: Multiple clones, subclones, and non-clonal alterations in 82 Midwestern patients. Genes Chromosom Cancer 4:273–280, 1992.

35. DF Callen, JH Ford. Chromosome abnormalities in chronic lymphocytic leukemia revealed by TPA as a mitogen. Cancer Genet Cytogenet 10:87–93, 1983.

36. H Van den Berghe, C Parloir, G David, JL Michaux, G Sokal. A new characteristic karyotypic anomaly in lymphoproliferative disorders. Cancer 44:188–195, 1979.

37. C Bloomfield, D Arthur, G Frizzera, E Levine, B Peterson, K Gajl-Peczalska. Nonrandom chromosome abnormalities in lymphoma. Cancer Res 43:2975–2984, 1983.

38. Y Ueshima, ML Bird, JW Vardiman, JD Rowley. A 14;19 translocation in B-cell chronic lymphocytic leukemia: a new recurring chromosome aberration. Int J Cancer 36:287–290, 1985.

39. M Raffeld, ES Jaffe. bcl-1, t(11;14), and mantle cell-derived lymphomas. Blood 78:259–263, 1991.

40. RA Weinberg. The retinoblastoma protein and cell cycle control. Cell 81:323–330, 1995.

41. Y Liu, D Grandér, S Söderhäll, G Juliusson, G Gahrton, S Einhorn. Retinoblastoma gene deletions in B-cell chronic lymphocytic leukemia. Genes Chrom Cancer 4:250–256, 1992.

42. S Stilgenbauer, H Döhner, M Bulgay-Mörschel, S Weitz, M Bentz, P Lichter. High frequency of monoallelic retinoblastoma gene deletion in B-cell chronic lymphoid leukemia shown by interphase cytogenetics. Blood 81:2118–2124, 1993.

43. H Döhner, T Pilz, K Fischer, G Cabot, D Diehl, T Fink, S Stilgenbauer, M Bentz, P Lichter. Molecular cytogenetic analysis of Rb-1 deletions in chronic B-cell leukemias. Leuk Lymphoma 16:97–103, 1994.

44. Y Liu, L Szekely, D Grandér, S Söderhäll, G Juliusson, G Gahrton, S Linder, S Einhorn. Chronic lymphocytic leukemia cells with allelic deletions at 13q14 commonly have one intact RB1 gene: Evidence for a role of an adjacent locus. Proc Natl Acad Sci USA 90:8697–8701, 1993.

45. AG Brown, FM Ross, EM Dunne, CM Steel, EM Weir-Thompson. Evidence for a new tumour suppressor locus (DBM) in human B-cell neoplasia telomeric to the retinoblastoma gene. Nat Genet 3:67–72, 1993.

46. RM Chapman, MM Corcoran, A Gardiner, LA Hawthorn, JK Cowell, DG Oscier. Frequent homozygous deletions of the D13S25 locus in chromosome region 13q14 defines the location of a gene critical in leukaemogenesis in chronic B-cell lymphocytic leukaemia. Oncogene 9:1289–1293, 1994.

47. MC Devilder, S François, C Bosic, A Moreau, MP Mellerin, D Le Paslier, R Bataille, JP Moisan. Deletion cartography around the D13S25 Locus in B cell chronic lymphocytic leukemia. Cancer Res 55:1355–1357, 1995.

48. S Stilgenbauer, E Leupolt, S Ohl, G Weiß, M Schröder, K Fischer, M Bentz, P Lichter, H Döhner. Heterogeneity of deletions involving RB-1 and the D13S25 locus in B-cell chronic lymphocytic leukemia revealed by FISH. Cancer Res 55:3475–3477, 1995.

49. Y Liu, M Hermanson, D Grandér, M Merup, X Wu, M Heyman, O Rasool, G Juliusson, G Gahrton, R Detlofsson, N Nikiforova, C Buys, S Söderhäll, N Yankovsky, E Zabarovsky, S Einhorn. 13q deletions in lymphoid malignancies. Blood 86:1911–1915, 1995.

50. F Bullrich, ML Veronese, S Kitada, J Jurlander, MA Caligiuri, JC Reed, CM Croce. Minimal region of loss at 13q14 in B-cell chronic lymphocytic leukemia. Blood 88:3109–3115, 1996.

51. S Kalachikov, A Migliazza, E Cayanis, NS Fracchiolla, MF Bonaldo, L Lawton, P Jelenc, X Ye, X Qu, M Chien, R Hauptschein, G Gaidano, U Vitolo, G Saglio, L Resegotti, V Brodjansky, N Yankovsky, P Zhang, MB Soares, J Russo, IS Edelman, A Efstratiadis, R Dalla-Favera, SG Fischer. Cloning and gene mapping of the chromosome 13q14 region deleted in chronic lymphocytic leukemia. Genomics 42:369–377, 1997.

52. Y Liu, M Corcoran, O Rasool, G Ivanova, R Ibbotson, D Grandér, A Iyengar, A Baranova, V Kashuba, M Merup, X Wu, A Gardiner, R Mullenbach, A Poltaraus, AL Hultström, G Juliusson, R Chapman, M Tiller, F Cotter, G Gahrton, N Yankovsky, E Zabarovsky, S Einhorn, D Oscier. Cloning of two candidate tumor suppressor genes within a 10 kb region on chromosome 13q14, frequently deleted in chronic lymphocytic leukemia. Oncogene 15: 2463–2473, 1997.

53. T Bouyge-Moreau, G Rondeau, H Avet-Loiseau, MT André, S Bézieau, M Chérel, S Saleün, E Cadoret, T Shaikh, MM De Angelis, S Arcot, M Batzer, JP Moisan, MC Devilder. Construction of a 780-kb PAC, BAC, and cosmid contig encompassing the minimal critical dele-

tion involved in B cell chronic lymphocytic leukemia at 13q14.3. Genomics 46:183–190, 1997.

54. MM Corcoran, O Rasool, Y Liu, A Iyengar, D Grander, RE Ibbotson, M Merup, X Wu, V Brodyansky, AC Gardiner, G Juliusson, RM Chapman, G Ivanova, M Tiller, G Gahrton, N Yankovsky, E Zabarovsky, DG Oscier, S Einhorn. Detailed molecular delineation of 13q14.3 loss in B-cell chronic lymphocytic leukemia. Blood 91:1382–1390, 1998.

55. S Stilgenbauer, J Nickolenko, J Wilhelm, S Wolf, S Weitz, K Döhner, T Böhm, H Döhner, P Lichter. Expressed sequences as candidates for a novel tumor suppressor gene at band 13q14 in B-cell chronic lymphocytic leukemia and mantle cell lymphoma. Oncogene 16: 1891–1897, 1998.

56. G Rondeau, I Moreau, S Bezieau, E Cadoret, JP Moisan, MC Devilder. Exclusion of Leu1 and Leu2 genes as tumor suppressor genes in 13q14.3-deleted B-CLL. Leukemia 10:1630–1632, 1999.

57. M Bentz, A Plesch, L Bullinger, S Stilgenbauer, G Ott, HK Müller-Hermelink, M Baudis, TFE Barth, P Möller, P Lichter, H Döhner. t(11;14) positive mantle cell lymphoma exhibit complex karyotypes and share similarities with B-cell chronic lymphocytic leukemia. Genes Chromosom Cancer 27:285–294, 2000.

58. J Shaughnessy, B Barlogie. Chromosome 13 deletion in myeloma. Curr Top Microbiol Immunol 246:199–203, 1999.

59. JA Garcia-Marco, C Caldas, CM Price, LM Wiedemann, A Ashworth, D Catovsky. Frequent somatic deletion of the 13q12.3 locus encompassing BRCA2 in chronic lymphocytic leukemia. Blood 88:1568–1575, 1996.

60. P Panayiotidis, K Ganeshaguru, C Rowntree, SAB Jabbar, VA Hoffbrand, L Foroni. Lack of clonal BRCA2 gene deletion on chromosome 13 in chronic lymphocytic leukaemia. Br J Haematol 97:844–847, 1997.

61. B Johansson, F Mertens, F Mitelman. Cytogenetic deletion maps of hematologic neoplasms: Circumstantial evidence for tumor suppressor loci. Genes Chromosom Cancer 8:205–218, 1993.

62. E Matutes, D Oscier, J Garcia-Marco, J Ellis, A Copplestone, R Gillingham, T Hamblin, D Lens, GJ Swansbury, D Catovsky. Trisomy 12 defines a group of CLL with atypical morphology: correlation between cytogenetic, clinical and laboratory features in 544 patients. Br J Haematol 92:382–388, 1996.

63. CH Geisler, P Philip, B Egelund Christensen, K Hou-Jensen, N Tinggaard Pedersen, O Myhre Jensen, K Thorling, E Andersen, HS Birgens, A Drivsholm, J Ellegard, JK Larsen, T Plesner, P Brown, P Kragh Andersen, M Mørk Hansen. In B-cell chronic lymphocytic leukaemia chromosome 17 abnormalities and not trisomy 12 are the single most important cytogenetic abnormalities for the prognosis: A cytogenetic and immunophenotypic study of 480 unselected newly diagnosed patients. Leuk Res 21:1011–1023, 1997.

64. JM Hernandez, C Mecucci, A Criel, P Meeus, L Michaux, A van Hoof, G Verhoef, A Louwagie, JM Scheiff, JL Michaux, M Boogaerts, H van den Berghe. Cytogenetic analysis of B cell chronic lymphoid leukemias classified according to morphologic and immunophenotypic (FAB) criteria. Leukemia 9:2140–2146, 1995.

65. C Fegan, H Robinson, P Thompson, JA Whittaker, D White. Karyotypic evolution in CLL. Identification of a new sub-group of patients with deletions of 11q and advanced or progressive disease. Leukemia 9:2003–2008, 1995.

66. JR Neilson, R Auer, D White, N Bienz, JJ Waters, JA Whittaker, DW Milligan, CD Fegan. Deletions at 11q identify a subset of patients with typical CLL who show consistent disease progression and reduced survival. Leukemia 11:1929–1932, 1997.

67. H Kobayashi, R III Espinosa, AA Fernald, C Begy, MO Diaz, MM Le Beau, JD Rowley. Analysis of deletions of the long arm of chromosome 11 in hematologic malignancies with fluorescence in situ hybridization. Genes Chromosom Cancer 8:246–252, 1993.

68. S Stilgenbauer, P Liebisch, MR James, M Schröder, B Schlegelberger, K Fischer, M Bentz,

P Lichter, H Döhner. Molecular cytogenetic delineation of a novel critical genomic region in chromosome bands 11q22.2–q23.1 in lymphoproliferative disorders. Proc Natl Acad Sci USA 93:11837–11841, 1996.

69. MR James, CW Richard III, JJ Schott, C Yousry, K Clark, J Bell, JD Terwilliger, J Hazan, C Dubay, A Vignal, M Agrapart, T Imai, Y Nakamura, M Polymeropoulos, J Weissenbach, DR Cox, GM Lathrop. A radiation hybrid map of 506 STS markers spanning human chromosome 11. Nat Genet 6:70–76, 1994.

70. Y Zhu, O Monni, W El-Rifai, SM Siitonen, L Vilpo, J Vilpo, S Knuutila. Discontinuous deletions at 11q23 in B cell chronic lymphocytic leukemia. Leukemia 13:708–712, 1999.

71. KK Wilgenbus, A Milatovich, U Franke, H Furthmayr. Molecular cloning, cDNA sequence and chromosomal assignment of the human radixin gene and two dispersed pseudogenes. Genomics 16:199–206, 1993.

72. C Barlow, S Hirotsune, R Paylor, M Liyanage, M Eckhaus, F Collins, Y Shiloh, JN Crawley, T Ried, D Tagle, A Wynshaw-Boris. Atm-deficient mice: A paradigm of ataxia telangiectasia. Cell 86:159–171, 1996.

73. S Stilgenbauer, C Schaffner, A Litterst, P Liebisch, S Gilad, A Bar-Shira, MR James, P Lichter, H Döhner. Biallelic mutations in the *ATM* gene in T-prolymphocytic leukemia. Nat Med 3:1155–1159, 1997.

74. I Vorechovsky, L Luo, MJS Dyer, D Catovsky, PL Amlot, JC Yaxley, L Foroni, L Hammarström, ADB Webster, MAR Yuille. Clustering of missense mutations in the ataxia-telangiectasia gene in a sporadic T-cell leukaemia Nat Genet 17:96–99, 1997.

75. P Starostik, T Manshouri, S O'Brien, E Freireich, H Kantarjian, M Haidar, S Lerner, M Keating, M Albitar. Deficiency of the ATM protein defines an aggressive subgroup of B-cell chronic lymphocytic leukemia. Cancer Res 58:4552–4557, 1998.

76. F Bullrich, D Rasio, S Kitada, P Starostik, T Kipps, M Keating, M Albitar, JC Reed, CM Croce. *ATM* mutations in B-cell chronic lymphocytic leukemia. Cancer Res 59:24–27, 1999.

77. T Stankovic, P Weber, G Stewart, T Bedenham, J Murray, PJ Byrd, PAH Moss, AMR Taylor. Inactivation of ataxia telangiectasia mutated gene in B-cell chronic lymphocytic leukaemia. Lancet 353:26–29, 1999.

78. C Schaffner, S Stilgenbauer, G Rappold, H Döhner, P Lichter. Somatic *ATM* mutations indicate a pathogenic role of ATM in B-cell chronic lymphocytic leukemia. Blood 94:748–753, 1999.

79. O Monni, Y Zhu, K Franssila, R Oinonen, P Höglund, E Elonen, H Joensuu, S Knuutila. Molecular characterisation of deletion at 11q22.1–23.3 in mantle cell lymphoma. Br J Haematol 104:665–671, 1999.

80. S Stilgenbauer, D Winkler, G Ott, C Schaffner, E Leupolt, M Bentz, P Möller, HK Müller-Hermelink, MR James, P Lichter, H Döhner. Molecular characterization of 11q deletions points to a pathogenic role of the ATM gene in mantle cell lymphoma. Blood 94:3262–3264, 1999.

81. C Schaffner, I Idler, S Stilgenbauer, H Döhner, P Lichter. Mantle cell lymphoma is characterized by inactivation of the ATM gene. Proc Natl Acad Sci U S A 97:2773–2778, 2000.

82. G Gahrton, KH Robèrt, K Friberg, G Juliusson, P Biberfeld, L Zech. Cytogenetic mapping of the duplicated segment of chromosome 12 in lymphoproliferative disorders. Nature 297:513–514, 1982.

83. S Einhorn, K Burvall, G Juliusson, G Gahrton, T Meeker. Molecular analysis of chromosome 12 in chronic lymphocytic leukemia. Leukemia 3:871–874, 1989.

84. A Perez Losada, M Wessman, M Tiainen, AHN Hopman, HF Willard, F Solé, MR Caballín, S Woessner, S Knuutila. Trisomy 12 in chronic lymphocytic leukemia: An interphase cytogenetic study. Blood 78:775–779, 1991.

85. J Anastasi, MM Le Beau, JW Vardiman, AA Fernald, RA Larson, JD Rowley. Detection of trisomy 12 in chronic lymphocytic leukemia by fluorescence in situ hybridization to interphase cells: A simple and sensitive method. Blood 79:1796–1801, 1992.

86. S Raghoebier, RE Kibbelaar, K Kleiverda, JC Kluin-Nelemans, JHJM van Krieken, F Kok, PM Kluin. Mosaicism of trisomy 12 in chronic lymphocytic leukemia detected by non-radioactive in situ hybridisation. Leukemia 6:1220–1226, 1992.

87. SM Escudier, JM Pereira-Leahy, JW Drach, HU Weier, AM Goodacre, MA Cork, JM Trujillo, MJ Keating, M Andreeff. Fluorescence in situ hybridization and cytogenetic studies of trisomy 12 in chronic lymphocytic leukemia. Blood 81:2702–2707, 1993.

88. TH Que, J Garcia Marco, J Ellis, E Matutes, V Brito-Babapulle, S Boyle, D Catovsky. Trisomy 12 in chronic lymphocytic leukemia detected by fluorescence in situ hybridization: Analysis by stage, immunophenotype, and morphology. Blood 82:571–575, 1993.

89. A Criel, I Wlodarska, P Meeus, M Stul, A Louwagie, A van Hoof, M Hidajat, C Mecucci, H van den Berghe. Trisomy 12 is uncommon in typical chronic lymphocytic leukaemias. Br J Haematol 87:523–528, 1994.

90. M Arif, K Tanaka, H Asou, R Ohno, N Kamada. Independent clones of trisomy 12 and retinoblastoma gene deletion in Japanese B cell chronic lymphocytic leukemia, detected by fluorescence in situ hybridization. Leukemia 9:1822–1827, 1995.

91. H Döhner, S Stilgenbauer, MR James, A Benner, T Weilguni, M Bentz, K Fischer, W Hunstein, P Lichter. 11q deletions identify a new subset of B-cell chronic lymphocytic leukemia characterized by extensive nodal involvement and inferior prognosis. Blood 89: 2516–2522, 1997.

92. M Merup, G Juliusson, X Wu, M Jansson, B Stellan, O Rasool, E Roijer, G Stenman, G Gahrton, S Einhorn. Amplification of multiple regions of chromosome 12, including 12q13-15, in chronic lymphocytic leukaemia. Eur J Haematol 58:174–180, 1997.

93. J Dierlamm, I Wlodarska, L Michaux, JR Vermeesch, P Meeus, M Stul, A Criel, G Verhoef, J Thomas, A Delannoy, A Louwagie, JJ Cassiman, C Mecucci, A Hagemeijer, H Van den Berghe. FISH identifies different types of duplications with 12q13-15 as the commonly involved segment in B-cell lymphoproliferative malignancies characterized by partial trisomy 12. Genes Chromosom Cancer 20:155–166, 1997.

94. S Solinas-Toldo, S Lampel, S Stilgenbauer, J Nickolenko, A Benner, H Döhner, T Cremer, P Lichter. Matrix-based comparative genomic hybridization: Biochips to screen for genomic imbalances. Genes Chromosom Cancer 20:399–407, 1997.

95. D Pinkel, R Segraves, D Sudar, S Clark, I Poole, D Kowbel, C Collins, WL Kuo, C Chen, Y Zhai, SH Dairkee, BM Ljung, JW Gray, DG Albertson. High resolution analysis of DNA copy number variation using comparative genomic hybridization to microarrays. Nat Genet 20:207–211, 1998.

96. K Offit, NZ Parsa, G Gaidano, DA Filippa, D Louie, D Pan, SC Jhanwar, R Dalla-Favera, RSK Chaganti. 6q deletions define distinct clinico-pathologic subsets of non-Hodgkin's lymphoma. Blood 82:2157–2162, 1993.

97. K Offit, DC Louie, NZ Parsa, D Filippa, M Gangi, R Siebert, RSK Chaganti. Clinical and morphologic features of B-cell small lymphocytic lymphoma with del(6)(q2l–q23). Blood 83:2611–2618, 1994.

98. M Merup, TC Moreno, M Heyman, K Rönnberg, D Grandér, R Detlofsson, O Rasool, Y Liu, S Söderhäll, G Juliusson, G Gahrton, S Einhorn. 6q deletions in acute lymphoblastic leukemia and non-Hodgkin's lymphomas. Blood 91:3397–4000, 1998.

99. G Gaidano, EW Newcomb, JZ Gong, V Tassi, A Neri, A Cortelezzi, R Calori, L Baldini, R Dalla-Favera. Analysis of alterations of oncogenes and tumor suppressor genes in chronic lymphocytic leukemia. Am J Pathol 144:1312–1319, 1994.

100. S Stilgenbauer, L Bullinger, A Benner, K Wildenberger, M Bentz, K Döhner, AD Ho, P Lichter, H Döhner. Incidence and clinical significance of 6q deletions in B-cell chronic lymphocytic leukemia. Leukemia 13:1331–1334, 1999.

101. Y Zhang, P Matthiesen, S Harder, R Siebert, G Castoldi, MJ Calasanz, KF Wong, A Rosenwald, G Ott, NB Atkin, B Schlegelberger. A 3-cM commonly deleted region in 6q21 in

leukemias and lymphomas delineated by fluorescence in situ hybridization. Genes Chromosom Cancer 27:52–58, 2000.

102. G Gaidano, P Ballerini, JZ Gong, G Inghirami, A Neri, EW Newcomb, IT Magrath, DM Knowles, R Dalla-Favera. p53 mutations in human lymphoid malignancies: Association with Burkitt lymphoma and chronic lymphocytic leukemia. Proc Natl Acad Sci USA 88:5413–5417, 1991.

103. P Fenaux, C Preudhomme, JL Laï, I Quiquandon, P Jonveaux, M Vanrumbeke, C Sartiaux, P Morel, MH Loucheux-Lefebvre, F Bauters, R Berger, P Kerckaert. Mutations of the p53 gene in B-cell chronic lymphocytic leukemia: A report on 39 cases with cytogenetic analysis. Leukemia 6:246–250, 1992.

104. S El Rouby, A Thomas, D Costin, CR Rosenberg, M Potmesil, R Silber, EW Newcomb. p53 gene mutation in B-cell chronic lymphocytic leukemia is associated with drug resistance and is independent of MDR1 MDR3 gene expression. Blood 82:3452–3459, 1993.

105. H Döhner, K Fischer, M Bentz, K Hansen, A Benner, G Cabot, D Diehl, R Schlenk, J Coy, S Stilgenbauer, M Volkmann, PR Galle, A Poustka, W Hunstein, P Lichter. p53 gene deletion predicts for poor survival and non-response to therapy with purine analogs in chronic B-cell leukemias. Blood 85:1580–1589, 1995.

106. CL Rosenberg, E Wong, EM Petty, AE Bale, Y Tsujimoto, NL Harris, A Arnold. PRADI, a candidate BCL1 oncogene: Mapping and expression in centrocytic lymphoma. Proc Natl Acad Sci USA 88, 9638–9642, 1991.

107. DA Withers, RC Harvey, JB Faust, O Melnyk, K Carey, TC Meeker. Characterization of a candidate bcl-1 gene. Mol Cell Biol 11:4846–4853, 1991.

108. F Bosch, P Jares, E Campo, A Lopez-Guilllermo, MA Piris, N Villamor, D Tassies, SE Jaffe, E Montserrat, C Rozman, A Cardesa. PRAD-1/Cyclin D1 gene overexpression in chronic lymphoproliferative disorders: a highly specific marker of mantle cell lymphoma. Blood 84:2726–2732, 1994.

109. Y Tsujimoto, J Yunis, L Onorato-Showe, J Erikson, PC Nowell, CM Croce. Molecular cloning of the chromosomal breakpoint of B-cell lymphomas and leukemias with the t(11;14) chromosome translocation. Science 224:1403–1406, 1984.

110. Y Tsujimoto, E Jaffe, J Cossman, J Gorham, PC Nowell, CM Croce. Clustering of breakpoints on chromosome 11 in human B-cell neoplasms with the t(11;14) chromosome translocation. Nature 315:343–345, 1985.

111. TC Meeker, JC Grimaldi, R O'Rourke, E Louie, G Juliusson, S Einhorn. An additional breakpoint in the BCL-1 locus associated with the t(11;14)(q13;q32) translocation of B-lymphocytic malignancy. Blood 74:1801–1806, 1989.

112. G Rechavi, N Katzir, F Brok-Simoni, F Holtzman, M Mandel, N Gurfinkel, D Givol, I Ben-Bassat, B Ramot. A search for bcl1, bcl2, and c-myc oncogene rearrangements in chronic lymphocytic leukemia. Leukemia 3:57–60, 1988.

113. J Medeiros, JH van Krieken, ES Jaffe, M Raffeld. Association of bcl-1 rearrangements with lymphocytic lymphoma of intermediate differentiation. Blood 76:2086–2090, 1990.

114. S Raghoebier, JHJM van Krieken, JC Kluin-Nelemans, A Gillis, GJB van Ommen, AM Ginsberg, M Raffeld, PM Kluin. Oncogene rearrangements in chronic B-cell leukemia. Blood 77:1560–1564, 1991.

115. RA Newman, B Peterson, FR Davey, C Brabyn, H Collins, VL Brunetto, DB Duggan, RB Weiss, I Royston, FE Millard, AA Miller, CD Bloomfield. Phenotypic markers and BCL1 rearrangements in B-cell chronic lymphocytic leukemia: a cancer and leukemia group B study. Blood 82:1239–1246, 1993.

116. International Workshop on Chronic Lymphocytic Leukemia. Chronic lymphocytic leukemia: recommendations for diagnosis, staging, and response criteria. Ann Intern Med 110:236–238, 1989.

117. BD Cheson, JM Bennet, K Rai, M Grever, N Kay, C Schiffer, M Oken, M Keating, D Boldt, S Kempin, K Foon. Guidelines for clinical protocols for chronic lymphocytic leukemia:

recommendations of the NCI sponsored working group. Am J Hematol 29:152–163, 1988.

118. M Adachi, J Cossmna, D Longo, CM Croce, Y Tsujimoto. Variant translocation of the bcl-2 gene to Ig in a chronic lymphocytic leukemia. Proc Natl Acad Sci USA 86:2771–2774, 1989.

119. M Adachi, A Tefferi, PR Greipp, TJ Kipps, Y Tsujimoto. Preferential linkage of bcl-2 to immunoglobulin light chain gene in chronic lymphocytic leukemia. J Exp Med 171:559–564, 1990.

120. M Hanada, D Delia, A Aiello, E Stadtmauer, JC Reed. bcl-2 gene hypomethylation and high-level expression in B-cell chronic lymphocytic leukemia. Blood 82:1820–1828, 1993.

121. PE Crossen, MJ Morrison. Lack of 5'*bcl2* rearrangements in B-cell leukemia. Cancer Genet Cytogenet 69:72–73, 1993.

122. MJS Dyer, VJ Zani, WZ Lu, A O'Byrne, S Mould, R Chapman, JM Heward, H Kayano, D Jadayel, E Matutes, D Catovsky, DG Oscier. BCL2 translocations in leukemias of mature B cells. Blood 83:3682–3688, 1994.

123. L Michaux, C Mecucci, M Stul, I Wlodarska, JM Hernandez, P Meeus, JL Michaux, JM Scheiff, H Noël, A Louwagie, A Criel, M Boogaerts, A Van Orshoven, JJ Cassiman, H Van Den Berghe. BCL3 rearrangements and t(14;19)(q32;q13) in lymphoproliferative disorders. Genes Chromosom Cancer 15:38–47, 1996.

124. TW McKeithan, JD Rowley, T Shows, M Diaz. Cloning of the chromosome translocation breakpoint junction of the t(14;19) in chronic lymphocytic leukemia. Proc Natl Acad Sci USA 84:9257–9260, 1987.

125. TW McKeithan, H Ohno, M Diaz. Identification of a transcriptional unit adjacent to the breakpoint in the 14;19 translocation of chronic lymphocytic leukemia. Genes Chromosom Cancer 1:247–255, 1990.

126. TW McKeithan, GS Takimoto, H Ohno, VS Bjorling, R Morgan, BK Hecht, I Dubé, AA Sandberg, JD Rowley. *BCL3* rearrangements and t(14;19) in chronic lymphocytic leukemia and other B-cell malignancies: A molecular and cytogenetic study. Genes Chromosom Cancer 20:64–72, 1997.

127. LD Kerr, CS Duckett, P Wamsley, Q Zhang, P Chiao, G Nabel, T McKeithan, P Baewerle, I Verma. The proto-oncogene bcl-3 encodes an I kappa B protein. Genes Dev 6:2352–2363, 1992.

128. TJ Hamblin, Z Davis, A Gardiner, DG Oscier, FK Stevenson. Unmutated Ig V_H genes are associated with a more aggressive form of chronic lymphocytic leukemia. Blood 94:1848–1854, 1999.

129. JN Damle, T Wasil, F Fais, F Ghiotto, A Valetto, SL Allen, A Buchbinder, D Budman, K Dittmar, J Kolitz, SM Lichtman, P Schulman, VP Vinciguerra, KR Rai, M Ferrarini, N Chiorazzi. Ig V gene mutation status and CD38 expression as novel prognostic indicators in chronic lymphocytic leukemia. Blood 94:1840–1847, 1999.

130. TJ Hamblin, JA Orchard, A Gardiner, DG Oscier, Z Davis, FK Stevenson. Immunoglobulin V genes and CD38 expression in CLL (letter). Blood 95:2455–2456, 2000.

131. JN Damle, T Wasil, SL Allen, P Schulman, KR Rai, N Chiorazzi, M Ferrarini. Updated data on V gene mutation status and CD38 expression in CLL (letter). Blood 95:2456–2457, 2000.

132. M Schröder, U Mathieu, MH Dreyling, SK Bohlander, A Hagemeijer, BH Beverloo, OI Olopade, S Stilgenbauer, K Fischer, M Bentz, P Lichter, H Döhner. *CDKN2* gene deletion is not found in chronic lymphoid leukemias of B- and T-cell origin but is frequent in acute lymphoblastic leukemia. Br J Haematol 91:865–870, 1995.

133. G Stranks, SE Height, P Mitchell, D Jadayel, MAR Yuille, C De Lord, RD Clutterbuck, JG Treleaven, RL Powles, E Nacheva, DG Oscier, A Karpas, GM Lenoir, SD Smith, JL Millar, D Catovsky, MJS Dyer. Deletions and rearrangement of CDKN2 in lymphoid malignancy. Blood 85:893–901, 1995.

134. B Quesnel, C Preudhomme, N Philippe, M Vanrumbeke, I Dervite, JL Lai, F Bauters, E Wat-

tel, P Fenaux. p16 gene homozygous deletions in acute lymphoblastic leukemia. Blood 85: 657–663, 1995.

135. S Ogawa, A Hangaishi, S Miyawaki, S Hirosawa, Y Miura, K Takeyama, N Kamada, S Ohtake, N Uike, C Shimazaki, K Toyama, M Hirano, H Mizoguchi, Y Kobayashi, S Furusawa, M Saito, N Emi, Y Yazaki, R Ueda, H Hirai. Loss of the cyclin-dependent kinase 4-inhibitor (p16; MTS1) gene is frequent in and highly specific to lymphoid tumors in primary human hematopoietic malignancies. Blood 86:1548–1556, 1995.

136. KH Robèrt, G Gahrton, K Friberg, L Zech, B Nilsson. Extra chromosome 12 and prognosis in chronic lymphocytic leukaemia. Scand J Haematol 28:163–168, 1982.

137. H Tilly, A Rossi, A Stamatoullas, B Lenormand, C Bigorgne, A Kunlin, M Monconduit, C Bastard. Prognostic value of chromosomal abnormalities in follicular lymphoma. Blood 84:1043–1049, 1994.

138. A Cuneo, R Bigoni, M Negrini, F Bullrich, ML Veronese, MG Roberti, A Bardi, GM Rigolin, P Cavazzini, CM Croce, G Castoldi. Cytogenetic and interphase cytogenetic characterization of atypical chronic lymphocytic leukemia carrying BCL1 translocation. Cancer Res 57:1144–1150, 1997.

139. E Matutes, P Carrara, L Coignet, V Brito-Babapulle, N Villamor, A Wotherspoon, D Catovsky. FISH analysis for BCL-1 rearrangements and trisomy 12 helps the diagnosis of atypical B cell leukemias. Leukemia 13:1721–1726, 1999.

140. V Levy, V Ugo, A Delmer, R Tang, S Ramond, JY Perrot, R Vrhovac, JP Marie, R Zittoun, F Ajchenbaum-Cymbalista. Cyclin D1 overexpression allows identification of an aggressive subset of leukemic lymphoproliferative disorder. Leukemia 13:1343–1351, 1999.

141. BD Cheson, JM Bennett, M Grever, N Kay, MJ Keating, S O'Brien, KR Rai. National Cancer Institute–Sponsored Working Group guidelines for chronic lymphocytic leukemia: Revised guidelines for diagnosis and treatment. Blood 87:4990–4997, 1996.

142. H Döhner, S Stilgenbauer, A Benner, E Leupolt, A Kröber, L Bullinger, K Döhner, M Bentz, P Lichter. Genomic aberrations and survival in chronic lymphocytic leukemia. N Engl J Med 343:1910–1916, 2000.

17

Developing Risk-Adapted Treatment Strategies for Chronic Lymphocytic Leukemia

EMILIO MONTSERRAT

University of Barcelona, Barcelona, Spain

I. INTRODUCTION

B-cell chronic lymphocytic leukemia (CLL), which is due to the accumulation of neoplastic CD5+ B lymphocytes, is the most frequent form of leukemia in the Western hemisphere, where it accounts for 20% to 40% of all leukemias. CLL predominates in the elderly, with the median age of patients at diagnosis being around 65 years. The course of the disease is heterogeneous. Thus, whereas in some patients survival is not affected by the disease, others die shortly after diagnosis (1–3).

For many years treatment of CLL revolved around the use of alkylating agents, particularly chlorambucil. This resulted in symptom palliation and a small proportion of transient responses but no definitive improvement of survival. These disappointing results were not ameliorated by combination chemotherapy regimens (4).

Over the last decade, new agents such as purine analogs or monoclonal antibodies have been introduced in the treatment of CLL; in addition, there are an increasing number of patients who are being transplanted [5, 6 and reviewed by Dyer and (Österborg) (see Chapter 15), Thomas et al. (see Chapter 14), and Krackhardt and (Gribben) see (Chapter 18)].

All these approaches are promising and it is likely will improve the outcome of patients with CLL. Nevertheless, the cost of most of these treatments is high, and, more importantly, some of them, particularly transplants, are associated with a high morbidity and even mortality. Furthermore, given the still limited follow-up of patients treated with these approaches, the potential long-term complications of these treatments are largely unknown.

The lack of a curative treatment for CLL, along with the heterogeneous course of the disease, its variable impact on patients's life expectancy, and the diversity of available treatments, demand the development of risk-adapted therapies for CLL. In this chapter, issues that should be considered when planning individual, risk-adapted therapies in CLL are reviewed (Table 1).

Table 1 Factors to Be Considered in Risk-Adapted Treatment Strategies for CLL

Patient-related
  Age
  Associated diseases
  Performance status
  Patient's expectations
Disease-related
  Diagnosis
    Exclude B-cell chronic lymphoproliferative disorders that can mimic CLL
  Symptomatic disease
    Exclude complications or disease transformation
  CLL-associated disturbances
    Hypogammaglobulinemia
    Autoimmune hemolytic anemia
    Infections
  Prognostic factors
    Classical
      Clinical stages
      Degree of bone marrow infiltration
      WBC count
      Percentage of atypical cells in peripheral blood
      Lymphocyte doubling time
    Other[a]
      Thymidin-kinase serum levels
      sCD23 serum levels
      β_2-microglobulin serum levels
      Cytogenetics
      Mutational status of the IgV gene
      CD38 expression
      BCL-2/BAX ratio
      MDR expression
Treatment-related
  Sensitivity of the disease to treatment
  Prior therapy
  Number of lines of previous treatment
  Degree and quality of the response
  Minimal disease status

---

[a] Although the prognostic value of these parameters has been shown in some studies, their independent prognostic significance should be further corroborated.

II. PATIENT CHARACTERISTICS

A. Age

CLL is a disease of the elderly. In recent series, the median age of patients at diagnosis is close to 70 years. Although CLL is not frequent in individuals younger than 40, the number of patients diagnosed at a younger age, and in asymptomatic phase, is increasing as a result of routine analyses. In a large group of patients from a single institution, about 20% of the patients were less than 56 years (7). In the series from the Postgraduate School of Hematology of Barcelona, 12% of the patients were 50 years or younger at diagnosis; overall, about one-third of the patients were younger than 60; another third, between 60 and 70; and the remaining third, older than 70 (Fig. 1).

The patient's age should be taken into consideration when making treatment decisions. However, the *biological* age, rather than the *chronological* should be assessed. Although age by itself should not be a criterion to initiate, or to modify, treatment, comorbidity and performance status are, as discussed later, important variables to be weighed in all patients.

Treatments totally warranted in younger people would be unrealistic, or even inappropriate, in elderly patients. A large proportion of older individuals have associated chronic illnesses and poor performance status, with this making tolerance to intensive treatments poor. On the other hand, in some patients, particularly those displaying asymptomatic, smoldering forms of CLL, life expectancy is not jeopardized by the disease.

As mentioned previously, CLL is increasingly being diagnosed in younger patients; this is not due to a real increment in the incidence of CLL in young people but to the growing practice of blood analyses for routine or trivial reasons.

Because CLL is not curable with conventional treatments, there is an increasing interest in the role of hematopoietic stem cell transplants in the management of this disease, particularly in those subjects for whom symptom palliation alone is not an acceptable goal of therapy (8–10).

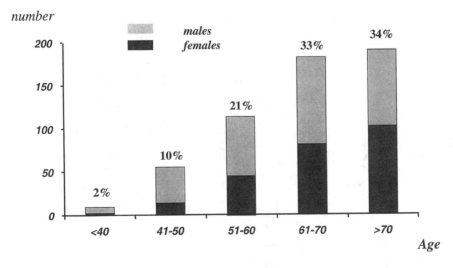

Figure 1 CLL: age and sex distribution.

However, transplants can only be offered to a reduced number of patients. A theoretical model of the proportion of patients that are potential candidates to transplants or to other experimental, intensive treatments is shown in Figure 2. This model assumes the age distribution mentioned earlier, as well as that about 70% of patients are currently diagnosed in the early, nonsymptomatic phases of their disease, thereby not requiring therapy. As can be seen, only about 10% of the total number of patients with CLL can potentially gain benefit from intensive approaches. Interestingly, this model fits well with actual data. Thus, at the Postgraduate School of Hematology of Barcelona, between 1991 and 1998, 334 patients with CLL have been diagnosed and followed up; of these patients, only 28 (8.3%) have received a transplant, a procedure that is offered to all patients less than the age of 60 requiring therapy (unpublished data). The use of nonmyeloablative regimens in allogeneic transplants is particularly appealing in CLL, because they could contribute to increasing the age limit of transplantable patients (11,12).

The aforementioned facts underscore the need to search effective treatments for all age groups, including the elderly, a group of patients clearly underrepresented in clinical trials or for whom clinical trials are rarely available, biases that should be corrected.

Furthermore, the notion that CLL is a "benign" disease, particularly in the elderly, is inappropriate. Although a proportion of patients may have a rather indolent course and eventually die from causes not directly related to the disease, some studies have shown that the relative survival (observed survival divided by expected survival for a control population) is reduced in all age groups. In a registry study based on about 25,000 cases of CLL, 5-year overall survival was 48.2%, and 10-year overall survival was 22.5%. The relative survival was 66.4% at 5 years from diagnosis. When broken down by age, relative survival was shortened in all age groups, including the elderly. Thus, the 5-year relative survival was 69.5%, 72.2%, 63.1%, and 41.7% for age groups <40, 40–59, 60–79, and 80 or more, respectively (13).

B. Associated Diseases and Performance Status

Older individuals tend to have numerous organ dysfunction (e.g., impairment in renal, hepatic, or cardiac function) or chronic illnesses. Although this issue has not been widely

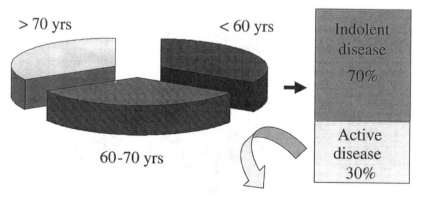

Figure 2 Experimental therapies in CLL.

investigated in CLL patients, in some studies focused on cancer patients, up to 70% had comorbid conditions (14–16). Moreover, chemotherapy schedules may require modification when renal or hepatic function is impaired, thus presenting an additional difficulty to treatment (14). On the other hand, performance status is another variable not necessarily related to associated diseases, that is important to prognosis (16).

C. Patient's Expectations About Treatment

Given the absence of a truly curative treatment, the different impact of the disease on overall survival, the fact that active disease is not incompatible with an active life, and the diversity of treatments available make it necessary to consider the patient's own expectations about the treatment and his or her disease when planing treatment.

III. DISEASE CHARACTERISTICS

A. Diagnosis

In most instances, the diagnosis of CLL is easy. The hallmark of the diagnosis is the presence of a monoclonal population of small, mature-appearing B lymphocytes with a characteristic immunophenotype in peripheral blood. Although most CLL cases have typical morphology, some patients display atypical features. In such cases, a relatively simple set of cell-surface markers is useful for diagnosis. Typical CLL cases are SmIg weak, CD5+, CD22 weak, CD23+, and FMC7− (17,18).

The detection of a CD5(+) B-cell proliferation should not be considered as tantamount to the diagnosis of CLL. Although atypical cases do exist, the diagnosis of atypical CLL should not be accepted without discarding other lymphoproliferative disorders (19–21). In this regard, not only the immunophenotype of the malignant cells but also cytogenetic and molecular findings can be of help [reviewed by Gascoyne (Chapter 11)]. The accurate diagnosis of the different types of chronic B cell malignancies with leukemic expression has important consequences in the prognosis and treatment of these disorders.

B. Complications Associated with the Disease

Patients with CLL frequently present immune disturbances. Autoimmune hemolytic anemia, which can be observed in 5% to 20% of the cases, can be triggered or aggravated by treatment, particularly purine analogs (22,23). This complication, which can be fatal, is more frequently observed in heavily pretreated patients. Patients who have this complication develop should not be rechallenged with purine analogs. Moreover, it seems advisable to spare purine analogs in patients with a past history of autoimmune hemolytic anemia or with a positive Coombs' test.

Infections, which are facilitated by hypogammaglobulinemia, imbalance in T-cell subsets, and neutropenia, are the most important cause of morbidity and mortality in CLL (24–28). Infections have to be treated with broad-spectrum antibiotics, antiviral, or antifungal agents as indicated. On the other hand, measures to prevent infections may be useful.

Hypogammaglobulinemia can occur in up to 60% of the patients, particularly when the disease is in advanced phase (29). In a placebo-controlled randomized study published several years ago, 400 mg/kg of immunoglobulin given intravenously at 3-week intervals for 1 year proved to be of some effectiveness in preventing infections, but survival was not prolonged (30). This fact, along with cost/benefit considerations, has limited the use of high-dose immunoglobulin to extremely selected patients with profound hypogammaglobulinemia and severe, life-threatening infections (31). When indicated, lower doses of immunoglobulin (e.g., 10 g every 3 weeks; 250 mg/kg every 4 weeks) can be as effective as higher doses (32,33).

Purine analogs induce a marked decrease in CD4(+) cells, which has been related to opportunistic infections [e.g., toxoplasmosis, listeriosis, *Pneumocystis carinii* pneumonia (PCP)] (26). Older age, advanced clinical stage, previous treatment, concomitant administration of corticosteroids, and elevated serum creatinine have been found to be associated with a high risk of infections in patients treated with fludarabine (26,27). Cotrimoxazole, acyclovir, and antifungal agents are potentially useful to prevent this type of infection. The impact of prophylactic measures, however, has not been investigated in prospective, randomized trials. Recommendations of strategies aimed at preventing infections are, therefore, based on retrospective studies. The agent most widely used is cotrimoxazole, given as prophylaxis of PCP, a complication that has occasionally been reported, especially in patients heavily pretreated before receiving purine analogs. In a retrospective study, fludarabine + chlorambucil resulted in a significantly more infections than treatment with either single agent; patients receiving fludarabine had more major infections and herpesvirus (HSV) infections compared with chlorambucil-treated patients (28). The role of acyclovir in preventing HSV infections is being prospectively investigated.

Absolute neutropenia is rare in untreated patients but may be induced by chemotherapy. In such cases, prophylactic antibiotics are usually given to prevent infections, although their effectiveness, as that of cotrimoxazole to prevent PCP, has not been formally demonstrated in randomized trials. Granulocyte colony-stimulating factor (G-CSF) and granulocyte-macrophage colony-stimulating factor (GM-CSF) have been effective in cases with severe neutropenia and decrease the number of infections in patients treated with fludarabine, although survival is not prolonged (34,35). Finally, in cases with profound anemia unresponsive to treatment, erythropoietin may be useful to increase the hemoglobin level and to avoid transfusions (36).

Although all the measures previously mentioned have not been found to prolong survival, reasonable use of them can substantially contribute to improving the quality of life of some patients and to limit the period of hospitalization.

IV. INDICATIONS FOR THERAPY

Patients with CLL should not be treated unless they present symptomatic or progressive disease. This concept, which applies to all patients with CLL regardless of their clinical stage, is based on the fact that there are patients who, despite their advanced stage, do not present symptoms and run a rather indolent course. Although most of these patients will eventually require therapy, a proportion of them remains stable for a long period of time.

A number of factors that justify therapy in CLL are generally accepted (17). Almost none of the features listed in the following is found isolated; rather, they are present altogether in the same patient:

1. *Disease-related symptoms* (i.e., weight loss, fever without infection, night sweats, weakness). Because systemic symptoms in uncomplicated CLL are not

very common, infection or the transformation of the disease to a more aggressive lymphoproliferative disorder (Richter's syndrome, CLL/PL) should be excluded before assuming that these symptoms are due to the disease.

2. *Development of anemia or thrombocytopenia caused by bone marrow infiltration.*
3. *Autoimmune hemolytic anemia or thrombocytopenia.* In such cases, treatment should be initiated with corticosteroids alone and cytotoxic agents added only if no response is achieved.
4. *Bulky lymphadenopathy and/or splenomegaly causing compressive problems.*
5. *Rapidly increasing blood lymphocytosis* (i.e., doubling time of less than 12 months).

V. PROGNOSIS

In recent series, the median survival of patients with CLL is 7 to 10 years, 3 to 5 years longer than that reported in series from the '70s. This prolongation in survival is basically because CLL is increasingly being diagnosed in early phases of the disease and, hence, with a better prognosis (37). The individual prognosis of patients with CLL is extremely variable. Thus, whereas in some cases the life expectancy is not modified by the disease, in others the median survival is less than 3 years. Therefore, the decision to treat, and, most importantly, *how* to treat, CLL patients cannot be made without considering the expected survival that, on the basis of prognostic factors, a given patient has. The outcome of patients with CLL can be determined quite accurately thanks to different prognostic parameters [reviewed by Molica (see Chapter 12)]. Among the many existing prognostic factors, clinical stages (38,39), WBC count (40), degree of bone marrow infiltration (41), peripheral blood morphology (42), and blood lymphocyte doubling time (43) are simple and reliable parameters that have proved useful in many studies (44).

Although clinical stages are essential tools for predicting prognosis and indicating therapy, the mechanisms accounting for the features, particularly the cytopenias, that define clinical stages are unfortunately not contemplated in any of the most extensively used staging systems (Rai, Binet). This is a setback, because cytopenias are not always due to bone marrow failure related to a high tumor burden. In such a context, immune-mediated cytopenias, particularly autoimmune hemolytic anemia, which can be observed in 5% to 20% of the patients, and immune thrombocytopenia (present in about 2% of the cases) are of special concern. Pure red-cell aplasia can also be rarely observed. Besides these, iron-deficiency anemia, anemia caused by nutritional deficiency, and hypersplenism should all be considered, and ruled out, before assuming that the cytopenia is related to the tumor burden. Clues to suspect such situations are the presence of an isolated cytopenia and the absence of features (e.g., lymphadenopathy, massive bone marrow infiltration) characteristic of a high tumor burden. Recognizing these situations is important, because their treatment is not the same as for CLL (Table 2).

On the other hand, disease transformation into large-cell lymphoma (Richter syndrome), or more rarely into Hodgkin's disease, occurs in 3% to 10% of patients with CLL (45). Disease transformation should be suspected whenever a patient has symptoms that can not be easily explained. These include fever for which an infectious origin can not be identified, night sweats, or weight loss, as well as an increase in the size of lymph nodes, augmentation of lactate dehydrogenase serum values, or the appearance of hyper-

Table 2   CLL—Situations that May Lead to Anemia or Thrombocytopenia Not Related
to Bone Marrow Failure

Situation	Diagnosis	Potential intervention
Autoimmune hemo-lytic anemia	Coombs' test Reticulocytes LDH Haptoglobin	Prednisone Cyclophosphamide Cyclosporine High-dose Ig Splenectomy
Thrombocytopenia of immune basis	Bone marrow aspirate and biopsy Platelet antibodies	Prednisone Cyclophosphamide Cyclosporine High-dose Ig Splenectomy
Iron-deficiency anemia	Serum iron, ferritin Bleeding lesions? (GI and other studies as indi-cated)	Correct cause Iron replacement
B_{12} or folic acid defi-ciency	B_{12} and folic acid measurements	Correct cause B_{12} or folic acid administration
Erythroblastopenia	Reticulocyte count Bone marrow aspirate and biopsy	Cyclosporine $\pm$ prednisone
Hypersplenism	Bone marrow biopsy Imaging studies	Splenectomy Irradiation of the spleen

calcemia or a M serum component. Disease transformation should be confirmed by taking biopsies of lymph nodes or other tissues suspicious of harboring transformed disease and has to be treated with aggressive lymphoma-type chemotherapy regimens.

Besides the classic prognostic parameters mentioned in the preceding paragraphs, other important predictors of the outcome do exist. These include serum levels of thymidin-kinase (46), sCD23 (47), β_2-microglobulin (48,49), and cytogenetic abnormalities (50,51). Cytogenetic alterations are important. Thus, patients with del(13q) as a single abnormality have an excellent prognosis (median survival, 133 months), whereas those with del(11q) or del(17p) respond poorly to therapy and have short survival (median survival, 79 and 32 months, respectively) (51).

On the other hand, CLL has long been considered a homogeneous disease of naïve CD5(+), pregerminal B cells not exposed to antigenic stimulation. Recently, it has been found that the mutational status of the IgV gene correlates with different disease subsets. Thus, those patients with unmutated IgV gene ("naïve" or "pregerminal" CLL) have a poorer prognosis than those displaying mutated IgV gene ("memory" or "postgerminal" CLL). Patients with mutated IgV gene forms appear to have a much better prognosis than those with unmutated IgV gene (52,53). Unfortunately, most laboratories are currently unable to isolate and characterize IgV gene sequences. To simplify the technique for studying IgV gene mutational status or to find a widely applicable surrogate for such an event would be, therefore, important for clinical practice. In one study, it has been found that CD38 expression on leukemic cells correlated with IgV gene mutations (i.e., CD38+

≥30%, unmutated IgV genes; CD38+ < 30%, mutated IgV genes) (52,54), but this was not confirmed in the other study in which this relationship has been investigated up to now (55). Although the value of CD38 expression as surrogate of IgV gene mutational status is controversial, CD38 expression may have prognostic value in itself.

In summary, prognostic factors allow the identification of different prognostic subgroups among CLL patients. Moreover, some prognostic parameters may help identifying indolent or smoldering forms of the disease, not likely to progress (54). Patients with smoldering CLL are characterized by having low WBC counts, typical lymphocyte morphology, Hb levels ≥12 g/dL, prolonged lymphocyte doubling time (>12 months), nondiffuse bone marrow involvement, and minor or absent lymphadenopathy. In addition, deletions at chromosome 13q, normal levels of serum β_2-microglobulin and TK, as well as mutated IgV gene, are other features that correlate with a smoldering course of the disease (46–53).

VI. TREATMENT-RELATED VARIABLES

In the setting of risk-adapted therapies, some treatment-related variables are worth considering. These include the likelihood of achieving response, the impact of initial therapy on subsequent treatments, and the identification of treatments to which a given patient is more likely to respond (Table 3). The relevance of these issues stems from the simple fact that response to therapy is an important prognostic factor by itself (55).

In patients treated with conventional chemotherapy, younger age, early disease, no prior exposure to therapy, and good performance status correlate with a high possibility of obtaining a response (56,57). In addition, serum levels of β_2-microglobulin, albumin, and creatinine also correlate with response achievement (56). Moreover, cytogenetic abnormalities such as del(11q) and del(17p) with $p53$ abnormalities have been associated with poor response to therapy (50,51). In addition, in some studies, BCL-2/BAX protein

Table 3 CLL—Variables Associated with Response to Therapy

Age <70 yr
No prior therapy
Low tumor burden
Good performance status
No associated diseases
No signs of disease transformation
Normal levels in serum of
   Albumin
   Creatinine
   β_2-Microglobulin
Prior response to therapy
No poor prognostic cytogenetic abnormalities [e.g., del(11q), del(17p)]
Short interval diagnosis-treatment[a,b]
No MDR gene expression[b]
Low BCL-2/BAX ratio[b]
Sensitivity in DiSC assay[c,b]

[a] In autologous stem-cell transplants.
[b] Requires further investigation.
[c] Differential staining cytotoxicity.

ratio and the expression of multiple drug resistance (MDR) genes have been found to be associated with response (58,59).

With respect to hematopoietic stem cell transplants, no extensive prognostic studies have been performed. In the autologous transplantation setting, the status of the disease immediately before transplant (complete remission or very good partial response) is the most important prognostic factor (9,10,60). Other variables correlating with prognosis are the number of previous lines of therapy (≤ 2 vs >2), response to purine analogs, degree of bone marrow infiltration pretransplant ($\leq 30\%$ vs $>30\%$ lymphocytes), and the interval between diagnosis and transplantation (≤ 36 vs >36 months). Interestingly, classic prognostic factors at CLL diagnosis such as clinical stage or degree of bone marrow involvement have no influence on the outcome after transplant (60). This would suggest that, rather than depending on factors related to the natural history of the disease, the success of the transplant depends primarily on the sensitivity of the disease to treatment. Type of conditioning regimen total body irradiation (TBI)-containing vs non TBI-containing), source of hematopoietic stem cells, and purging did not correlate with outcome. The achievement of a MRD ($-$) status, as measured by cytofluorometry and IgH gene rearrangements, correlates with a longer disease-free interval, particularly in the autologous setting (10,61,62). Because several studies indicate that achieving an MRD ($-$) status is critical to the outcome, the investigation of strategies (e.g., purine analoges in combination with other drugs, monoclonal antibodies) that have the potential to improve not only the response rate but also to eradicate MRD seems warranted. Nonetheless, studies of prognostic factors in patients with CLL receiving transplants should be interpreted with caution, given possible biases in patient selection. On the other hand, variables such as the number of lines of therapy before transplantation, sensitivity of the disease to treatment, degree of the response, and interval between diagnosis and transplant might be mutually related.

Of note, transplants produce substantial morbidity and mortality, with the transplant-related mortality in different series being between 5% and 19% for autologous transplants and 25% to 50% for allogeneic transplants, respectively (10). Transplants, therefore, should only be indicated in patients with high-risk disease and should not be performed outside trials.

Finally, when planning individually designed, risk-adapted therapies, the impact of front-line treatment on subsequent therapies should be carefully considered. In this regard, patients refractory to, or relapsing after, purine-analogs are difficult to rescue by means of other treatments, particularly in totally refractory cases. The same applies to patients who have hematopoietic stem-cell transplants fail (10). On the other hand, treatment with purine analogs, particularly in heavily pretreated patients, has been associated with a lower possibility of obtaining enough hematopoietic stem cells for autotransplantation (9,10). The fact that treatment with purine analogs can jeopardize autologous transplantation, particularly in heavily pretreated patients, should be carefully considered when the necessity of performing an autograft at some point during the course of the disease is envisaged.

For obvious reasons, the possibility of predicting the response to different treatment modalities in in vitro models is appealing. Among several in vitro cytotoxicity tests, the nonclonogenic 3-(4,5-dimethylthiazol-2-yl)-2,5-diphenyl tetrazolium bromide (MTT) assay and the differential staining cytotoxicity (DISC) assay are the most extensively used (63–67). Although these techniques are not widely used, several studies have analyzed the correlation between in vitro and in vivo results. A direct relationship has been found, among other agents, for chlorambucil, fludarabine, and cladribine.

These results suggest that in vitro assays might help identify patients not likely to respond to a given therapy, thereby avoiding unnecessary exposure to noneffective drugs and the appearance of cross-resistance. Although an in vitro sensitivity may not always be indicative of a clinical response, in vitro resistance often correlates with a lack of clinical response (64). Pretreatment in vitro assays might enable the toxic, clinical, and financial costs of some treatments to be avoided in resistant cases. This is an interesting venue that is deserving prospective investigation.

VII. GOALS OF THERAPY

The most important goals of therapy are to prolong survival and to improve quality of life. Given the different impact of the disease on survival, these goals can be achieved by different means. In some cases, no therapy or the sound use of gentle treatment aimed at palliating symptoms and slowing down the pace of the disease will be enough to achieve these goals. In other cases, however, an attempt to cure the disease by using experimental, intensive treatments will be totally warranted. The latter, however, should not be performed outside clinical trials. The physician taking care of patients with CLL should keep in mind that treatment end points such as complete response, disease-free interval, or the achievement of a MRD ($-$) status, potentially useful in clinical trials, do not constitute per se the *goals* of therapy: to ameliorating the quality of life and to prolonging the life span of the patient (ideally, matching the expected survival by age and sex).

VIII. CONCLUSION

The task of making treatment decisions in CLL was easy in those years in which the only treatments for this form of leukemia were alkylating agents. Nowadays, deciding when and how to treat a patient with CLL is much more complex, given the existence of new, potentially more active, and also potentially more toxic, agents and procedures. In the

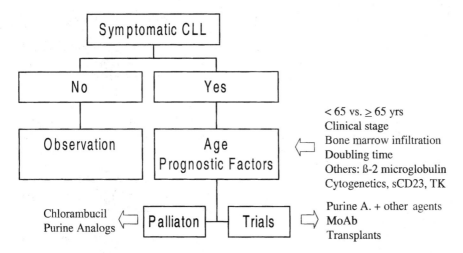

Figure 3 Risk-adapted treatment strategies for CLL.

challenging process of advising treatment for patients with CLL, patient's age and general status, symptoms related to the disease, and prognostic factors are all essential. A step-by-step procedure that considers the accuracy in the diagnosis, patient and disease characteristics, and prognostic factors is shown in (Fig. 3). Furthermore, because most of the new and most promising agents to treat CLL are still in investigational phase, patients should be encouraged to enter into clinical trials based on risk factors. Although the ultimate goals of therapy are to improve quality of life and to prolong survival, the means for achieving these goals not only may, but should, vary according the characteristics of the patient and the disease. Finally, in no case should risks outweigh potential benefits of a given treatment.

REFERENCES

1. E Montserrat, F Bosch, C Rozman. B-cell chronic lymphocytic leukemia: Recent progress in biology, diagnosis, and therapy. Ann Oncol 8(suppl 1):93–101, 1997.
2. WG Wierda, TJ Kipps. Chronic lymphocytic leukemia. Curr Opin Hematol 6:253–261, 1999.
3. F Caligaris-Cappio, TJ Hamblin. B-cell chronic lymphocytic leukemia: a bird of a different feather. J Clin Oncol 17:399–408, 1999.
4. CLL Trialists's Collaborative Group. Chemotherapeutic options in chronic lymphocytic leukemia: a meta-analysis of the randomized trials. J Natl Cancer Inst 91:861–868, 1999.
5. BD Cheson, Guest Ed. Future strategies toward the cure of indolent B-cell malignancies. Semin Hematol 36(suppl 5):1–33, 1999.
6. MJ Keating. Chronic lymphocytic leukemia in the next decade: Where do we go from here? Semin Hematol 35(suppl 3):27–33, 1998.
7. FR Mauro, R Foa, D Giannarelli, I Cordone, S Crescenzi, E Pescarmona, R Sala, R Cerretti, F Mandelli. Clinical characteristics and outcome of young chronic lymphocytic leukemia patients: A single institution study of 204 patients. Blood 94:448–454, 1999.
8. A Gratwohl, J Passweg, H Baldomero, J Hermans. Blood and marrow transplantation activity in Europe 1997. European Group for Blood and Marrow Transplantation (EBMT). Bone Marrow Transplant 24:231–245, 1999.
9. P Dreger, Michallet, N Schmitz. Stem-cell transplantation for chronic lymphocytic leukemia. The 1999 perspective. Ann Oncol 11(suppl 1):S49–S53, 2000.
10. E Montserrat, J Esteve. Hematopoietic stem-cell transplants for chronic lymphocytic leukemia: Current status. Rev Clin Exp Hematol. 4:167–178, 2000.
11. R Champlin, I Khouri, S Kornblau, F Marini, P Anderlini, NT Ueno, J Molldrem, S Giralt. Allogeneic hematopoietic transplantation as adoptive immunotherapy: induction of graft-versus-malignancy as primary therapy. Hematol/Oncol Clin North America 13:1041–1057, 1999.
12. IF Khouri, M Keating, M Korbling, D Przepiorka, P Anderlini, S O'Brien, S Giralt, C Ippoliti, B von Wolff, J Gajewski, M Donato, D Claxton, N Ueno, B Andersson, A Gee, R Champlin. Transplant-lite: induction of graft-versus-malignancy using fludarabine-based nonablative chemotherapy and allogeneic blood progenitor-cell transplantation as treatment for lymphoid malignancies. J Clin Oncol 16:2817–2824, 1998.
13. LF Diehl, LH Karnell, HR Menck. The national cancer data base on age, gender, treatment, and outcomes of patients with chronic lymphocytic leukemia. Cancer 86:2684–2692, 1999.
14. RJ McKenna Sr. Clinical aspects of cancer in the elderly: Treatment decisions, treatments choices, and follow-up. Cancer 75:2107–2117, 1994.
15. KS Ogle, GM Swanson, N Woods, F Azzouz. Cancer and comorbidity: redifining chronic diseases. Cancer 88:653–655, 2000.
16. M Extermann, J Overcash, GH Lyman, J Parr, L Balducci. Comorbidiy and functional status are independent in older cancer patients. J Clin Oncol 16:1582–1587, 1998.

17. BD Cheson, JM Bennett, M Grever, N Kay, MJ Keating, S O'Brien, KR Rai. National Cancer Institute-sponsored Working Group guidelines for chronic lymphocytic leukemia: revised guideliness for diagnosis and treatment. Blood 87:4990–4997, 1996.

18. International Workshop on Chronic Lymphocytic Leukemia: Chronic lymphocytic leukemia: recommendations for diagnosis, staging, and response criteria. Ann Intern Med 110:236–238, 1989.

19. A Criel, L Michaux, C De Wolf-Peeters. The concept of typical and atypical chronic lymphocytic leukaemia. Leuk Lymphoma 33:33–45, 1999.

20. JC Huang, WG Finn, CL Goolsby, D Variakojis, LC Peterson. CD5-small B-cell leukemias are rarely classifiable as chronic lymphocytic leukemia. Am J Clin Pathol 111:123–130, 1999.

21. GA Pangalis, MK Angelopoulou, TP Vassilakopoulos, MP Siakantaris, C Kittas. B-chronic lymphocytic leukemia, small lymphocytic lymphoma, and lymphoplasmacytic lymphoma, including Waldenstrom's macroglobulinemia: a clinical, morphologic, and biologic spectrum of similar disorders. Semin Hematol 36:104–114, 1999.

22. FR Mauro, R Foa, R Cerretti, D Giannarelli, S Coluzzi, S Mandelli, G Girelli. Autoimmune hemolytic anemia in chronic lymphocytic leukemia: clinical, therapeutic, and prognostic features. Blood 95:2786–2792, 2000.

23. RB Weiss, J Freiman, SL Kweder, LF Diehl, JC Byrd. Hemolytic anemia after fludarabine therapy for chronic lymphocytic leukemia. J Clin Oncol. 16:1885–1889, 1998.

24. S Molica. Infections in chronic lymphocytic leukemia: Risk factors, an impact on survival, and treatment. Leuk Lymphoma 13:203–214, 1994.

25. VA Morrison. The infectious complications in chronic lymphocytic leukemia. Semin Oncol 25:98–106, 1998.

26. BD Cheson. Infectious and immunosuppressive complications of purine analog therapy. J Clin Oncol 13:2431–2448, 1995.

27. EJ Anaissie, DP Kontoyiannis, S O'Brien, H Kantarjian, L Robertson, S Lerner, MJ Keating. Infections in patients with chronic lymphocytic leukemia treated with fludarabine. Ann Intern Med 129:559–566, 1998.

28. VA Morrison. The infectious complications of chronic lymphocytic leukemia. Semin Oncol 25:98–106, 1998.

29. C Rozman, E Montserrat, N Viñolas. Serum immunoglobulins in B-chronic lymphocytic leukemia. Natural history and prognostic significance. Cancer 61:279–283, 1988.

30. Cooperative Group for the Study of Immunoglobulin in Chronic Lymphocytic Leukemia: Intravenous immune globulin in chronic lymphocytic leukemia. N Engl J Med 319:902–907, 1988.

31. JC Weeks, ER Tierney, MC Weinstein. Cost effectiveness of prophylactic intravenous immunoglobulin in chronic lymphocytic leukemia. N Engl J Med 325:81–86, 1991.

32. H Chapel, M Dicato, H Gamm, V Brennan, F Ries, C Bunch, M Lee. Immunoglobulin replacement in patients with chronic lymphocytic leukaemia: a comparison of two dose regimes. Br J Haematol 88:209–212, 1994.

33. J Jurlander, C Hartmann Geisler, MM Hansen. Treatment of hypogammaglobulinaemia in chronic lymphocytic leukaemia by low-dose intravenous gammaglobulin. Eur J Haematol 53:114–118, 1994.

34. S O'Brien, H Kantarjian, M Beran, et al. Fludarabine and granulocyte colony-stimulating factor (G-CSF) in patients with chronic lymphocytic leukemia. Leukemia 11:1631–1635, 1997.

35. T Südhorff, M Arning, W Schneider. Prophylactic strategies to meet infectious complications in fludarabine-treated CLL. Leukemia 11(suppl 2):S38–S41, 1997.

36. CH Pozpoulos, MK Panayotidis, Angelopoulos, GA Pangalis. Treatment of anaemia in B-chronic lymphocytic leukaemia (B-CLL) with recombinant human erythropoietin (r-HuEPO) (abstract). Br J Haematol 87 (suppl 1):232, 1994.

37. C Rozman, F Bosch, E Montserrat. Chronic lymphocytic leukemia: a changing natural history?. Leukemia 11:775–778, 1997.

38. KR Rai, A Sawitsky, EP Cronkite, A Chanana, R Levy, B Pasternack. Clinical staging of chronic lymphocytic leukemia. Blood 46:219, 1975.

39. JL Binet, A Auquier, G Dighiero, C Chastang, H Piguet, J Goasguen, G Vaugier, G Potron, P Colona, F Oberling, M Thomas, G Tchernia, C Jacquillat, P Boivin, C Lesly, MT Duault, M Monconduit, S Belabbes, F Gremy. A new prognostic classification of chronic lymphocytic leukemia derived from a multivariate survival analysis. Cancer 48:198, 1981.

40. C Rozman, E Montserrat, E Feliu, A Grañena, P Marin, B Nomdedeu, JL Vives-Corrons. Prognosis of chronic lymphocytic leukemia: a multivariate survival analysis of 150 cases. Blood 59:1001–1005, 1982.

41. E Montserrat, N Villamor, JC Reverter, RM Brugués, D Tassies, F Bosch, JL Aguilar, JL Vives Corrons, M Rozman, C Rozman. Bone marrow assessment in chronic lymphocytic leukemia: Aspirate or biopsy?. A comparative study in 258 patients. Br J Haematol 57:292–300, 1996.

42. T Vallespí, MA Sanz, E Montserrat. Chronic lymphocytic leukaemia: Prognostic value of lymphocyte morphological subtypes. A multivariate survival analysis in 146 patients. Br J Haematol 77:478–485, 1991.

43. E Montserrat, J Sánchez-Bisonó, N Viñolas, C Rozman. Lymphocyte doubling time in chronic lymphocytic leukemia: Analysis of its prognostic importance. Br J Haematol 62:567–573, 1986.

44. M Hallek, I Kuhn-Hallek, B Emmerich. Prognostic factors in chronic lymphocytic leukemia. Leukemia 11(suppl 2):S4–S13, 1997.

45. FJ Giles, SM O'Brien, MJ Keating. Chronic lymphocytic leukemia in Richter's transformation. Semin Oncol, 25:117–125, 1998.

46. M Hallek, I Langenmayer, C Nerl, W Knauf, H Dietzfelbinger, D Adorf, M Ostwald, R Busch, I Kuhn-Hallek, E Thiel, B Emmerich. Elevated serum thymidine kinase levels indentify a subgroup at high risk of disease progression in early, nonsmoldering chronic lymphocytic leukemia. Blood 93:1732–1737, 1999.

47. M Sarfarti, S Chevret, C Chastang, G Biron, P Stryckman, G Delespesse, JL Binet, H Merle-Beral, D Bron. Prognostic importance of serum soluble CD23 in chronic lymphocytic leuke-mia. Blood 88:4259–4264, 1996.

48. B Simonsson, L Wibell, K Nilsson. β2-microglobulin in chronic lymphocytic leukaemia. Scand J Haematol 24:174–180, 1980.

49. M Keating, S Lerner, H Kantarjian, E Freireich, S O'Brien. The serum beta2-microglobulin is more powerful than stage in predicting response and survival in chronic lymphocytic leuke-mia (abst). Blood 86:606a, 1995.

50. D Döhner, S Stilgenbauer, K Döhner, M Bentz, P Lichter. Chromosome aberrations in B-cell chronic lymphocytic leukemia: reassessment based on molecular cytogenetic analysis. J Mol Med 77:266–281, 1999.

51. S Stilgenbauer, E Leupolt, A Kröbe, K Döhner, M Bentz, A Benner, P Lichter, H Döhner. Molecular cytogenetic analysis of B-CLL: Incidence and prognostic significance of the most frequent chromosome aberrations (abstr). Blood 94(suppl 1):543, 1999.

52. RN Damle, T Wasil, F Fais, F Ghiotto, A Valetto, SL Allen, A Buchbinder, D Budman, K Dittmar, J Kolitz, SM Lichtman, P Schulman, VP Vinciguerra, KR Rai, M Ferrarini, N Chiorazzi. IgV gene mutation status and CD38 expression as novel prognostic indicators in chronic lymphocytic leukemia. Blood 94:1840–1847, 1999.

53. TJ Hamblin, Z Davis, A Gardiner, DG Oscier, FK Stevenson. Unmutated immunoglobulin V_H genes are associated with a more aggressive form of chronic lymphocytic leukemia. Blood 94:1848–1854, 1999.

54. R Damle, T Wasil, S Allen, P Schulman, KR Rai, N Chiorazzi, M Ferrarini. Updated data on V gene mutation status and CD38 expression in B-CLL. Blood 95:2456–2457, 2000.

55. TJ Hamblin, JA Orchard, A Gardiner, DG Oscier, Z Davis, FK Stevenson. Immunoglobulin V genes and CD38 expression in CLL. Blood 95:2455–2456, 2000.

56. E Montserrat, N Viñolas, JC Reverter, C Rozman. Natural history of chronic lymphocytic leukemia: On the progression and prognosis of early clinical stage. Nouv Rev Fr Hematol 30: 359–361, 1988.

57. D Catovsky, J Fooks, S Richard. Prognostic factors in chronic lymphocytic leukaemia—the importance of age, sex, and response to treatment in survival. A report from the MRC CLL 1 Trial. Br J Haematol 72:141–149, 1989.

58. S O'Brien, H Kantarjian, M Beran, T Smith, C Koller, E Estey, LE Robertson, S Lerner, M Keating. Results of fludarabine and prednisone therapy in 264 patients with chronic lympho-cytic leukemia with multivariate analysis-derived prognostic model for response to treatment. Blood 82:1695–1700, 1993.

59. MJ Keating, S O'Brien, S Lerner, C Koller, M Beran, LE Robertson, EJ Freireich, E Estey, H Kantarjian. Long-term follow-up of patients with chronic lymphocytic leukemia (CLL) re-ceiving fludarabine regimens as initial therapy. Blood 92:1165–1171, 1998.

60. WR Friedenberg, SK Spencer, C Musser, TF Hogan, KA Rodvold, DA Rushing, JJ Mazza, DA Tewksbury, JJ Marx. Multi-drug resistance in chronic lymphocytic leukemia. Leuk Lymphoma 34:171–178, 1999.

61. C Pepper, A Thomas, J Hidalgo de Quintana, S Davies, Y Hoy, P Bentley. Pleiotropic drug resistance in B-cell chronic lymphocytic leukaemia-the role of Bcl-2 family disregulation. Leuk Res 23:1007–1014, 1999.

62. E Montserrat, J Esteve, N Schmitz, P Dreger, G Meloni, S Pavletic, B Coiffier, G Juliusson, J Besalduch, E del Potro, D Caballero, M Michallet. Autologous stem-cell transplantation (ASCT) for chronic lymphocytic leukemia (CLL): results in 107 patients (abstract). Blood 94 (suppl 1):397, 1999.

63. J Mattson, M Uzuel, M Remberger, P Ljungman, E Kimby, O Ringden, H Zetterquist. Minimal residual disease is common after allogeneic stem cell transplantation in patients with B cell chronic lymphocytic leukemia and may be controlled by graft-versus-host disease. Leukemia 14:247–254, 2000.

64. ZS Pavletic, ER Arrowsmith, PJ Bierman, SA Goodman, JM Vose, SR Tarantolo, RS Stein, G Bociek, JP Greer, CD Wu, JP Kollath, D Weisenburger, A Kessinger, SN Wolff, JO Armi-tage, MR Bishop. Outcome of allogeneic stem cell transplantation for B cell chronic lympho-cytic leukemia. Bone Marrow Transpl 25:717–722, 2000.

65. AG Bosanquet, MI Bosanquet. Ex vivo assessment of drug response by differential staining cytotoxicity (DiSC) assay suggests a biological basis for equality of chemotherapy irrespective of age for patients with chronic lymphocytic leukaemia. Leukemia 14:712–715, 2000.

66. AG Bosanquet, JA Coppleston, SA Johnson, AG Smith, SJ Povey, JA Orchard, DG Oscier. Response to cladribine in previously treated patients with chronic lymphocytic leukaemia iden-tified by ex vivo assessment of drug sensitivity by DiSC assay. Br J Haematol 106:474–476, 1999.

67. AG Bosanquet, SA Johnson, SM Richards. Prognosis for fludarabine therapy of chronic lymphocytic leukaemia based on ex vivo drug response by DiSC assay. Br J Haematol 106: 71–77, 1999.

68. B Bellosillo, N Villamor, D Colomer, G Pons, E Montserrat, J Gil. In vitro evaluation of fludarabine in combination with cyclophosphamide and/or mitoxantrone in B-cell chronic lymphocytic leukemia. Blood 94:2836–2843, 1999.

69. Y Kano, M Akutsu, S Tsunoda, K Suzuki, A Ichikawa, Y Furukawa, L Bai, K Kon. In vitro cytotoxic effects of fludarabine (2-F-ara-A) in combination with commonly used antileukemic agents by isobologram analysis. Leukemia 14:379–388, 2000.

18

High-Dose Therapy and Stem Cell Support in Chronic Lymphocytic Leukemia

ANGELA M. KRACKHARDT and JOHN G. GRIBBEN

Dana-Farber Cancer Institute, Harvard Medical School, Boston, Massachusetts

I. INTRODUCTION

Chronic lymphocytic leukemia (CLL) is the most common leukemia in the Western World, and the incidence of this disease is increasing yearly. CLL generally follows an indolent clinical course affecting mainly elderly patients, with a median age at presentation of greater than 65 years. Many such patients will not require therapy. However, the disease is heterogeneous, and some patients have a more aggressive clinical course. A number of clinical and biochemical features can be used to identify patients likely to have a more aggressive clinical course. In addition, 40% of patients with CLL are younger than age 60, and 12% are younger than age 50. These patients almost invariably die of their disease or its complications. In the last 10 years, several new drugs have been shown to be effective in CLL, and in the United States, fludarabine has emerged as the treatment of choice. However, to date, no evidence exists that conventional chemotherapy approaches are curative in CLL. Despite the high initial response rates reported with effective agents such as fludarabine, patients invariably relapse, and subsequently resistance to chemotherapy develops. The role of fludarabine in combination with other chemotherapy and/or monoclonal antibody therapy appears promising and is currently under investigation. At present, the only potentially curative treatment for CLL is high-dose (HD) ablative therapy with hematopoietic stem cell support. However, there are many unanswered questions about the different treatment modalities of stem cell transplantation (SCT), and their roles in the management of CLL remain to be established. In particular, patient selection for consideration of SCT, the timing of SCT in the clinical course of CLL, autologous versus allogeneic SCT, use of nonmyeloablative regimens, and exploitation of the graft versus leukemia effect are currently under investigation.

II. ROLE OF STEM CELL TRANSPLANTATION IN CLL

Stem cell transplantation has become an important treatment option for an increasing number of selected patients with hematological and solid tumors. However, this treatment has not been extensively investigated for patients with CLL. Several reasons exist for a reserved use of this procedure in patients with CLL. First, CLL is largely a disease of the elderly, with a median age at diagnosis of greater than 65 years. Most of these more elderly patients may not be able to tolerate the toxicity associated with high-dose myeloablative treatment approaches. Second, the disease often has a very long natural history, and under these circumstances there has been a reluctance to subject patients who may have long survival despite their disease to a treatment approach with a significant morbidity and potential mortality. Third, most patients do not have a suitable allogeneic donor, and the use of autologous bone marrow (BM) or peripheral blood stem cells (PBSC) has been hampered by the extensive leukemic infiltration of the bone marrow and peripheral blood involvement that is invariable with this disease. Last, many of these patients have been heavily pretreated, so that by the time of referral for SCT they have chemoresistant disease and decreased stem cell reserve develop.

However, several rational reasons exist for more aggressive treatment options in CLL. Although the disease is incurable using standard doses of chemotherapy, the disease is characterized by chemosensitivity at least early in the disease course, making investigation of the role of chemotherapy dose escalation attractive in CLL. Forty percent of CLL patients are younger than 60 years, and conventional therapy has not been shown to be curative in this disease (1,2). These younger patients should largely be able to tolerate HD chemotherapy approaches. The disease has a variable course, and patients with poor prognostic factors have a median survival of less than 5 years (1). Established poor prognosis features include advanced stage disease, diffuse bone marrow infiltration, short lymphocyte doubling time, unfavorable cytogenetics, and high leukocyte count. In particular, 60% of the younger patient group have a poor prognosis with a median survival probability of 5 years after therapy (3).

Stem cell transplantation in CLL must therefore maintain a balance between the risk of this procedure and the risk of dying from the disease. Therefore, the decrease in morbidity and mortality that have resulted from improvements in transplantation procedures and supportive care have led to an increase in the use of SCT in CLL, often with promising results. Moreover, the identification of patients with CLL, who have a sufficiently poor prognosis to merit more experimental treatment approaches with curative intent, is of crucial relevance with regard to the morbidity and mortality risks of this procedure.

III. IDENTIFICATION OF PATIENTS AT POOR RISK

As described earlier, the clinical course of CLL shows a marked heterogeneity, with a median survival ranging from 2 to more than 20 years. This range in clinical course has led clinicians to examine the clinical and biological factors that predict overall survival and disease progression. The most important factor that determines prognosis is stage at diagnosis. Several staging systems have been proposed, two of which, the Rai and Binet staging systems, have become widely accepted because of their simplicity (4,5). The International Workshop on CLL recommends an integrated system incorporating the Binet criteria with the Rai criteria, defining three prognostic categories: ''low risk,'' with a median survival of greater than 8 years, "medium risk," with median survival of 5 to 6 years; and "high risk," with median survival less than 3 years.

However, the staging systems do not provide sufficient information to determine the likelihood of disease progression in an individual patient. For this, other prognostic factors have to be examined. A number of additional prognostic factors, in addition to clinical stage, have also been shown to have an impact on survival. Many factors have been examined, including lymphocyte doubling time, pattern of bone marrow infiltration, lymphocyte and prolymphocyte count, cytogenetics, biological markers of disease, (β_2-microglobulin, thymidine kinase, sCD23) immunophenotype, and pattern of immunoglobulin gene rearrangement. Of these factors, the lymphocyte doubling time and the pattern of bone marrow infiltration have provided the most clinically useful information (6–10). Using with these prognostic factors in addition to the absolute lymphocyte and prolymphocyte count (11) and cytogenetics (12–14) it is possible to identify patients with a shortened median survival (15,16). The role of cytogenetics has been intensively investigated recently. Cytogenetic abnormalities have a high frequency in patients with CLL (17), and specific cytogenetic abnormalities identify special subgroups with different clinical courses (12–17). Deletion at 13q is the most common form of cytogenetic abnormality occurring in up to 55% of patients and is associated with a favorable outcome (18,19). In contrast, 17p deletion and 11q deletion have been reported to be associated with poor prognosis (20–23).

Recent studies have assessed the prognostic significance of the pattern of immunoglobulin (Ig) gene rearrangements, immunophenotype, and biological features. It was previously thought that the rearranged immunoglobulin genes in CLL remained in germline configuration. This was in keeping with the naïve immunophenotype of these cells, and the malignancy was therefore believed to be derived from a pregerminal center B-cell precursor. Recently, it has been reported that a significant proportion of cases of CLL have undergone somatic hypermutation, more in keeping with a postgerminal center cell of origin of this disease (24). This may have prognostic significance, because cases with somatic mutation tend to be lower stage disease and have better prognosis, whereas unmutated Ig genes seem to be associated with a more aggressive form of CLL (25,26). A poor prognosis has also been observed in patients with a high level of CD38 expression on CLL cells, and these patients were found to have an unmutated Ig pattern (26). In addition, elevated levels of β_2-microglobulin and serum thymidine kinase have been identified as independent prognostic parameters of disease (27), and the level of bcl-2 protein also has prognostic significance (28). Last, once patients are unresponsive to therapy, they have poor survival. In a recent study examining the role of fludarabine in patients who had become refractory to alkylating agents, the median survival of patients was approximately 1 year (29,30).

Unlike more elderly patients who often die of other causes, younger patients with unfavorable prognostic factors will likely die of their disease or its complications (31). Despite the high initial response rates with conventional chemotherapy, patients invariably relapse and subsequently have resistance to chemotherapy develop. These younger patients with aggressive disease are candidates for more experimental treatment approaches, including SCT (3,32–35). A significant concern in the use of HD therapy in CLL is the morbidity and mortality associated with this approach. This is especially the case in treating patients who may have prolonged natural history without aggressive treatment. For this reason, only patients determined to have sufficiently adverse prognostic factors to severely limit their life expectancy should be eligible for this approach. Criteria that can

Table 1   Selection Criteria to Define Eligibility of CLL Patients to Undergo Stem Cell
Transplantation

Essential factors	Age	Younger age
	Rai classification	III–IV
	Binet classification	B or C
	IWCLL integrated staging system	High risk
	Performance status	Good
Established risk factors	Lymphocyte doubling time	< 12 mo
	Pattern of bone marrow infiltration	Diffuse
	Cytogenetics	17p and 11q deletion
Additional risk factors	Immunophenotype	CD38 Expression
	Immunoglobuline gene rearrangement	Unmutated
	Others	High β_2-microglobulin
		High thymidine kinase
		High sCD23

be used for the selection of patients with CLL who are suitable for SCT are shown in
Table 1. Caution should be used when directing a patient with CLL toward SCT simply
because of younger age at presentation, and several additional poor prognostic factors
should be established before directing patients toward transplantation.

IV. MOLECULAR MONITORING OF DISEASE

Although SCT is performed with curative intent in CLL and in other malignancies, the
long natural history of CLL means that very long-term follow-up is required. Investigators
have therefore been examining whether laboratory investigation might provide surrogate
measurements that will be useful to predict which patients are likely to relapse. If such
surrogate measurements can be established, we would be able to establish more rapidly
whether alterations to treatment strategies are likely to result in improvement in outcome,
as well as to identify those patients who will require additional therapy for cure. Considerable attention has focused on whether detection of minimal residual disease (MRD) will
provide such a surrogate for subsequent relapse. A number of techniques can be used to
increase the sensitivity of detection of MRD in patients with CLL, including flow cytometric analysis, restriction fragment analysis with Southern blotting, and polymerase chain
reaction (PCR) analysis. The most sensitive of these techniques is PCR analysis. Human
lymphoid malignancies, including CLL, are characterized by proliferation of cells that
have undergone transformation with subsequent clonal expansion. The underlying principle for the application of molecular biological techniques to the diagnosis and detection
of these cancers is the detection of such clonal proliferation. In B cells, clonal immunoglobulin gene (Ig) diversity is generated by rearrangement of the germline sequences of
the Ig heavy chain (IgH) region on chromosome 14. The most hypervariable region of
the Ig molecule is the third complementarity determining region (CDRIII). The CDRIII
is generated early in B-cell development by the rearrangement of germline variable (V),
diversity (D), and joining (J) region elements. The initial event joins the D segment with
the J segment. The resulting D-J segment then joins one V region sequence, producing a
V-D-J complex. In a mechanism common to Ig and TCR gene assembly, the enzyme
terminal deoxynucleotidyl transferase (TdT) inserts random nucleotides at both the V-D

and D-J junctions. Further diversity is generated by random excision of nucleotides by exonucleases. Antibody diversity is further increased by subsequent somatic mutation of V, D, J, and N region nucleotides. The final V-N-D-N-J sequence that comprises the CDRIII is unique to that cell. CLL cells usually rearrange either the Ig heavy or light genes or both, and their clonal progeny bear the identical antigen receptor rearrangement.

PCR amplification of the CDR III region is possible due to the presence of highly conserved sequences within the V (Vcon) and J (Jcon) regions. Although the large number of V regions makes it difficult to design a single oligonucleotide primer pair capable of amplifying all Ig rearrangements, a combined approach with Vcon and primers specific to each family of V regions will amplify most rearrangements. The strategy used to amplify the CDRIII region by is shown in Figure 1. The amplified rearrangements serve as clonal markers for detection of MRD when they are sequenced. Clone allele-specific oligonucleotides (ASO) can be constructed and used as oligonucleotide probes for the subsequent detection of MRD or as primers for second round or nested PCR amplification (36,37). This strategy successfully amplifies and allows sequencing of the CDRIII to design patient ASO probes for the detection of MRD in almost 90% of patients with poor prognosis CLL who are referred for autologous and allogeneic HSCT.

The clinical usefulness of PCR detection of MRD after HSCT has previously been suggested by studies from Dana-Farber Cancer Institute (38). The aim of this study was to determine whether HD therapy was capable of eradicating PCR-detectable MRD in patients with B-cell CLL undergoing SCT and to determine whether detection of MRD might act as a surrogate end point for subsequent clinical relapse of disease. PCR amplification was performed on patient samples at the time of and after autologous (21 patients) and allogeneic (10 patients) SCT in whom serial bone marrow samples obtained after SCT were available for analysis. Persistence of MRD after SCT was associated with increased probability of relapse. In all cases that have relapsed to date, the IgH CDRIII region was

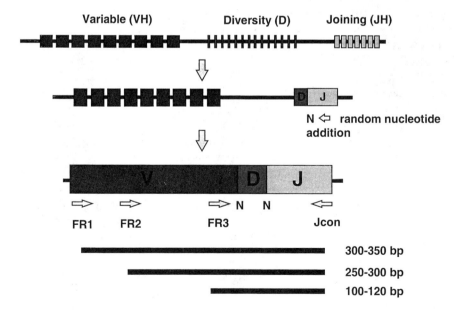

Figure 1 IgH structure and PCR strategy.

identical at the time of initial presentation and at relapse, suggesting that clonal evolution of the IgH locus is unusual in this disease. The finding that a significant number of patients remain disease free and with no evidence of PCR-detectable MRD after SCT suggests that HD therapy may contribute to improved outcome in selected patients with CLL.

The results of the PCR analysis are in keeping with our previous findings using restriction fragment analysis to assess MRD after ABMT (32). The finding that so many patients had eradication of PCR detectable disease was surprising. Although all of the patients reported here had persistence of MRD at the time of SCT and most of the patients had received fludarabine, all of the patients in this study had advanced stage, aggressive disease. However, all patients were also selected in that they had chemosensitive disease and may well have excellent response to HD therapy. Patients may continue to harbor MRD below the limit of detection using the strategy outlined here. If this were the case, then on further follow-up it would be expected that with further follow-up more patients will have evidence of PCR-detectable leukemia cells. A third possibility is that the technique is not capable of detecting MRD in these patients because there has been clonal evolution at the IgH locus. This may arise when subclones emerge that predominate over the original clone, or alteration to the IgH sequence such the leukemic clone can now no longer be detected by the PCR strategy. This has proved to be a significant problem in studies of MRD detection in acute lymphoblastic leukemia. However, CLL is regarded as a stable and indolent malignancy, and sequence analysis confirmed identity of the leukemia clone in all at presentation and subsequent relapse in all of the CLL patients who have relapsed to date. Ongoing studies are using quantitative PCR strategies that use real-time PCR analysis. Methods have been developed that are capable of quantifying MRD using rearranged IgH genes as clonal markers (39–41).

V. NEW THERAPIES TO IMPROVE STATUS OF MRD

Monoclonal antibodies have been demonstrated to be effective in non-Hodgkin's lymphoma. Rituximab, the humanized anti-CD20 antibody, has a 46% response rate in previously treated low-grade non-Hodgkin's lymphoma (42–44). Anti-CD20 monoclonal antibodies with the radiolabeled conjugate yttrium-90 have been also shown to be effective in recurrent B-cell lymphoma (45). Anti-CD20 monoclonal antibody therapy has not been systematically evaluated for CLL so far, although many clinical trials are currently ongoing. Although CLL cells express CD20, they do so at a lower surface density than other low-grade lymphomas, and it appears that response rates to such therapy are significantly lower in CLL and small lymphocytic lymphoma than in follicular lymphomas (44). Campath-1H, a humanized anti-CD52 monoclonal antibody, results in a 42% response rate in pretreated CLL patients (46). The question whether these therapies are able to improve eradication of MRD before SCT is currently under investigation. These agents are also being investigated for their potential to decrease tumor contamination at the time of collection of stem cells using an "in-vivo purging" approach. This approach also has the advantage that they can be applied in multi-institutional studies, unlike many of the ex vivo purging strategies that use reagents available only at individual academic institutions.

VI. AUTOLOGOUS AND ALLOGENEIC BMT FOR B-CELL CLL

A. Timing of SCT in CLL

In a number of disease settings it is clear that timing of SCT appears crucial, and patients have the best outcome when they are treated relatively early in their disease course and at a time when they have little tumor bulk. Fundamental for the improved outcome in early treated patients is the achievement of a state of MRD especially in the autologous setting (47,48), whereas relapses have been observed more frequently in patients with large tumor burden (33). In addition, of considerable interest with the use of PBSC in autologous SCT is whether previous therapy with stem cell–toxic agents impairs the ability to mobilize progenitor cells or impairs engraftment potential. In a recent study marrow and blood hematopoietic progenitor cells of patients with CLL were investigated before and after chemotherapy (49). In this study the number of circulating $CD34^+$ cells was significantly lower in patients treated with fludarabine or chlorambucil before stem cell mobilization compared with previously untreated patients. The type of previous chemotherapy seems to have a major effect on the number of $CD34^+$ cells that can be collected by leukopheresis, as well as on the time to platelet recovery after PBSC transplantation (50). In a feasibility study, 20 patients were enrolled with intent to proceed to autologous SCT; 12 of these patients were not eligible for transplantation because of the lack of sufficient mobilization of CD34+ cells, disease progression or pretransplant therapy-related deaths (51). Therefore, there appears to be significant advantages in considering SCT early in the treatment course of selected patients with CLL, especially if autologous SCT is the intended treatment.

B. Autologous SCT in CLL

For patients with intermediate grade non-Hodgkin's lymphoma (NHL) autologous SCT has been offered as the treatment of choice rather than allogeneic SCT because of the reduced treatment-related mortality of autologous compared with allogeneic SCT. In this setting, autologous SCT has been shown to result in improved outcome compared with salvage therapy for patients with chemosensitive disease (52). In CLL, several studies for autologous SCT have been reported to date, and the major studies reported are summarized in Table 2. The pilot study from Dana-Farber Cancer Institute reported 12 patients who underwent autologous SCT (32). These patients had been heavily pretreated and received an intensive conditioning regimen. Eligibility criteria for entry into this study included documented chemosensitivity at the time of SCT, and patients had to achieve protocol-eligible MRD before SCT. Complete remission after a median follow-up of 12 months

Table 2 Overview of Results of Autologous Stem Cell Transplantation in CLL at Different Centers

	Patients transplanted	Treatment-related deaths	Ongoing complete remission	Median follow-up (mo)
Rabinowe et al. 1993 (32)	12	1	6	12
Khouri et al. 1994 (33)	11	1	2	10
Itaelae et al. 1997 (53)	5	0	4	9
Dreger et al. 1998 (55)	13	0	12	19
Esteve et al. 1998 (56)	5	0	2	15
Pavletic et al. 1998 (54)	16	2	5	37
Sutton et al. 1998 (51)	8	0	6	30
Schey et al. 1999 (57)	10	0	5	11
DFCI (unpublished data)	154	6	132	49

was achieved in six of nine patients. Initial results of autologous SCT from the M. D. Anderson Cancer Center were less encouraging (33). These patients were also heavily pretreated and underwent autologous SCT not at a time of minimal tumor burden but after subsequent relapse. Seven patients received stem cells purged by immunomagnetic depletion; however, in five patients, residual clonal B cells were detectable. The outcome of these patients was poor. Three underwent a Richter's transformation, two died in complete remission (CR), and two relapsed. Only two achieved a complete remission and one a partial remission. In a Finnish study, eight patients received autologous SCT with partially purged CD34+ PBSC. These patients were also heavily pretreated. Although, four patients were in complete remission, the median follow-up is very short at only 9 months (53). In the study of Sutton et al., 20 heavily pretreated patients with advanced CLL were evaluated for autologous SCT (51). Most of patients were not eligible for SCT because of the lack of sufficient mobilization of CD34+ cells, disease progression, or pretransplant therapy-related deaths. Of the remaining eight patients, six achieved a complete remission with a median duration of 33 months. A high relapse rate after autologous SCT in CLL has been also observed by Pavletic and colleagues (54). After a median follow-up of 41 months, 8 of 16 patients have relapsed, and 6 have died (three from progressive malignancy). Other groups observed better results. Dreger et al. (55) investigated 18 patients with CLL including early stage disease. Transplantation was performed in 13 patients. Only one patients had relapsed at the time of publication. In this study and in the following studies, the authors used PCR analysis to follow MRD. In a study of Esteve and colleagues (56), five patients underwent autologous SCT. Four of these patients achieved a complete molecular remission. The median follow-up in this study was 13 months. In another recent study 10 patients undergoing autologous SCT were investigated (57). At a follow-up of 22 months, five patients remained in complete molecular remission.

At Dana-Farber Cancer Institute, SCT has emerged as the treatment of choice for younger patients with poor prognosis CLL. Studies investigating the role of SCT in this disease have been ongoing since 1989 and have focused on the use of autologous compared with allogeneic SCT. The treatment approach for younger poor-risk patients is shown in Figure 2. To be eligible for autologous SCT such patients must achieve a protocol-eligible low disease burden after induction or salvage therapy with largest nodal masses less than 2.5 cm, bone marrow involvement less than 20%, and no splenomegaly. Patients with high-risk CLL who achieve a protocol-eligible low tumor burden state have been offered allogeneic SCT if they have an HLA-matched sibling donor. If no suitable HLA-matched sibling donor is available, patients receive B cell purged autologous SCT. Results to date have demonstrated an improved overall and event-free survival advantage of autologous compared with allogeneic BMT because of the higher treatment-related mortality associated with graft-versus-host disease in those patients undergoing allogeneic BMT. Those patients who do not achieve a protocol-eligible disease state are still eligible for allogeneic SCT, either form matched sibling donors or from unrelated donors. The outcome of these two latter groups of patients is not compared with those patients who have undergone autologous SCT, because these patients are taken to SCT with larger tumor burden and without demonstrated chemosensitivity of their disease. To date more than 150 patients have now undergone autologous SCT for CLL. Treating patients with chemosensitive disease at a time of achieving a minimal disease state appears to be associated with a low treatment-related mortality of less than 5%. With a median follow-up of more than 4 years, the 5-year estimated overall survival for these patients is more than 80%, with event-free survival estimated at 65%. In this study, a number of patients with heavily pretreated poor

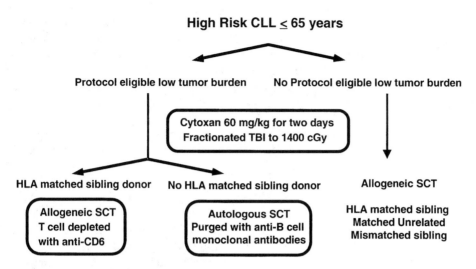

Figure 2   Stem cell transplantation for CLL.

prognosis CLL have now remained disease free for more than 10 years after-autologous SCT. Patients with poor prognosis CLL in first complete or partial remission became eligible for consideration of this approach in 1994. These patients are demonstrating excellent disease-free survival to date, but clearly further follow-up will be required to determine whether autologous SCT in this setting improves outcome in CLL. These patients are all followed using PCR to assess the impact of MRD on outcome (38).

Clearly larger randomized studies and longer follow-up are warranted, and from the published data it is premature to make a final assessment of the role of autologous SCT in CLL. A number of problems occur in assessing the published studies. Preselection of patients in these single-institution studies makes full assessment of the potential role of SCT problematic. However, these studies have demonstrated several specific features and obstacles of autologous SCT in CLL. Although treatment-related deaths were relatively rare after autologous SCT, the outcome of heavily pretreated patients with larger tumor bulk at the time of autologous SCT was poor. Better results were obtained in patients with documented chemosensitivity who were taken to SCT after pretreatment and achievement of a low tumor burden and in patients undergoing SCT earlier in their disease course. Whether SCT is superior to conventional chemotherapy remains to be demonstrated and would require a randomized clinical trial. An obstacle to this approach is the lack of an effective salvage regimen in poor-risk patients with advanced stage CLL.

Morbidity and mortality of patients appears to be considerably lower for patients with CLL undergoing autologous SCT compared with allogeneic SCT. However, there does appear to be a higher incidence of opportunistic infections in patients undergoing autologous SCT for CLL compared with other patient populations. Whether this is due to a higher incidence of infections in patients with CLL or is secondary to the immune suppressive effects of fludarabine therapy remains to be determined (58–60). However, the use of prophylactic antimicrobial therapy appears to be indicated in CLL patients after SCT (61).

A major concern with autologous stem cell transplant (SCT) is the risk of secondary malignancies, and in particular the increased risk of development of myelodysplastic syndrome (MDS) and secondary leukemias (62). Attempts have been made to identify patients at high risk for this complication (63). A significant proportion of patients have clonal hematopoiesis at the time of autologous SCT, and clonal hematopoiesis after autologous SCT is predictive for the development of MDS and acute myeloid leukemia (AML) (64). In some series the incidence of MDS after autologous SCT approaches 15%, and after relapse this is now the most important cause of failure (63). Outcome for these patients is dismal, even after salvage therapy with allogeneic SCT (65). Because MDS rarely occurs after allogeneic SCT, the risk of graft-versus-host disease can now be weighed against the risk of MDS to determine for an individual patient whether allogeneic rather than autologous SCT should be performed. Although the actuarial risk of development of MDS after autologous SCT for non-Hodgkin's lymphoma is high and approaches 20% at 10 years, in studies at Dana-Farber Cancer Institute, to date, only one case of secondary leukemia or MDS has been observed in more than 150 patients who have undergone autologous SCT for CLL at this center. The reasons for this are not clear, because the HD induction regimen used for SCT was identical for both CLL and NHL patients and consisted of HD cyclophosphamide and hyperfractionated total body irradiation to a total dose of 1400 cGy. It may be that the CLL patients will require additional follow-up, although a large number of the CLL patients have now been followed for more than 5 years and are being watched closely for the emergence of this complication. Whether the disease itself or the different induction or salvage regimens used for treatment of CLL patients contributes to the lower incidence of MDS in CLL patients remains unknown.

C. Source of Autologous Stem Cells

Historically BM has been used as the source of stem cells. However, stem cells are mobilized into peripheral blood (PB) after chemotherapy, and this stem cell mobilization is increased with concomitant use of hematopoietic growth factors, particularly with recombinant granulocyte-colony stimulating factor (G-CSF). Most centers now use peripheral blood stem cells (PBSC) rather than BM. A number of advantages exist with the use of PBSC rather than BM. It is easier, cheaper, and safer to collect stem cells by pheresis than to harvest BM. Mobilized PBSC hastens engraftment compared with BM. In a randomized prospective trial, use of PBSC rather than BM decreased the number of platelet transfusions, time to neutrophil and platelet engraftment, and earlier discharge from the hospital (66). In a recent study, 17 patients with advanced stage CLL were enrolled in a multicenter study assessing the use of PBSC transplantation in this disease (67). Patients were mobilized with HD cyclophosphamide and G-CSF. The PSBC were then further tumor depleted by CD34$^+$ selection. Three patients failed to mobilize sufficient numbers of stem cells, but sufficient CD34$^+$ cells were obtained in the remaining 14 patients. However, in this study PCR analysis of immunoglobulin gene rearrangements demonstrated persistence of tumor cells in the CD34$^+$-selected cells. This study demonstrates that PBSC are not necessarily free of tumor contamination and that the question of purging of *autologous* stem cells remains an important issue that may have to be addressed to improve outcome after autologous SCT. Several other small single-center studies are investigating the role of autologous PBSCT in CLL. However, the results concerning the yield of CD34$^+$ cells for transplantation and the relapse rates are divergent (51,54,55). A possible explanation for these differences could be the different stage of disease and pretreatment at time of transplantation and the different median follow-up. PCR monitoring of the peripheral blood after transplantation revealed PCR-negative stem cell collections in several of these studies, suggesting that this might provide a method to obtain a source of stem cells relatively free of tumor contamination. A recent report suggested that in CLL the CD34$^+$ cells contain trisomy 12 and deletions of the retinoblastoma gene (68). However, a subsequent larger analysis of patients from the same groups revealed no involvement of cytogenetic abnormalities in CD34-positive cells of CLL patients (69).

D. Contribution of Reinfused CLL Cells to Relapse after Autologous SCT

The major obstacle to the use of autologous SCT is that the reinfusion of occult tumor cells harbored within the marrow may result in more rapid relapse of disease. A variety of methods have therefore been developed to ''purge'' malignant cells from the stem cell collection. The aim of purging is to eliminate any contaminating malignant cells and leave intact the hematopoietic stem cells that are necessary for engraftment. Because of their specificity, monoclonal antibodies are ideal agents for selective elimination of malignant cells or for positive selection of stem cells (Figure 3). Polymerase chain reaction amplification of grafts can be used to detect residual lymphoma cells in the stem cell collection before and after purging in patients undergoing autologous SCT to assess whether the efficiency of purging had any impact on disease-free survival (70,71). The combination of CD34-positive selection of CD34$^+$ cells and negative selection of malignant B cells seems to be superior to positive selection alone and has been tested in clinical studies. (72) Results of clinical trials assessing immunologic purging are outlined in Table 3. However, malignant cells were detectable by PCR using available strategies in all investigations, demonstrating that improvements in method are required if infusion of contaminating tumor cells is as seems likely, contributing to subsequent relapse in these patients.

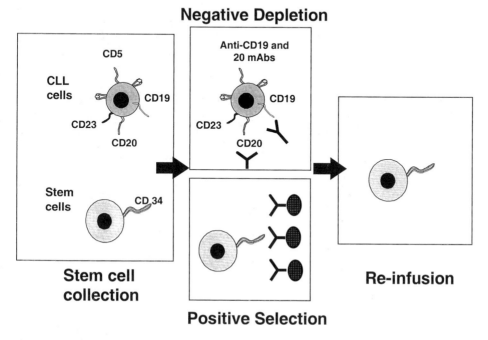

Figure 3 Tumor depletion from autologous stem cells.

Table 3 Purging Procedures and Results for Autologous Stem Cell Transplantation in CLL at Different Centers

	Selection type	Device	Median % malignant cells by FACS —preselection	Median % malignant cells by FACS —postselection	PCR-negative result
Khouri et al. 1994 (33)	Positive/negative combined	Not indicated	19.57	5.2	—
Paulus et al. 1997 (72)	Positive/negative combined	Isolex/magnetic beads	15.9	0	—
Scime et al. 1998 (67)	Positive	Ceprate/isolex	6.4	1.55	—
DFCI (unpublished data)	Negative	Complement	12	0	50%

The use of purging procedures to deplete tumor cells from autologous stem cells remains experimental and this is being investigated in a number of ongoing clinical and preclinical settings.

E. Allogeneic SCT in CLL

Allogeneic SCT is associated with increased morbidity and mortality and for this reason has been studied even less extensively in CLL. Nonetheless, it remains a potentially curative procedure that provides a tumor-free source of stem cells that may ultimately allow assessment of whether there is a graft-versus-tumor effect in this disease. The studies reported are shown in Table 4. It might be assumed that the relative risk of allogeneic versus autologous SCT will be in the balance of the increased morbidity and mortality of allogeneic SCT with the complication of GVHD versus the increased risk of disease relapse after autologous SCT. Fundamental for this better outcome might be a graft versus tumor effect. In the pilot study reported by Rabinowe et al., eight heavily pretreated patients with advanced disease received allogeneic SCT (32). Six patients were in complete clinical remission, and the median follow-up was only 11 months. Similar results were reported from the M. D. Anderson Cancer Center (33). Eleven heavily pretreated patients with advanced disease received allogeneic SCT. Seven of these patients achieved complete remission. Ten of the 11 patients were alive, although the median follow-up was also very short at only 10 months. Patients who have undergone allogeneic SCT for CLL and whose outcome had been registered with the European or International Bone Marrow Transplant Registry (EBMT/IBMTR) were reported (34). Fifty four patients had undergone allogeneic SCT, 38 achieved hematologic remission, and 24 were alive after a median follow-up of 27 months. Unfortunately, treatment-related mortality was unacceptably high with 46%, particularly because this study included patients with early stage disease. Before allogeneic SCT is more widely accepted in this disease, the treatment-related morbidity and mortality will have to be improved significantly. Of note, however, for those patients surviving the procedure, response rates were high. Recent studies have demonstrated lower treatment-related deaths after allogeneic SCT with high response rates, perhaps because of selection of better risk patients (73–75).

Interestingly with regard to improved outcome, a reduced incidence of GVHD has been observed in patients with CLL compared with other malignancies (76). The authors

Table 4 Overview of Results of Allogeneic Stem Cell Transplantation in CLL at Different Centers

	Patients transplanted	Treatment-related deaths	Severe acute/chronic GVHD (%)	Ongoing complete remission	Median follow-up (mo)
Rabinowe et al. 1993 (32)	8	0	24	7	12
Michallet et al. 1996 (34)	54	25	18	24	27
Khouri et al. 1997 (76)	15	5	26	8	35
Esteve et al. 1998 (56)	7	2	42	5	21
Mattsson et al. 2000 (74)	6	0	1	4	24
Pavletic et al. 2000 (73)	23	8	47	14	24
Toze et al. 2000 (75)	7	1	n.s.	4	28
DFCI (unpublished data)	47	12	28	21	52

n.s., not stated.

suggest that the immunosuppressive effect of fludarabine used to treat the underlying disease might be responsible for the lower incidence of GVHD. However, in studies at the Dana-Farber Cancer Institute, the incidence and severity of GVHD after T cell–depleted allogeneic SCT appears to be higher in CLL than in other disease settings, despite the fact that all of the patients who had GVHD develop had received previous therapy with fludarabine. Therefore, whether fludarabine prevents or diminishes the severity of GVHD remains controversial, and further studies are warranted to examine this issue. Other attempts have been made to reduce the toxicity of allogeneic SCT by steps such as T-cell depletion of allogeneic SCT in the hope that this might therefore improve outcome (77,78). Such steps appear capable of reducing the short-term toxicity associated with allogeneic SCT and, in particular, in reducing the incidence of acute GVHD. However, whether this will also decrease the potential for a graft versus lymphoma (GVL) effect remains to be seen. New agents are currently under investigation to reduce the incidence of GVHD (79– 81). Promising results have been achieved using CTLA-4–treated allografts (79). Although this approach has been tested to date only in the setting of mismatched allogeneic SCT, induction of tolerance is an attractive approach that might reduce morbidity and mortality associated with GVHD.

Patients who relapse after SCT for non-Hodgkins lymphoma do so because of the persistence of small numbers of lymphoma cells that survive HDT. Eradication of such "minimal residual" disease might be mediated by immune recognition of these lymphoma cells by the host immune system. One particular problem with this approach is that the host immune system is severely compromised by the SCT procedure itself. The major potential advantage of the use of allogeneic rather than autologous SCT is the potential for a graft-versus-tumor effect. In the same way that donor T cells can recognize the host and induce GVHD, they are also capable of recognizing host tumor cells. The clearest demonstration of the power of the graft versus tumor effect has been the demonstration that donor lymphocyte infusions (DLI) are capable of inducing remission in patients in frank relapse after allogeneic SCT (82,83).

In our studies and in those of others, such a graft-versus-leukemia effect has been observed in CLL. In patients who have relapsed after allogeneic SCT, infusion of DLI as the only therapy has induced a number of such patients back into clinical complete remission. Results in an individual patient are shown in Figure 4, in which quantitative PCR analysis of the clonal Ig gene rearrangement is used to follow the malignant clone after therapy. Allogeneic SCT in this patient led to a marked reduction in disease but did not eradicate PCR-detectable disease. Quantitative PCR analysis showed a marked increase in tumor burden that preceded subsequent clinical relapse. After infusion of DLI, this patient demonstrated a rapid return to clinical CR despite receiving no additional therapy. Of note, it took several years for this patient to eradicate the PCR-detectable disease, demonstrating that the antileukemic effect can be ongoing for long periods after infusion of donor lymphocytes.

F. Nonmyeloablative SCT for CLL

A major advance in reducing the short-term morbidity and mortality has been with the introduction of nonmyeloablative conditioning regimens to allow engraftment of allogeneic stem cells. Frequently, these regimens include fludarabine in the conditioning regimen and exploit the immunosuppressive and antileukemic properties of this agent (Figure 5). In this setting most of the antilymphoma effect results from the graft-versus-lymphoma

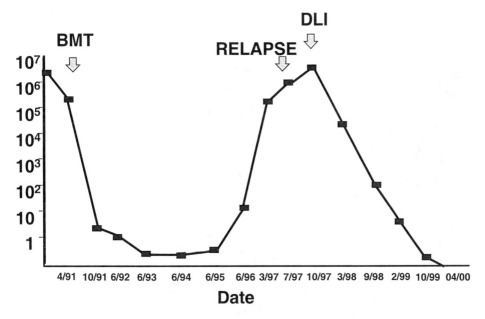

Figure 4 Quantitative PCR analysis after allogeneic BMT and DLI for CLL.

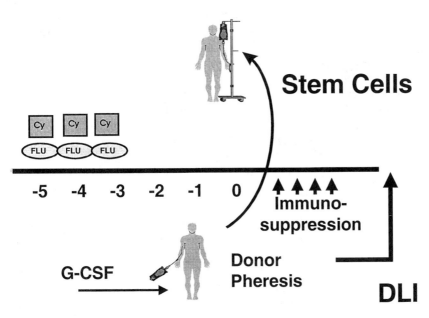

Figure 5 Nonmyeloablative SCT.

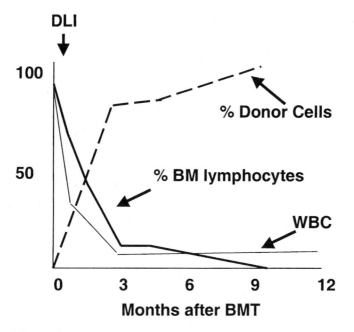

Figure 6   Response to DLI.

effect and not from the chemotherapy. Outcome after this "transplant-lite" procedure was performed in 15 patients. The patients were heavily pretreated and partially therapy refractory. Eleven of 15 patients had donor cell engraftment, and eight patients achieved complete remission. Survival was better in patients with sensitive disease. Only limited acute GVHD was observed, and two cases of chronic GVHD with one of those was fatal. This study provides perhaps the strongest direct evidence to date for a graft-versus-lymphoma effect and most certainly demonstrates the presence of a potentially powerful graft-versus-leukemia effect in CLL. The results demonstrate that these procedures are most effective in patients with chemotherapy-responsive disease and those with low tumor burden. However, within this study there was also clear demonstration that DLI are capable of inducing remission in patients with CLL in frank relapse at the time of infusion of the donor cells. An example of the clinical course of a patient who underwent a nonmyeloablative SCT is shown in Figure 6. A major focus of ongoing research is the amount of pretransplant and posttransplant immunosuppression required to establish stable mixed chimerism and eventual full donor chimerism after nonmyeloablative SCT, (84–86). Finally, it should be stressed that these procedures are currently investigational in nature, and although the acute morbidity and mortality appear significant compared with HD conditioning regimens with allogeneic transplantation, the longer term results with regard to morbidity of chronic GVHD and disease control are currently lacking. Although these procedures are commonly known as "mini-SCT," this misnomer significantly underestimates the risks of such procedures because of GVHD.

VII.   CONCLUSIONS

High-dose therapy autologous HSCT is feasible in the many younger patients with poor-risk CLL. Allogeneic SCT is associated with increased morbidity and mortality and should be restricted to patients with very poor prognoses. High-dose therapy is associated with a very high CR rate and results in long-term event-free survival and eradication of PCR detectable MRD in a cohort of these patients. Clearly in terms of assessing whether the use of SCT can cure CLL, the follow-up of clinical trials is short. However, the median time to relapse after fludarabine therapy for previously untreated patients with advanced stage CLL patients is reported to be from 12 to 26 months and is significantly shorter in previously treated patients (87–89). It is therefore possible that autologous HSCT will result in significant prolongation of overall and disease-free survival compared with conventional therapy.

Approaches to further improve DFS after SCT include immunological approaches to attempt to eradicate MRD. Use of biological response modifiers have generally resulted in no improvement in outcome in CLL, (90), but studies are underway examining the role of monoclonal antibody therapy or infusion of allogeneic donor lymphocytes (46,91,92). Future approaches to the management of this disease should take into account the balance between the increased morbidity and mortality of HD chemotherapy in CLL with the curative potential that this approach may potentially offer. In the absence of any other treatment modalities currently capable of improving outcome in this disease, we conclude that the treatment of choice for younger patients with poor-risk CLL should be allogeneic or autologous SCT. Such treatment should be considered only in the setting of well-designed clinical trials assessing the impact of this treatment on outcome in these patients.

REFERENCES

1. C Rozman, E Montserrat. Chronic lymphocytic leukemia. N Engl J Med 333:1052–1057, 1995.
2. D Catovsky, RL Murphy. Key issues in the treatment of chronic lymphocytic leukemia. Eur J Cancer 31A:2146–2154, 1995.
3. FR Mauro, R Foa, D Giannarelli, I Cordone, S Crescenzi, E Pescarmona, R Sala, R Cerretti, F Mandelli. Clinical characteristics and outcome of young chronic lymphocytic leukemia patients: a single institution study of 204 cases. Blood 94:448–454, 1999.
4. KR Rai, A Sawitsky, EP Cronkite, AD Chanana, RN Levy, BS Pasternack. Clinical staging of chronic lymphocytic leukemia. Blood 46:219–234, 1975.
5. JL Binet, A Auquier, G Dighiero, C Chastang, H Piguet, J Goasguen, G Vaugier, G Potron, P Colona, F Oberling, M Thomas, G Tchernia, C Jacquillat, P Boivin, C Lesty, MT Duault, M Monconduit, S Belabbes, F Gremy. A new prognostic classification of chronic lymphocytic leukemia derived from a multivariate survival analysis. Cancer 48:198–206, 1981.
6. E Montserrat, J Sanchez-Bisono, N Vinolas, C Rozman. Lymphocyte doubling time in chronic lymphocytic leukaemia: analysis of its prognostic significance. Br J Haematol 62:567–575, 1986.
7. S Molica, A Alberti. Prognostic value of "total tumor mass score" (TTM): a retrospective analysis of 130 patients with chronic lymphocytic leukemia. Tumori 72:559–564, 1986.
8. MD Lipshutz, R Mir, KR Rai, A Sawitsky. Bone marrow biopsy and clinical staging in chronic lymphocytic leukemia. Cancer 46:1422–1427, 1980.
9. C Rozman, E Montserrat, JM Rodriguez-Fernandez, R Ayats, T Vallespi, R Parody, A Rios, D Prados, M Morey, F Gomis. Bone marrow histologic pattern—the best single prognostic parameter in chronic lymphocytic leukemia: a multivariate survival analysis of 329 cases. Blood 64:642–648, 1984.
10. C Geisler, E Ralfkiaer, MM Hansen, K Hou-Jensen, SO Larsen. The bone marrow histological pattern has independent prognostic value in early stage chronic lymphocytic leukaemia. Br J Haematol 62:47–54, 1986.
11. T Vallespi, E Montserrat, MA Sanz. Chronic lymphocytic leukaemia: prognostic value of

lymphocyte morphological subtypes. A multivariate survival analysis in 146 patients. Br J Haematol 77:478–485, 1991.

12.   G Juliusson, DG Oscier, M Fitchett, FM Ross, G Stockdill, MJ Mackie, AC Parker, GL Castoldi, A Guneo, S Knuutila. Prognostic subgroups in B-cell chronic lymphocytic leukemia defined by specific chromosomal abnormalities. N Engl J Med 323:720–724, 1990.

13.   DG Oscier. Cytogenetic and molecular abnormalities in chronic lymphocytic leukaemia. Blood Rev 8:88–97, 1994.

14.   E Matutes, D Oscier, J Garcia-Marco, J Ellis, A Copplestone, R Gillingham, T Hamblin, D Lens, GJ Swansbury, D Catovsky. Trisomy 12 defines a group of CLL with atypical morphology: correlation between cytogenetic, clinical and laboratory features in 544 patients. Br J Haematol 92:382–388, 1996.

15.   JS Lee, DO Dixon, HM Kantarjian, MJ Keating, M Talpaz. Prognosis of chronic lymphocytic leukemia: a multivariate regression analysis of 325 untreated patients. Blood 69:929–936, 1987.

16.   M Dhodapkar, A Tefferi, J Su, RL Phyliky. Prognostic features and survival in young adults with early/intermediate chronic lymphocytic leukemia (B-CLL): a single institution study. Leukemia 7:1232–1235, 1993.

17.   H Dohner, S Stilgenbauer, K Dohner, M Bentz, P Lichter. Chromosome aberrations in B-cell chronic lymphocytic leukemia: reassessment based on molecular cytogenetic analysis. J Mol Med 77:266–281, 1999.

18.   F Bullrich, ML Veronese, S Kitada, J Jurlander, MA Caligiuri, JC Reed, CM Croce. Minimal region of loss at 13q14 in B-cell chronic lymphocytic leukemia. Blood 88:3109–3115, 1996.

19.   S Kalachikov, A Migliazza, E Cayanis, NS Fracchiolla, MF Bonaldo, L Lawton, P Jelenc, X Ye, X Qu, M Chien, R Hauptschein, G Gaidano, U Vitolo, G Saglio, L Resegotti, V Brodjansky, N Yankovsky, P Zhang, MB Soares, J Russo, IS Edelman, A Efstratiadis, R Dalla-Favera, SG Fischer. Cloning and gene mapping of the chromosome 13q14 region deleted in chronic lymphocytic leukemia. Genomics 42:369–377, 1997.

20.   H Dohner, K Fischer, M Bentz, K Hansen, A Benner, G Cabot, D Diehl, R Schlenk, J Coy, S Stilgenbauer. p53 gene deletion predicts for poor survival and non-response to therapy with purine analogs in chronic B-cell leukemias. Blood 85:1580–1589, 1995.

21.   S el Rouby, A Thomas, D Costin, CR Rosenberg, M Potmesil, R Silber, EW Newcomb. p53 gene mutation in B-cell chronic lymphocytic leukemia is associated with drug resistance and is independent of MDR1/MDR3 gene expression. Blood 82:3452–3459, 1993.

22.   CH Geisler, P Philip, BE Christensen, K Hou-Jensen, NT Pedersen, OM Jensen, K Thorling, E Andersen, HS Birgens, A Drivsholm, J Ellegaard, JK Larsen, T Plesner, P Brown, PK Andersen, MM Hansen. In B-cell chronic lymphocytic leukaemia chromosome 17 abnormalities and not trisomy 12 are the single most important cytogenetic abnormalities for the prognosis: a cytogenetic and immunophenotypic study of 480 unselected newly diagnosed patients. Leuk Res 21:1011–1023, 1997.

23.   JR Neilson, R Auer, D White, N Bienz, JJ Waters, JA Whittaker, DW Milligan, CD Fegan. Deletions at 11q identify a subset of patients with typical CLL who show consistent disease progression and reduced survival. Leukemia 11:1929–1932, 1997.

24.   F Fais, F Ghiotto, S Hashimoto, B Sellars, A Valetto, SL Allen, P Schulman, VP Vinciguerra, K Rai, LZ Rassenti, TJ Kipps, G Dighiero, H Schroeder, M Ferrarini, N Chiorazzi. Chronic lymphocytic leukemia B cells express restricted sets of mutated and unmutated antigen receptors. J Clin Invest 102:1515–1525, 1998.

25.   TJ Hamblin, Z Davis, A Gardiner, DG Oscier, FK Stevenson. Unmutated Ig V(H) genes are associated with a more aggressive form of chronic lymphocytic leukemia. Blood 94:1848–1854, 1999.

26.   RN Damle, T Wasil, F Fais, F Ghiotto, A Valetto, SL Allen, A Buchbinder, D Budman, K Dittmar, J Kolitz, SM Lichtman, P Schulman, VP Vinciguerra, KR Rai, M Ferrarini, N Chiora-

zzi. Ig V gene mutation status and CD38 expression as novel prognostic indicators in chronic lymphocytic leukemia. Blood 94:1840–1847, 1999.

27. M Hallek, L Wanders, M Ostwald, R Busch, R Senekowitsch, S Stern, HD Schick, I Kuhn-Hallek, B Emmerich. Serum beta(2)-microglobulin and serum thymidine kinase are independent predictors of progression-free survival in chronic lymphocytic leukemia and immunocytoma. Leuk Lymphoma 22:439–447, 1996.

28. LE Robertson, W Plunkett, K McConnell, MJ Keating, TJ McDonnell. Bcl-2 expression in chronic lymphocytic leukemia and its correlation with the induction of apoptosis and clinical outcome. Leukemia 10:456–459, 1996.

29. JM Sorensen, DA Vena, A Fallavollita, HG Chun, BD Cheson. Treatment of refractory chronic lymphocytic leukemia with fludarabine phosphate via the group C protocol mechanism of the National Cancer Institute: five-year follow-up report. J Clin Oncol 15:458–465, 1997.

30. MJ Keating, TL Smith, S Lerner, S O'Brien, LE Robertson, H Kantarjian, EJ Freireich. Prediction of prognosis following fludarabine used as secondary therapy for chronic lymphocytic leukemia. Leuk Lymphoma 37:71–85, 2000.

31. E Montserrat, F Gomis, T Vallespi, A Rios, A Romero, J Soler, A Alcala, M Morey, C Ferran, J Diaz-Mediavilla. Presenting features and prognosis of chronic lymphocytic leukemia in younger adults. Blood 78:1545–1551, 1991.

32. SN Rabinowe, RJ Soiffer, JG Gribben, H Daley, AS Freedman, J Daley, K Pesek, D Neuberg, G Pinkus, PR Leavitt, NA Spector, ML Grossbard, K Anderson, MJ Robertson, P Mauch, K Chayt-Marcus, J Ritz, LM Nadler. Autologous and allogeneic bone marrow transplantation for poor prognosis patients with B-cell chronic lymphocytic leukemia. Blood 82:1366–1376, 1993.

33. IF Khouri, MJ Keating, HM Vriesendorp, CL Reading, D Przepiorka, YO Huh, BS Andersson, KW van Besien, RC Mehra, SA Giralt, RE Champlin. Autologous and allogeneic bone marrow transplantation for chronic lymphocytic leukemia: preliminary results. J Clin Oncol 12:748–758, 1994.

34. M Michallet, E Archimbaud, G Bandini, PA Rowlings, HJ Deeg, E Gahrton, C Rozman, A Gratwohl, RP Gale. HLA-identical sibling bone marrow transplantation in younger patients with chronic lymphocytic leukemia. European Group for blood and marrow transplantation and the International bone marrow transplant registry. Ann Intern Med 124:311–315, 1996.

35. M Michallet, A Thiebaut, P Dreger, K Remes, N Milpied, G Santini, M Hamon, B Bjorkstrand, E Kimby, A Belhabri, ML Tanguy, JF Apperley. Peripheral blood stem cell (PBSC) mobilization and transplantation after fludarabine therapy in chronic lymphocytic leukaemia (CLL): a report of the European Blood and Marrow Transplantation (EBMT) CLL subcommittee on behalf of the EBMT Chronic Leukaemias Working Party (CLWP). Br J Haematol 108:595–601, 2000.

36. OG Jonsson, RL Kitchens, FC Scott, RG. Smith. Detection of minimal residual disease in acute lymphoblastic leukemia using immunoglobulin hypervariable region specific oligonucleotide probes. Blood 76:2072–2079, 1990.

37. D Billadeau, M Blackstadt, P Greipp, RA Kyle, MM Oken, N Kay, NB Van. Analysis of B-lymphoid malignancies using allele-specific polymerase chain reaction: a technique for sequential quantitation of residual disease. Blood 78:3021–3029, 1991.

38. D Provan, L Bartlettpandite, C Zwicky, D Neuberg, A Maddocks, P Corradini, R Soiffer, J Ritz, LM Nadler, JG Gribben. Eradication of polymerase chain reaction-detectable chronic lymphocytic leukemia cells is associated with improved outcome after bone marrow transplantation. Blood 88:2228–2235, 1996.

39. MJ Pongers-Willemse, OJ Verhagen, GJ Tibbe, AJ Wijkhuijs, V de Haas, E Roovers, CE van der Schoot, JJ van Dongen. Real-time quantitative PCR for the detection of minimal residual disease in acute lymphoblastic leukemia using junctional region specific TaqMan probes. Leukemia 12:2006–2014, 1998.

40. JW Donovan, M Ladetto, G Zou, D Neuberg, C Poor, D Bowers, JG Gribben. Immunoglobulin

heavy-chain consensus probes for real-time PCR quantification of residual disease in acute lymphoblastic leukemia. Blood 95:2651–2658, 2000.

41. M Ladetto, JW Donovan, S Harig, A Trojan, C Poor, R Schlossnan, KC Anderson, JG Gribben. Real-time polymerase chain reaction of immunoglobulin rearrangements for quantitative evaluation of minimal residual disease in multiple myeloma. Biol Blood Marrow Transplant 6: 241–253, 2000.

42. DG Maloney, AJ Grillo-Lopez, DJ Bodkin, CA White, TM Liles, I Royston, C Varns, J Rosenberg, R Levy. IDEC-C2B8: results of a phase I multiple-dose trial in patients with relapsed non-Hodgkin's lymphoma. J Clin Oncol 15:3266–3274, 1997.

43. DG Maloney, AJ Grillo-Lopez, CA White, D Bodkin, RJ Schilder, JA Neidhart, N Janakiraman, KA Foon, TM Liles, BK Dallaire, K Wey, I Royston, T Davis, R Levy. IDEC-C2B8 (Rituximab) anti-CD20 monoclonal antibody therapy in patients with relapsed low-grade non-Hodgkin's lymphoma. Blood 90:2188–2195, 1997.

44. P McLaughlin, AJ Grillo-Lopez, BK Link, R Levy, MS Czuczman, ME Williams, MR Heyman, I Bence-Bruckler, CA White, F Cabanillas, V Jain, AD Ho, J Lister, K Wey, D Shen, BK Dallaire. Rituximab chimeric anti-CD20 monoclonal antibody therapy for relapsed indolent lymphoma: half of patients respond to a four-dose treatment program. J Clin Oncol 16:2825–2833, 1998.

45. SJ Knox, ML Goris, K Trisler, R Negrin, T Davis, TM Liles, A Grillo-Lopez, P Chinn, C Varns, SC Ning, S Fowler, N Deb, M Becker, C Marquez, R Levy. Yttrium-90-labeled anti-CD20 monoclonal antibody therapy of recurrent B-cell lymphoma. Clin Cancer Res 2:457–470, 1996.

46. A Osterborg, MJ Dyer, D Bunjes, GA Pangalis, Y Bastion, D Catovsky, H Mellstedt. Phase II multicenter study of human CD52 antibody in previously treated. Clin Oncol 15:1567–1574, 1997.

47. Y Bastion, P Brice, C Haioun, A Sonet, G Salles, JP Marolleau, D Espinouse, F Reye, C Gisselbrecht, B Coiffier. Intensive therapy with peripheral blood progenitor cell transplantation in 60 patients with poor-prognosis follicular lymphoma. Blood 86:3257–3262, 1995.

48. R Haas, M Moos, R Mohle, H Dohner, B Witt, H Goldschmidt, S Murea, M Flentje, M Wannermacher, W Hunstein. High-dose therapy with peripheral blood progenitor cell transplantation in low-grade non-Hodgkin's lymphoma. Bone Marrow Transplant 17:149–155, 1996.

49. R Sala, FR Mauro, R Bellucci, MS De Propris, I Cordone, A Lisci, R Foa, P de Fabritiis. Evaluation of marrow and blood haemopoietic progenitors in chronic lymphocytic leukaemia before and after chemotherapy. Eur J Haematol 61:14–20, 1998.

50. HT Hassan, T Hinz, N Kroger, W Zeller, AR Zander. Factors influencing platelet recovery after autologous transplantation of G-CSF-mobilized peripheral blood stem/progenitor cells following myeloablative therapy in 50 heavily pretreated lymphoma patients. Clin Lab Haematol 21:21–27, 1999.

51. L Sutton, K Maloum, H Gonzalez, H Zouabi, N Azar, C Boccaccio, F Charlotte, JM Cosset, J Gabarre, V Leblond, H Merle-Beral, JL Binet. Autologous hematopoietic stem cell transplantation as salvage treatment for advanced B cell chronic lymphocytic leukemia. Leukemia 12:1699–1707, 1998.

52. T Philip, JO Armitage, G Spitzer, F Chauvin, S Jagannath, J-P Cahn, D Maraninchi, J Pico, A Bosly, C Andersonn, R Schots, P Biron, F Cabanillas, K Dicke. High-dose therapy and autologous bone marrow transplantation after failure of conventional chemotherapy in adults with intermediate-grade or high-grade non-Hodgkin's lymphoma. N Engl J Med 316:1493–1498, 1987.

53. M Itala, TT Pelliniemi, A Rajamaki, K Remes. Autologous blood cell transplantation in B-CLL: response to chemotherapy prior to mobilization predicts the stem cell yield. Bone Marrow Transplant 19:647–651, 1997.

54. ZS Pavletic, PJ Bierman, JM Vose, MR Bishop, CD Wu, JL Pierson, JP Kollath, DD Weisenburger, A Kessinger, JO Armitage. High incidence of relapse after autologous stem-cell trans-

plantation for B-cell chronic lymphocytic leukemia or small lymphocytic lymphoma. Ann Oncol 9:1023–1026, 1998.

55. P Dreger, N von Neuhoff, R Kuse, R Sonnen, B Glass, L Uharek, R Schoch, H Loffler, N Schmitz. Early stem cell transplantation for chronic lymphocytic leukaemia: a chance for cure? Br J Cancer 77:2291–2297, 1998.
56. J Esteve, N Villamor, D Colomer, F Bosch, A Lopez-Guillermo, M Rovira, A Urbano-Ispizua, J Sierra, E Carreras, E Montserrat. Hematopoietic stem cell transplantation in chronic lymphocytic leukemia: a report of 12 patients from a single institution. Ann Oncol 9:167–172, 1998.
57. S Schey, G Ahsan, R Jones. Dose intensification and molecular responses in patients with chronic lymphocytic leukaemia: a phase II single centre study. Bone Marrow Transplant 24: 989–993, 1999.
58. H Griffiths, J Lea, C Bunch, M Lee, H Chapel. Predictors of infection in chronic lymphocytic leukaemia (CLL). Clin Exp Immunol 89:374–377, 1992.
59. LE Robertson, YO Huh, JJ Butler, WC Pugh, C Hirsch-Ginsberg, S Stass, H Kantarjian, MJ Keating. Response assessment in chronic lymphocytic leukemia after fludarabine plus prednisone: clinical, pathologic, immunophenotypic, and molecular analysis. Blood 80:29–36, 1992.
60. A Zomas, J Mehta, R Powles, J Treleaven, T Iveson, S Singhal, B Jameson, B Paul, S Brincat, D Catovsky. Unusual infections following allogeneic bone marrow transplantation for chronic lymphocytic leukemia. Bone Marrow Transplant 14:799–803, 1994.
61. J Mehta, R Powles, S Singhal, U Riley, J Treleaven, D Catovsky. Antimicrobial prophylaxis to prevent opportunistic infections in patients with chronic lymphocytic leukemia after allogeneic blood or marrow transplantation. Leuk Lymphoma 26:83–88, 1997.
62. JS Miller, DC Arthur, CE Litz, JP Neglia, WJ Miller, DJ Weisdorf. Myelodysplastic syndrome after autologous bone marrow transplantation: An additional late complication of curative cancer therapy. Blood 83:3780–3786, 1994.
63. RM Stone. Myelodysplastic syndrome after autologous transplantation for lymphoma: the price of progress? Blood 83:3437–3440, 1994.
64. S Mach-Pascual, RD Legare, D Lu, M Kroon, D Neuberg, R Tantravahi, RM Stone, AS Freedman, LM Nadler, JG Gribben, DG Gilliland. Predictive value of clonality assays in patients with non-Hodgkin's lymphoma undergoing autologous bone marrow transplant: a single institution study. Blood 91:4496–4503, 1998.
65. JW Friedberg, D Neuberg, RM Stone, E Alyea, H Jallow, A LaCasce, PM Mauch, JG Gribben, J Ritz, LM Nadler, RJ Soiffer, AS Freedman. Outcome in patients with myelodysplastic syndrome after autologous bone marrow transplantation for non-Hodgkin's lymphoma. J Clin Oncol 17:3128–3135, 1999.
66. N Schmitz, DC Linch, P Dreger, AH Goldstone, MA Boogaerts, A Ferrant, HM Demuynck, H Link, A Zander, A Barge. Randomized trial of filgrastim-mobilized peripheral blood progenitor cell transplantation versus autologous bone-marow transplantation in lymphoma patients. Lancet 347:353–357, 1996.
67. R Scime, A Indovina, A Santoro, M Musso, A Olivieri, S Tringali, A Crescimanno, M Montanari, R Felice, P Catania, G Mariani, P Leoni, I Majolino. PBSC mobilization, collection and positive selection in patients with chronic lymphocytic leukemia. Bone Marrow Transplant 22:1159–1165, 1998.
68. B Gahn, C Schafer, J Neef, C Troff, M Feuring-Buske, W Hiddemann, B Wormann. Detection of trisomy 12 and Rb-deletion in CD34+ cells of patients with B-cell chronic lymphocytic leukemia. Blood 89:4275–4281, 1997.
69. B Gahn, B Wendenburg, C Troff, J Neef, D Grove, T Haferlach, W Hiddemann, B Wormann. Analysis of progenitor cell involvement in B-CLL by simultaneous immunophenotypic and genotypic analysis at the single cell level. Br J Haematol 105:955–959, 1999.
70. JG Gribben, AS Freedman, D Neuberg, DC Roy, KW Blake, SD Woo, ML Grossbard, SN Rabinowe, F Coral, GJ Freeman, JK Ritz, LM Nadler. Immunologic purging of marrow as-

sessed by PCR before autologous bone marrow transplantation for B-cell lymphoma. N Engl J Med 325:1525–1533, 1991.

71. M Moos, R Schulz, F Cremer, C Sucker, D Schmohl, H Dohner, H Goldschmidt, R Haas, W Hunstein. Detection of minimal residual disease by polymerase chain reaction in B cell malignancies. Stem Cells 13 (suppl 3):42–51, 1995.

72. U Paulus, N Schmitz, K Viehmann, N von Neuhoff, P Dreger. Combined positive/negative selection for highly effective purging of PBPC grafts: towards clinical application in patients with B-CLL. Bone Marrow Transplant 20:415–420, 1997.

73. ZS Pavletic, ER Arrowsmith, PJ Bierman, SA Goodman, JM Vose, SR Tarantolo, RS Stein, G Bociek, JP Greer, CD Wu, JP Kollath, DD Weisenburger, A Kessinger, SN Wolff, JO Armitage, MR Bishop. Outcome of allogeneic stem cell transplantation for B cell chronic lymphocytic leukemia. Bone Marrow Transplant 25:717–722, 2000.

74. J Mattsson, M Uzunel, M Remberger, P Ljungman, E Kimby, O Ringden, H Zetterquist. Minimal residual disease is common after allogeneic stem cell transplantation in patients with B cell chronic lymphocytic leukemia and may be controlled by graft-versus-host disease. Leukemia 14:247–254, 2000.

75. CL Toze, JD Shepherd, JM Connors, NJ Voss, RD Gascoyne, DE Hogge, HG Klingemann, SH Nantel, TJ Nevill, GL Phillips, DE Reece, HJ Sutherland, MJ Barnett. Allogeneic bone marrow transplantation for low-grade lymphoma and chronic lymphocytic leukemia. Bone Marrow Transplant 25:605–612, 2000.

76. IF Khouri, D Przepiorka, K van Besien, S O'Brien, JL Palmer, S Lerner, RC Mehra, HM Vriesendorp, BS Andersson, S Giralt, M Korbling, MJ Keating, RE Champlin. Allogeneic blood or marrow transplantation for chronic lymphocytic leukaemia: timing of transplantation and potential effect of fludarabine on acute graft-versus-host disease. Br J Haematol 97:466–473, 1997.

77. RJ Soiffer, AS Freedman, D Neuberg, DC Fisher, EP Alyea, J Gribben, RL Schlossman, L Bartlett-Pandite, C Kuhlman, C Murray, A Freeman, P Mauch, KC Anderson, LM Nadler, J Ritz. CD6+ T cell-depleted allogeneic bone marrow transplantation for non-Hodgkin's lymphoma. Bone Marrow Transplant 21:1177–1181, 1998.

78. M Juckett, P Rowlings, M Hessner, C Keever-Taylor, W Burns, B Camitta, J Casper, WR Drobyski, G Hanson, M Horowitz, C Lawton, J Margolis, D Peitryga, D Vesole. T cell-depleted allogeneic bone marrow transplantation for high-risk non-Hodgkin's lymphoma: clinical and molecular follow-up. Bone Marrow Transplant 21:893–899, 1998.

79. EC Guinan, VA Boussiotis, D Neuberg, LL Brennan, N Hirano, LM Nadler, JG Gribben. Transplantation of anergic histoincompatible bone marrow allografts. N Engl J Med 340:1704–1714, 1999.

80. PA Taylor, A Panoskaltsis-Mortari, RJ Noelle, BR Blazar. Analysis of the requirements for the induction of CD4+ T cell alloantigen hyporesponsiveness by ex vivo anti-CD40 ligand antibody. J Immunol 164:612–622, 2000.

81. D Przepiorka, NA Kernan, C Ippoliti, EB Papadopoulos, S Giralt, I Khouri, JG Lu, J Gajewski, A Durett, K Cleary, R Champlin, BS Andersson, S Light. Daclizumab, a humanized anti-interleukin-2 receptor alpha chain antibody, for treatment of acute graft-versus-host disease. Blood 95:83–89, 2000.

82. HJ Kolb, J Mittermuller, C Clemm, E Holler, G Ledderose, G Brehm, M Heim, W Wilmanns. Donor leukocyte transfusions for treatment of recurrent chronic myelogenous leukemia in marrow transplant patients. Blood 76:2462–2465, 1990.

83. S Mackinnon, EB Papadopoulos, MH Carabasi, L Reich, NH Collins, RJ O'Reilly. Adoptive immunotherapy using donor leukocytes following bone marrow transplantation for chronic myeloid leukemia: is T cell dose important in determining biological response? Bone Marrow Transplant 15:591–594, 1995.

84. IF Khouri, M Keating, M Korbling, D Przepiorka, P Anderlini, S O'Brien, S Giralt, C Ippoliti, B von Wolff, J Gajewski, M Donato, D Claxton, N Ueno, B Andersson, A Gee, R Champlin.

Transplant-lite: induction of graft-versus-malignancy using fludarabine-based nonablative chemotherapy and allogeneic blood progenitor cell transplantation as treatment for lymphoid malignancies. J Clin Oncol 16:2817–2824, 1998.

85. M Sykes, F Preffer, S McAfee, SL Saidman, D Weymouth, DM Andrews, C Colby, R Sackstein, DH Sachs, TR Spitzer. Mixed lymphohaemopoietic chimerism and graft-versus-lymphoma effects after non-myeloablative therapy and HLA-mismatched bone-marrow transplantation. Lancet 353:1755–1759, 1999.

86. BM Sandmaier, P McSweeney, C Yu, R Storb. Nonmyeloablative transplants: preclinical and clinical results [in process citation]. Semin Oncol 27:78–81, 2000.

87. MJ Keating, S O'Brien, H Kantarjian, W Plunkett, E Estey, C Koller, M Beran, EJ Freireich. Long-term follow-up of patients with chronic lymphocytic leukemia treated with fludarabine as a single agent. Blood 81:2878–2884, 1993.

88. SB Gjedde, MM Hansen. Salvage therapy with fludarabine in patients with progressive B-chronic lymphocytic leukemia. Leuk Lymphoma 21:317–320, 1996.

89. S Johnson, AG Smith, H Loffler, E Osby, G Juliusson, B Emmerich, PJ Wyld, W Hiddemann. Multicentre prospective randomised trial of fludarabine versus cyclophosphamide, doxorubicin, and prednisone (CAP) for treatment of advanced-stage chronic lymphocytic leukaemia. The French Cooperative Group on CLL. Lancet 347:1432–1438, 1996.

90. S O'Brien, A del Giglio, M Keating. Advances in the biology and treatment of B-cell chronic lymphocytic leukemia. Blood 85:307–318, 1995.

91. G Rondon, S Giralt, Y Huh, I Khouri, B Andersson, M Andreeff, R Champlin. Graft-versus-leukemia effect after allogeneic bone marrow transplantation for chronic lymphocytic leukemia. Bone Marrow Transplant 18:669–672, 1996.

92. MJ Dyer, SM Kelsey, HJ Mackay, E Emmett, P Thornton, G Hale, H Waldmann, AC Newland, D Catovsky. In vivo 'purging' of residual disease in CLL with Campath-1H. Br J Haematol 97:669–672, 1997.

19

Finding New Therapies for Patients with Chronic Lymphocytic Leukemia

JOHN C. BYRD and MICHAEL R. GREVER

The Ohio State University, Columbus, Ohio

Chronic lymphocytic leukemia (CLL) is one of the most common types of leukemia diagnosed in the Western Hemisphere, with 8100 projected new cases in the United States for the year 2000 (1). CLL is a disease of the elderly with a median age at diagnosis of approximately 64. The impact on overall survival in young and elderly patients with CLL is quite substantial. In the patient diagnosed younger than the age of 50, Montserrat and colleagues (2) have demonstrated that the median expected life span is 12.3 years compared with 31.2 years in the age-matched control group. Several studies have identified elderly patients at high risk for poor survival in treatment studies (3,4). A recent report of the United States SEER database comparing outcome of elderly patients with CLL to age- and sex-matched healthy controls demonstrated that CLL has the greatest impact on survival in the most elderly group of patients (5). Thus, CLL is a significant health problem that has an impact on young and older patients alike.

Even though the impact of CLL on young and elderly patients alike is substantial, only two classes of drugs have been introduced and approved for marketing by regulatory groups in the United States or Europe for the treatment of this disease. Alkylator agents (chlorambucil or cyclophosphamide) ± predisone have been used for the treatment of CLL for many years and are effective at palliating cytopenias or symptoms of organomegaly attributed to this disease (6). In the early 1980s the adenosine deaminase inhibitor

The opinions or assertions contained herein are the private views of the authors and are not to be construed as official or as reflecting the views or any government agency.

This work in part supported by the CLL Research Consortium (P01 CA81534-02) to which JCB and MG are members and the Sidney Kimmel Cancer Research Foundation (JCB).

pentostatin (7) and related nucleosides (8–13) were introduced with demonstrable activity in alkylator-refractory CLL. Subsequent studies demonstrated that these were also highly effective in previously untreated CLL patients. Fludarabine has emerged from these trials as the most widely used nucleoside analog, and three phase III trials have demonstrated its superiority to alkylator-based therapy, (14–16). Although a multiple number of other agents have been brought into the clinic by the National Cancer Institute and industry alike for the treatment of cancer, few have been examined in CLL. Indeed, the greatest degree of drug development relevant to patients with CLL in the 1980s outside of the nucleoside and adensosine deaminase inhibitors relates to biological agents, such as murine monoclonal antibodies (17–19) and cytokines (20). Why despite the numerous books, chapters, and review articles on the disease CLL does this chapter represent one of the first summaries written about preclinical to clinical drug development specific to this disease?

I. DISEASE-SPECIFIC DRUG DEVELOPMENT: A NEW EVOLVING APPROACH

Drug development for the treatment of cancer over the past 30 years has focused mainly on chemical modification of already successful drug classes and identifying new agents through in vivo or in vitro screening processes. The initial screening efforts of the National Cancer Institute used a murine leukemia in vivo model that best facilitated agents that inhibit cell growth (DNA damaging agents, antimetabolites, etc). This pattern of drug screening was modified in 1985 because of the failure of this screening mechanism to identify new therapies for the more common solid tumors. Since 1985, the National Cancer Institute has used 60 disease-specific human tumor cell lines for in vitro testing of new compounds. Included in this panel are a variety of leukemia/lymphoma cell lines including the CCRF-CEM, HL-60, K562, MOLT-4, RPMI-8226, and SR. Unfortunately, none of these are relevant to the model of slow growth observed clinically in CLL cells. The end point of the assay is the sulfurhodamide-B protein stain, which quantifies the viable tumor remaining at the end of a 48-hour incubation. Response patterns to the different cell lines are subsequently compared with other agents with known mechanisms of action that use the COMPARE program, which facilitates insight into whether the agent has a novel mechanism of action or is similar to other agents currently used in the clinic. Agents with selective and unique patterns of response relative to other agents are seen as potentially novel targets and are generally moved forward.

Once identified as promising in preliminary in vitro screens, isolation of sufficient drug supply and subsequent in vivo studies to determine the therapeutic index in mice are performed. The effectiveness of the respective agent is assessed against the three most sensitive tumor cell lines using an in vivo nude mouse xenograft model. An agent with a promising in vivo profile is tested further and has detailed animal pharmacology and toxicology studies (usually two to three different species). In addition, attempts to make structural analogs of the lead compound are often pursued in hopes of improving tumor efficacy before full transition to the clinic. Indeed, it is this period of development, including in vivo testing of different schedules of drug administration, formulation, pharmacology, and toxicology, that is quite costly and time consuming. This component of drug development ultimately limits the number of therapies that can be transitioned to clinical trials. Until most recently, if a respective agent passed through each of these development phases, two phase I studies in patients with solid tumors were performed, with almost certain exclusion of most hematological malignancies (particularly CLL). Phase II studies of these new compounds were often driven by clinical responses noted in phase I trials for which the CLL patients had previously been excluded. Furthermore, until recently, many physicians were less likely to refer CLL patients for phase I trials because of the misconceived perception that this was a disease that did not require investigational therapy. Fortunately for CLL patients, the focus of drug development has been favorably altered by success noted early with the purine analogs.

Advances in both the basic biology and pathophysiology of cancer have fostered a second approach to drug discovery. Rather than broadly screening agents for activity in cell lines for lead compounds with potentially different response profiles and then empirically bringing agents forward without the knowledge of its particular mechanism of action, an emerging focus is to work backwards. That is, a specific molecular or cellular feature that is either mutated, overexpressed, or selectively expressed on a particular tumor type is identified. At this point, potential lead structures for this particular aberration are then identified on the basis of several pathways. If the aberration is well characterized, computerized modeling (21) can be applied and specific inhibitory molecules (small compounds, antisense molecules, neutralizing antibodies, or receptors, etc.) are identified, and efforts to advance these to clinical trials ensues. In a similar fashion, lead compounds previously studied by the National Cancer Institutes broad screening program that may work against tumors that have specific molecular aberrations can be identified by working backwards. Specifically, the 60 cell line screening panel currently used by the National Cancer Institute is examined for the presence or absence of this specific aberration, and then patterns of response for this select group of cell lines are examined with attention to agents that selectively inhibit growth. Once identified, compounds can then be further characterized to determine whether their cytotoxic action is specific to this molecular aberration or others. Once lead compounds are identified for a specific target, they must then go through all of the secondary steps of development. Such a development approach with specific targeting makes nonselect toxicity (i.e., myelosuppression) less likely and mandates that the specific aberration be present in the tumor tested if therapeutic success is to be appreciated. In such studies, identifying if the molecular target is being favorably altered in the tumor cell is quite important. Indeed, with this development approach, a new clinical paradigm has emerged that focuses on the minimally effective pharmacological dose (provided tumor can be serially sampled) rather than the often nonspecific maximally tolerated dose to test in subsequent phase II trials. It is at this development point in experimental therapeutics that CLL and other hematological malignancies represent the ideal diseases to test new agents, because tumor cells can be sampled serially before and during therapy with direct assessment of change of the molecular target.

It is therefore not surprising that disease-specific drug development with a number of agents summarized in Table 1 is occurring in CLL. Development of new therapies for patients with CLL will clearly require both an understanding of the biology of CLL and then how to actively affect factors that give these tumor cells a growth or survival advantage. These particular issues have been covered elsewhere and therefore will not be reviewed with exception to therapeutic approaches discussed later to exemplify advantages and pitfalls of both in vitro and in vivo drug testing in CLL. Once in the clinic, important pharmacological, pharmacodynamic, and in vivo validation studies of the target must occur to ensure the agent is being given its optimal chance of working.

II. BIOLOGY OF CLL RELEVANT TO DRUG DEVELOPMENT

A variety of findings related to the molecular biology of CLL are relevant to therapeutics. These can be subdivided into factors associated with poor response to therapy (e.g., p53

Table 1 Novel Therapies Currently Being Tested or Soon Coming to the Clinic for CLL

A. Previously untreated combination approaches
    Fludarabine + cyclophosphamide versus fludarabine
    Fludarabine followed by campath-1H
    Fludarabine + cyclophosphamide + rituximab
    Fludarabine + cyclophosphamide + rituximab followed by IDEC-Y2B8
B. Chemical compounds
    Compound GW506U78
    Depsipeptide
    Flavopiridol
    KRN5500
    Phosphodiesterase inhibitors
    Clofarabine
    Bryostatin
    Decitabine
    Thalidomide
    LDP-341
C. Monoclonal antibodies and radioimmune conjugates
    Rituximab (anti-CD22)
    Campath-1H (anti-CD52)
    Hu1D10 (anti-1D10, a HLA DR antibody)
    Humanized anti-CD22 antibody
    Yttrium-90 ibritumomab tiuxetan (IDEC-Y2B8)
    Iodine (131)I tositumomab
D. Miscellaneous biological agents
    CD154 adenovirus mediated gene therapy
    Genasense™ (formerly known as G3139)

mutations) and those that distinguish CLL cells from normal cells (e.g., antigen expression). Each of these has immediate relevance to drug development. Specifically, once a molecular marker is associated with drug resistance, it can be incorporated into an in vitro system to determine their dependence on the marker for inducing tumor apoptosis. On a similar note, antigens or proteins that are overexpressed by the leukemia cell, a dependent stromal cell, or isolated to one compartment (e.g., B cells) can be targeted with biological therapies (monoclonal antibodies or antisense compounds) that produce relatively selective leukemia cell killing. Although discussed elsewhere in this text, a brief review of several such features (chromosomal abnormalities, cell surface antigens, and chromatin status) will be discussed for which references to specific therapeutic approaches occur later.

Chromosomal abnormalities or gene mutations in a variety of hematological malignancies have generated insight into the pathogenesis of the underlying disease and subsequently lead to new treatment strategies. Chromosomal abnormalities are seen in at least half of all cases of B-CLL by traditional karyotype analysis (22,23), with the most common findings in CLL being deletions at 13q14, trisomy 12, translocations and deletions of 17p13, and 11q22-23 deletions. Of the genetic markers most relevant for targeting therapeutics are aberrations of the p53 gene for which karyotype analysis measures only a proportion. Inactivation of the p53 gene can occur as a consequence of a deletion, mutation, or possibly from functional inactivation of the protein product by the mdm2 protein. Mutations of the p53 gene are relatively frequent (10%–20%) in B-CLL, become more frequent as the disease progresses, and predict for aggressive disease unresponsive to alkylator or purine analog-based therapy (24–28). Genes, which regulate p53, may also play an important role in the clinical progression of B-CLL. The human mdm-2 gene, on chromosome 12, is up-regulated by p53 and then binds to p53 to inactivate it as part of an intracellular negative feedback loop. Developing new therapeutics in CLL that do not rely on intact p53 function to induce apoptosis therefore remains a top priority.

How can abnormalities such as p53 inactivation be modeled in a system similar to CLL to predict whether new therapies will work independent of this resistance mechanism? Unlike many diseases, there are few CLL cell lines and by virtue of growth in culture, their relevance to the disease can be called into question. The advent of knock-out mice has provided the opportunity to study the consequences of deleted genes for which this species is not dependent for viability. This removes other genetic variables that are often present in cell lines that could cocontribute to p53 inactivation and drug resistance. Murine lymphocytes from both the spleen and lymph nodes can be obtained from p53 knock-out mice and matched mice with an intact p53 gene. These nondividing lymphocytes can be cultured in vitro with parallel doses of a particular agent and concentration curves generated that either demonstrate dependence or independence on an intact p53 pathway. Use of such an assay by our group (29) and others (30) has been subsequently used as preclinical validation of an agent being both p53 dependent or independent. Indeed, this assay correctly identified that inactivation of p53 drastically affects fludarabine sensitivity. This finding correlates with the known clinical association of p53 mutations in CLL cells with resistance to fludarabine-based therapy (24–28).

Cell surface antigens, extracellular cytokines, and intracellular antiapoptotic proteins that promote CLL cell survival are other targets exploitable by modern technologies not previously available for phase I/II studies in CLL. This can be facilitated by passive direct and indirect serotherapy with unconjugated monoclonal antibodies. These are made less immunogenic by incorporating either a partial (chimeric) or almost complete (humanized) backbone. Monoclonal antibodies are targeted; many do not produce significant cytopenias or extramedullary toxicity. Targeted therapy directed at the leukemia cell could occur with several cell surface antigens on CLL cells, including CD20, CD52, CD22, HLA-DR, CD23, CD25, and CD47. In addition, a variety of neutralizing chimeric or humanized antibodies or receptors toward cytokines (TNF-α, IFN-γ, IL-8, IL-4, and CD40 ligand) might promote CLL survival in their free form. Other novel biological agents such as the bcl-2 antisense molecule (G3139) that directly inhibits production of bcl-2 protein offer the promise for targeted therapy. With each of these biological agents comes one or more unique developmental problems, including infusion-toxicity, unexplained shortened drug half-life, increased susceptibility to infection, and impaired delivery to the target cell mandating detailed preclinical and clinical translational studies to avoid abandonment of a potential effective therapy.

An additional recently identified exploitable target in CLL is removal of transcriptional gene silencing induced by histone acetylation. In most tumor types and normal cells, transcriptional silencing of the genome can occur through a variety of mechanisms, including DNA promoter region hypermethylation or acetylation of nuclear histone proteins (31–36). Recent studies have shown that DNA methylation effectively overrides changes in histone acetylation with respect to gene silencing (37). Unlike normal hematopoietic cells and a variety of neoplasms, CLL remains unique in that the genomic DNA

Table 2   Ideal Features for New Drugs in Chronic Lymphocytic Leukemia

Selective cytotoxicity toward CLL cells compared with normal mononuclear cells
Nonmyelosuppressive
Oral administration
Ability to abrogate classic drug resistance factors associated with CLL
Synergy with fludarabine and/or monoclonal antibodies

is hypomethylated (38–40). This laboratory finding provides the basis for the hypothesis that CLL cells might be more reliant on the presence of this class of enzymes that regulate histone acetylation (histone deacetylase) for tumor-specific gene silencing. Disruption of this enzyme's activity may therefore induce selective cytotoxicity toward CLL cells through activation of a variety of genes and subsequent protein products whose absence prevents apoptosis in CLL cells.

Testing of compounds in CLL that abrogate the effect of a particular bad molecular aberration, target a cell membrane or intracellular protein that ultimately results in destruction of a chemotherapy-resistant cell, or inhibits an enzyme such as histone deacetylase is among many approaches that are desirable. Table 2 summarizes desirable features of an ideal new agent for the treatment of CLL. A detailed discussion of both in vitro and in vivo testing methods specific to CLL follows, by which disease-specific drug development can occur with these and other agents.

III. INITIAL IN VITRO DRUG TESTING

Once a particularly interesting therapy is identified for testing in CLL, the usual approach is to validate the agent's in vitro activity against human tumor cells. A variety of in vitro testing approaches have been used for identifying novel anticancer therapies as part of drug discovery efforts. Many of these broad preclinical screening tests have used immortalized cell lines that do not approximate the natural history of CLL tumor cells. Specifically, these cell lines often have high proliferative rates, whereas CLL is predominately a nonproliferating disease of impaired apoptosis. Attempts at generating CLL-specific cell lines from patients with CLL with low proliferative rates in the absence of Ebstein Barr virus transformation has also been relatively unsuccessful. Furthermore, CLL cells derived from patients undergo spontaneous apoptosis to a variable degree in culture, making long-term culture approaches problematic. Adaptation using short culture techniques of CLL cells therefore occurred to facilitate screening of novel compounds.

Several efforts for screening new drugs in CLL rely on tumor cells derived from the blood of patients with CLL. These cells are best immediately transferred to the reference laboratory at room temperature. Isolation of the CLL cells in the mononuclear cell compartment after density gradient centrifugation often occurs and depends on the purity of the isolated cells, negative selection of T cells (with sheep red cell rosetting, antibody/complement depletion, or antibody tagged magnetic beads) and monocytes. No studies to date have examined the affect of T-cell or monocyte depletion on the frequency of spontaneous apoptosis, although studies in which depletion has been done have often noted a high rate of spontaneous apoptosis after 1 to 2 days of culture. Because accessory T cells and their cytokines (such as IL-2 and IL-4) help promote survival of CLL cells (41–44), our approach is not to deplete these effector cells. CLL cells are cultured in standard media (with glutamine) with either heat-inactivated fetal calf serum or heat-inactivated human serum/plasma. Only one trial has examined the benefit of human to fetal calf serum relative to spontaneous apoptosis and failed to demonstrate a difference between the two culture techniques (45). Although considerably more expensive, human serum/plasma is ideal for specific types of in vitro studies. Studies with cytokines or other biological molecules that seek to promote proliferation of CLL cells are generally more successful when performed with human serum, (46). Similarly, when performing preclinical studies with drugs for which a large proportion of drug is protein bound and the status of species variable binding (e.g., is human plasma protein binding the same as calf plasma protein binding) is not known, use of human plasma is probably better. This avoids underestimating the in vitro concentration of a drug that produces apoptosis in vivo (47).

Several nonclonogenic assays such as the dye exclusion assay, differential staining cytotoxicity (DiSC) assay, and tetrazolium dye assay (MTT) have been used to screen new drugs for CLL. Both the MTT (48–53) and DiSC (54–57) assays are quite applicable to testing nondividing cells such as CLL cells in culture. The DiSC assay has been used predominately by investigators in Europe to predict response to therapy, as opposed to identifying new therapies for CLL. The DiSC assay distinguishes live from dead cells by changes in the cell color, because membrane integrity is lost during the late phase of apoptosis. This assay adds a mixture of fast green/nigrosin stain with an absolute standard number of permanently fixed duck red blood cells to the tumor cells immediately after incubation at each of the experimental conditions. The mixture is then placed on a slide, fixed with methanol, and stained with a secondary stain that allows identification of each cell type on the basis of morphology. Viable tumor cells are counted and expressed as a ratio of viable morphologically identified tumor cells/morphologically identified duck red blood cells by a skilled morphologist. Although ideal for examining loss of tumor cell viability when the cell population is heterogeneous and variable (as in acute leukemia or multiple myeloma), this assay is quite time consuming and has the potential for interperson variability. In contrast, the MTT assay depends on viable cells to reduce the water-soluble yellow tetrazolium salt to an insoluble purple formazan product. The absorbance of the formazan product is read at a fixed wavelength (usually 540 nm) and then the ratio of absorbance between the control cells to drug-exposed cells is compared. This assay can rarely be confounded by T-cell proliferation, which under rare circumstances can convert the tetrazolium salt to formazan and give a falsely negative result (e.g., demonstrate findings consistent with no drug activity). Because most cells derived from CLL patients' blood separation are tumor cells and these are generally nondividing, this assay is quite appropriate and less technically demanding than the DiSC assay. A comparison of the two assays has demonstrated similar results (51), thereby justifying either (or variant assays thereof) for preclinical in vitro screening of new agents. Indeed, both are quite adaptable to examining both different drug concentrations and times of incubation, which is critical to modeling ideal schedules of administration before bringing new agents into in vivo testing or actual phase I/II trials.

Before beginning in vitro studies on human CLL cells, careful examination of preclinical (and clinical) pharmacology, toxicology, and concentrations previously demonstrated to produce the selected targeted effect in other tumor systems (if available) should be assessed. For example, if prolonged incubation with an agent produced irreversible (cardiac toxicity with depsipeptide in mice) or reversible but dose-limiting (diarrhea with flavopiridol in dogs) toxicity, an attempt to identify shorter, clinically feasible schedules of administration should be pursued. In addition, characterization of the target enzyme concentration, antigen, or biological protein expression relative to other normal cells should be performed if feasible. This is particularly relevant if the agent irreversibly inhibits the proposed target, when overexpression of the target in the tumor cell relative to normal cells might produce excessive toxicity. An example of this is the excessive toxicity that was observed when pentostatin, an adenosine deaminase inhibitor, was tested in acute lymphoblastic leukemia with the goal of inhibiting the target enzyme (58,59). This type of leukemia has a very high level of adenosine deaminase relative to normal cells and therefore produced excessive toxicity. When CLL, a cell type that has less adenosine deaminase activity relative to normal mononuclear cells, was targeted in a similar fashion, favorable activity without prohibitive toxicity was noted (7). The range of drug concentrations examined should fall within that attainable in animals or humans, because cytotoxicity in excess of pharmacologically attainable levels rarely translates into an agent that moves forward into the clinic to benefit CLL patients.

Once the ideal schedule of administration is identified, investigation of the proposed agent's ability to promote selective toxicity in the normal lymphocyte/monocyte compartment is assessed using primarily the schedule of administration that produces the most optimum cytotoxicity in vitro. This is performed most often with natural or synthetic products, because preclinical in vivo testing done on dogs does identify granulocytopenia or thrombocytopenia but does not characterize the effect on normal immune effector cells. Because the signaling pathways and cell surface markers of normal T cells, B cells, and CLL cells are sometimes similar, agents that are effective in CLL in vitro and in vivo can also have an impact on the normal immune system. The value of this is best demonstrated with fludarabine. This agent (60) has a greater effect on normal mononuclear cells (including T cells) than CLL cells, producing a cellular immune defect in vivo. Manifestation of this was reflected in the higher incidence of opportunistic infections observed after this agents' use (61–63). Early identification of such side effects allows use of prophylactic approaches for opportunistic infections, particularly in phase I testing of CLL patients who are generally fludarabine refractory and already predisposed to opportunistic infections.

Several additional factors must be considered when performing an in vitro evaluation of a new therapeutic agent using human CLL cells. If prolonged exposure to the drug is desired, structural stability must be determined, because some small molecules lose biological activity over time when placed in aqueous solution. Our approach is to use a hematopoetic tumor cell line for which the compound demonstrates inhibitory activity and to measure the relative growth inhibitory concentration over time after incubation in aqueous solution. If change is noted at a given time, then stability of the compound is not assumed beyond this time. In addition, if a prodrug is converted in vivo to an active metabolite (e.g., 2-F-ara-A monophosphate [fludarabine] to 2-F-ara-A or cyclophosphamide to 4-hydroperoxycyclophosphamide), this should be used in the in vitro culture. With biological agents such as monoclonal antibodies, it might be necessary to use an anti-human Fc-specfic cross-linking antibody to evoke evidence of biological activity in vitro in the absence of effector cells (64). Finally, if the particular drug of interest is highly protein bound and there is a potential variability between species, it is best to use human serum/plasma or parallel human/fetal calf serum for the initial experiments. This avoids the potential over- or underestimation of the ideal drug concentration necessary for in vivo apoptosis.

With the transition to later phases of drug development, attention to combination strategies should be considered. Elegant methods for establishing synergy in tumor cell lines exists but generally mandate that a fixed concentration of drug produces known cytotoxicity at a given time. Applying this to human CLL cells is problematic because of the interpatient variability and response (65). However, when a rationale for combining therapies exists, it is possible to administer each agent at a subtherapeutic approach, in which additive versus synergistic activity can be ascertained. Indeed, although sufficient cell line data substantiated both fludarabine's and pentostatins' (as DNA repair inhibitors) ability to synergistically work with DNA-damaging agents such as mafosfamide, cisplatin, or radiation in cell lines or normal human lymphocytes (66–69). Performance of in vitro synergy studies (70) in human CLL cells subsequently validated this approach. An extensive discussion of combination approaches is discussed elsewhere in this text.

IV. IN VIVO DRUG TESTING IN CLL

Once a chemical agent demonstrates promising in vitro activity, testing often proceeds to in vivo xenograft models. This allows assessment of factors such as drug metabolism, distribution, and a preliminary assessment of the contribution active metabolites might contribute to the agent's total activity. Up until recently, there have been very few in vivo models of CLL because of the limited number of CLL cell lines. Mohammed and colleagues (71) described the isolation of a non-EBV immortalized CLL cell line (WSUCLL) from a terminal patient with CLL that maintained many of the immunophenotypical features of CLL, with exception to losing CD5 expression. This same group successfully demonstrated tumor formation after fixed cell inoculation in the severe combined immunodeficiency (SCID) mouse (72,73). The immunophenotypical features of the tumor were preserved in vivo, and the authors were subsequently able to validate the synergistic benefit of combining bryostatin with cladribine (72) or auristatin PE (73). With the former combination (bryostatin and cladribine), the authors were also able to validate the optimal sequence of administration (bryostatin followed by cladribine). With the later combination, the authors were able to select the best microtubule-inhibiting agent (e.g., auristatin PE over dolastatin 10) and to demonstrate that auristatin combined with bryostatin cured most animals of CLL tumors. On the basis of these observations, this group is testing the former combination in an ongoing phase I/II trial. Other CLL cell lines (JOK-1) have recently been shown to successfully yield tumors in SCID mice (74), and it is likely that application of such in vivo testing in the future will be used more frequently as novel combination approaches are developed.

V. EARLY CLINICAL TRIALS IN CLL: CONTINUOUS LABORATORY TO CLINIC INTERFACE

Once all of the preclinical features are completed, time for clinical trial design begins. Indeed, several of the agents listed in Table 1 have entered or completed phase I/II testing in CLL disease-specific trials. It is at this point for the respective agent that laboratory-clinic interface becomes most important, because the pathway from the laboratory to the clinic can be easily reversed to understand new observations seen in the clinic. These can subsequently be studied in the laboratory and returned to the clinic for additional testing. Specific examples relevant to some of the agents actively being investigated in the clinic for CLL are summarized below.

A. Flavopiridol: Altered Pharmacokinetics and Varied Species Plasma Protein Binding

Flavopiridol is a synthetic flavone that is a potent inhibitor of several cyclin-dependent kinases. Three independent groups (29,75,76) have demonstrated that flavopiridol has marked in vitro activity against both human CLL cells and CLL cell lines. Scheduling studies were performed to examine a shorter infusion schedule (4 and 24 hours comparison with 96 hours) of flavopiridol on the basis of other preclinical data showing that prolonged infusion (72 hour) in dogs produced more diarrhea compared with the shorter (24-hour) infusion schedules. These studies substantiated that the LC$_{50}$ of CLL cells was similar with a shortened as opposed to more prolonged flavopiridol administration. Furthermore, all of the in vitro schedules of flavopiridol examined lacked selectivity for normal mononuclear cells. Additional preclinical work by our group demonstrated that flavopiridol induces cytotoxicity independent of the p53 status (29). Work by Kitada and colleagues (75) also demonstrated that flavopiridol favorably down-modulated mcl-1, independent of caspase activation. These studies substantiated studying flavopiridol in CLL.

After long delays because of lack of drug supply, a corporate-designed phase II study using a biweekly shorter infusion schedule (24 hours) was initiated in patients with fludarabine-refractory CLL. The initial dose selected (80 mg/m^2) for this portion of the trial failed to produce notable toxicity or efficacy. A modification to the trial was performed to allow intrapatient dose escalation with successive cycles to a maximum dose of 140 mg/m^2 if no dose-limiting toxicity was observed. Although the 140 mg/m^2 dose administered over 24 hours biweekly produced some biological activity, episodes of grade III toxicity were also observed, suggesting the dose-limiting toxicity would soon be exceeded. Furthermore, true efficacy as defined by the modified National Cancer Institute (NCI) criteria was lacking. Examination of the initial pharmacokinetics performed from this trial was informative, because it demonstrated that the target dose of flavopiridol had been reached, drug protein binding was high (approximately 95%), and the terminal half-life far exceeded that observed on any NCI-sponsored trial to date (47,77). Given the high plasma protein binding observed with flavopiridol, additional in vitro experiments comparing incubation with fetal calf serum and human plasma were performed. These data demonstrated an unexpected marked difference in the LC$_{50}$ between fetal calf serum at early and late time points (47). These studies demonstrated that the concentration of flavopiridol required to induce apoptosis in vitro using human plasma had not been obtained in the patients enrolled on the previously completed trial. Concurrent experiments demonstrated that while flavopiridol was highly protein bound (>90%) with human serum, its binding in fetal calf serum was markedly less (47). Pharmacokinetic modeling from this CLL study demonstrated that a short bolus schedule followed by a 4-hour infusion would provide the higher target concentration identified from these new in vitro studies with human plasma. On the basis of these data, a phase I/II study will be initiated by the CLL Research Consortium to determine whether flavopiridol warrants further study in this disease.

The lessons to learn from the above-mentioned trial are many. These include the importance of defining the ideal dose before embarking on a phase II trial and including pharmacokinetics in all early trials (phase I and II) to ensure previous studies are correct and relevant to the patient population examined. The importance of assessing the plasma protein binding of these drugs in vivo along with species variability is extremely important. This was also demonstrated with another phase I agent, UCN-01 (78). Most important, however, is always performing a detailed analysis of discordant laboratory and clinic data. In the particular case of flavopiridol, careful assessment of data derived from the trial in conjunction with additional experiments provides a scientific rationale for an additional trial before abandoning what still may be an active drug for this disease.

B. Rituximab: An Inactive Agent Before Testing in CLL

Rituximab is an anti-CD20 chimeric antibody that has been extensively studied in low-grade non-Hodgkins lymphoma (NHL). Indeed, responses in low-grade NHL are noted in approximately 50% of the patients (79). The CD20 antigen is present in approximately 95% of patients with CLL, but its expression is dim compared with follicular lymphoma (80–82). Data derived from both phase II NHL studies that included patients with small lymphocytic lymphoma (SLL, tissue variant of CLL) without peripheral blood lymphocytosis (79,83,84) demonstrated that rituximab had marginal activity. Specifically, the response rates in these studies ranged from 12% to 13% when administered once weekly for 4 weeks at a dose of 375 mg/m^2. These data prompted many investigators to conclude that rituximab was not active in CLL before a single patient with this disease was treated. Indeed, many investigators were surprised when CLL investigators and CTEP scientists alike pushed for early monotherapy and combination trials with this agent in patients with CLL.

Why did these initial studies demonstrate poor response to rituximab in patients with SLL/CLL? When developing new biological therapies, one must consider that follicular NHL and SLL/CLL are not the same disease. Specifically, toxicity and pharmacokinetics might be quite different with biological agents between the subgroups of patients with low-grade follicular lymphoma and CLL/SLL. In the pivotal multiple-dose study (79) in which rituximab was administered once weekly for four treatments, a significantly lower response was noted in the 33 patients with SLL (12% vs 58%; $p < 0.001$) compared with those with patients with International Working Formulation B, C, or D histology. Pharmacokinetic studies were performed as part of this study and demonstrated a strong correlation of mean pretreatment (trough) plasma antibody concentration with response (85). Patients with SLL demonstrated a significantly lower pretreatment plasma trough concentration of rituximab compared with other low-grade histological findings (85).

Given the unfavorable pharmacokinetics of the once-weekly 375 mg/m^2 dosing schedule of rituximab in CLL, two phase I/II studies examining dose escalation of rituximab with the same weekly schedule of administration used in the pivotal study (86) or a more frequent (thrice weekly) administration (87) were undertaken. In both studies, rituximab therapy was initiated with caution in patients with CLL, because these individuals seemed to have more severe infusion-related toxicity (88–91). These infusion-related side effects were subsequently demonstrated to be secondary to release of cytokines. Diminution of these side effects by use of a ''stepped-up'' dosing approach in which rituximab is administered at low doses (100 mg over 4 hours without dose escalation) on day 1 and then dose-escalated thereafter was observed in one trial. The therapeutic results of these two studies are quite similar, with both demonstrating significant activity of rituximab in patients with CLL. Indeed, response rates of 39% (86) and 45% (87) were observed. Limited analysis of the pharmacokinetics from the thrice-weekly study demonstrated sustained trough concentration of rituximab after the first week of treatment similar to those seen in the pivotal study of the follicular lymphoma subset. Translational studies accompanying this trial (92) identified in vivo apoptosis by means of a caspase-9 pathway immediately after completion of the rituximab treatment in responding patients concurrent with down-regulation of the mcl-1 protein in most patients examined. These laboratory studies may in part explain why rituximab sensitizes CLL cells to the effects of chemotherapy. Indeed, combination trials of rituximab with fludarabine or fludarabine and cyclophosphamide have been initiated for which initial response data appear promising.

The lessons to learn from the above-mentioned trial are several. Foremost is recognizing that biological agents might have very different pharmacokinetic and side effect profiles among different diseases. In addition, translational bedside to laboratory studies can greatly enhance our understanding of how new therapies with potentially unknown mechanisms of action are working in patients with CLL.

C. Depsipeptide: To Find the CLL-Specific Biologically Effective Dose

Depsipeptide is a novel bicyclic depsipeptide structure and has selective cytotoxicity toward drug-resistant P388 leukemia cell lines compared with nonresistant p388 cell lines (93–95). Depsipeptide causes down-regulation of c-myc and morphologic normalization of ras-transformed cells (96). Recent studies have identified that this agent also effectively inhibits the enzyme histone deacetylase in human tumor cell lines (97). Animal pharmacology and toxicology studies with depsipeptide demonstrated marked animal lymphoid depletion in all schedules examined. Our group was the first to report the activity of depsipeptide in human chronic lymphocytic leukemia cells (98). These data demonstrate that depsipeptide induces selective cytotoxicity in CLL cells compared with both normal mononuclear cells and bone marrow progenitor cells with maximal cytotoxicity observed after a 4-hour drug exposure. Specifically, all of the CLL patients treated (previously untreated, treated, and fludarabine refractory) demonstrated an in vitro response to depsipeptide. The average concentration of depsipeptide required to produce 50% cytotoxicity (LC_{50}) after 4 hours of agent exposure followed by incubation in fresh media for 4 days was 0.038 μM (range, 0.003–0.1; 95% CI $\pm$ 0.046). Contrasting with this, peripheral mononuclear cells from four healthy volunteers had a significantly higher ($p = 0.03$) LC_{50} of 3.44 μM (range, 0.5–6.99; 95% CI $\pm$ 2.61) when incubated in a similar fashion. Studies with bone marrow mononuclear cell isolates from three healthy volunteers exposed for 4 hours to varying concentrations of depsipeptide ranging from 0.0015 to 3.44 μM demonstrated that even at the highest concentration of depsipeptide, greater than 50% suppression of CFU-GM was not observed. In addition to this impressive selective cytotoxic advantage of depsipeptide against CLL cells, additional studies have been performed demonstrating that depsipeptide both favorably modulates p27 protein expression and alters the bcl-2/bax ratio favoring apoptosis in human CLL cells. Recent efforts have demonstrated a direct relationship of depsipeptide acetylation of H3 and H4 histone proteins in human CLL cells with a decreased bcl-2/bax ratio and induction of apoptosis. On the basis of these observations, a novel study design, targeting a minimally effective biological dose will be initiated in collaboration with scientists at CTEP.

In the past, attempts to define the maximally tolerated dose were targeted to DNA damaging agents or antimetabolites. In the current era of molecularly targeted therapy, searching for the optimally pharmacologic or biologically relevant dose appears attractive. The concept of the biologically effective dose as a trial end point also facilitates rapid transition to combination strategies. For depsipeptide this approach is justified, because laboratory data demonstrate that plasma concentrations attained in the initial phase I trials of this agent exceed those that cause in vitro histone acetylation, favorable alteration in the bcl-2/bax ratio, and apoptosis in human CLL cells. It is hoped that identification of the biologically effective dose will facilitate early combination of depsipeptide with other chromatin remodeling agents (decitabine) in CLL and other diseases. Indeed, the authors feel privileged to be part of developing new strategies for phase I studies in CLL.

VI. THE FUTURE FOR CLL DRUG DEVELOPMENT

The advances in understanding the molecular biology of CLL and technology outside of this field are beginning to direct our therapeutic direction. Indeed, microarrays have identified profiles of diseases within the pathological entity of diffuse large-cell lymphoma (99) and are now being applied to CLL. Complex computer modeling of protein-binding sites such as that described by Wang and colleagues (21) leads to identification of novel small molecules that can inhibit function of important antiapoptotic proteins such as bcl-2. Furthermore, perfecting the humanization process for monoclonal antibodies has led to an awakening of new and exciting therapy in a therapeutic field that previously had become stagnated. But all does not come from the laboratory. The fact that we observe only a small proportion of serious reactions with monoclonal antibody administration (Campath-1H or rituximab) without predisposing clinical features directs us back to the laboratory to genetically profile those patients having serious reactions compared with those not having serious reactions. Targeted drug development focused on establishing either a pharmacologically or biologically effective dose of new agents will hopefully facilitate combination approaches that can cure patients with CLL in the future.

REFERENCES

1. RT Greenlee, T Murray, S Bolden, et al. Cancer Statistics 2000. Ca Cancer J Clin 50:7–33, 2000.
2. E Montserrat, F Gomis, T Vallespi, et al. Presenting features and prognosis of chronic lymphocytic leukemia in younger adults. Blood 78:1545–1551, 1991.
3. B Jaksic, B Vitale, E Hauptmann, et al. The roles of age and sex in the prognosis of chronic leukaemias. A study of 373 cases. Br J Cancer 64:345–8, 1991.
4. D Catovsky, J Fooks, S Richards. Prognostic factors in chronic lymphocytic leukaemia: the importance of age, sex and response to treatment in survival. A report from the MRC CLL 1 trial. MRC Working Party on Leukaemia in Adults. Br J Haematol 72:141–149, 1989.
5. JM Flynn, JC Byrd, LF Diehl. The causes of death and the impact of age on the survival of patients with chronic lymphocytic leukemia. Blood 94:298b, 1999.
6. JC Byrd, KR Rai, EA Sausville, et al. New and old treatments of chronic lymphocytic leukemia: It's time for a treatment reassessment. Semin Oncol 25:65–73, 1998.
7. MR Grever, JM Leiby, EH Kraut, et al. Low-dose deoxycoformycin in lymphoid malignancy. J Clin Oncol 3:1196–201, 1984.
8. MR Grever, KJ Kopecky, CA Coleman, et al. Fludarabine monophosphate: A potentially useful agent in chronic lymphocytic leukemia. Nouv Rev Fr Hematol 30:457–459, 1988.
9. MJ Keating, H Kantarjian, S O'Brien, et al. Fludarabine: A new agent with marked cytoreductive activity in untreated chronic lymphocytic leukemia. J Clin Oncol 9:44–49, 1991.
10. MJ Keating, H Kantarjian Talpaz, et al. Fludarabine: A new agent with major activity against chronic lymphocytic leukemia. Blood 74:19–25, 1989.
11. LD Piro, CJ Carrera, E Beutler, et al. 2-Chlorodeoxyadenosine: an effective new agent for the treatment of chronic lymphocytic leukemia. Blood 72:1069–1073, 1988.

12. S O'Brien, H Kantarjian, M Beran, et al. Results of fludarabine and prednisone therapy in 264 patients with chronic lymphocytic leukemia with multivariate analysis-derived prognostic model for response to treatment. Blood 82:1695–700, 1993.

13. C Pott, W Hiddemann. Purine analogs in the treatment of chronic lymphocytic leukemia. Leukemia 11:25–28, 1997.

14. KR Rai, B Peterson, J Kolitz, et al. A randomized comparision of fludarabine and chlorambucil for patients with previously untreated chronic lymphocytic leukemia. A CALGB, SWOG, CTG/NCI-C, and ECOG Inter-Group Study (abstr). Blood 88:141a, 1996.

15. The French Cooperative Group on CLL, S Johnson, AG Smith, et al. Multicentre prospective randomized trial of fludarabine versus cyclophosphamide, doxorubicin, and prednisone (CAP) for treatment of advanced-stage chronic lymphocytic leukemia. Lancet 347:1432–1438, 1996.

16. M Leporrier, S Chevret, B Cazin, et al. Randomized comparison of fludarabine CAP and CHOP, in 696 previously untreated stage B and C chronic lymphocytic leukemia (CLL) (abstr). Early stopping of the CAP accrual. Blood 90:529a, 1997.

17. RO Dillman, J Beauregard, DL Shawler, et al. Continuous infusion of T101 monoclonal antibody in chronic lymphocytic leukemia and cutaneous T-cell lymphoma. J Biol Response Mod 5:394–410, 1986.

18. RW Schroff, MM Farrell, RA Klein, et al. T65 antigen modulation in a phase I monoclonal antibody trial with chronic lymphocytic leukemia patients. J Immunol 133:1641–1648, 1984.

19. RO Dillman, DL Shawler, JB Dillman, et al. Therapy of chronic lymphocytic leukemia and cutaneous T-cell lymphoma with T101 monoclonal antibody. J Clin Oncol 2:881–891, 1984.

20. MJ O'Connell, JP Colgan, MM Oken, et al. Clinical trial of recombinant leukocyte A interferon as initial therapy for favorable histology non-Hodgkin's lymphomas and chronic lymphocytic leukemia. An Eastern Cooperative Oncology Group pilot study J Clin Oncol 4: 128–136, 1986.

21. JL Wang, D Liu, ZJ Zhang et al. Structure-based discovery of an organic compound that binds Bcl-2 protein and induces apoptosis of tumor cells. Proc Natl Acad Sci USA 97:7124–7129, 2000.

22. H Dohner, S Stilgenbauer, K Dohner, et al. Chromosome aberrations in B-cell chronic lymphocytic leukemia: reassessment based on molecular cytogenetic analysis. J Mol Med 77:266–281, 1999.

23. G Juliusson, M Murup. Cytogenetics in chronic lymphocytic leukemia. Semin Oncol 25:19–26, 1998.

24. S El Rouby, A Thomas, D Costin, et al. p53 gene mutation in B-cell chronic lymphocytic leukemia is associated with drug resistance and is independent of MDR1/MDR3 gene expression. Blood 82:3452–3459, 1993.

25. E Wattel, C Preudhomme, B Hecquet, et al. p53 Mutations are associated with resistance to chemotherapy and short survival in hematologic malignancies. Blood 84:3148–3157, 1994.

26. P Fenaux, C Preudhomme, JL Lai, et al. Mutations of the p53 gene in B-cell chronic lymphocytic leukemia: a report on 39 cases with cytogenetic analysis. Leukemia 6:246–250, 1992.

27. H Dohner, K Fischer, M Bentz, et al. p53 Gene deletion predicts for poor survival and nonresponse to therapy with purine analogs in chronic B-cell leukemias. Blood 85:1580–1589, 1995.

28. I Cordone, S Masi, FR Mauro, et al. p53 Expression in B-cell chronic lymphocytic leukemia: A marker for disease progression and poor prognosis. Blood 91:4132–4349, 1998.

29. JC Byrd, C Shinn, A Bedi, et al. Flavopiridol induces apoptosis in chronic lymphocytic leukemia cells via activation of caspase-3 without evidence of bcl-2 modulation or dependence upon functional p53 Blood 92:3804–3816, 1998.

30. AR Pettitt, AR Clarke, JC Cawley, et al. Purine analogues kill resting lymphocytes by p53-dependent and -independent mechanisms Br J Haematol 105:986–988, 1999.

31. S Baylin. Tying it all together: epigenetics, genetic, cell cycle, and cancer. Science 288:1948–1949, 1997.

32. S Baylin, J Herman, J Graff, et al. Alteration in DNA methylation: a fundamental aspect of neoplasia. Adv Cancer Res 72:141–196, 1998.

33. JP Issa, BA Zehnbauer, SH Kaufmann, et al. H1C1 hypermethylation is a late event in hematopoetic neoplasms. Cancer Res 57:1678–1681, 1997.

34. CA Hassig, JK Tong, TC Fleischer, et al. A role for histone deacetylase activity in HDAC1-mediated transcriptional repression. Proc Nat Acad Sci USA 95:3519–3524, 1998.

35. L Nagy, KY Kao, D Chakravarti, et al. Nuclear receptor repression mediated by a complex containing SMRT, mSin3A and histone deacetylase. Cell 89:373–380, 1998.

36. B Quesnel, G Guillerm, R Vereecque, et al. Methylation of p15 (INK4b) gene in myelodysplastic syndromes is frequent and acquired during disease progression. Blood 91:2985–2990, 1998.

37. E Cameron, KE Bachman, S Myohanen, et al. Synergy of demethylation and histone deacetylase inhibition in the re-expression of genes silenced in cancer. Nat Genet 21:103–107, 1999.

38. PJ Browett, JD Norton. Analysis of ras gene mutations and methylation state in human leukemias. Oncogene 4:1029–1036, 1989.

39. S Kochanek, A Radbruch, H Tesch, et al. DNA methylation profiles in the human genes for tumor necrosis factors afla and beta in sub-populations of leukocytes and in leukemias. Proc Nat Acad Sci USA 88:5759–5763, 1991.

40. J Wahlfors, H Hiltunen, KE Heinonen, et al. Genomic hypomethylation in human chronic lymphocytic leukemia. Blood 80:2074–2080, 1992.

41. P Panayiotidis, K Ganeshaguru, SA Jabbar, et al. Interleukin-4 inhibits apoptotic cell death and loss of the bcl-2 protein in B-chronic lymphocytic leukaemia Br J Haematol 85:439–442, 1993.

42. M Dancescu, M Rubio-Trujillo, et al. Interleukin 4 protects chronic lymphocytic leukemic B cells from death by apoptosis and upregulates Bcl-2 expression. J Exp Med 176:1319–1326, 1992.

43. R Castejon, JA Vargas, Y Romero, et al. Modulation of apoptosis by cytokines in B-cell chronic lymphocytic leukemia. Cytometry 38:224–230, 1999.

44. X Mu, NE Kay, MP Gosland, et al. Analysis of blood T-cell cytokine expression in B-chronic lymphocytic leukaemia: evidence for increased levels of cytoplasmic IL-4 in resting and activated CD8 T cells. Br J Haematol 96:733–735, 1997.

45. RJ Collins, LA Verschuer, BV Harmon, et al. Spontaneous programmed death (apoptosis) of B-chronic lymphocytic leukaemia cells following their culture in vitro. Br J Haematol 71: 343–350, 1989.

46. MG Goodman, SB Wormsley, JC Spinosa, et al. Loxoribine induces chronic lymphocytic leukemia B cells to traverse the cell cycle. Blood 84:3457–3464, 1984.

47. CA Shinn, MA Pearson, V Buj, et al. Marked difference in sensitivity of human CLL cells to flavopiridol based upon culture conditions: A consequence of different interspecies plasma protein binding. Blood (abstract submitted).

48. MR Muller, J Thomale, C Lensing, et al. Chemosensitisation of alkylating agents by pentoxifylline, O6-benzylguanine and ethacrynic acid in haematological malignancies. Anticancer Res 6:2155–2159, 1993.

49. F Morabito, G Messina, B Oliva, et al. In vitro chemosensivity of chronic lymphocytic leukemia B-cells to multidrug regimen (CEOP) compounds using the MTT colorimetric assay. Haematological 78:213–218, 1993.

50. E Lambert, JK Rees, PR Twentyman. In vitro chemosensivity of chronic lymphocytic leukemia B-cells to multidrug regimen (CEOP) compounds using the MTT colorimetric assay 6: 1063–1071, 1992.

51. JA Hanson, DP Bentley, EA Bean, et al. In vitro chemosensitivity testing in chronic lymphocytic leukaemia patients. Leuk Res 15:565–569, 1991.

52. DP Cohen, DJ Adams, JL Flowers, et al. Pre-clinical evaluation of SN-38 and novel camptothecin analogs against human chronic B-cell lymphocytic leukemia lymphocytes. 23:1061–1070, 1999.

53. R Silber, B Degan, D Costin, et al. Chemosensitivity of lymphocytes from patients with B-cell chronic lymphocytic leukemia to chlorambucil, fludarabine, and camptothecin analogs. Blood 84:3440–3446, 1994.

54. AG Bosanquet, MI Bosanquet. Ex vivo assessment of drug response by differential staining cytotoxicity (DiSC) assay suggests a biological basis for equality of chemotherapy irrespective of age for patients with chronic lymphocytic leukaemia. Leukemia 14:712–715, 2000.

55. AG Bosanquet, SA Johnson, SM Richards. Prognosis for fludarabine therapy of chronic lymphocytic leukaemia based on ex vivo drug response by DiSC assay. Br J Haematol 106: 71–77, 1999.

56. AG Bosanquet, PB Bell. Novel ex vivo analysis of nonclassical, pleiotropic drug resistance and collateral sensitivity induced by therapy provides a rationale for treatment strategies in chronic lymphocytic leukemia. Blood 87:1962–1971, 1986.

57. AG Bosanquet, SR McCann, et al. Methylprednisolone in advanced chronic lymphocytic leukaemia: rationale for, and effectiveness of treatment suggested by DiSC assay. Acta Haematol 93:73–79, 1995.

58. HG Prentice, NH Russell, N Lee, et al. Therapeutic selectivity of and predication of response to 2′-deoxycoformycin in acute leukaemia. Lancet 2:1250–1254, 1981.

59. DG Poplack, SE Sallan, G Rivera, et al. Phase I study of 2′-deoxycoformycin in acute lymphoblastic leukemia. Cancer Res 41:3343–3346, 1981.

60. JC Byrd, CA Shinn, A Bedi, et al. UCN-01: A new agent for chronic lymphocytic leukemia that induces apoptosis independent of p53 status. (submitted)

61. JC Byrd, JB Hargis, KM Kester, et al. Opportunistic pulmonary infections with fludarabine in previously treated patients with low-grade lymphoid malignancies: A role for *Pneumocytis carinii* pneumonia prophylaxis. Am J Hematol 49:135–142, 1995.

62. EJ Anaissie, DP Kontoyiannis, S O'Brien, et al. Infections in patients with chronic lymphocytic leukemia treated with fludarabine. Ann Intern Med 129:559–566, 1998.

63. JC Byrd, LL Houde-McGrail, DR Hospenthal, et al. Herpes virus infections occur frequently following treatment with fludarabine: Results of a prospective natural history study. Br J Haematol 105:445–447, 1999.

64. MD Pearson, C Shinn, MR Grever, et al. Rituximab induces in vitro apoptosis In human chronic lymphocytic leukemia cells (cll) independent of complement mediated lysis but requires Fcγ receptor ligation. Blood 94:313b, 1999.

65. Y Kano, M Akutsu, S Tsunoda, et al. In vitro cytotoxic effects of fludarabine (2-F-ara-A) in combination with commonly used antileukemic agents by isobologram analysis. Leukemia 14:379–388, 2000.

66. A Sandoval, U Consoli, W Plunkett. Fludarabine-mediated inhibition of nucleotide excision repair induces apoptosis in quiescent human lymphocytes. Clin Cancer Res 2:1731–1741, 1996.

67. L Li, X Liu, AB Glassman, et al. Fludarabine triphosphate inhibits nucleotide excision repair of cisplatin-induced DNA adducts in vitro. Cancer Res 57:1487–1494, 1997.

68. A Begleiter, L Pugh, LG Israels, et al. Enhanced cytotoxicity and inhibition of DNA damage repair in irradiated murine L5178Y lymphoblasts and human chronic lymphocytic leukemia cells treated with 2′-deoxycoformycin and deoxyadenosine in vitro. Cancer Res 48:3981–3986, 1988.

69. S Seto, CJ Carrera, DB Wasson, et al. Inhibition of DNA repair by deoxyadenosine in resting human lymphocytes. J Immunol 136:2839–2843, 1986.

70. B Bellosillo, N Villamor, D Colomer, et al. In vitro evaluation of fludarabine in combination with cyclophosphamide and/or mitoxantrone in B-cell chronic lymphocytic leukemia. Blood 94:2836–2843, 1999.

71. RM Mohammad, AN Mohamed, MY Hamdan, et al. Establishment of a human B-CLL xenograft model: utility as a preclinical therapeutic model. Leukemia 10:130–137, 1996.

72. RM Mohammad, K Katato, VP Almatchy, et al. Sequential treatment of human chronic

lymphocytic leukemia with bryostatin 1 followed by 2-chlorodeoxyadenosine: preclinical studies. Clin Cancer Res 4:445–453, 1998.

73. RM Mohammad, ML Varterasian, et al. Successful treatment of human chronic lymphocytic leukemia xenografts with combination biological agents auristatin PE and bryostatin. Clin Cancer Res 4:1337–1343, 1998.

74. L Bai, K Kon, M Tatsumi, et al. A human B-cell CLL model established by transplantation of JOK-1 cells into SCID mice and an anti-leukemia efficacy of fludarabine phosphate. Oncol Rep 7:33–38, 2000.

75. S Kitada, JM Zapata, M Andreeff, et al. Protein kinase inhibitors flavopiridol and 7-hydroxy-staurosporine down-regulate antiapoptosis proteins in B-cell chronic lymphocytic leukemia. Blood 96:393–397, 2000.

76. A Konig, GK Schwartz, RM Mohammad, et al. The novel cyclin-dependent kinase inhibitor flavopiridol downregulates Bcl-2 and induces growth arrest and apoptosis in chronic B-cell leukemia lines. Blood 90:4307–4312, 1997.

77. L Levasseur, JC Byrd, JL Binet, et al. Interim population pharmacokinetic/pharmacodyamic analysis of flavopiridol administered as a 24-hour infusion with fludarabine-refractory or intolerant B-cell chronic lymphocytic leukemia (abstr). (Submitted).

78. E Fuse, H Tanii, K Takai, et al. Altered pharmacokinetics of a novel anticancer drug, UCN-01, caused by specific high affinity binding to alpha1-acid glycoprotein in humans. Cancer Res 59:1054–1060, 1999.

79. P McLaughlin, AJ Grillo-Lopez, BK Link, et al. Rituximab chimeric anti-CD20 monoclonal antibody therapy for relapsed indolent lymphoma: Half of patients respond to a four-dose treatment program. J Clin Oncol 16:2825–2833, 1998.

80. L Ginaldi, M De Martinis, E Matutes, et al. Levels of expression of CD19 and CD20 in chronic B cell leukaemias. J Clin Pathol 51:364–369, 1998.

81. S Molica, D Levato, A Dattilo, et al. Clinico-prognostic relevance of quantitative immunophenotyping in B-cell chronic lymphocytic leukemia with emphasis on the expression of CD20 antigen and surface immunoglobulins. Eur J Haematol 60:47–52, 1998.

82. A Tefferi, BJ Bartholmai, TE Witzig, et al. Heterogeneity and clinical relevance of the intensity of CD20 and immunoglobulin light-chain expression in B-cell chronic lymphocytic leukemia. Am J Clin Pathol 106:457–461, 1996.

83. JM Foran, AZ Rohatiner, D Cunningham, et al. European phase II study of rituximab (chimeric anti-CD20 monoclonal antibody) for patients with newly diagnosed mantle-cell lymphoma and previously treated mantle-cell lymphoma, immunocytoma, and small B-cell lymphocytic lymphoma. J Clin Oncol 18:317–324, 2000.

84. DT Nguyen, JA Amess, H Doughty, et al. IDEC-C2B8 anti-CD20 (rituximab) immunotherapy in patients with low-grade non-Hodgkin's lymphoma and lymphoproliferative disorders: evaluation of response on 48 patients Eur J Haematol 62:76–82, 1999.

85. N Berinstein, A Grillo-Lopez, CA White, et al. Association of serum rituximab concentration and anti-tumor response in the treatment of recurrent low-grade or follicular non-Hodgkin's lymphoma. Ann Oncol 9:1–7, 1998.

86. S O'Brien, E Freireich, M Andreeff, et al. Phase I/II study of rituxan in chronic lymphocytic leukemia. Blood 92:105a, 1998.

87. JC Byrd, MR Grever, B Davis, et al. Phase I/II study of thrice weekly rituximab in chronic lymphocytic leukemia/small lymphocytic lymphoma: A feasible and active regimen. Blood 94:704a, 1999.

88. JC Byrd, JK Waselenko, T Maneatis, et al. Rituximab therapy in hematologic malignancy patients with circulating blood tumor cells: Association with increased infusion-related side effects and rapid blood tumor clearance. J Clin Oncol 17:791–795, 1999.

89. M Jensen, U Winkler, O Manzke, et al. Rapid tumor lysis in a patient with B-cell chronic lymphocytic leukemia and lymphocytosis treated with an anti-CD20 monoclonal antibody (IDEC-C2B8, rituximab). Ann Hematol 77:89–91, 1998.

90. LC Lim, LP Koh, P Tan. Fatal cytokine release syndrome with chimeric anti-CD20 mono-
     clonal antibody rituximab in a 71-year-old patient with chronic lymphocytic leukemia. J Clin
     Oncol 17:1958, 1999.
91. U Winkler, M Jensen, O Manzke, et al. Cytokine-release syndrome in patients with B-cell
     chronic lymphocytic leukemia and high lymphocyte counts after treatment with an anti-CD20
     monoclonal antibody (rituximab, IDEC-C2B8). Blood 94:2217–24, 1999.
92. S Kitada, M Pearson, IW Flinn, et al. The mechanism of in vivo tumor clearance by rituximab
     n patines with CLL involves apoptosis by a caspase 9 pathway (abstr). Blood (submitted).
93. N Shigematsu, H Ueda, S Takase, et al. Depsipeptide: A novel antitumor bicyclic depsipeptide
     produced by Chromobacterium violaceum No. 968. Structural determination. J Antibiot 47:
     311–314, 1994.
94. N Shigematsu, H Ueda, S Takase, et al. Depsipeptide: A novel antitumor bicyclic depsipeptide
     produced by *Chromobacterium violaceum* No. 968. Structural determination. J Antibiot 47:
     311–314, 1994.
95. H Ueda, Y Nakajima, Y Hori, et al. Action of FR901228 a novel antitumor bicyclic depsipep-
     tide produced by *Chromobacterium violaceium*, No. 968, I. Taxonomy, fermentation, isolation,
     physico-chemical and biologic properties, and antitumor activity. J Antibiot 47:301–310,
     1994.
96. H Ueda, H Nakajima, Y Hori. Action of depsipeptide, a novel antitumor bicyclic depsipeptide
     produced by *Chromobacterium violaceum* No. 968, on Ha-*ras* transformed NIH3T3 cells.
     Biosci Bioltech Biochem 58:1579–1583, 1994.
97. H Nakajima, YB Kim, H Terano, et al. FR901228, a potent antitumor antibiotic, is a novel
     histone deacetylase inhibitor. Exp Cell Res 241:126–133, 1998.
98. JC Byrd, CA Shinn, R Raji, et al. Depsipeptide (FR901228): A novel therapeutic agent with
     selective in vitro activity against human B-cell chronic lymphocytic leukemia cells. Blood 94:
     1401–1408, 1999.
99. AA Alizadeh, MB Eisen, RE Davis, et al. Distinct types of diffuse large B-cell lymphoma
     identified by gene expression profiling. Distinct types of diffuse large B-cell lymphoma identi-
     fied by gene expression profiling. Nature 403:503–511, 2000.

20

Autoimmune Disease and Its Management in Chronic Lymphocytic Leukemia

TERRY HAMBLIN

Royal Bournemouth Hospital, Bournemouth, England

I. INTRODUCTION

It has long been understood that chronic lymphocytic leukemia (CLL) is associated with autoimmune disease, almost as a counterpoint to the profound hypogammaglobulinemia that also accompanies it. This chapter takes a fresh look at the original literature and assesses to what extent that understanding reflects the true facts. It recognizes that many of the defining articles were written at a time when CLL was not well distinguished from a number of similar lymphomas. It also attempts to derive an explanation of why autoimmunity occurs in this context and asks what insights into the pathogenesis of both CLL and autoimmunity the association provides. Finally, it looks at management and considers how secure is current advice.

II. HISTORY

Winifred Ashby carried out her pioneering work into the life span of red cells at the Mayo Clinic between 1917 and 1921. Her technique (1) involved the transfusion of red cells that were compatible but serologically distinct from those of the recipient and then tracking their survival by differential agglutination. Berlin (2) used this technique in nine patients with CLL. All had a shortened red cell survival, even though only one had a reticulocytosis. This was probably the first demonstration that the anemia of CLL might be hemolytic in nature.

It was shortly after Ehrlich (3) published the concept of "horror autotoxicus," the idea that the body would not make an antibody that destroyed its own tissues, that Donath and Lansteiner (4) described an antibody that did just that. Shortly afterwards, Fernand

Widal (5) was probably the first to recognize acquired hemolytic anemia with red cell agglutination. Thirty years later, Dameshek and Schwartz (6) in Boston stressed the importance of "hemolysins" in the most common type of acquired hemolytic anemia. It was not clear quite what these "hemolysins" were until the development of the direct antiglobulin test (DAT) by Robin Coombs (7) and its application to hemolytic anemia (8). Wasserman (9) found hemolytic anemia to be present in 9 of 58 consecutive patients with CLL; 5 of 7 tested had a positive Coombs' test. A series of studies suggested that autoimmune hemolytic anemia (AIHA) occurs at some time in the course of CLL in between 10% and 26% of cases (9–14).

It is often forgotten that the "I" in ITP originally stood for "idiopathic" and not "immune." Harrington and his colleagues (15) first demonstrated that the plasma of patients with chronic ITP transfused into a normal recipient (himself) would produce thrombocytopenia. Later Shulman et al. (16) showed that this plasma factor was present in the 7S gamma globulin fraction and was absorbed by human platelets.

Thrombocytopenia is quite common in CLL. Minot and Buckman (17) found it in half their patients at presentation and in virtually all those whose white count rose above 175×10^9/L. Harrington and Arimura (18) reported seven cases of autoimmune thrombocytopenia occurring in CLL. Ebbe et al. (19) reported five more, but because of the unsatisfactory nature of platelet antibody tests the true prevalence of immune thrombocytopenia in CLL is unknown. Increase in bone marrow megakaryocytes remains the surest touchstone, but in a marrow full of small lymphocytes they may be difficult to estimate.

Reporting autoimmunity in CLL then became a popular sport. Immune neutropenia (20), pure red cell aplasia (21), Sjögren's syndrome (22), nephrotic syndrome (23), bullous pemphigoid (24) and Graves' disease (25) have all been associated with CLL. Reviews by Miller (26) and Dameshek (27) also mentioned systemic lupus erythematosus, rheumatoid arthritis, ulcerative colitis, allergic vasculitis, and pernicious anemia.

III. WHAT IS THE TRUE PREVALENCE OF AUTOIMMUNITY IN CLL?

Several difficulties exist in establishing the true prevalence of autoimmunity in CLL. First, in the early literature authors were unable to distinguish between CLL and other types of lymphoma with a leukemic phase. Second, non-Hodgkin's lymphoma, but not CLL, is well established as a secondary complication of autoimmune diseases such as rheumatoid arthritis and Sjögren's syndrome. Third, many published series contain only the most severe forms of CLL, such as would be referred to a tertiary referral center. Fourth, there is a publication bias in favor of interesting associations. Because of these difficulties, I will examine each autoimmune disease in turn and try to establish whether there is an association, and if there is, just how commonly it is seen.

A. Autoimmune Hemolytic Anemia

No one doubts that warm-antibody AIHA is more common in CLL than in the general population. The highest reported prevalence is 35% (28). Conversely, a positive antiglobulin test at diagnosis was found in only 1.8% of patients entered into the French Co-operative Group's CLL 1980 and CLL 1985 trials (29). The truth behind the disparity is that the prevalence is closely related to stage and progression. In stable stage A disease, Hamblin et al. (30) found a prevalence of 2.9% compared with 10.5% in stage B and C disease and 18.2% in progressive stage A disease.

Looking at the problem from another point of view, CLL is the most common known cause of AIHA. In a large series of patients with AIHA, Engelfriet et al. (31) found that 14% were associated with CLL, roughly twice as common as the next known cause, systemic lupus erythematosus. However, in about half the cases of AIHA no cause is found. AIHA is often thought of as a problem with lymphomas generally, but, from Engelfriet's figures, it is possible to calculate that AIHA occurs about eight times more commonly in CLL than in other forms of non-Hodgkin's lymphoma and about two and a half times more commonly than in Hodgkin's disease.

B. Immune Thrombocytopenia

Ebbe et al. (19) suggested that the prevalence of ITP in CLL was 2%, and this was confirmed by Hamblin et al. (30) and Duhrsen et al. (32). However, in all three series the numbers were small and the reliability of the diagnoses suspect. Diagnosis of ITP in CLL depends on the presence of isolated thrombocytopenia, normal or increased bone marrow megakaryocytes with an excess of early forma, increased mean platelet volume (MPV) and platelet distribution width, and detection of platelet antibodies in the serum or on the platelet membrane.

Unfortunately, tests for platelet antibodies are still unsatisfactory. Hegde et al. (33) found increased levels of platelet associated IgG in 3 of 10 thrombocytopenic patients with CLL and 1 of 10 nonthrombocytopenic patients. Even higher rates were found in non-Hodgkin's lymphomas. This test is known to have a high false-positive rate. Using an ELISA for the detection of serum antibodies and radioimmunoassay for platelet-bound antibodies, Kuznetsov et al. (34) found antibodies in the serum in 7 of 54 thrombocytopenic patients with CLL, and platelet bound antibodies in 21 of 27. Clearly, these assays are oversensitive.

Platelet kinetic studies using radiolabeled platelets are seldom performed, and in any case demonstrate a shortened survival in splenomegaly. Bone marrows heavily infiltrated with CLL make megakaryocyte numbers difficult to assess. The diagnoses is often made by exclusion and confirmed by response to therapy. The fact that ITP occurs together with AIHA in CLL as Evans' syndrome reinforces the belief that the thrombocytopenia seen in these circumstances has an autoimmune basis. About a third of patients with ITP resulting from CLL also have a positive direct antiglobulin test, a much higher rate than for primary ITP (35).

C. Autoimmune Neutropenia

Neutropenia may occur in CLL because of marrow infiltration or treatment. I have yet to be convinced that it occurs as an autoimmune phenomenon. There is a well-recognized syndrome of large granular lymphocytic (LGL) leukemia that is regularly associated with neutropenia (36), and perhaps some of the earlier reports and impressions mistook this for CLL. A study from Crete (37) reported higher numbers of CD3+, CD8+, and CD57+ cells in neutropenic patients with CLL and demonstrated that CD8+ cells from neutropenic patients exerted a greater suppressive effect on CFU-GM colony growth than similar cells from nonneutropenic patients. However, this has not been a consistent finding, and a recent hypothesis implicates the secretion of high levels of Fas-ligand in the cause of the neutropenia that is sometimes seen in B-CLL (38). Antineutrophil antibodies do not seem to be involved.

D. Pure Red Cell Aplasia

Like neutropenia, pure red cell aplasia (PRCA) is a frequent complication of LGL leukemia; indeed, this is probably its most common cause (39). Nevertheless, by 1986 (40) PRCA had been recognized in as many as 23 cases of B-CLL, and it has subsequently been reported on at least five occasions (35). From their own cases Chikkappa et al. (40) suggest that the prevalence is about 6%, but this is either an exaggeration borne of underestimating the denominator or the prevalence has been seriously underestimated. In our series, about 1% of our 800 unselected patients with CLL have had PRCA develop. It is not possible to estimate how many of these had an autoimmune cause.

E. Nonhemic Autoimmunity

In an elderly population autoantibodies are found quite commonly. Hamblin et al. (30) found that a control population of individuals older than 60 had tissue-specific autoantibodies detected by immunofluorescence in 21.5%. In an age-matched series of 195 patients with CLL, the prevalence of autoantibodies was exactly the same. In this series there were two cases of rheumatoid arthritis; two of cryptogenic cirrhosis; two of immune vasculitis; and one each of pulmonary fibrosis, nephrotic syndrome, polymyositis, and polymyalgia rheumatica. Dührsen et al. (32) reported one case each of Graves' disease, Hashimoto's thyroiditis, myasthenia gravis, ankylosing spondylitis, and iritis among 104 cases of CLL. Given that patients with active disease are more likely to have a blood test, which would uncover occult CLL, it is probable that all these are chance associations. However, there are three conditions with a considerable literature that should be looked at more closely.

1. Nephrotic Syndrome and Glomerulonephritis

It could be argued that nephrotic syndrome occurs more commonly in CLL than would be expected by chance. In 1974 Dathan et al. (23) reported two cases of CLL in which nephrotic syndrome developed, caused by an immune complex glomerulonephritis. In the letters column of the same journal, Cameron and Ogg (41) reported a further three cases, but subsequent letters, including my own, were turned down with the excuse that there were so many. A MEDline search reveals a total of 48 cases, mostly in the form of single case reports. The histological lesion may be either membranous glomerulonephritis or membranoproliferative glomerulonephritis. Although there are two reports of antineutrophil cytoplasmic antibodies, one of which followed treatment with fludarabine (42,43), a more likely explanation for the renal disease is the deposition of monoclonal immunoglobulin (sometimes in the form of a cryoglobulin) secreted by the leukemic cells (44,45). In most cases the glomerulonephritis remits on successful treatment of the leukemia.

2. Acquired Angioedema

The syndrome of acquired angioedema is characterized by late onset of recurrent bouts of angioedema and abdominal pain and is caused by an acquired deficiency of the inhibitor if the first component of complement (C1-INH). Type I is associated with lymphoproliferative diseases, including CLL and type II with autoantibodies. The normal C1-INH molecule has a molecular weight (MW) of 105 kD with a binding site for the serine protease C1s. The autoantibodies recognize two synthetic peptides (peptides 2 and 3) that span the reactive site of the molecule. A study of six cases of AAE demonstrated that the autoantibodies were monoclonal whether they were associated with a lymphoproliferative disease or not (46). In both types of AAE a nonfunctional C1-INH molecule of MW 95 kD is found in the serum. The mechanism of action of the antibody is to cause or allow the cleavage of the C1-INH molecule and so render it inactive (47).

Although this syndrome is well recorded as a complication of CLL, it seems to be a consequence of the antibody activity of the tumor immunoglobulin. It is not confined to CLL and is more common among lymphoproliferative diseases that secrete more immunoglobulin, including monoclonal gammopathy of undetermined significance (MGUS). A serum paraprotein is an unusual feature of CLL but seen in two thirds of patients with splenic lymphoma with villous lymphocytes (SLVL). This syndrome, which is probably the same as splenic marginal zone lymphoma, is frequently mislabeled as CLL (particularly CD5 negative CLL), because, despite the name, the tumor cells often lack villi. In our series the only patient with AAE had SLVL and an IgM paraprotein.

3. Autoimmune Blistering Skin Disease

Possibly the first patient with CLL and a pemphigoid-like skin disease was reported in 1910 (48), although the two patients reported by Sachs in 1921 (49) had a more certain diagnosis of CLL. A clear diagnosis of antibody-proven bullous pemphigoid in association with CLL was not achieved until 1974, when Cuni et al. (24) described a single case. In their review of the literature, they discovered 16 other cases of CLL with either bullous or vesicular skin lesions. Goodnough and Muir (50) reported the next case 6 years later, but in the same year Laskaris et al. (51) reported two cases of CLL associated with oral pemphigus.

The question as to whether pemphigus or pemphigoid is associated with CLL was resolved when Anhalt et al. (52) described paraneoplastic pemphigus. The clinical features were of painful erosions of the oropharynx and vermilion borders of the lips that were resistant to conventional treatment. There was a severe pseudomembranous conjunctivitis. Pruritic, polymorphous cutaneous lesions included confluent erythema with skin denudation and papules on the trunk and extremities forming target lesions with central blistering. Cases had often been previously diagnosed as pemphigus vulgaris or erythema multiforme. Histologically, three elements were observed: suprabasilar intraepithelial acantholysis, necrosis of individual keratinocytes, and vacuolar interface change. Immunofluorescence studies revealed the presence in the serum of antibodies that reacted with the intracellular spaces, such as is seen in pemphigus vulgaris or foliaceus. However, direct immunofluorescence studies of the skin also demonstrated complement deposition along the basement membrane typical of bullous pemphigoid.

The serum from all the patients immunoprecipitated an identical complex of four polypeptides from keratinocyte extracts with MWs of 250, 230, 210, and 190 kD, respectively. Subsequently several groups have confirmed this pattern of autoantibodies (53–55), but two groups have also found an antibody against a 130-kD component (56,57). Most of these antigenic components have subsequently been identified. The 130-kD glycoprotein is characteristically involved in pemphigus vulgaris. It has been cloned and sequenced (58) and termed desmoglein-3. It belongs to the cadherin family of cell adhesion molecules. Antibodies to the 230-kD polypeptide are characteristically found in the sera of patients with bullous pemphigoid. The protein is known as BPAG2 (53) and is an intracellular protein that localizes to the hemidesmsomal plaque. The 250-kD protein is desmoplakin I (53), the 210-kD protein is envoplakin (59), and the 190-kD protein is periplakin (60).

Although it is rare, paraneoplastic pemphigus is a discrete autoimmune blistering skin disease with characteristic clinical features, a pathognomonic pattern of antibody specificity, and an association with lymphoid tumors. It may occur in an array of lymphoid tumors, and especially in Castleman's disease, but about 30% of cases occur in CLL (61).

IV. PATHOGENESIS OF AUTOIMMUNITY IN CLL

A. Do Tumor Cells Secrete Autoantibody?

Perhaps the simplest explanation for autoimmune disease in CLL would be that the autoantibodies were the product of the tumor. Older series of patients with CLL suggested that serum paraproteins occurred in 5% to 10% of cases (62,63). However, it is likely that patients with splenic marginal zone lymphoma (SMZL) contaminated these series. The peripheral lymphocytes from this condition are morphologically similar to those of CLL, and although they are CD5 negative, the two conditions are nevertheless frequently confused. In SMZL a monoclonal protein is found on serum electrophoresis in more than 60% of cases.

However, the CLL cell should not be thought of as nonsecretory. By use of a sensitive radioimmunoassay, Stevenson et al. (64) were able to demonstrate secretion of 19S idiotypic IgM in most cases. Baume et al. (65) used a very sensitive immunoblotting technique to find monoclonal immunoglobulins in the sera of 80% of CLLs. However, the light chain type was the same as that of the surface immunoglobulin in only half the cases. Apparently, in CLL serum monoclonal immunoglobulins cannot be assumed to have been produced by the tumor.

Some evidence exists that CLL lymphocytes may be committed to produce autoantibodies. Cells from 12 of 14 CLLs could be induced by stimulation with phorbol ester to secrete IgM that reacted with a variety of autoantigens, including the Fc portion of IgG, both single- and double-stranded DNA, histones, cardiolipin, and cytoskeletal proteins (66). Many reacted with more than one antigen. Similar polyreactive antibodies have been described by Sthoeger et al. (67). By demonstrating that the antibodies were of the same light chain types as the surface Ig of the CLL cells, they established that the autoantibodies were not the product of contaminating normal B cells. The also demonstrated the production of IgG autoantibodies from CLL cells expressing surface IgG.

These findings appeared to give weight to the hypothesis that CLL is derived from a B cell of separate lineage akin to the Ly-1 (CD5) B cell of mice. This subset, which is particularly enriched in the peritoneal cavity, comprises 5% of circulating B cells in mice but is markedly expanded in strains such as NZB and MeV, which are prone to autoimmunity (68–71). The link between CD5 and autoimmunity appeared as an important buttress supporting unifying theories of CLL (72). However, some facts weigh against it. CD5-positive B cells are not augmented in other strains of mice prone to autoimmunity (73), whereas Xid mice, which do not express the CD5 marker at all on B cells, have a similar incidence of autoimmunity as other strains (74). It has also become clear that CD5 is an activation antigen, because negative B cells can be induced to express the antigen on stimulation with phorbol ester (75).

Perhaps the clinching argument is the realization that in both mice and man the germline configuration of many V_H gene products tends to favor weak reactions with autoantigens irrespective of whether they are carried by CD5-positive or CD5-negative B cells (76–78). Hybridomas made from fusing CD5-negative lymphoma cells with nonsecreting murine myeloma cells also secrete autoantibodies (79). Thirty percent of monoclonal IgMs found in patients' sera are accounted for by only four specificities: rheumatoid factor, cold agglutinins, polyreactivity, and myelin-associated glycoproteins (80). In the light of this information, the CD5 B cell: autoimmunity hypothesis seems in want of sufficient support.

Cold agglutination syndrome is perhaps the best described disease in which the antibody activity of a monoclonal protein is responsible for the clinical manifestations. The molecular basis for this reaction is now understood. A rat monoclonal antibody, 9G4, raised against the surface IgM of a B-cell lymphoma recognized a shared idiotypic determinant on all anti-I or anti-i cold agglutinins (81). Tumor cells from patients with cold agglutination syndrome were immortalized with Epstein Barr virus. The 9G4-positive lines were investigated for the use of immunoglobulin V_H genes and found exclusively to use the V_{4-34} gene (82,83). This specificity was retained whether the V_H gene was in germline configuration or showed evidence of somatic mutation.

A comparison of eight sequences of cold agglutinins reacting with I or i demonstrated that neither complementarity determining region (CDR) 3 or light chain sequences were required for binding either to 9G4 or to red cells. Other V_H4 genes do not react with the anti-idiotype or with red cells in the cold. Three sections of V_{4-34} are distinct compared with other V_H gene segments: framework region (FR) 1, CDR1, and the first amino acids of CDR2. Experiments that generated recombinant mutants with changed sequences in all of these areas have demonstrated that the 9G4 idiotope is determined by the motif AVY at amino acid positions 23 to 25 in FR1 (84).

FR1 of V_{4-34} is also essential for binding to the I or i antigens, but other parts of the V_H gene are permissive for binding and determine specificity (85). Anti-I antibodies almost exclusively use V_κ III light chains, whereas anti-i antibodies make use of a much broader array of κ and λ light chains (86). The CDR3 must also be permissive for red cell binding. For example, antibodies with V_{4-34}-encoded heavy chains associated with CDR3s with a predominance of basic amino acids bind preferentially to DNA and lipid A, and only weakly if at all to red cells (87,88).

Do patients with CLL develop cold agglutination syndrome? Among 78 patients with persistent cold agglutinins reported by Crisp and Pruzanski in 1982 (89), 6 had CLL. It is difficult to be sure whether cases of CLL in series of this era were truly cases of CLL as we would now recognize it, and the same is true of the single case report from Feizi et al. (90). Indeed, the single case of CLL with cold agglutination syndrome reported by us (30), in retrospect, had a spillover lymphoma. A more recent case was also CD5 negative (91), an almost certain indication that this also was a different type of lymphoma (92). In this case also the heavy chain gene used by the surface immunoglobulin was DP54 and not V_{4-34}, an indication that the cold agglutinin was not the product of the tumor. In the last year we have seen a patient with long-standing cold agglutination syndrome who developed definite CLL during his last illness. The relationship between his tumor and cold agglutinins awaits determination. We have, however, seen 11 other cases of CLL that made use of the V_{4-34} Ig heavy chain gene, none of whom developed cold agglutination syndrome (93).

As far as other autoimmune syndromes are concerned, there is little evidence that the autoantibodies are the product of the CLL cell. It is believed that CLL-associated angioedema (46) and possibly CLL-associated glomerulonephritis (44,45) may be caused in this way. On the other hand, a recent publication suggests that the anti-230-kD autoantibody associated with paraneoplastic pemphigus is not synthesized by the CLL cells (94). A study by Sikora et al. (95) demonstrated that the monoclonal Ig rescued from CLL cells was not responsible for a concurrent warm antibody AIHA. In contrast, Sthoeger et al.

(96) have reported two cases of CLL in whom it was claimed that immunoglobulin eluted from direct antiglobulin-positive red cells reacted with anti-κ but not anti-λ antibodies. In addition, the CLL cells produced in culture a monoclonal IgM that reacted with red cells, although more strongly at 4°C than at 37°C. Despite this claim, most workers agree that the antibody in AIHA is polyclonal and the product of the residual lymphoid tissue and not of the tumor cells.

B. The V Gene Hypothesis

Recently, Efremov and co-workers (97) produced a startlingly different hypothesis for the pathogenesis of AIHA in CLL. They suggested that AIHA was particularly associated with the use by the tumor of the V_H genes DP10 and DP50 (modern nomenclature V_{1-69} and V_{3-33}), the D segment gene DXP4 (modern nomenclature D3-3), and J_H6. Such a combination of genes would code for a particularly shaped antibody combining site on the surface of the CLL cells, which, it was hypothesised, would engender an immune attack on red cells, perhaps by invoking idiotype networks in an unspecified way.

It is likely that because of small numbers, this apparent association was a chance finding despite the statistics. Only 12 cases of AIHA were included in the study, 5 using V_{1-69} and 4 using V_{3-33}, neither being used in 12 controls. In two much larger studies (98,99) comprising 40 with AIHA and 166 controls, only 7 (17.5%) with AIHA used the V_{1-69} gene, close to usage in controls. There was similarly no excess use of V_{3-33} or D3-3. The only association with AIHA found in CLL was with progressive disease. Because the use of V_{1-69} is also associated with progressive disease (93), it is likely that this is a case of guilt by association.

C. Autoimmunity Triggered by Treatment

More than 30 years ago, Damashek suggested that hemolysis might be triggered by treatment with x-rays or alkylating agents (100). Two such case reports have subsequently appeared in the literature (101,102), but among 37 hemolytic episodes in his large series of patients followed for a long time, Hansen found only 5 in which treatment with x-rays or alkylating agents had been given in the previous 2 months (103). Interestingly, paraneoplastic pemphigus may also be triggered by radiotherapy (104,105). Recently, it has become apparent that hemolysis after treatment with the purine analogs is much more common than after other forms of treatment (106).

The first report appeared as a letter in 1992 (107). Two cases of AIHA occurred after treatment of CLL with fludarabine, although one had been DAT positive before treatment and did not start hemolysing until 5 weeks after the twelfth course of treatment. The association remained in doubt, especially as the M. D. Anderson group, who had the most experience in the world of the new drug, argued that the cases they had seen represented the natural prevalence of AIHA in CLL (108). Among 112 patients treated with fludarabine, they found 5 patients without preexisting AIHA who had hemolysis develop after between one and six courses and a further 4 patients whose preexisting AIHA deteriorated after fludarabine treatment. In four further patients with preexisting AIHA, fludarabine was given safely.

At the 1994 ASCO meeting, Byrd et al. (109) reported a further case and stated that the association had been reported to the FDA on 30 occasions. In 1995 Myint et al. (106) reported that of 52 heavily pretreated patients 12 had AIHA develop after between two and six courses of fludarabine. Since then, many reports have confirmed the association.

Table 1 lists a total of 98 patients reported. It is difficult to ascertain exactly how common this association is. Table 2 lists the series in which some attempt has been made to provide a denominator. Only about 2% of patients treated for the first time have AIHA develop, compared with about 5% of patients who have received some previous treatment and more than 20% of heavily pretreated patients.

Autoimmune thrombocytopenia may also be triggered by fludarabine. Montillo first reported relapse of CLL-associated ITP after exposure to fludarabine (136). A total of 25 cases of fludarabine-related ITP have now been reported (116,120,127,129,130,136–138). Only one possible case of immune neutropenia has been reported (139) and three cases of PRCA (108,140,141). Paraneoplastic pemphigus has been reported in five cases (142–144). There have been two cases of post fludarabine glomerulonephritis (145,146).

The other purine analogs, cladribine and pentostatin, are also capable of triggering autoimmune complications (111,118,124,147,148). Because the best-known toxicity of the purine analogs is their profound T cell suppression, it is interesting to note that treatment with CAMPATH-1 (149) can trigger autoimmune disease in CLL.

Table 1 98 Cases of AIHA After Treatment with Fludarabine

Article	Previous DAT+	Previous DAT−	Previous DAT?	Relapse after retreatment
Bastion 1992 (107)	1	1		
Di Raimondo 1993 (108)	4	5		
Myint 1995 (106)	3	9		6/8 FDA 1/1 CDA
Montillo 1995 (110)			1	
Byrd 1995 (111)				1/1 DCF
Maclean 1996 (112)	1			
Crozat-Grosleron 1996 (113)			1	
Tertian 1996 (114)		1		
Longo 1997 (115)		1		
Shvidal 1997 (116)			1	
Lopez 1997 (117)			1	
Robak 1997 (118)		2		
Tsiara 1997 (119)			1	
Weiss 1998 (120)	6	7	11	7/8 FDA
Gonzalez 1998 (121)	3	5		
Nathwani 1998 (122)		1		
Orchard 1998 (123)				1/1 CHL
Hamblin 1998 (124)		2		
Taha 1998 (125)	1	3		
Vick 1998 (126)			1	
Sen 1999 (127)			1	
Sanmugarajah 1999 (128)		2		
Montillo 1999 (129)			8	
Spiriano 1999 (130)			4	
Boogaerts 1999 (131)			4	
Aguirre 1999 (132)			6	
Total	19	39	40	

DAT = direct antiglobulin test; CDA = cladribine; CHL = chlorambucil; DCF = pentostatin; FDA = fludarabine.

Table 2 Establishing a Denominator

Series	No. of cases	Outcome	Percentage
Di Raimondo 1993 Montillo 1999 Houston Series (108,129)	307 patients treated with FDA	17 DAT neg > AIHA 1 with DAT+ AIHA deteriorated 10 with DAT+ AIHA resolved	5.5
Myint/Orchard/Hamblin 1995/1998 Bournemouth Series (106,123,124)	66 patients with FDA All heavily pretreated Older than most patients with CLL	11 DAT neg > AIHA 3 DAT+ > AIHA 1 DAT+ > no change	21.2
Montillo 1995 Nacona, Italy (110)	16 heavily pretreated patients	1 DAT neg > AIHA	6.25
Fenaux 1996 European Registration Series (133)	100 untreated patients 96 previously treated patients	Randomized between FDA (2 AIHA) & CAP (0 AIHA)	2
Leporrier/Gonzales 1997/1998 French Series (121,134)	695 untreated patients randomized between FDA/CHOP/CAP	<2% AIHA no difference between groups	<2
	36 previously treated patients Rx FDA	3 DAT+ > AIHA 5 DAT neg > AIHA	22.2
Aguirre 1999 Argentinian trial (132)	106 patients 74 pretreated 32 untreated	6 cases of AIHA	5.6
Spriano 1999 Genoa trial (130)	16 heavily pretreated patients	4 cases of AIHA	25
Boogaerts 1999 Schering AG trial (131)	78 patients treated with oral FDA. All alkylator resistant	4 cases of AIHA	5.1
Mauro 1997 Rome series (135)	1155 patients with CLL retrospectively studied Mainly first-line treatment	55 cases of AIHA 38 at initial diagnosis Chl + P 13/470 (2.9%) FDA 3/105 (2.8%)	2.8

From these observations some general conclusions can be drawn. Most cases of postfludarabine autoimmunity have occurred in heavily pretreated patients. Usually patients have previously received an alkylating agent. The complication is severe and often difficult to treat. In many cases it has been fatal. If control is achieved, reexposure to any of the purine analogs retriggers the complication. Even alkylating agents may retrigger it. The recurrence is likely to be even more virulent. Although most common in CLL, autoimmunity may also be induced in other low-grade lymphoproliferative diseases.

D. The T Cell Hypothesis

Because of the known, almost AIDS-like, CD4 T cell suppression that occurs after treatment with fludarabine (150), Myint et al. (106) suggested autoimmunity in CLL is caused by loss of T cell regulatory control of autoreactive T cells. Is there any evidence for such a mechanism? In the mouse there is.

Autoreactive T cells can readily be identified in the peripheral lymphocyte pool of both humans and mice (151). Shevach and his colleagues (152) have identified a population of CD4+ CD25+ T cells that maintain peripheral tolerance. Mice thymectomized on the third day of life develop a wide spectrum of organ-specific autoimmune diseases. Reconstitution of these mice with CD4+ CD25+ T cells from normal mice prevents the development of disease. These cells can also prevent the transfer of disease by autoantigen-specific cloned T cells derived from neonatally thymectomized mice. Elimination of CD4+ CD25+ T cells, which constitute 5% to 10% of peripheral CD4+ T cells, leads to spontaneous development of various autoimmune diseases (153). They suppress autoreactive T cells by specifically inhibiting the production of IL-2, an action remarkably like that of cyclosporin (154). This subset of T cells is susceptible to killing with chemotherapeutic agents compared with the CD4+ CD25 negative subset.

Thymic function declines with age (155), and T cell function is known to be impaired in CLL. Surprisingly, T cell numbers are increased in CLL, especially in early cases (156). The greatest increase is in the CD8-positive cells, so that the CD4/CD8 ratio is often reversed. At least in part this is explained by a redirection of CD4-positive cells to the bone marrow (157). However, circulating T cells are functionally impaired, showing a reduced proliferative response to mitogens and antigens (158), reduced stimulation in the mixed lymphocyte reaction (159), and poor T cell colony formation (160). They also show diminished helper activity for B cells (161). All of these functions deteriorate with increased stage of the disease.

Human studies of autoregulatory T cells have concentrated on the CD4+ CD45RA+ subset. It is not clear whether they represent the same subset as the CD4+ CD25+ subset in the mouse. CD4+ CD45RA+ cells have been shown to be selectively lost in the more advanced stages of CLL, especially in those with autoimmune hemolytic anemia (162).

E. Summary

Autoimmune disease is more common than should be expected in CLL. In the main, autoimmunity is confined to AIHA and ITP. If neutropenia and PRCA occur in CLL, it is more likely that they are mediated through a T cell or NK cell mechanism than through autoantibodies. Cells may secrete immunoglobulin of the same idiotype as that on the surface of the cells. Usually it is present in the serum in amounts undetectable by serum electrophoresis. Nevertheless, such secreted immunoglobulin may be responsible for the rare cases of cold agglutination syndrome, glomerulonephritis, and acquired angioedema that are seen in CLL. In common with other lymphoid tumors, CLL may be accompanied by paraneoplastic pemphigus, a recently described autoimmune disease. The cause of autoimmunity in CLL is unknown, but its frequent triggering by treatment with purine analogs suggests that it may be related to defects in T cell function. The recent discovery of a subset of T cells in mice that is able to suppress autoreactive T cells is an invitation to study these cells in CLL.

V. TREATMENT OF AUTOIMMUNITY IN CLL

Few data address the problem of how to treat the autoimmune complications of CLL. In general, treatment has been the same as when the disease occurs spontaneously. However, some treatments are less appropriate, and there is also the question of whether and how to treat the CLL itself. The possibility that the immunosuppression caused by the disease or its treatment has triggered the autoimmunity has to be weighed against the prospect that treating the disease will eliminate the complication.

A. Autoimmune Hemolytic Anemia

There are no controlled trials of treatment of AIHA secondary to CLL. It is important to note that transfusion of red cells is often vital. Autoimmune destruction of blood cells in CLL is frequently vigorous, especially when triggered by purine analogs, and some patients have died because of the mistaken belief that because transfused cells will also be destroyed by the immune process, they are of no value. It is important also to replenish folic acid. Specific treatment follows what has been established for idiopathic AIHA.

1. Corticosteroids and Cytotoxic Drugs

Prednisolone, 1 mg/kg for 10 to 14 days, is the standard treatment for acute hemolysis (163). The dose is then reduced slowly over the next 3 months. Most patients will respond. The usual steroid side effects, gastric erosions, hypertension, and diabetes, should be looked for, and especially in immunodeficient patients, prophylaxis against fungal infections should be given. The mode of action of steroids is multifarious and includes decreased lymphocyte proliferation, decreased IL-2 production, decreased T-cell activation and T-helper function, impaired NK function, monocyte maturation and handling of antigen by macrophages, and deficient macrophage chemotaxis (164).

Because most cases occur in progressive CLL, it would be usual to also treat the CLL, either with chlorambucil or fludarabine, but this carries a risk. In patients in whom the AIHA has been triggered by fludarabine, further exposure to purine analogs (106,110,126) or even to any other cytotoxic drug may be hazardous (123). Conventionally, patients failing to respond to prednisolone, or relapsing when the dose is reduced, are offered azathioprine or cyclophosphamide. In the case of AIHA or ITP complicating CLL, the most appropriate cytotoxic drug should be exhibited.

2. Splenectomy

Few data exist on splenectomy in this condition. In a series of 113 splenectomies for AIHA only 4 were for hemolysis secondary to CLL (165). The hazards of splenectomy are well known and are certainly increased in frail, elderly, immunodeficient patients. Nevertheless, it may be lifesaving. In our experience, laparoscopic splenectomy extends the possibility of operation to a less healthy population. Patients with AIHA with IgG alone and no complement components on their red cells respond better (166). Before elective splenectomy vaccination against pneumococcus, meningococcus, and *Hemophilus influenza* is recommended, and some groups also recommend long-term prophylactic penicillin or equivalent.

3. Intravenous Immunoglobulin

A review of the literature (167) details 73 cases of AIHA treated with IvIg; 40% responded. Doses of 0.4 g/kg/day for 5 days were effective. Only 18 of the 73 also had CLL. In these, reduction of the size of lymph nodes and spleen was noted, response was transient, lasting only 3 to 4 weeks, but retreatment was effective (35).

4. Cyclosporin

Cyclosporin is used in AIHA when other modalities have failed. When these conditions complicate CLL, failure is a common experience, and cyclosporin has been used most

frequently in this situation (168). The dosage is 5 to 8 mg/kg/day, tapering to a maintenance dosage of about 3 mg/kg/day. We aim to keep the blood level at about 100 μg/L.

5. Other Treatments

Splenic irradiation may substitute for splenectomy in patients too sick for surgery (169).
It may be more appropriate when the spleen is large. Danazol may have a role in steroid
sparing, although its use in CLL is unreported (35). Plasma exchange is less fashionable
than it was. Although successful in a few reports of idiopathic AIHA, there are no reports
in cases secondary to CLL (35). However, the author is aware of one patient so treated
who died while attached to the cell separator. Immunoadsorption is an adjunct to plasma
exchange, in which IgG is adsorbed onto a column containing protein A. At least one
patient has been successfully treated in this way (170). The infusion of vincristine-loaded
platelets aims at destroying macrophages. One patient whose CLL-related AIHA was unresponsive to other modes of treatment responded to this heroic measure (171).

B. Autoimmune Thrombocytopenia

This complication is so rarely diagnosed that there is next to no guidance in the literature
on treatment. It therefore seems wise to follow the Clinical Guidelines of the American
Society of Hematology (172) for the treatment of ITP and treat the CLL independently
as required. Thus, asymptomatic thrombocytopenia should only be treated when the platelet count is $<30 \times 10^9$/L. Hospitalization should be confined to patients with mucous
membrane or other severe bleeding. Conventional dose oral prednisolone is the treatment
of choice for those who need any treatment, (those with severe bleeding or a platelet count
$<30 \times 10^9$/L).

 Prednisolone is given in the same dose as for AIHA. Patients failing to respond are
treated with IvIg, 0.4 g/kg/day for 5 days. The response rate is higher than for AIHA.
Splenectomy is also more effective than in AIHA with response rates of more than 70%
in patients unresponsive to steroids (173). Other treatments found to be successful in
AIHA may also be tried. Unique to autoimmune thrombocytopenia is treatment with vinca
alkaloids. Vincristine, 1 mg IV weekly $\times$6, is often effective, but vinblastine has also
been used. The drugs may be given as boluses or by slow infusion (174).

 ITP complicating CLL may be severe, causing intractable bleeding such as to constitute a medical emergency. Special measures may need to be taken to control the bleeding.
IvIg is followed immediately by platelet transfusion (175). Alternatively, methylprednisolone, 1 g/day IV $\times$3, followed by platelet transfusion may be effective. Tranexamic acid
is worth trying.

C. The Management of Postfludarabine Autoimmunity

The severity of hemolysis or thrombocytopenia after fludarabine is often extreme, and
several reports detail fatalities. It is important not to stint on transfusions of red cells or
platelets. Patients who have these complications develop are often immunosuppressed and
prone to infection. Further immunosuppressive treatment will intensify this risk. We have
patients who, despite successful control of the autoimmune complication, have died from
cytomegalovirus or *Aspergillus* infections (106).

 Anticipating that the complication will be difficult to control, we move rapidly to
secondary treatments. When steroids have failed, we have found success with IvIg and

splenectomy, but many of our patients have required cyclosporin, and because responses are often delayed, we move rapidly to prescribing it.

A special risk is the retriggering of autoimmunity by reexposure to fludarabine (106), cladribine (106), or pentostatin (111). Even chlorambucil may retrigger the complication (123). In a small number of patients it has been possible to reintroduce fludarabine while the patient is maintained on cyclosporin. Whether it is safe to use fludarabine in patients with a positive DAT or evidence of preexisting AIHA is a vexing question. Certainly, some patients have had an exacerbation of their hemolysis or thrombocytopenia when treated this way. Nevertheless, there are reports of both fludarabine and cladribine being used successfully in these circumstances (129,176). There is little to guide us. Probably purine analogs should be avoided in older, heavily treated patients, and they should always be used with caution.

D. Pure Red Cell Aplasia

Treatment for pure red cell aplasia has been reviewed by Diehl and Ketchum (35). On the basis of literature reports of 41 treatments in 33 patients, they recommend instituting treatment to control the CLL, because this will be necessary to achieve long-term remission of the PRCA. At the same time, the PRCA is treated with prednisolone, 1 mg/kg/day. If there is no response, cyclosporin is added. The reticulocyte count should increase within 2 to 3 weeks, and the hemoglobin normalize in 1 to 2 months. At this point, the steroid dose can be reduced and stopped. Cyclosporin should be continued for 6 to 7 months and then gradually withdrawn.

E. Paraneoplastic Pemphigus

This syndrome is frequently fatal; four of the original five patients died (52), and two patients who had it develop after fludarabine also succumbed (142,177). One patient has survived postfludarabine paraneoplastic pemphigus after having been treated with prednisolone, 500 mg/day, cyclophosphamide, 100 mg/day for several weeks, together with IvIg, 120 mg over the first 3 days (143). Other patients with a similar syndrome, unrelated to malignancy, have responded to IvIg (178,179). Three British patients responded to the combination of high-dose steroids and cyclosporin or cyclophosphamide, although one later died of sepsis (144).

F. Rapidly Progressive Glomerulonephritis

Treatment for glomerulonephritis has to involve intense immunosuppression with high-dose intravenous methylprednisolone and cyclophosphamide. Plasma exchange has a role in those cases that are seen with renal failure requiring dialysis (180). Aggressive immunosuppression has the added benefit of suppressing the CLL. It is moot whether control of the CLL or control of the autoimmune process is responsible for the beneficial effect of such treatment.

G. Acquired Angioedema

Treatment of this disorder has been recently reviewed by Markovic et al. (181). They recommend treatment of the CLL as the most important element of the management. Otherwise, the androgens, stanozolol and danazol, have been widely used for both the hereditary and acquired form of the disease and are generally successful. They act by increasing the production of C1 esterase inhibitor by the liver. Not all patients are happy taking androgenic steroids, and for many years I have been using tranexamic acid, 0.5 g three times daily, in the hereditary form. It has been uniformly successful and without side effects. In the one patient with the acquired form that I have seen, it has been equally as effective.

REFERENCES

1. W Ashby. Determination of the length of life of transfused blood corpuscles in man. J Exp Med 29:267–281, 1919.
2. R Berlin. Red cell survival studies in normal and leukaemic subjects; latent haemolytic syndrome in leukaemia with splenomegaly—nature of anaemia in leukaemia—effect of splenomegaly. Acta Med Scand 139(suppl 252):1–141, 1951.
3. P Ehrlich, J Morgenroth, Ueber Hämolysine. V. Berlin Klin Wschr 38, 251, 1901.
4. J Donath, K Landsteiner. Ueber paroxysmale Hämoglobinurie. Münchenr Medzin Wochenschr 51:1590–1593, 1904.
5. F Widal, P Abrami, M Brulé. Les ictères d'origine hémolytique. Arch Mal Coeur, 1:193–231, 1908.
6. W Dameshek, SO Schwartz. Hemolysins as the cause of clinical and experimental hemolytic anemias. With particular reference to the nature of spherocytosis and increased fragility. Am J Med Sci 1938; 196:769–792, 1938.
7. RRA Coombs, AE Mourant, RR Race. A new test for the detection of weak and "incomplete" Rh agglutinins. Br J Exp Pathol 26:255–266, 1945.
8. KE Boorman, BE Dodd, JF Loutit. Haemolytic icterus (acholuric jaundice) congenital and acquired. Lancet i:812–814, 1946.
9. LR Wasserman, D Stats, L Schwartz, H Fudenberg. Symptomatic and hemopathic hemolytic anemia. Am J Med 18:961–989, 1955.
10. AV Pisciotta, JS Hirschboeck. Therapeutic considerations in chronic lymphocytic leukemia. Arch Intern Med 99:334–335, 1957.
11. A Beickert. Die hämolytische Verlausform der chronischen lymphatischen Leukämie. München Medizin Woschenschr 101:2067–2072, 1959.
12. W Dameshek, RS Schwartz. Leukemia and auto-immunization. Some possible relationships. Blood 14:1151–1158, 1959.
13. SB Troup, SN Swisher, LE Young. The anemia of leukemia. Am J Med 28:751–763, 1960.
14. AA Videbæk. Auto-immune haemolytic anaemia in some malignant systemic diseases. Acta Med Scand 171:463–476, 1962.
15. J Harrington, V Minnich, JW Hollingsworth, CV Moore. Demonstration of a thrombocytopenic factor in the blood of patients with thrombocytopenic purpura. J Lab Clin Med 38:1–10, 1951.
16. NR Shulman, VJ Marder, RS Weinrach. Similarities between known anti-platelet antibodies and the factor responsible for thrombocytopenia in idiopathic purpura: physiologic serologic and isotopic studies. Ann NY Acad Sci 124:499, 1965.
17. GR Minot, TE Buckman. The blood platelets in the leukemias. Am J Med Sci 169:477–485, 1925.
18. WJ Harrington, G Arimura. Immune reactions of platelets. In: SA Johnson, RW Monto, JW Rebuck, RC Horn, eds. Blood Platelets. Boston: Little, Brown & Co, 1961.
19. S Ebbe, B Wittels, W Dameshek. Autoimmune thrombocytopenic purpura ("ITP type") with chronic lymphocytic leukemia. Blood 19:23–27, 1962.
20. S-A Killman. Auto-aggressive leukocyte agglutinins in leukaemia and chronic leukopenia. Acta Med Scand 163:207–222, 1959.

21. MD Abeloff, MD Waterbury. Pure red cell aplasia and chronic lymphocytic leukemia. Arch Intern Med 134:721–724, 1974.

22. G Lehner-Netsch, A Barry, JM Delage. Leukemias and autoimmune diseases: Sjøgren's syndrome and hemolytic anemia associated with chronic lymphocytic anemia. Can Med Assoc J 100:1151–1154, 1969.

23. JRE Dathan, MF Heyworth, AG MacIver. Nephtotic syndrome in chronic lymphocytic leukaemia. BMJ 3:655–657, 1974.

24. LJ Cuni, H Grünwald, F Rosner. Bullous pemphigoid in chronic lymphocytic leukemia with the demonstration of anti-basement membrane antibodies. Am J Med 57:987–992, 1974.

25. A Haubenstock, R Zalusky. Autoimmune hyperthyroidism and thrombocytopenia in a patient with chronic lymphocytic leukemia. Am J Hematol 19:281–283, 1985.

26. DG Miller. Patterns of immunological deficiency in lymphomas and leukemias. Ann Intern Med 57:703–715, 1962.

27. W Dameshek. Chronic lymphocytic leukemia—an accumulative disease of immunologically incompetent lymphocytes. Blood 24:566–584, 1967.

28. DE Bergsagel. The chronic leukemias: a review of disease manifestations and the aims of therapy. Can Med Assoc J 96:1615–1620, 1967.

29. G Dighiero. Hypogammaglobulinemia and disordered immunity in CLL. In: BD Cheson, ed. Chronic Lymphocytic Leukemia: Scientific Advances and Clinical Developments. New York: Marcel Dekker, 1993, pp 167–180.

30. TJ Hamblin, DG Oscier, BJ Young. Autoimmunity in chronic lymphocytic leukaemia. J Clin Pathol 39:713–716, 1986.

31. CP Engelfriet, MAM Overbeeke, AEGK von dem Borne. Autoimmune hemolytic anemia. Semin Hematol 29:3–12, 1992.

32. U Dührsen, W Augener, T Zwingers, G Brittinger. Spectrum and frequency of autoimmune derangements in lymphoproliferative disorders: analysis of 637 cases and comparison with myeloproliferative diseases. Br J Haematol 67:235–239, 1987.

33. UM Hegde, K Williams, S Devereux, A Bowes, D Powell, D Fisher. Platelet associated IgG and immune thrombocytopenia in lymphoproliferative and autoimmune disorders. Clin Lab Haemat 5:9–15, 1983.

34. AI Kuznetsov, LI Idel'son, AL Ivanov, AV Mazurov. Antithrombocyte antibodies in the serum and on the surface of the thrombocytes in patients with chronic lymphoproliferative diseases. Ter Arkh 63:26–30, 1991.

35. LF Diehl, LH Ketchum. Autoimmune disease and chronic lymphocytic leukemia: autoimmune hemolytic anemia, pure red cell aplasia and autoimmune thrombocytopenia. Sem Hematol 25:80–97, 1998.

36. TP Loughran, ME Kardin, G Starkebaum, JL Abkowitz, EA Clark, C Disteche, LG Lum, SJ Slichter. Leukemia of parge granular lymphocytes: association with clonal chromosomal abnormalities and autoimmune neutropenia, thrombocytopenia, and hemolytic anemia. Ann Intern Med 102:169–175, 1985.

37. G Katrinakis, D Kyriakou, M Alexandrakis, D Sakellariou, A Foudoulakis, GD Eliopoulos. Evidence for involvement of activated CD8+/HLA-DR+ cells in the pathogenesis of neutropenia in patients with B-cell chronic lymphocytic leukaemia. Eur J Haematol 55:33–41, 1995.

38. T Lamy, TP Loughran. Current concepts: large granular lymphocyte leukaemia. Blood Rev 13:230–240, 1999.

39. MQ Lacy, PJ Kurtin, A Tefferi. Pure red cell aplasia: association with large granular lymphocytic leukemia and the prognostic value of cytogenetic abnormalities. Blood 87:3000–3006, 1996.

40. G Chikkappa, MH Zarrabi, MF Tsan. Pure red cell aplasia in patients with chronic lymphocytic leukemia. Medicine (Baltimore) 65:339–351, 1986.

41. S Cameron, CS Ogg. Nephrotic syndrome in chronic lymphocytic leukaemia. BMJ 3:164, 1974.
42. B Dussol, P Brunet, H Vacher-Coponat, R Bouabdallah, P Chetaille, Y Berland. Crescentic glomerulonephritis with antineutrophil cytoplasmic antibodies associated with chronic lymphocytic leukaemia. Nephrol Dial Transplant 12:785–786, 1997.
43. A Tisler, A Pierratos, JH Lipton. Crescentic glomerulonephritis with p-ANCA positivity in fludarabine-treated chronic lymphocytic leukaemia. Nephrol Dial Transplant 11:2306–2308, 1996.
44. D Gouet, R Marechaud, G Touchard, JC Abadie, O Pourrat, Y Sudre. Nephrotic syndrome associated with chronic lymphocytic leukaemia. Nouv Presse Med 11:3047–3049, 1982.
45. B Moulin, PM Ronco, B Mougenot, A Francois, JP Fillastre, F Mignon. Glomerulonephritis in chronic lymphocytic leukaemia and related B cell lymphomas. Kidney Int 42:127–135, 1992.
46. S He, S Tsang, J North, N Chohan, RB Sim, K Whaley. Epitope mapping of C1 inhibitor autoantibodies from patients with acquired C1 inhibitor deficiency. J Immunol 156:2009–2013, 1996.
47. A Chevailler, G Arlaud, D Ponard, M Pernollet, F Carrere, G Renier, M Drouet, D Hurez, J Gardais. C-1-inhibitor binding monoclonal immunoglobulins in three patients with acquired angioneurotic edema. J Allergy Clin Immunol 97:998–1008, 1996.
48. M Oppenheim. Verhandlungen Der Weiner Dermatologischen Gesellschaft. Arch Dermatol Syphiligr 101:379–382, 1910.
49. O Sachs. Ueber Pemphigoide Hauteruption in Einem Falle von Lymphatischer Leukaemie. Wien Klin Wochenschr 34:317, 1921.
50. LT Goodnough, A Muir. Bullous pemphigoid as a manifestation of chronic lymphocytic leukemia. Arch Interm Med 140:1526–1527, 1980.
51. GC Laskaris, SS Papavasilou, OD Bovopoulou, GD Nicolis. Association of oral pemphigus with chronic lymphocytic leukemia. Oral Surg Oral Med Oral Pathol 50:244–249, 1980.
52. GJ Anhalt, SC Kim, JR Stanley, NJ Korman, DA Jabs, M Kory, H Izumi, H Ratrie, D Mutasim, L Ariss-Abda, RS Labib. Paraneoplastic pemphigus. An autoimmune mucocutaneous disease associated with neoplasia. N Engl J Med 323:1729–1735, 1990.
53. C Camisa, TN Helm, YC Liu, R Valenzuela, C Allen, S Bona, N Larrimer, NJ Korman. Paraneoplastic pemphigus: a report of three cases including one long term survivor. J Am Acad Dermatol 27:547–553, 1992.
54. WP Su, JR Oursler, SA Muller. Paraneoplastic pemphigus: a case with high titer of circulating anti-basement membrane zone antibodies. J Am Acad Dermatol 30:841–844, 1994.
55. S Rodot, V Botcazou, JP Lacour, JF Dor, I Bodokh, P Joly, JP Ortonne. Paraneoplastic pemphigus: review of the literature, apropos of a case associated with chronic lymphocytic leukemia. Rev Med Interne 16:938–943, 1995.
56. P Joly, E Thomine, D Gilbert, S Verdier, A Delpech, C Prost, C Iebbe, P Iauret, F Tron. Overlapping distribution of autoantibody specificities in paraneoplastic pemphigus and pemphigus vulgaris. J Invest Dermatol 103:65–72, 1994.
57. T Hashimoto, M Amagai, W Ning, T Nishikawa, T Karashima, O Mori, S Jablonska, TP Chorzelski. J Dermatol Sci 17:132–139, 1998.
58. M Amagai, V Klaus-Kovtun, JR Stanley. Autoantibodies against a novel cadherin in pemphigus vulgaris, a disease of call adhesion. Cell 67:869–877, 1991.
59. SC Kim, YD Kwon, IJ Lee, SN Chang, TG Lee. cDNA cloning of the 210-kDa paraneoplastic pemphigus antigen reveals that envoplakin is a component of the antigen complex. J Invest Dermatol 109:365–369, 1997.
60. C Ruhrberg, MA Hajibagheri, DA Parry, FM Watt. Periplakin, a novel component of cornified envelopes and desmosomes that belongs to the plakin family and forms complexes with envoplakin. J Cell Biol 39:1835–1849, 1997.

61. GJ Anhalt, HC Nousari. Paraneoplastic autoimmune syndromes. In: NR Rose, IR Mackay, eds. The Autoimmune Diseases. 3rd ed. San Diego: Academic Press, 1998, pp 795–804.
62. R Alexanian. Monoclonal gammapathy in lymphoma. Arch Intern Med 135:62–66, 1975.
63. TJ Hamblin. Chronic lymphocytic leukaemia. Balliere's Clin Haematol 1:449–491, 1987.
64. FK Stevenson, TJ Hamblin, GT Stevenson, A Tutt. Extracellular idiotypic immunoglobulin arising from human leukemia B lymphocytes. J Exp Med 152:1484–1496, 1980.
65. A Beaume, A Brizard, B Dreyfus, JL Preud'homme. High incidence of serum monoclonal Igs detected by a sensitive immunoblotting technique in B-cell chronic lymphocytic leukemia. Blood 84:1216–1219, 1994.
66. BM Broker, A Klajman, P Youinou, J Jouquan, CP Worman, J Murphy, L Mackenzie, R Quarty-Papafio, M Blaschek, P Collins. Chronic lymphocytic leukemis (CLL) cells secrete multispecific autoantibodies. J Autoimmune 1:469–481, 1988.
67. ZM Sthoeger, M Wakai, DB Tse, VP Viciguerra, SL Allen, DR Budman, SM Lichtman, P Schulman, LR Weiselberg, N Chiorazzi. Production of autoantibodies by CD5-expressing B lymphocytes from patients with chronic lymphocytic leukemia. J Exp Med 169:255–268, 1989.
68. V Manohar, E Brown, WM Leiserson, TM Chused. Expression of Ly-1 by a subset of B lymphocytes. J Immunol 129:532–538, 1982.
69. K Hayakawa, RR Hardy, DR Parks, LA Herzenberg. The Ly-1 B cell subpopulation in normal, immunodefective and autoimmune mice. J Exp Med 157:202–218, 1983.
70. LA Herzenberg, AM Stall, PA Lalor, C Sidman, WA Moore, DR Pards. The Ly1-B cell lineage. Immunol Rev 93:81–102, 1986.
71. K Hayakawa, RR Hardy, LA Herzenberg. Peritoneal Ly1-B cells: genetic control, autoantibody production, increased lambda light chain expression. Euro J Immunol 16:450–456, 1986.
72. F Caligaris-Cappio. B-chronic lymphocytic leukemia: a malignancy of anti-self B cells. Blood 87:2615–2620, 1996.
73. G Dighiero. Relevance of murine models in elucidating the origin of B-CLL lymphocytes and related immune associated phenomena. Semin Hematol 24:240–251, 1987.
74. G Dighiero, P Poncet, S Rouyre, JC Mazie. Newborn Xid mice carry the genetic information for the production of natural autoantibodies. J Immunol 136:4000–4005, 1986.
75. RA Miller, J Gralow. The induction of Leu-1 antigen expression in human malignant and normal B cells by phorbolmyristic acetate (PMA). J Immunol 133:3408–3412, 1984.
76. D Holmberg, S Forsgren, F Ivars, A Coutinho. Reactions among IgM antibodies derived from normal neonatal mice. Eur J Immunol 14:435–440, 1984.
77. P Lymberi, G Dighiero, T Ternyck, S Avrameas. A high incidence of cross reactive idiotypes among murine natural autoantibodies. Eur J Immunol 5:702–707, 1985.
78. JF Kearney, M Vakil. Idiotype directed interactions during ontogeny play a major role in the establishment of the adult B cell repertoire. Immunol Rev 94:39–62, 1986.
79. G Dighiero, S Hart, A Lim, L Borche, R Levy, RA Miller. Autoantibody activity of immunoglobulins isolated from B cell follicular lymphomas. Blood 78:581–585, 1991.
80. K Dellagi, JC Brouet, F Danon. Cross reacting idiotypic antigens among monoclonal immunoglobulin M from patients with Waldenström's macroglobulinemia and polyneuropathy. J Clin Invest 64:1530–1539, 1979.
81. FK Stevenson, M Wrightham, MJ Glennie, DB Jones, T Cattan, T Feizi, TJ Hamblin, GT Stevenson. Antibodies to shared idiotypes as agents for analysis and therapy for human B cell tumours. Blood 68:430–436, 1986.
82. V Pascual, K Victor, D Lelsz, MB Spellerberg, TJ Hamblin, KM Thompson, I Randen, J Natvig, JD Capra, FK Stevenson. Nucleotide sequence analysis of the V regions of two IgM cold agglutinins. Evidence that the V$_H$4-21 gene segment is responsible for the major cross-reactive idiotype. J Immunol 146:4385–4391, 1991.
83. V Pascual, K Victor, M Spellerberg, TJ Hamblin, FK Stevenson, JD Capra. VH restriction

among human cold agglutinins: The VH4-21 gene segment is required to encode anti-I and anti-i specificities. J Immunol 149:2337–2344, 1992.

84. KN Potter, Y Li, V Pascuel, RC Williams, LA Byres, M Spellerberg, FK Stevenson, JD Capra. Molecular characterization of a cross-reactive idiotope on human immunoglobulins utilizing the V_H4-21 gene segment. J Exp Med 178:1419–1428, 1993.

85. Y Li, M Spellerberg, FK Stevenson, JD Capra, KN Potter. The I binding specificity of V_H4-34 (V_H4-21) encoded antibodies is determined by both V_H framework region 1 and complementarity determining region 3. J Mol Biol 256:577–589, 1996.

86. LE Silberstein, LC Jefferies, J Goldman, D Friedman, JS Moore, PC Nowell, D Roelcke, W Pruzanski, J Roudier, GJ Silverman. Variable region gene analysis of pathologic human autoantibodies related to the i and I red blood cell antigens. Blood 78:2372–2388, 1991.

87. FK Stevenson, C Longhurst, CJ Chapman, M Ehrenstein, MB Spellerberg, TJ Hamblin, C Ravirajan, D Isenberg. Utilization of the VH4-21 gene segment by anti-DNA antibodies from patients with SLE. J Autoimmunity 6:809–825, 1993.

88. MB Spellerberg, C Chapman, TJ Hamblin, F Stevenson. Dual recognition of lipid A and DNA by human antibodies encoded by the VH4-21 gene. A possible link between infection and lupus. Ann NY Acad Sci, 764:427–432, 1995.

89. D Crisp, W Pruzanski. B-cell neoplasms with homogenous cold-reacting antibodies (cold agglutinins). Am J Med 72:915–922, 1982.

90. T Feizi, P Wernet, HG Kunkel, SD Douglas. Lymphocytes forming red cell rosettes in the cold in patients with chronic cold agglutinin disease. Blood 42:753–762, 1973.

91. F Ishida, H Saito, K Kitano, K Kiyosawa. Cold agglutinin disease by auto-i blood type antibody associated with B cell chronic lymphocytic leukemia. Int J Hematol 67:69–73, 1998.

92. JC Huang, WG Finn, CL Goolsby, D Variakojis, LC Peterson. CD5-small B-cell leukemias are rarely classifiable as chronic lymphocytic leukemia. Am J Clin Pathol 111:123–130, 1999.

93. TJ Hamblin, Z Davis, A Gardiner, DG Oscier, GT Stevenson. Unmutated Ig V_H genes are associated with a more aggressive form of chronic lymphocytic leukemia. Blood 94:1848–1854, 1999.

94. L Lisery, F Cambazard, R Rimokh, R Ghohestani, JP Magaud, A Gaudillere, JL Perot, F Berard, A Claudy, D Guyotat, D Schmitt, C Vincent. Bullous pemphigoid associated with chronic B-cell lymphatic leukemia: the anti-230-kDa autoantibody is not synthesized by leukemia cells. Br J Dermatol 141:155–157, 1999.

95. K Sikora, J Kirkorian, R Levy. Monoclonal immunoglobulin rescued from a patient with chronic lymphocytic leukemia and autoimmune hemolytic anemia. Blood 54:513–518, 1979.

96. ZM Sthieger, D Stoeger, M Shtalrid, E Sigler, D Geltner, A Berrebi. Mechanism of autoimmune hemolytic anemia in chronic lymphocytic leukemia. Am J Hematol 43:259–264, 1993.

97. DG Efremov, M Ivanovski, N Siljanovski, G Pozzato, L Cevreska, F Fais, N Chiorazzi, FD Batista, OR Burrone. Restricted immunoglobulin V_H regopn repertoire in chronic lymphocytic leukemia patients with autoimmune hemolytic anemia. Blood 87:3869–3876, 1996.

98. A Bessudo, A Chen, LZ Rassenti, A Savin, TJ Kipps. Autoimmune hemolytic anemia in patients with chronic lymphocytic leukemia apparently is not associated with leukemia cell expression of Ig V_H 1-69 (51p1) genes (abstr 3672). Blood 90:(suppl 1:209b), 1997.

99. TJ Hamblin, Z Davies, D Oscier, F Stevenson. In chronic lymphocytic leukaemia (CLL) autoimmune haemolytic anaemia (AIHA) is not related to any particular immunoglobulin V gene usage. Br J Haematol 105:(suppl 1):88, 1999.

100. FB Lewis, RS Schwarz, W Damashek. X-irradiation and alkylating agents as possible trigger mechanisms in autoimmune complications of malignant lymphoproliferative diseases. Clin Exp Immunol 1:3–11, 1966.

101. D Catovsky, R Foa. B-cell chronic lymphocytic leukaemia. In: D Catovsky, R Foa, eds. The Lymphoid Leukaemias. London: Butterworths, 1990, pp 73–112.

102. L Thompson-Moya, T Martin, HG Heuft, A Neubaur, R Herrmann. Allergic reaction with immune hemolytic anemia arising from chlorambucil. Am J Hematol 32:230–231, 1989.

103. MM Hansen. Chronic lymphocytic leukaemia: clinical studies based on 189 cases followed for a long time. Scand J Haematol 18:(suppl 1):1–282, 1973.

104. R Fried, Y Lynfield, P Vitale, G Anhalt. Paraneoplastic pemphigus appearing as a bullous pemphigoid eruption after palliative radiation therapy. J Am Acad Dermatol 29:815–817, 1993.

105. MS Lee, S Kossard, KK Ho, RS Barnetson, RB Ravich. Paraneoplastic pemphigus triggered by radiotherapy. Austalas J Dermatol 36:206–210, 1995.

106. H Myint, JA Copplestone, J Orchard, V Craig, D Curtis, AG Prentice, MD Hamon, DG Oscier, TJ Hamblin. Fludarabine-related autoimmune haemolytic anaemia in patients with chronic lymphocytic leukaemia. Br J Haematol 91:341–344, 1995.

107. Y Bastion, B Coiffier, C Dumontet, D Espinouse, PA Bryon. Severe autoimmune hemolytic anemia in two patients treated with fludarabine for chronic lymphocytic leukemia. Ann Oncol 3:171–172, 1992.

108. F Di Raimondo, R Guistolisi, E Caccioia, S O'Broen, H Kantarjian, LB Robertson, MJ Keating. Autoimmune hemolytic anemia in chronic lymphocytic leukemia patients treated with fludarabine. Leukemia and Lymphoma. 11:63–68, 1993.

109. JC Byrd, RB Weiss, SL Kweeder, LF Deihl. Fludarabine therapy with lymphoid malignancies is associated autoimmune hemolytic anemia. Proceedings of ASCO 13:304a, 1994.

110. M Montillo, A Tedeschi, C Delfini, A Olivieri, F D'Adamo, P Leoni. Effectiveness of fludarabine in advanced B-cell chronic lymphocytic leukemia. Tumori 81:419–423, 1995.

111. JC Byrd, AA Hertler, RB Weiss, J Freiman, SL Kweder, LF Diehl. Fatal recurrence of autoimmune hemolytic anemia following pentostatin therapy in a patient with a history of fludarabine-associated hemolytic anemia. Ann Oncol 6:300–301, 1995.

112. R Maclean, D Meiklejohn, R Soutar. Fludarabine-related autoimmune haemolytic anaemia in patients with chronic lymphocytic leukaemia. Br J Haematol 92:768–769, 1996.

113. S Crozat-Grosleron, D Reynaud, S Yeche, JF Rossi, A Dubois. Fludarabine and severe autoimmune hemolytic anemia: a new case. Rev Med Interne 17:701–702, 1996.

114. G Tertian, J Cartron, C Bayle, A Rudent, T Lambert, G Tchernia. Fatal intravascular autoimmune hemolytic anemia after fludarabine treatment for chronic lymphocytic leukemia. Hematol Cell Therap 38:359–369, 1996.

115. G Longo, G Gandini, L Ferrara, U Torelli, G Emilia. Fludarabine and autoimmune hemolytic anemia in chronic lymphocytic leukemia. Eur J Haematol 59:124–125, 1997.

116. L Shvidel, M Shtarlid, A Klepfish, E Sigler, A Berrebi. Evans syndrome complicating fludarabine treatment for advanced B-CLL. Br J Haematol 99:706, 1997.

117. L Lopez, V del Villar, T Pascual. Fludarabine and fatal hemolytic anemia. Sangre (Barc) 40:335–336, 1995.

118. T Robak, M Blasinska-Morawiec, E Krykowski, A Hellmann, L Konopka. Autoimmune haemolytic anaemia in patients with chronic lymphocytic leukaemia treated with 2-chlorodeoxyadenosine (cladribine). Eur J Haematol 58:109–113, 1997.

119. S Tsiara, L Christou, P Konstantinidou, A Panteli, E Briasoulis, KL Bourantas. Severe autoimmune hemolytic anemia following fludarabine therapy in a patient with chronic lymphocytic leukemia. Am J Hematol 54:342, 1997.

120. RB Weiss, J Freiman, SL Kweder, LF Diehl, JC Byrd. Hemolytic anemia after fludarabine therapy for chronic lymphocytic leukemia. J Clin Oncol 16:1885–1889, 1998.

121. H Gonzalez, V Leblond, N Azar, L Sutton, J Gabarre, JL Binet, JP Vernant, G Dighiero. Severe autoimmune hemolytic anemia in eight patients treated with fludarabine. Hematol Cell Ther 40:113–118, 1998.

122. A Nathwani, K Nulty, K Patterson. Fatal auto-immune haemolytic anaemia in chronic lymphocytic leukaemia treated with fludarabine, A case report. CME Bull Haematol 1:59–60, 1998.

123. J Orchard, S Bolam, H Myint, DG Oscier, TJ Hamblin. In patients with lymphoid tumours recovering from the autoimmune complications of fludarabine, relapse may be triggered by conventional chemotherapy. Br J Haematol 102:1112–1113, 1998.

124. TJ Hamblin, JA Orchard, H Myint, DG Oscier. Fludarabine and hemolytic anemia in chronic lymphocytic leukemia. J Clin Oncol 16:3209, 1998.

125. HM Taha, P Narasihman, L Venkatesh, M Cawley, B Kaplan. Fludarabine-related hemolytic anemia in chronic lymphocytic leukemia and lymphoproliferative disorders. Am J Hematol 59:316, 1998.

126. DJ Vick, JC Byrd, CL Beal, DJ Chaffin. Mixed-type autoimmune hemolytic anemia following fludarabine treatment in a patient with chronic lymphocytic leukemia/small cell lymphoma. Vox Sang 74:122–126, 1998.

127. K Sen, M Kalaycio. Evan's syndrome precipitated by fludarabine therapy in a case of CLL. Am J Hematol 61:219, 1999.

128. J Sanmugarajah, G Hematillake, JM Schwartz, G Fernandez. Fludarabine (FAMP)-linked Coombs-negative hemolysis associated with CLL and mantle cell lymphoma (MCL) (abstr 3171). Blood 94:6b, 1999.

129. M Montillo, A Tedeschi, S O'Brien, S Lerner, E Morra, MJ Keating. Autoimmune phenomena against hematopoietic cells and myelosuppression in CLL treated with fludarabine-including regimens as front-line therapy IWCLL VIII workshop on CLL (abstr P091). 54, 1999.

130. M Spriano, M Clavio, F Ballerini, G Samtini, M Gobbi, E Damasio. Fludarabine plus cyclophosphamide in the treatment of previously treated CLL. IWCLL VIII workshop on CLL (abstr P114). 62, 1999.

131. M Boogaerts, A Van Hoof, D Catovsky, M Kovacs, M Montillo, SS Tura, JL Binet, W Feremans, R Marcus, E Montserrat, G Verhoet, M Klein. Treatment of alkylator resistant CLL with oral fludarabine. IWCLL VIII workshop on CLL (abstr P113). 61, 1999.

132. R Aguirre, A Anselmo, A Basso, R Bengio, F Bezares, E Bullorsky, R Campestri, L Celebrin, J Cicco, M Dragowsky, C Dufour, D Fantl, G Flores, G Garate, S Goldztein, A Huberman, J Korin, M Marquez, H Murro, E Nucifora, L Palmer, S Pavlovsky, D Pechansky, A Peiro, E Ruberto, S Rudoy, A Sanchez, N Tartas, M Zerga. A multicentre trial in CLL with fludarabine—third interim analysis. IWCLL VIII workshop on CLL (abstr P135). 70, 1999.

133. P Fenaux, JL Binet, M Leporrier, P Travade, H Piguet, C Linassier, B Desablens, B Dreyfus, CP Brizatd, B Murgue, T Russet, P Souteyrand, S Johnson, MJ Phillips, W Hiddemann, A Smith, S Roath, H Loffler, M Bjorkholm, E Osby, B Emmerich, B Coiffier, E Thiel, W Knauf, G Juliusson, R Marcus, AG Prentice, JA Copplestone, M Freund, DW Milligan, D Winfield, J Yin, KP Hellriegel, DK Hossfeld, E Kimbey, AK Burnett, TA Lister, N Lucie, L Kanz, R Lerner, C Lindemalm, A Child, T Hamblin, D Oscier, JG Smith, C Singer, A Parker, J Whittaker, P Wyld. Multicentre prospective randomised trial of fludarabine versus cyclophosphamide, doxorubicin and prednisolone (CAP) for treatment of advanced stage chronic lymphocytic leukaemia. Lancet 347:1432–1438, 1996.

134. M Leporrier, S Chevret, P Feugier, MJ Rapp, N Boudjerra, C Autrand, B Dreyfus, B Desablens, G Dighiero, Ph Travade, CI Chastang, JL Binet. Randomized comparison of fludarabine, CAP and ChOP, in 695 previously treated stage B and C chronic lymphocytic leukemia. Early stopping of CAP accrual (abstr 2357). Blood 90 (suppl 1):529a, 1997.

135. FR Mauro, F Mandelli, R Foa, S Coluzzi, R Sala, R Crescenzi, G Girelli. Autoimmune hemolytic anemia in chronic lymphocytic leukemia (CLL): A retrospective study of 55 cases (abstr 4137). Blood 90 (suppl 1):308b, 1997.

136. M Montillo, A Tedeschi, P Leoni. Recurrence of autoimmune thrombocytopenia after treatment with fludarabine in a patient with chronic lymphocytic leukemia. Leuk Lymphoma 15: 187–188, 1994.

137. JO Bay, M Fouassier, D Beal, L Alcaraz, H Cure, P Chollet, R Plagne, P Travade. Autoim-

mune thrombocytopenia after six cycles of fludarabine phosphate in a patient with chronic lymphocytic leukemia. Hematol Cell Ther 39:209–212, 1997.

138. R Hall, S Bolam, J Orchard, D Oscier, T Hamblin, H Myint. Autoimmune thrombocytopenia (ITP) following fludarabine therapy in low grade lymphoproliferative disorders. Brit J Haematol 105 (suppl 1):88a, 1999.

139. SC Stern, S Shah, C Costello. Probable autoimmune neutropenia induced by fludarabine treatment for chronic lymphocytic leukaemia. Br J Haematol 106:836–837, 1999.

140. J Antich Rojas, H Balaguer, A Cladera. Selective aplasia of the red-cell series after fludarabine administration in a patient with chronic B-cell lymphatic leukemia. Sangre (Barc) 42: 254–256, 1997.

141. M Leporier, O Reman, X Troussard. Pure red cell aplasia with fludarabine for chronic lymphocytic leukemia. Lancet 342:555, 1993.

142. A Bazarbachi, H Bachelez, L Dehen, A Delmer, R Zittoun, L Dubertret. Lethal paraneoplastic pemphigus following treatment of chronic lymphocytic leukemia with fludarabine Ann Oncol 6:730–731, 1995.

143. J Braess, K Reich, S Willert, F Strutz, C Neumann, W Hiddemann, B Wormann. Mucocutaneous autoimmune syndrome following fludarabine therapy for low-grade non-Hodgkin's lymphoma of B-cell type (B-NHL). Ann Hematol 75:227–230, 1997.

144. TJ Littlewood, C Gooplu, CC Lyon, AJ Carmichael, S Oliwiecki, A McWhannel, N Amagai, T Nishikawa, T Hashimoto, F Wojnarowska. Paraneoplastic pemhigus—an association with fludarabine (abstr 4207). Blood 92:(suppl 1):280b, 1998.

145. MP Macheta, LA Parapia, DR Gouldesbrough. Renal failure in a patient with chronic lymphocytic leukaemia treated with fludarabine J Clin Pathol 48:181–182, 1995.

146. A Tisler, A Pierratos, JH Lipton. Crescentic glomerulonephritis associated with p-ANCA positivity in fludarabine-treated chronic lymphocytic leukaemia. Nephrol Dial Transplant 11: 2306–2308, 1996.

147. RA Fleischman, D Croy. Acute onset of severe autoimmune hemolytic anemia after treatment with 2-chlorodeoxyadenosine for chronic lymphocytic leukemia. Am J Hematol 48:293, 1995.

148. RC Chasty, H Myint, DG Oscier, J Orchard, DP Busuttil, MD Hamon, AG Prentice, JA Copplesone. Autoimmune haemolysis in patients with B-CLL treated with chlorodeoxyadenosine (CDA). Leuk Lymphoma 29:391–398, 1998.

149. SH Otton, DL Turner, R Frewin, SV Davies, SA Johnson. Autoimmune thrombocytopenia after treatment with Campath 1H in a patient with chronic lymphocytic leukaemia Br J Haematol 106:261–262, 1999.

150. DH Boldt, DD Van Hoff, JG Kuhn, M Hersh. Effect on human peripheral lymphocytes of the in vivo administration of 9-β-D-arabinofuranosyl-5'-monophosphate (NSC312887) a new purine antimetabolite. Cancer Res 44:4661–4666, 1984.

151. K Rosenkrantz, B Dupont, N Flomenberg. Relevance of autocytotoxic and autoregulatory lymphocytes in the maintenance of self tolerance. Concepts Immunipathol 4:22–41, 1987.

152. EM Shevach, A Thornton, E Suri-Payer. T lymphocyte-mediated control of autoimmunity. Novartis Found Symp 215:200–211, 1998.

153. T Takahashi, Y Kuniyasu, M Toda, N Sakaguchi, M Itoh, M Iwata, J Shimizu, S. Sakaguchi. Immunologic self-tolerance maintained by CD25+ CD4+ naturally anergic and suppressive T cells: induction of autoimmune disease by breaking their anergic/suppressive state. Int Immunol 19:1969–1980, 1998.

154. AM Thornton, EM Shevach. CD4+ CD25+ immunoregulatory T cells suppress polyclonal T cell activation by inhibiting interleukin 2 production. J Exp Med 188:287–296, 1998.

155. K Winberg, R Parkman. Age, the thymus and T lymphocytes. N Engl J Med 332:182–183, 1995.

156. NE Kay. Abnormal T cell subpopulation function in CLL: excessive suppressor and deficient helper activity with respect to B cell proliferation. Blood 57:418–420, 1981.

157. G Pizzolo, M Chilosi, A Ambrozetti, A Semenzato, L Fiore-Donati, AG Peron. Immunohisto-logic study of bone marrow involvement in B chronic lymphocytic leukemia. Blood 62: 1289–1296, 1983.

158. BA Bouroncle, KP Klausen, JR Aschenbrand. Studies of the delayed response to phytohae-magglutinin (PHA) stimulated lymphocytes in 25 chronic lymphocytic leukemias before and after therapy. Blood 34:166–178, 1969.

159. T Han, ML Bloom, B Dadey, et al. Lack of autologous mixed lymphocyte reaction in patients with chronic lymphocytic leukemia: evidence for autoreactive T cell dysfunction not corre-lated with phenotype, karyotype or clinical status. Blood 60:1075–1081, 1982.

160. R Foa, D Catovsky. T lymphocyte colonies in normal blood, bone marrow and lymphoprolif-erative disorders. Clin Exp Immunol 36:488–495, 1979.

161. N Chiorazzi, S Fu, M Ghodrat, HG Kunkel, K Rai, T Gee. T cell helper defect in patients with chronic lymphocytic leukemia. J Immunol 122:1087–1090, 1979.

162. S Peller, S Kaufman. Decreased CD45RA T cells in B-cell chronic lymphatic leukemia pa-tients: correlation with disease stage. Blood 78:1569–1573, 1991.

163. W Dameshek, ZP Komninos. The present status of treatment of autoimmune hemolytic ane-mia with ACTH and cortisone. Blood 11:648–664, 1956.

164. PW Collins, AC Newland. Treatment modalities of autoimmune blood disorders. Semin Hematol 29:64–74, 1992.

165. WW Coon. Splenectomy in the treatment of hemolytic anemia. Arcg Surg 120:625–628, 1985.

166. JV Dacie. Autoimmune hemolytic anemia. Arch Intern Med 135:1293–1300, 1975.

167. G Flores, C Cunningham-Rundles, AC Newland, J Bussel. Efficacy of intravenous immuno-globulin in the treatment of autoimmune hemolytic anemia: results in 73 patients. Am J Hematol 44:237–242, 1993.

168. MA Ruess-Borst, HD Waller, CA Muller. Successful treatment of steroid resistant hemolysis in chronic lymphocytic leukemia with cuclosporine A. Am J Hematol 9:357–359, 1994.

169. MJ Guinet, KH Liew, GG Quong, IA Cooper. A study of splenic irradiation in chronic lymphocytic leukemia. Int J Rad Oncol Biol Phys 16:225–229, 1989.

170. EC Esa, PK Ray, VK Swami, A Iddiculla, JE Jr Rhoades, JG Bassett, RR Joseph, DR Cooper. Specific immunoadsorption of IgG antibody in a patient with chronic lymphocytic leukemia and autoimmune hemolytic anemia. Am J Med 71:1035–1040, 1981.

171. E Sigler, M Shtalrid, S Goland, ZM Stoeger, A Berrebi. Intractable acute autoimmune hemo-lytic anemia in B-cell chronic lymphocytic leukemia successfully treated with vincristine loaded platelet infusion. Am J Hematol 50:313–315, 1995.

172. The American Society of Hematology ITP Practice Guideline Panel. Diagnosis and treatment of idiopathic thrombocytopenic purpura: recommendations of the American Society of He-matology. Ann Intern Med 126:319–326, 1997.

173. R McMillan. Therapy for adults with refractory chronic immune thrombocytopenic purpura. Ann Intern Med 126:307–314, 1997.

174. YS Ahn, WJ Harrington, R Mylvagnam, LM Allen, LM Pall. Slow infusion of vinca alkaloids in the treatment of idiopathic thrombocytopenic purpura. Ann Intern Med 100:192–196, 1984.

175. MA Baumann, JE Menitove, RH Aster, T Anderson. Urgent treatment of idiopathic thrombo-cytopenic purpura with single dose gammaglobulin infusion followed by platelet transfusion. Ann Intern Med 104:808–809, 1986.

176. S Tosti, R Caruso, F D'Adamo, A Picardi, M Ali-Ege, G Girelli, FR Mauro, L Marillo, S Amadori. Severe autoimmune hemolytic anemia in a patient with chronic lymphocytic leuke-mia responsive to fludarabine responsive treatment. Ann Hematol 65:238–239, 1992.

177. C Pott-Hoeck, W Hiddemann. Purine analogues in the treatment of low grade lymphomas and chronic lymphocytic leukemias. Ann Hematol 6:421–433, 1995.

178. F Meir, K Sonnichsen, G Schaumburg-Lever, R Dopfer, G Rassner. Epidermolysis bullosa

acquisita: efficiency of high dose intravenous immunoglobulins. J Am Acad Dermatol 29:
334–337, 1993.

179. C Mohr, C Sunderkottewr, A Hildebrand, K Biel, A Rutter, G Rutter, T Luger, G Kolde.
      Successful treatment of epidermolysis bullosa acquisita using intravenous immunoglobulins.
      Br J Dermatol 132:824–826, 1995.

180. JB Levy, CD Pusey. Still a role for plasma exchange in rapidly progressive glomerulonephri-
      tis? J Nephrol 10:7–13, 1997.

181. SN Marcovic, DJ Inwards, EA Frigas, RP Phyliky. Acquired C1 esterase inhibitor deficiency.
      Ann Intern Med 132:144–150, 2000.

21

Richter's Syndrome

JOHN SEYMOUR and JANINE CAMPBELL

Peter MacCallum Cancer Institute, East Melbourne, Victoria, Australia

I. HISTORY AND INTRODUCTION

The use of the term "Richter's syndrome" to denote the secondary development of a histologically aggressive lymphoid malignancy in a patient with preexisting chronic lymphocytic leukemia (CLL) is relatively recent. The first use of the term is attributed to Lortholary et al. (1) in their 1964 publication, although Richter's original description of the simultaneous occurrence of a "reticulum-cell sarcoma" and CLL in a 46-year-old male shipping clerk was published 36 years earlier in 1928 (2). Since this initial description, the issue of chance occurrence versus clonal progression of the underlying CLL has been debated with only recent resolution being obtained.

Although the term was initially restricted in its application to the development of a large-cell lymphoma, the spectrum of secondary lymphoid malignancies complicating CLL has expanded in recent years to now include prolymphocytic leukemia (PLL), Hodgkin's disease (HD), acute lymphoblastic leukemia (ALL), and multiple myeloma (Table 1). The term "Richter's syndrome" can equally justifiably be applied to these disorders, although such an expanded use does then require an additional descriptor in these rarer subtypes; for example, "Richter's syndrome of Hodgkin's disease type." Rarely, patients with CLL may be noted to have features of other indolent lymphoid malignancies develop, such as hairy-cell leukemia, Waldenström's macroglobulinemia, or follicular lymphoma, but these associations have not been adequately studied in a sufficient number of patients to justify consideration of clonal relatedness and will not be considered further.

The clinical features, histological types, incidence, treatment options, and pathogenesis of this spectrum of diseases now encompassed within the term "Richter's syndrome" will be reviewed and discussed in the context of our current understanding of clonal evolu-

Table 1 Entities Considered To Be Covered by the Term
"Richter's Syndrome" and Their Relative Frequency

Entity	Relative frequency (%)
Diffuse large-cell lymphoma	65–70
Hodgkin's disease	15
Prolymphocytic leukemia	15–20
Acute lymphoblastic leukemia	<1
Multiple myeloma	<1

See text for references.

tion and the role of immunosuppression in the development and progression of lymphoid malignancies.

II. CLINICAL, LABORATORY, AND RADIOLOGICAL FEATURES

In the past, histological confirmation of the development of Richter's syndrome was often only sought in the setting of a significant change in the apparent natural history of the underlying CLL. This practice can tend to create a self-perpetuating situation, in which such circumstances may then be considered to be the only context in which a risk of such transformation can occur. Unfortunately, the available large autopsy series of patients with CLL does not distinguish the histological features of involved sites (3,4) and so cannot yield information on the frequency of clinically unsuspected transformation. The more recent practice of obtaining repeat biopsy specimens of discordantly responding sites or dominant disease sites at relapse is likely to provide a more representative profile of the clinical manifestations of this syndrome, as well as a more accurate estimate of its true incidence.

A. Non-Hodgkin's Lymphoma

The development of diffuse large-cell lymphoma either during the course of the underlying CLL, or at the time of diagnosis, is the most frequently reported form of Richter's syndrome, constituting 67% of all transformation events in the U.S. Intergroup study cohort (5). The clinical features at the time of recognition have been similar across the larger reviews and series (Table 2) (6–11). Trump et al. (10) described five of their own cases from Johns Hopkins in 1980 and thoroughly reviewed the features of 41 previously reported cases of Richter's syndrome. They found a male/female ratio of 2:1, a median interval of 24 months from the diagnosis of CLL, fever in 65%, rapidly progressive adenopathy in 46%, weight loss in 29%, and abdominal pain in 26% of patients. Some earlier case reports had noted the phenomenon of a progressive reduction in lymphocyte counts preceding transformation (12), but this has not been confirmed to be a reproducible feature (10). Later series have described a less dominant male preponderance of 1.3:1 (6,8,9,11), more closely reflecting the gender ratio seen in uncomplicated CLL, but the other features noted in this early review have not changed substantially. From the largest published series of 39 patients by Robertson et al. from M. D. Anderson (11), the median time from diagnosis of CLL was 48 months, with progressive lymphadenopathy noted in 64%, the systemic symptoms of fever and weight loss in 54%, and a symptomatic abdominal mass evident in 23%. Extranodal manifestations of lymphoma were common, occurring in 38% of pa-

Table 2 Clinical and Laboratory Features of Patients with
Richter's Syndrome of Large-Cell Lymphoma Type

Entity	Relative frequency
Median interval from diagnosis of CLL	24–48 mo
Fever ± weight loss	50–65%
Progressive lymphadenopathy	50–65%
Symptomatic abdominal mass	20–30%
Involvement of extranodal sites	30–40%
Elevated serum LDH ($\geq 2 \times$ ULN)	80%
Hypercalcemia	~5%
Median survival	2–5 mo

See text for references.

tients, with involved sites including the pleura, oropharynx, skin, gastrointestinal tract, bone, and pulmonary parenchyma. Ott and co-workers (13) described localized gastric diffuse large cell lymphoma in three patients with CLL, with molecular evidence for independent clonal origin of the lymphoma in each case. *Helicobacter pylori* was detected in the gastric mucosa in each instance, although the role that this may have played in the development of the lymphoma was not discussed. Other sites of extranodal involvement described in other series include liver, spleen, and peritoneum (6,8,14–16). Other unusual manifestations reported include isolated cutaneous lymphomatous deposits (17) and central nervous system involvement (11,18–20), although other possible causes for such neurological symptoms need to be considered, including opportunistic infections and progressive multifocal leukoencepahalopathy (21).

Laboratory abnormalities associated with the development of aggressive NHL are also common; approximately 80% of patients have marked elevations of serum LDH disproportionate to that anticipated in uncomplicated CLL in the absence of hemolysis (11). Serum or urine paraproteins are found in a significant minority of patients (~40%), but this frequency does not appear to differ from a well-studied population of patients with uncomplicated CLL (22). Hypercalcemia has been reported to herald the onset of transformation (6,23,24), because this complication is extremely uncommon in uncomplicated CLL (25), in contrast to its frequency of up to 15% in patients with NHL (26).

Hematological disorders including anemia, neutropenia, and thrombocytopenia have been described in varying frequencies in the preceding series, but no evidence exists that these features are any more frequent than could be attributed to the extent of the underlying CLL. Robertson et al. (11), noted a median CD4+ T-lymphocyte count of 224/μL at the time of transformation in their series but it is unknown whether this differs from that which would be found in a similar group of heavily pretreated patients in the absence of histological transformation.

In a number of cases, it has been difficult to accurately stage the lymphomatous component of the disease separate from that of the CLL, but localized transformation appears to be relatively uncommon with just 16% of cases in one series having stage I/II disease (8) and a similar low frequency in the M. D. Anderson series (11).

The investigation of a patient with symptoms suggestive of transformation of their CLL should begin with a thorough clinical examination, the processing of appropriate microbiological samples to exclude possible opportunistic or occult infections (this should incorporate formal consultation with an infectious diseases specialist experienced in the field), and structural imaging such as computed tomography (CT) or ultrasonography. As with other investigators (27), we have found functional imaging with high-dose gallium-67 citrate scanning to be useful in recognizing differential uptake by areas involved by transformed disease, and positron emission tomography (PET) scanning may also be similarly useful. Although the presence of symptoms or suggestive radiological findings may be suspicious for transformation, a tissue biopsy specimen should always be obtained before specific therapy is instituted.

B. Prolymphocytic Leukemia

In 1978, Enno and colleagues described seven patients with CLL in whom a progressive rise in circulating prolymphocytes occurred and was accompanied by increasing refractoriness to treatment (28). This was followed in the mid-1980s by a series of carefully documented studies by Melo, Catovsky, and Galton, which further examined the relationship between CLL and PLL and provided a rational basis for the classification of CLL, PLL, and CLL in prolymphocytic transformation (CLL/PLL) (29–31).

   The usually insidious onset of prolymphocytic transformation of CLL contrasts with the relatively abrupt onset of the syndrome in most patients with "Richter's syndrome" of DLCL type described earlier (Table 3). As with other forms of Richter's syndrome, the development of PLL is likely to be underreported, because the very careful morphological study of Melo et al. (29) found a significant proportion of prolymphocytes in 15% of cases. Few publications have specifically dealt with this manifestation of Richter's syndrome (32–36), but even with relatively short follow-up, the U.S. Intergroup study (CALGB 9011) suggests that PLL develops in 2% of all CLL patients and may comprise as much as 20% of all forms of Richter's syndrome (5). The median time to development was 14.8 months, although the maximum follow-up of the whole cohort was only ~5 years. Thus, this figure is somewhat earlier than the few published series (32–36), in which the median time to development of PLL was 24 to 36 months.

   The most frequent clinical features associated with transformation are dominant splenomegaly with an increasing rate of rise of the peripheral lymphocyte count and, by definition, an increased proportion of prolymphocytes. These resemble the clinical features of de novo B-cell PLL. Lymphadenopathy is usually moderate in extent. Serum LDH may

Table 3   Clinical and Laboratory Features of Patients with Richter's Syndrome of Prolymphocytic Type

Entity	Relative frequency
Median interval from diagnosis of CLL	24–36 mo
Insidious disease progression	>75%
Systemic symptoms	~30%
Dominant splenomegaly	~65%
Progressive adenopathy	~35%
Involvement of extra-nodal sites	? relatively uncommon
Elevated serum LDH ($\geq 2 \times$ ULN)	? probably common
Hypercalcemia	Rare
Median survival	6–12 mo

Figures are estimates based on available data, see text for references.

be elevated (36), and as with other forms of Richter's syndrome B-symptoms are present in ~30% (33) and hypercalcemia may rarely be encountered (36). The almost universal presence of splenomegaly in patients with both CLL/PLL and PLL has led to the suggestion that the site of origin of the prolymphocyte is the spleen (29). This remains unsubstantiated, and we have anecdotally seen instances of prolymphocytic transformation of CLL in patients who have undergone prior splenectomy (unpublished observations).

C. Hodgkin's Disease

Hodgkin's disease is one of the most frequent "second malignancies" in patients with CLL. Travis et al. (37) reported a relative risk of 7.69. Although some early reports of "Richter's syndrome" included some cases of Hodgkin's disease (1), the features of these patients having Hodgkin's disease develop in the setting of underlying CLL have only more recently begun to be scrutinized (Table 4). From the U.S. Intergroup study described earlier, just 1% of all CLL patients have Hodgkin's disease develop, and these constituted 15% of all cases of Richter's syndrome. From a summary of the larger recent series (38–42) describing 28 cases (Table 4), the median age at diagnosis of Hodgkin's disease was 65 years (range, 51–83), and 82% of cases were among men. Five of the 28 cases were recognized at the time of diagnosis of the CLL, and overall the median time from diagnosis of CLL to Hodgkin's disease was similar to other forms of histological transformation at 44 months (up to 180 months). The Hodgkin's disease tended to be quite widespread when recognized, with 13 of 15 adequately staged patients having disseminated disease (stage III/IV). Quite characteristically, persistent unexplained high fevers, often with significant weight loss, were present in 55% of cases, and many patients manifest progressive generalized adenopathy. In the M. D. Anderson series, two of seven cases had the new onset of autoimmune hemolytic anemia as part of their presentation of Hodgkin's disease (40).

D. Myeloma and Acute Lymphoblastic Leukemia

The available reports of the few patients described who had myeloma develop (43,44) suggest that the underlying features of the myeloma may differ from those of de novo myeloma. In the largest published series of such cases, Brouet et al. (43) performed a retrospective analysis of the clinical and laboratory features of 11 patients with CLL and multiple myeloma. CLL preceded the development of myeloma by 2 to 15 years in six cases and was diagnosed simultaneously in the remaining five patients. Extraosseus

Table 4 Clinical and Laboratory Features of Patients with Richter's Syndrome of Hodgkin's Disease Type

Entity	Relative frequency
Median interval from diagnosis of CLL	44 mo
Progressive adenopathy	50–75%
Dominant splenomegaly	10–20%
Systemic symptoms	~60%
Autoimmune hemolytic anemia	~10%
Median survival	13 mo

Figures are estimates based on available data, see text for references.

involvement by the myeloma occurred in six patients, and B symptoms were observed in another five. Conversely, no specific features seem to distinguish secondary ALL in patients with CLL from de novo disease.

III. THE CONCEPT OF CLONAL EVOLUTION

In immature B cells, the immunoglobulin heavy and light chain genes exist in a germline configuration. As the cells mature, these genes are rearranged, beginning with the IgH gene. This is followed by rearrangement of the κ light chain gene; if this cannot successfully be accomplished, the λ light chain gene then undergoes rearrangement. The ordered nature of these recombination events allows the point at which a clonal population of cells emerges to be determined and provides a means of identifying the degree of clonal relatedness between different cells. The degree of homology between clonally related cells should then vary, according to the point at which the clonal population develops. A number of different methods have been used to examine the clonal relatedness of CLL and Richter's syndrome, including comparison of immunoglobulin heavy and light chain isotypes and determination of immunoglobulin idiotypes (45,46). More recently, cytogenetics, detection, and comparison of immunoglobulin gene rearrangements and direct sequencing of immunoglobulin heavy chain genes have also been used (45,46). The results of these approaches as they have been applied to exploring the potential clonal relatedness of the phenotypically distinct lymphoid populations in patients with CLL complicated by "Richter's syndrome" are summarized in the following.

A. Immunoglobulin Isotypes

Concordance between the immunoglobulin isotypes of CLL cells and NHL cells in Richter's syndrome is consistent with but is insufficient to prove their common clonal origin. Data from "sporadic" lymphoid malignancies across the population generally have established that most B-CLL and NHL cells demonstrate a μ/κ isotype (47), so that the finding of a concordant isotype among CLL and NHL cells in a single patient is still likely to have occurred by chance. Conversely, the demonstration of discordant immunoglobulin isotypes does not exclude the possibility of clonal relatedness, because CLL and NHL cells with identical IgH gene rearrangements may express different light chains (48,49). Similarly, postrearrangement modifications of IgH genes may result in different IgH isotypes in cells that can be shown to be clonally related (50). Analysis of light chain rearrangements are useful in this regard because postrearrangement mutations are much less likely to occur (50). Finally, although the use of large panels of monoclonal antibodies for immunophenotyping may be more reliable than the use of immunoglobulin isotypes alone in determining clonal relatedness, this method can indicate only whether the two populations are of the same cell lineage and developmental stage but not of the same clonal origin (50).

B. Idiotype

The observation that the cells in CLL and Richter's syndrome share a common idiotype provides more conclusive evidence of clonal relatedness between the two cell populations. This approach has been used to support the clonal evolution of multiple myeloma from CLL (43,51) and to confirm the clonal origin of Richter's syndrome in a patient with discordant immunophenotypical features but identical IgH gene rearrangement (16). However, this method is time consuming and labor intensive, and care must be exercised when interpreting the results of idiotype analysis, because cross-reactivity between anti-idiotype antibodies directed against B-CLL and B cell lymphomas may occur (52).

C. Cytogenetics

The use of various mitogens to induce cell division has increased the number of cases of CLL in which cytogenetic analysis is possible. In general, the cytogenetic abnormalities commonly seen in CLL are uncommonly encountered in NHL, multiple myeloma, or ALL (see Chapter 16). The demonstration of identical cytogenetic abnormalities in CLL and Richter's syndrome cells is therefore relatively reliable evidence that the two populations of cells are clonally related. This approach was used by Koduru et al. (53), who observed secondary, tertiary, and quaternary cytogenetic evolution in specimens obtained from a patient during the transformation from CLL to diffuse large cell lymphoma, and by Nakamine et al. (49), who observed trisomy 12 in both cell populations in a similar case of Richter's syndrome.

D. Immunoglobulin Gene Rearrangements

Detection of clonal immunoglobulin gene rearrangements by Southern blotting is currently the most frequently applied means of examining the clonal origins of Richter's syndrome. Identical immunoglobulin heavy and/or light chain rearrangements in CLL and Richter's syndrome cell populations have been reported in a number of cases, including transformation of CLL to NHL, Hodgkin's disease, and multiple myeloma (50,53–59). This approach has also been used to demonstrate the independent origin of diffuse large cell lymphoma in several patients with CLL (14,15,60), suggesting that the pathogenesis of Richter's syndrome is a heterogeneous process. Although this method provides a valuable tool for the investigation of clonality in Richter's syndrome, it is subject to a number of limitations, reviewed by Foon et al. (45) and Bessudo and Kipps (46). A clonal Ig gene rearrangement may not be detected if the clonal population comprises fewer than 5% of the cells tested. Somatic mutations, random nucleotide insertions or imprecise joining of immunoglobulin gene segments may alter restriction enzyme cleavage sites and change the pattern of bands seen on the Southern blot. If the clonal event occurred at a very early stage of B cell maturation (early pro-B cell), different Ig rearrangements may be detected despite the common origin of the two cell populations (60). Because analysis of the genetic relatedness between CLL and the subsequent transformation to Richter's syndrome is largely limited to case reports, the frequency and significance of such events is unclear. However, in a small number of carefully studied cases, Matolcsy and colleagues (56,60,61) have provided evidence that somatic mutation of IgH genes in most cases of CLL/SLL is a relatively uncommon event (see Chapter 5).

E. Frequency of Clonal Relatedness

It is apparent from the studies cited earlier that Richter's syndrome may arise either from the same clonal population as the antecedent CLL or as an independent second malignancy. In their review of 27 cases of Richter's syndrome examined for IgH rearrangement, Bessudo and Kipps (46) reported evidence for a common clonal origin of the CLL and lymphoma in 22 patients (81%). This proportion is supported by the data of Matolcsy and coworkers who used direct nucleic acid sequencing of the unique complementary determinant region 3 (CDR3) of the lgH gene to demonstrate clonal evolution of DLCL from CLL/SLL in seven of nine cases (78%), including one case with disparate lgH gene rearrangements (56,60,61). In two of their nine cases, the CDR3 sequence differed in the CLL and DLCL cell populations, indicating their independent clonal origins. In summary, it therefore appears that approximately three quarters of cases of Richter's syndrome occur as a consequence of clonal evolution from the initial original CLL cells.

IV. HISTOLOGICAL SUBTYPES OF RICHTER'S SYNDROME

A. Non-Hodgkin's Lymphoma

The transformation from CLL to a histologically aggressive NHL is the most common manifestation of Richter's syndrome. In most cases, the histopathology is that of diffuse large B-cell lymphoma; however, transformation to pleomorphic or "high-grade" lymphomas as well as T-cell lymphomas has also been described. Subsequent development of diffuse large-cell lymphoma is reported to occur in approximately 3% to 5% of patients with CLL (6,11) and accounted for 76% of cases of Richter's syndrome in one study (8). The cells are large, moderately irregular or round, with vesicular nuclei, prominent nucleoli and a moderate amount of cytoplasm (6,8,46). In some cases, a more pleomorphic cell population is observed and can be intimately admixed with the background CLL cells (6,8,46). The lymph node may be totally effaced by large cell lymphoma or CLL, and DLCL may coexist as a composite lymphoma in the same specimen.

Detailed immunophenotypical studies using contemporary antibody panels that compare antigen expression profiles of the CLL cells, and their transformed NHL counterparts are largely limited to case reports. However, evidence suggests that in some cases the transformed cells essentially retain their original immunophenotype (48,50,56), whereas in others differential antigen expression is noted (15,16,18). As discussed in detail earlier, although immunophenotypical concordance may support a common clonal origin of two cell populations; on its own it is insufficient proof that such a relationship exists. The possible relationship of such transformed lymphomas to the recently described entity of de novo CD5+ large B-cell lymphoma is unclear, but the two disorders appear to be distinct (62,63).

1. High-grade NHL

Rarely, CLL has been observed to transform to a high-grade B-cell lymphoma of either Burkitt's or lymphoblastic type. In a case described by Litz et al. (64) and Estrov et al. (65), mature B-cell blastic transformation of Burkitt's type with cytogenetic abnormalities involving the *myc* locus were diagnosed in two patients with prior CLL. In the first case (64), both the CLL and transformed tumor cells were CD10 negative, and in the second case (65) the Burkitt cells were CD5+. Both of these immunophenotypical features are somewhat unusual for Burkitt's lymphoma and provide circumstantial support for the suggestion of a common clonal origin of the two tumors. Similarly, evidence of the clonal relatedness of the underlying CLL and Burkitt's cells was provided by the finding of identical immunoglobulin gene rearrangements by Klepfish et al. (66), although in this case the Burkitt cells lacked any clear cytogenetic abnormality involving the *c-myc* locus. In another case report, lymphoblastic lymphoma occurred in a patient with CLL (67). The two cell populations demonstrated discordant expression of CD5 but identical karyotypic abnormalities, again suggesting clonal evolution of CLL to a high-grade lymphoma.

2. T-cell NHL

Another rare manifestation of Richter's syndrome is the development of a T-cell lympho-proliferative disorder. Cutaneous T-cell lymphoma, pleomorphic T-cell lymphoma, diffuse large T-cell lymphoma, T-cell anaplastic large cell lymphoma, and T-cell immunoblastic lymphoma have all been reported (68–72). In our own institution we have treated a patient with B-CLL who had peripheral T-cell lymphoma and hemophagocytic syndrome develop (unpublished observation). Although currently no evidence to supports the contention that these T-cell tumors are clonally related to the B-CLL, it is theoretically possible that a single defect at the lymphoid stem cell level could result in the development of both T- and B-cell malignant proliferation.

No clinical or laboratory features seem to be able to distinguish between patients with B-, versus T-lineage DLCL complicating CLL. Although the number of cases is small, the outlook for those patients with T-cell DLCL as their manifestation of Richter's syndrome appears to be even more grim than for those with B-cell disease.

B. Prolymphocytic Leukemia

The prolymphocyte is morphologically identified by its large size, round nucleus, prominent single nucleolus, condensed nuclear chromatin, and intermediate nuclear/cytoplasmic ratio (29,73). Patients with <10% circulating prolymphocytes are classified as having "typical" CLL, whereas those with >55% prolymphocytes are defined as having PLL. Patients with the composite entity CLL/PLL occupy an intermediate position (11% to 55% prolymphocytes), sharing features of each condition (29,73). The immunophenotypic features of CLL/PLL may vary, with approximately two thirds showing the CD5+, FMC7−, weak slg-staining profile of typical CLL, and one third demonstrating the CD5−, FMC7+, strong slg-staining profile characteristic of PLL (73).

C. Hodgkin's Disease

The pathological features of Hodgkin's variant of Richter's syndrome can be broadly divided into two groups. In the first group, Reed-Sternberg–like cells are present within a background of CLL. In the second, the appearances are those of typical Hodgkin's disease (59).

The presence of Reed-Sternberg–like cells in otherwise typical CLL is a well-documented phenomenon (8,58,74) and until recently was considered to be of uncertain significance. It now appears that the Reed-Sternberg–like cells in CLL can at times herald a transformation to frank Hodgkin's disease and that this process may be mediated by Epstein-Barr virus (EBV) (41,42,58,59,74). The evidence regarding the role of EBV in the pathogenesis of Hodgkin's variant Richter's syndrome is discussed in the following.

Momose and colleagues have described 13 cases of Reed-Sternberg–like cells in CLL (58). In five cases, the Reed-Sternberg–like cells were CD20 positive and CD15 negative. In two cases, CD20 and CD15 were coexpressed, whereas in six cases the cells were CD15 positive and CD20 negative. Three patients in the latter group subsequently had disseminated Hodgkin's disease develop. Similar findings were reported by Williams et al. (74) and Ohno et al. (59) in three additional patients with Hodgkin's variant Richter's syndrome.

Now increasing molecular evidence exists for the clonal relatedness of CLL and Hodgkin's variant Richter's syndrome. The initial report of two cases by Ohno et al. (59)

described sequencing of the hypervariable region of the lgH gene, which demonstrated that the Reed-Sternberg cells were derived from the CLL clone. Similarly, identical immunoglobulin V-region gene rearrangements were found in one of three patients in a second study (75).

Taken together, these results support the contention that Reed-Sternberg–like cells are clonally derived from the CLL population and that expression of a typical Reed-Sternberg cell immunophenotype may predispose to the development of fully fledged Hodgkin's disease.

All subtypes of classical Hodgkin's disease have been reported, with mixed cellularity and nodular sclerosing Hodgkin's disease occurring in approximately 60% and 25% of published cases, respectively (40–42,76). Nodular lymphocyte-predominant Hodgkin's disease has also been reported, including one case in which diffuse large cell lymphoma later developed (41). Another patient is described who had both DLCL and nodular sclerosing Hodgkin's disease develop simultaneously 3 years after the diagnosis of CLL (77), although no information on the possible clonal relatedness of these three malignant clones was available.

D. Acute Leukemia

The development of acute leukemia in patients with CLL is a rare but well-recognized phenomenon. Such cases were initially attributed to the use of radioactive phosphorous and/or radiation in the treatment of the underlying disease, although instances of blastic transformation of CLL in patients who had received little or no therapy for their CLL were also reported (78,79). In an early, but well-researched, review of the literature, Zarrabi et al. (78) identified 31 cases of acute leukemia in patients with CLL. Of the 20 cases in which the lineage of the transformed cells was documented, 10 were of lymphoid and 7 were of myeloid origin.

The development of acute myeloid leukemia has generally been assumed to be either secondary to the use of mutagens in the treatment of CLL or to a chance occurrence. In contrast, immunophenotypical, cytogenetic, and molecular evidence from a small number of case reports suggests that acute B cell lymphoblastic leukemia may very rarely arise as a consequence of clonal evolution (65,80–82), with a total of approximately 15 well-documented cases reported. We have also had a case of pre-B ALL developing after a 13-year history of CLL but have no data available to confirm the clonal relatedness of the two diseases in this instance (unpublished observations). Acute T-cell lymphoblastic leukemia has also been reported in patients with B-CLL (80,83). In these cases a lineage switch at the level of the common lymphoid progenitor has been proposed in an attempt to explain the anomalous development of a T-cell malignancy from a B-cell clone, although currently no objective evidence supports this assertion, and the development of a clonally unrelated disorder is more likely.

The development of ALL is usually a late event in the natural history of CLL, but three instances of simultaneous diagnosis of both disorders have been reported and should be considered where apparently dimorphic features are seen in patients with ALL (65).

E. Multiple Myeloma

The observation that phorbol ester can induce B-CLL cells to differentiate into plasma cells (84) raises the possibility that the rare cases of multiple myeloma reported in patients with CLL may potentially have occurred as a consequence of clonal evolution from the leukemic cell population. As discussed earlier, analysis of immunoglobulin heavy and light chain isotypes provides insufficient evidence to determine the clonal relatedness of two B cell populations. This is illustrated by Brouet et al. (43), who reported different immunoglobulin idiotypes despite identical immunoglobulin light chain isotypes in two patients with CLL and multiple myeloma. In contrast, identical idiotypes were demonstrated in a patient whose CLL and myeloma cells showed discordant immunoglobulin heavy chain expression (51). Studies using immunoglobulin gene rearrangements as a marker of clonality have provided evidence that both supports (57) and refutes (85) a shared clonal origin of multiple myeloma in CLL patients. It is therefore probable that, like NHL, the pathogenesis of multiple myeloma in these patients is a heterogeneous process.

V. INCIDENCE, RISK FACTORS, AND EPIDEMIOLOGY

The earliest series of Richter's syndrome usually suggested an overall incidence rate of 3% to 5.4% among CLL patients (6,9,11), but with more careful scrutiny of relapsing patients, the incidence may be somewhat higher. More recent series have cited estimated cumulative incidence rates of 8% (86), ~10% (87), and 19% (88). Within the largest prospectively analyzed cohort, the 544 U.S. Intergroup study patients, there has been an incidence of transformation of just less than 1% (5), but this is certain to increase in the future, because the median follow-up of the cohort is currently less than 5 years, and more mature data (88) suggest a median time to development of just less than 10 years with an apparently consistent rate through until 20 years after diagnosis.

Many investigators consider the development of Richter's syndrome to be a random or stochastic event with a relatively consistent rate throughout the natural history of the underlying CLL. This is consistent with the observations of the Amiens group cited earlier (88) and is also consistent with the approximately 10% of instances of Richter's syndrome that are diagnosed coincidentally with the recognition of the CLL. In a number of ways this model parallels the paradigm for the development of an accelerated or blastic phase of CML. Using this same analogy, it may be hoped that the risk of transformation may be reduced by the application of therapies that are able to attain durable molecular suppression of the underlying CLL clone. The confirmation of this hypothesis awaits the development of such therapies. However, the emerging data suggesting a role for immunosuppression in the development of at least a portion of instances of Richter's transformation (discussed later) need to be incorporated into such a model, and it may be more accurate to consider two separate pathways, a dominant stochastic path and a less frequent immunosuppression-dependent path. The relative proportion of these two modes of transformation may vary depending on the treatments used.

No recognized risk factors are predictive of the development of subsequent transformation in patients with CLL. The initial mode of treatment does not appear to alter the risk (5), but one group has suggested that patients with more aggressive disease requiring the subsequent use of nucleoside analogs may have a greater risk (87,88). Conversely, the analysis of the patients from M. D. Anderson did not find any increased risk among those patients treated with fludarabine or 2-CdA (11). Initial disease stage, age, or gender are not predictive (5). It will be of great interest in the future to determine whether the distinction between cases of CLL with or without somatic hypermutation of the IgH genes is associated with a differential risk of subsequent histological transformation (89,90), as suggested by the preliminary work of Aoki et al. (127).

VI. TREATMENT OPTIONS AND PROGNOSIS

A. Non-Hodgkin's Lymphoma

The available series has most frequently described the use of anthracycline-based combination chemotherapy such as CHOP after the recognition of histologically aggressive NHL (6–10,91). However, in these series, up to 20% of patients have not been treated, presumably because of severe debilitation at the time of diagnosis. With such therapies, approximately 40% of patients will obtain an objective response (11), but these responses are transient, with reported median survival figures remarkably consistent at 2 to 5 months (6–8,10,11). The small series of seven patients from Yugoslavia (9) is somewhat more optimistic, with three patients surviving at 32+, 36+, and 120+ months, which they attribute to the use of more intensive chemotherapy containing both ara-C and methotrexate. The largest series of Robertson et al. had only one of 39 patients alive beyond 2 years despite the use of MACOP-B or DHAP therapy in a significant proportion of cases (11).

This dismal outlook with standard large-cell lymphoma therapies has led the M. D. Anderson investigators to explore the usefulness of specifically designed regimens in patients with Richter's syndrome. The first report described results with fludarabine-based combination therapies coupled with either cisplatin/ara-C or cyclophosphamide/ara-C based on the known capacity of fludarabine to potentiate the cytotoxicity of both these DNA-damaging agents (92). A total of 12 patients were treated (six with each regimen), one died from complications of therapy (8%), and 5 of 11 evaluable patients responded (45%), without differences evident between the regimens (128). Median survival was 17 months, which appeared superior to the historical experience of 5.1 months from the institution with conventional therapies (11).

Subsequently, they have modified the successful ALL regimen on the basis of the delivery of fractionated doses of the alkylating agent (HyperCVAD) (93) by substituting liposomal daunorubicin for adriamycin (94). This regimen was associated with significant myelosuppression, moderate infectious complications, but a 24% treatment-related death rate among a group of 29 patients. Despite the difficulties of safely delivering the therapy, efficacy was noteworthy, with an overall response rate of 34% (31% CR). Although follow-up was short, there had been no relapses observed among the CR patients at 12 months. Although associated with significant toxicity in such a poor prognosis group of patients, such aggressive therapies may be justifiable in selected patients, given the uniformly dismal outlook of the underlying disease. Obviously, means to improve the tolerance of such therapies are needed. There are no other available studies of specific therapies targeting patients with Richter's syndrome. The anti-B-cell monoclonal antibodies (naked and conjugated) would be appropriate components to consider integrating into future therapeutic strategies. Allogenic transplantation also shows some promise in preliminary studies (129).

As discussed earlier, transformed disease is usually widespread at the time of recognition. In such circumstances radiation therapy has no major role when the goal of treatment is durable systemic disease control. However, its local application can provide palliative benefit if individual nodal masses or extranodal disease sites are symptomatic. No accurate data are available on the level of CNS risk in patients with Richter's syndrome, although anecdotal reports clearly demonstrate the risk is present (18,19), and the series of Robertson et al. (11) noted CNS involvement at diagnosis in 13% of patients. Given the dominant risk of systemic failure in most cases, it may be reasonable to reserve CNS prophylaxis for those patients believed to be at high risk on the basis of conventional predictive indices (95) who attain a systemic CR with their initial treatment.

B. Prolymphocytic Leukemia

No studies specifically examine the efficacy of various treatments for PLL arising from CLL, but it is clear that alkylator-based therapies in conventional doses are inadequate with a median survival of approximately 6 to 12 months described (32–34,36). Of note, there is a single report of a patient treated with high-dose ara-C and an anthracycline who responded well and survived for 3.5 years, suggesting that there may be benefit in intensifying conventional chemotherapy agents. Most investigators would now attempt to use allogeneic-transplant–based therapies (conventional or nonmyeloablative) given the grim outlook with established therapies and the likelihood of preservation of the ''graft-versus-leukemia'' effect. In the absence of such options, nucleoside analog-based combination strategies as proposed for high-risk CLL or de novo PLL are most promising.

C. Hodgkin's Disease

The natural history and optimal treatment of Hodgkin's-type Richter's syndrome is difficult to determine, because the literature is limited to case reports and small series. Most reports have used conventional Hodgkin's-type combination chemotherapy (MOPP, ABVD, or variants thereof), and there are no prospective studies to guide decision making. When disease has been localized, radiation therapy has usually been incorporated into treatment strategies.

To explore the outlook for these patients, the features of 28 patients from recent series have been extracted and analyzed (38–42). Patients with CLL and Hodgkin's disease appear to be first seen at a more advanced stage but are also more resistant to therapy and die more quickly than those with de novo Hodgkin's disease. The summary of outcomes from these series (Figure 1) reveals a median survival of 13 months, which is also

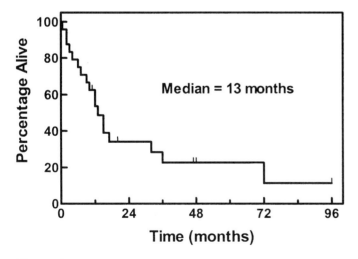

Figure 1   Overall survival of 28 patients with Richter's syndrome of Hodgkin's disease type. (Compiled from Refs. 38–42.)

consistent with the smaller individual reports of Fayad (40) and Brecher (42). However, although these patients have poor survival compared with those with de novo Hodgkin's disease, it remains considerably better than the dismal prognosis typically afforded to those with non-Hodgkin's Richter's syndrome; there are 34% ± 10% of patients surviving beyond 2 years. Also it is unclear whether this adverse outlook is an inherent biological property of the Hodgkin's disease developing in these patients or simply reflects the adverse consequences of delayed diagnosis. We have recent experience of a patient with Hodgkin's-type Richter's transformation who successfully underwent a matched unrelated myeloablative bone-marrow transplant and remains alive and well 24 months later (Jeff Szer, personal communication, December 2000), suggesting that intensification of therapy and allogeneic transplantation, where available, may be beneficial for those patients able to tolerate such treatments.

D. Acute Lymphoblastic Leukemia

The small number of described cases makes any cogent treatment recommendations impossible. It is clear that the hematological tolerance of conventional ALL-type chemotherapy is relatively poor in these patients, and even where applied, the prognosis for this form of Richter's syndrome is again extremely poor with just one of the described patients surviving beyond 1 year from the diagnosis of ALL (96).

E. Myeloma

As with the other rare manifestations of Richter's transformation, there are no specific data to guide the treatment of patients who have multiple myeloma develop, but the observation of Brouet et al. (43) that 3 of 11 such patients had prolonged remissions of 3 to 7 years with conventional therapies, suggests that the outlook may be less dismal than other forms of Richter's syndrome, even in the absence of intensified therapy.

VII. PATHOGENESIS OF RICHTER'S SYNDROME

A. Cytogenetics

The advent of B-cell mitogens and techniques such as interphase fluorescent in situ hybridization (FISH) have improved the detection of abnormal karyotypes in CLL. Trisomy 12 is a common cytogenetic abnormality, occurring in 12% to 54% of interphase FISH studies, either singly or in combination with other abnormalities (reviewed by Dierlamm et al. [97]). Other common anomalies include structural abnormalities of chromosomes 13q, 11q, 6q, and 14q (97). The presence of trisomy 12 is strongly correlated with the presence of an increasing proportion of prolymphocytes, atypical lymphocytes, and an abnormal immunophenotype, including CD5 negativity, FMC7 positivity, and strong staining for surface immunoglobulin (98–102). The additional chromosome 12 is usually only detected in a subpopulation of cells (97,99), but it has not been established whether the trisomic cells are those with atypical features. However these studies suggest that trisomy 12 may be a marker for prolymphocytic transformation of CLL and may play a role in the pathogenesis of this condition. The molecular consequences of chromosome 12 overexpression are unknown, but studies examining CLL cases with partial trisomy 12 have defined a "minimal duplicated region" on the long arm of the chromosome at 12q13-12q22 (97).

The role of trisomy 12 in the development of Richter's syndrome has been examined in a small number of cases by several authors. In a cytogenetic study of 77 patients with CLL, Richter's syndrome was diagnosed in four of nine patients subjected to autopsy, three of whom had trisomy 12 (103). The significance of this finding is questionable, because all three patients had other chromosomal abnormalities in addition to trisomy 12. Similarly, trisomy 12 was detected by interphase FISH in five of five cases of Richter's syndrome but in only one of the five specimens collected before transformation occurred (104). The additional chromosome 12 was detected in only a subpopulation of cells, ranging from 11% to 43%, and the possible presence of other karyotypic abnormalities was not examined. Finally, in a separate study using standard cytogenetic analysis, trisomy 12 was not detected in any of the six cases of Richter's syndrome analyzed (105). These results suggest that trisomy 12 is unlikely to be of primary importance in the transformation of CLL to aggressive lymphoma, but may play a secondary role in a small proportion of patients.

A further link between specific karyotypic abnormalities and prolymphocytic transformation of CLL was suggested by Cuneo and coworkers, who investigated the significance of t(11;14)(q13;q32) in 7 of 72 patients with CLL (106). Those patients with t(11;14)(q13;q32) were more likely to have atypical morphology, and all progressed to either atypical CLL (two patients) or PLL (five patients) during follow-up periods ranging from 6 to 60 months. Although the association of specific chromosomal abnormalities with prolymphocytic transformation of CLL has therefore been proposed, there is a scarcity of information regarding the presence of karyotypic anomalies in other forms of Richter's syndrome. Further more, given our current knowledge of the strength of association between the t(11;14)(q13;q32) and mantle cell lymphoma, it is possible that at least a proportion of these cases may now be considered to represent diseases other than CLL.

B. Immunosuppression

In a population-based study of 9456 patients with CLL, Travis and coworkers (37) demonstrated that CLL patients have a 1.3-fold increased risk of a second primary malignancy developing. The increased risk was independent of the initial therapy and constant over time, suggesting that impaired immune function related to the disease itself may have contributed to the development of malignancy in these patients. However, patients with NHL were specifically excluded from this study because of the difficulty in differentiating between CLL and the leukemic phase of certain types of NHL.

The advent of nucleoside analogs for the treatment of CLL has led to concerns that the immunosuppression that results from these therapies may facilitate the development of Richter's syndrome. Pocock et al. (107) reported the development of DLCL or CLL/PLL in 8 of 58 (14%) heavily pretreated patients who received one to nine courses of fludarabine, compared with 7 of 90 (8%) patients with follicular lymphoma who received similar therapy. Similarly, Desablens et al. (87) observed a greater than twofold increase in the rate of Richter's syndrome (14% versus 5%) in 42 CLL patients treated with fludarabine compared with those who had never received the drug. Unfortunately, such a design cannot clearly distinguish the role of fludarabine therapy from that of the intrinsic biology of the more aggressive or refractory disease, which is considered to require nucleoside-analog therapy. A large study of second malignancies in 791 patients with CLL who had received fludarabine found no increase in the rate of second tumors above that previously reported for patients who had never received a nucleoside analog (108). However, patients who had lymphoma develop were excluded from the analysis, and the median follow-up period was only 1.1 years, thereby limiting the conclusions that can be drawn from this study. Although it appears possible that CLL patients who have received fludarabine may be at increased risk of disease transformation, the causative role of the therapy per se remains to be determined. Long-term follow-up of the currently ongoing prospective randomized studies exploring the role of nucleoside-analog therapy, which include all manifestations of Richter's syndrome, will be required before the role of fludarabine-related immunosuppression in the development of Richter's syndrome can be determined.

C. p53

The p53 tumor suppressor gene encodes a transcriptional activator that has important functions in the regulation of the cell cycle and in induction of apoptosis in response to DNA damage. Depending on the method used, p53 mutations can be detected in 10% to 17% of patients with CLL (reviewed by Meinhardt et al. [109]) and are correlated with resistance to therapy, advanced stage of disease, and shortened survival (110–113). Even when present, p53 mutations have been reported to occur in only a subpopulation of cells, which suggests that such mutations may occur as a consequence of clonal evolution (110,112).

Like trisomy 12, p53 abnormalities in CLL are correlated with the presence of an increased proportion of prolymphocytes (111,112). In a study of 27 patients with CLL and p53 mutations, 41% of patients with CLL/PLL demonstrated p53 mutations compared with 15% of patients with classical CLL ($p = 0.002$) (112). However, the authors were unable to show an association between the percentage of cells with p53 mutations and the percentage of prolymphocytes. Similarly, in a study by Lens et al. (111) p53 mutations were detected in 8 of 15 patients with CLL/PLL compared with 3 of 17 cases with classical CLL. In this study, all of the CLL cases had only one p53 allele affected, whereas four of six CLL/PLL patients tested showed biallelic inactivation, suggesting that accumulation of p53 abnormalities may accompany the progression of CLL to CLL/PLL. Interestingly, trisomy 12 was more frequent in those patients without p53 mutations, raising the possibility that these abnormalities may represent independent pathways in the prolymphocytic transformation of CLL.

A scarcity of literature exists regarding the presence of p53 mutations in Richter's syndrome. Cuneo et al. (106) report a case of blastic transformation of CLL, with careful documentation of cumulative cytogenetic abnormalities, including del(17p), which corresponded to the development of Richter's syndrome. Direct sequencing of the p53 gene (located on chromosome 17p) demonstrated an exon 7 mis-sense point mutation that was not present in cells from the CLL phase. In another study, p53 mutations were detected in 3 of 7 patients with Richter's syndrome compared with 6 of 40 patients with CLL (114).

D. p16

The cyclin-dependent kinase-4 inhibitor p16 is a tumor suppressor gene involved in the negative regulation of the cell cycle. Deletions of p16 have been observed in numerous solid tumors and tumor cell lines. In hematological malignancies, p16 deletion is highly specific for lymphoid tumors, including ALL of both B and T cell lineage. NHL, and CLL (115–119) and is a poor prognostic indicator in T-cell acute lymphoblastic leukemia (119). Deletion of p16 has been reported to occur in between 7% and 13% of cases of CLL (115,118) and usually occurs as a heterozygous gene deletion, in contrast to the predominantly homozygous deletions in seen in ALL (115,118). Although the incidence of p16 gene deletions in Richter's syndrome has not been examined, it is interesting to speculate whether sequential deletions of p16 may underline the blastic transformation that has been reported in some patients with CLL.

It is likely that many other events can similarly lead to disturbed cell-cycle control and resulting disease transformation. Another potential pathway was reported by Qian et al. (120), who demonstrated the evolution of a translocation involving the promoter region of the cyclin D2 gene.

E. *c-myc*

The nuclear proto-oncogene *c-myc* is constitutively activated in a number of tumors with a high mitotic index. In B-CLL, *c-myc* expression is correlated with the stage of differentiation and the proliferative activity of the cells (121). In resting CLL cells, *c-myc* is generally not detected but can be induced using mitogens that result in lymphoblastic or plasmablastic differentiation (121,122). This raises the possibility that aberrant expression of *c-myc* in patients with CLL could play a role in the transformation to Richter's syndrome.

The investigation of *c-myc* abnormalities in Richter's syndrome is limited to case reports. Torelli and coworkers (123) have described an eightfold increase in *c-myc* gene expression over baseline levels in a patient with blastic transformation of CLL. Using a combination of modified comparative genomic hybridization and FISH, increased *c-myc* gene copy number was observed in the transformed cells from a patient with CLL and diffuse large cell lymphoma (124). In contrast, no evidence of *c-myc* gene rearrangement was found in six patients with Richter's syndrome; however, overexpression of *c-myc* has been observed in the absence of gene rearrangement (123). Although these reports are interesting, systematic examination of larger numbers of patients with Richter's syndrome is required before the role of *c-myc*, p53, and p16 in the pathogenesis of this process can be determined.

F. Epstein-Barr Virus

The human herpesvirus Epstein-Barr virus (EBV) is implicated in the pathogenesis of a number of lymphoproliferative disorders, including endemic Burkitt's lymphoma, post-transplantation lymphoproliferative disease, X-linked lymphoproliferative disease, AIDS-related NHL, peripheral T cell lymphoma, and Hodgkin's disease (reviewed by Lyons and Liebowitz [125]). In patients with CLL, EBV has been associated with transformation to both NHL and Hodgkin's disease (39,58,72,75,126). In-situ hybridization studies have shown EBV in the Reed-Sternberg–like cells of patients with CLL, with subsequent development of Hodgkin's disease and/or DLCL in some cases (39,58,75,126). Amplification of the virus from peripheral blood lymphoid cells before the development of Richter's syndrome has also been reported (126); however, in-situ hybridization and immunohistochemical studies have repeatedly demonstrated EBV in the Reed-Sternberg–like cells, but not the surrounding lymphocytes (39,58,75,126).

EBV appears to be of particular pathogenic importance in the development of Hodgkin's-type Richter's syndrome, with viral RNA present in the Reed-Sternberg–like cells in 12 of 13 patients, 3 of whom subsequently had frank Hodgkin's disease develop (58). In contrast, in a study of 25 patients with diffuse large-cell lymphoma transformation of CLL, EBV, RNA, and/or latent membrane protein (LMP) was detected in just 4 patients, 1 of whom had T-lineage DLCL (72). In this study, the median survival of EBV-positive patients was 3 months compared with 9 months in those not expressing LMP, although this difference was not statistically significant ($p = 0.4$). Interestingly, recent data suggest that those cases of Hodgkin's disease harboring EBV that develop in patients with CLL may not be clonally related to the underlying CLL. Of the three cases studied by Kanzler et al. (75), the two with evidence of EBV infection harbored different immunoglobulin V-region gene rearrangements to the CLL clone.

The means by which EBV acts to transform the lymphocytes in CLL has not been determined but is likely to be mediated by the viral membrane protein LMP1. LMP1 transforms fibroblast cell lines and can activate human lymphoma cell lines (reviewed by Lyons and Liebowitz [125]). LMP1 can alter intracellular processes by binding members of the TNF-associated factor (TRAF) family. TRAF molecules mediate activation of NF-κB, a transcription factor that in turn can induce the expression of a number of genes.

VIII. CONCLUSIONS

There has been a great fascination with the pathogenesis of Richter's syndrome over the years, out of proportion to the frequency of the events. Exploring the clonal relatedness of these disorders has shed a great deal of light on the process of lymphoid cell development and regulation of the immunoglobulin gene cluster. It is now clear that most instances of Richter's transformation are truly manifestations of clonal progression of the underlying CLL, with data emerging that different precipitating events may contribute to the various histological manifestations of such transformation.

Although there has been significant progress in the treatment of the "indolent" phase of CLL, the efficacy of treatment of the various manifestations of Richter's syndrome remains inadequate. The focused work of the M.D. Anderson group and others in developing specific therapeutic strategies for patients with Richter's syndrome is beginning to show promise that improvements are likely to emerge from intensified treatments, when they can be tolerated. In the interim, clinicians must remain wary of any apparent changes in the natural history of the disease in their patients, with a high index of suspicion and a willingness to obtain adequate tissue biopsy specimens from areas of concern.

REFERENCES

1. P Lortholary, M Boiron, P Ripault, JP Lvey, A Manus, J Bernard. Leucémie lymphoide chronique secondairement associée à une reticulopathie maligne, syndrome de Richter. Nouv Rev Fr Hematol 78:621–644, 1964.
2. MN Richter. Generalized reticular cell sarcoma of lymph nodes associated with lymphocytic leukemia. Am J Pathol 4:285–292, 1928.
3. M Barcos, W Lane, GA Gomez, T Han, A Freeman, H Preisler, E Henderson. An autopsy study of 1206 acute and chronic leukemias (1958 to 1982). Cancer 60:827–837, 1987.
4. E Viadana, IDJ Bross, JW Pickren. An autopsy study of the metastatic patterns of human leukemias. Oncology 35:87–96, 1978.
5. VA Morrison, KR Rai, BL Peterson, JE Kolitz, L Elias, JD Hines, L Shepherd, RA Larson, CA Schiffer. Transformation to Richter's syndrome or prolymphocytic leukemia (PLL), and other second hematologic malignancies in patients with chronic lymphocytic leukemia (CLL): an Intergroup Study (CALGB 9011)(abstr). Blood 94(suppl. 1):539a, 1999.
6. JO Armitage, FR Dick, MP Corder. Diffuse histiocytic lymphoma complicating chronic lymphocytic leukemia. Cancer 41:422–427, 1978.
7. K Foucar, RE Rydell. Richter's syndrome in chronic lymphocytic leukemia. Cancer 46:118–134, 1980.
8. JL Harousseau, G Flandrin, G Tricot, JC Brouet, M Seligmann, J Bernard. Malignant

lymphoma supervening in chronic lymphocytic leukemia and related disorders. Richter's syndrome: a study of 25 cases. Cancer 48:1302–1308, 1981.

9. C Jelic, V Jovanovic, N Milanovic, M Marinkovic, V Kovcin, D Milosevic, M Vlajic. Richter syndrome with emphasis on large-cell non-Hodgkin lymphoma in previously unrecognized subclinical chronic lymphocytic leukemia. Neoplasma 44:63–68, 1997.

10. DL Trump, RB Mann, R Phelps, H Roberts, CL Conley. Richter's syndrome: diffuse histiocytic lymphoma in patients with chronic lymphocytic leukemia. A report of five cases and review of the literature. Am J Med 68:539–548, 1980.

11. LE Robertson, W Pugh, S O'Brien, H Kantarjian, C Hirsch-Ginsberg, A Cork, P McLaughlin, F Cabanillas, M. Keating. Richter's syndrome: a report on 39 patients. J Clin Oncol 11: 1985–1989, 1993.

12. JC Long, AC Aisenberg. Richter's syndrome. A terminal complication of chronic lymphocytic leukemia with distinct clinicopathologic features. Am J Clin Pathol 63:786–795, 1975.

13. MM Ott, G Ott, U Roblick, B Linke, M Kneba, F de Leon, HK Muller-Hermelink. Localized gastric non-Hodgkin's lymphoma of high-grade malignancy in patients with pre-existing chronic lymphocytic leukemia or immunocytoma. Leukemia 9:609–614, 1995.

14. S Tohda, T Morio, T Suzuki, K Nagata, T Kamiyama, Y Imai, N Nara, N Aoki. Richter syndrome with two B cell clones possessing different surface immunoglobulins and immunoglobulin gene rearrangements. Am J Hematol 35:32–36, 1990.

15. JJ van Dongen, H Hooijkaas, JJ Michiels, G Grosveld, A de Klein, TH van der Kwast, ME Prins, J Abels, A Hagemeijer. Richter's syndrome with different immunoglobulin light chains and different heavy chain gene rearrangements. Blood 64:571–575, 1984.

16. PM van Endert, G Mechtersheimer, P Moller, B Dorken, GJ Hammerling, G Moldenhauer. Discordant differentiation antigen pattern in a case of Richter's syndrome with monoclonal idiotype expression and immunoglobulin gene rearrangement. Br J Cancer 62:248–252, 1990.

17. C Jiminez, JM Ribera, J Junca, F Milla, M Vaquero, E Feliu. Richter syndrome with exclusively cutaneous involvement. Sangre 38:67–69, 1993.

18. KM Bayliss, BD Kueck, CA Hanson, WG Matthaeus, UA Almagro. Richter's syndrome presenting as primary central nervous system lymphoma. Transformation of an identical clone. Am J Clin Pathol 93:117–123, 1990.

19. PK Lane, RM Townsend, JH Beckstead, L Corash. Central nervous system involvement in a patient with chronic lymphocytic leukemia and non-Hodgkin's lymphoma (Richter's syndrome) with concordant cell surface immunoglobulin isotypic and immunophenotypic markers. Am J Clin Pathol 89:254–259, 1988.

20. BP O'Neill, TM, Habermann, PM Banks, JR O'Fallon, JD Earle. Primary central nervous system lymphoma as a variant of Richter's syndrome in two patients with chronic lymphocytic leukemia. Cancer 64:1296–1300, 1989.

21. ED Saad, DA Thomas, S O'Brien, GN Fuller, LJ Mederios, A Forman, M Albitar, D Schomer, HM Kantarjian, MJ Keating. Progressive multifocal leukoencephalopathy with concurrent Richter's syndrome. Leuk Lymphoma 38:183–190, 2000.

22. P Noel, RA Kyle. Monoclonal proteins in chronic lymphocytic leukemia. Am J Clin Pathol 87:385–388, 1987.

23. J Beaudreuil, O Lortholary, A Martin, J Feuillard, L Guillevin, P Lortholary, M Raphael, P Casassus. Hypercalcemia may indicate Richter's syndrome. Report of four cases and review. Cancer 79:1211–1215, 1997.

24. J Briones, F Cervantes, E Montserrat, C Rozman. Hypercalcemia in a patient with chronic lymphocytic leukemia evolving into Richter's syndrome. Leuk Lymphoma 21:521–523, 1996.

25. JF Seymour, IF Khouri, RE Champlin, MJ Keating. Refractory chronic lymphocytic leukemia complicated by hypercalcemia treated with allogeneic bone marrow transplantation. Case report and review. Am J Clin Oncol 17:360–368, 1994.

26. JF Seymour, RF Gagel. Calcitriol: the major humoral mediator of hypercalcemia in Hodgkin's disease and non-Hodgkin's lymphoma. Blood 82:1383–1394, 1993.

27. S Partyka, S O'Brien, D Podoloff, H Kantarjian, MJ Keating. The usefulness of high dose (7–10 mci) Gallium (^{67}Ga) scanning to diagnose Richter's transformation. Leuk Lymphoma 36:151–155, 1999.

28. A Enno, D Catovsky, M O'Brien, M Cherchi, TO Kumaran, DA Galton. 'Prolymphocytoid' transformation of chronic lymphocytic leukaemia. Br J Haematol 41:9–18, 1979.

29. JV Melo, D Catovsky, WM Gregory, DA Galton. The relationship between chronic lymphocytic leukaemia and prolymphocytic leukaemia. IV. Analysis of survival and prognostic features. Br J Haematol 65:23–29, 1987.

30. JV Melo, D Catovsky, DA Galton. The relationship between chronic lymphocytic leukaemia and prolymphocytic leukaemia. II. Patterns of evolution of 'prolymphocytoid' transformation. Br J Haematol 64:77–86, 1986.

31. JV Melo, D Catovsky, DA Galton. The relationship between chronic lymphocytic leukaemia and prolymphocytic leukaemia. I. Clinical and laboratory features of 300 patients and characterization of an intermediate group. Br J Haematol 63:377–387, 1986.

32. CR Kjeldsberg, J Marty. Prolymphocytic transformation of chronic lymphocytic leukemia. Cancer 48:2447–2457, 1981.

33. AN Stark, HJ Limbert, BE Roberts, DB Jones, CS Scott. Prolymphocytoid transformation of CLL: a clinical and immunological study of 22 cases. Leuk Res 10:1225–1232, 1986.

34. AM Ghani, JR Krause, JP Brody. Prolymphocytic transformation of chronic lymphocytic leukemia. A report of three cases and review of the literature. Cancer 57:75–80, 1986.

35. JD Roberts, BH Tindle, BR MacPherson. Prolymphocytic transformation of chronic lymphocytic leukemia: a case report of lengthy survival after intensive chemotherapy. Am J Hematol 31:131–132, 1989.

36. D Lerner, C Esteves, MS De Oliveira. B-CLL in PLL transformation associated with hypercalcemia. Leuk Lymphoma 12:321–325, 1994.

37. LB Travis, RE Curtis, BF Hankey, JF Fraumeni, Jr. Second cancers in patients with chronic lymphocytic leukemia. J Natl Cancer Inst 84:1422–1427, 1992.

38. SK Juneja, D Carney, D Ellis, E Januszewicz, M Wolf, HM Prince. Hodgkin's disease type Richter's syndrome in chronic lymphocytic leukemia. Leukaemia 13:826–827, 1999.

39. T Petrella, N Yaziji, F Collin, G Rifle, F Morlevat, L Arnould, P Fargeot, O Depret. Implication of the Epstein-Barr virus in the progression of chronic lymphocytic leukemia/small lymphocytic lymphoma to Hodgkin-like lymphomas. Anticancer Res 17:3907–3913, 1997.

40. L Fayad, LE Robertson, S O'Brien, JT Manning, S Wright, F Hagemeister, F Cabanillas, M Keating. Hodgkin's disease variant of Richter's syndrome: experience at a single institution. Leuk Lymphoma 23:333–337, 1996.

41. E Weisenberg, J Anastasi, M Adenyanju, D Variakojis, J Vardiman. Hodgkin's disease associated with chronic lymphocytic leukemia. Am J Clin Pathol 103:479–484, 1995.

42. M Brecher, PM Banks. Hodgkin's disease variant of Richter's syndrome. Report of eight cases. Am J Clin Pathol 93:333–339, 1990.

43. JC Brouet, JP Fermand, G Laurent, MJ Grange, A Chevalier, C Jacquillat, M Seligmann. The association of chronic lymphocytic leukaemia and multiple myeloma: a study of eleven patients. Br J Haematol 59:55–66, 1985.

44. O Shpilberg, Z Mark, M Biniaminov, E Rosner, E Rosenthal, N Gipsh, V Rubanov, E Rachmilewitz, F Brok-Simoni, G Rechavi, I Ben-Bassat. Transformation of chronic lymphocytic leukemia to multiple myeloma: clonal evolution of second malignancy? Leukemia 9:1974–1978, 1995.

45. KA Foon, MD Thiruvengadam, A Saven, ZP Bernstein, RP Gale. Genetic relatedness of lymphoid malignancies. Ann Intern Med 119:63–73, 1993.

46. A Bessudo, TJ Kipps. Origin of high-grade lymphomas in Richter syndrome. Leuk Lymphoma 18:367–372, 1995.

47. AC Aisenberg, BM Wilkes, JC Long, NL Harris. Cell surface phenotype in lymphoproliferative disease. Am J Med 68:206–213, 1980.
48. K Miyamura, H Osada, T Yamauchi, M Itoh, Y Kodera, T Suchi, T Takahashi, R Ueda. Single clonal origin of neoplastic B-cells with different immunoglobulin light chains in a patient with Richter's syndrome. Cancer 66:140–144, 1990.
49. H Nakamine, AS Masih, WG Sanger, RS Wickert, DW Mitchell, JO Armitage, DD Weisenburger. Richter's syndrome with different immunoglobulin light chain types. Molecular and cytogenetic features indicate a common clonal origin. Am J Clin Pathol 97:656–663, 1992.
50. T Sun, M Susin, M Desner, R Pergolizzi, J Cuomo, P Koduru. The clonal origin of two cell populations in Richter's syndrome. Hum Pathol 21:722–728, 1990.
51. JP Fermand, JM James, P Herait, JC Brouet. Associated chronic lymphocytic leukemia and multiple myeloma: origin from a single clone. Blood 66:291–293, 1985.
52. M Chatterjee, M Barcos, T Han, XL Liu, Z Bernstein, KA Foon. Shared idiotype expression by chronic lymphocytic leukemia and B-cell lymphoma. Blood 76:1825–1829, 1990.
53. PKR Koduru, SM Lichtman, TF Smilari, T Sun, JC Goh, L Karp, W Hall, S Hashimoto, N Chiorazzi, JD Broome. Serial phenotypic, cytogenetic and molecular genetic studies in Richter's syndrome: demonstration of lymphoma development from the chronic lymphocytic leukaemia cells. Br J Haematol 85:613–616, 1993.
54. JJ Michiels, JJ van Dongen, A Hagemeijer, P Sonneveld, RE Ploemacher, HJ Adriaansen, TH van der Kwast, P Brederoo, J Abels. Richter's syndrome with identical immunoglobulin gene rearrangements in the chronic lymphocytic leukemia and the supervening non-Hodgkin lymphoma. Leukemia 3:819–824, 1989.
55. DJ Bernard, YJ Bignon, J Pauchard, F Ramos, Y Fonck, F Courja, P Chollet, R Plagne. Genotypic analyses of Richter's syndrome. Cancer 67:997–1002, 1991.
56. A Matolcsy, EJ Schattner, DM Knowles, P Casali. Clonal evolution of B cells in transformation from low- to high-grade lymphoma. Eur J Immunol 29:1253–1264, 1999.
57. DL Saltman, JA Ross, RE Banks, FM Ross, AM Ford, MJ Mackie. Molecular evidence for a single clonal origin in biphenotypic concomitant chronic lymphocytic leukemia and multiple myeloma. Blood 74:2062–2065, 1989.
58. H Momose, ES Jaffe, SS Shin, YY Chen, LM Weiss. Chronic lymphocytic leukemia/small lymphocytic lymphoma with Reed-Sternberg-like cells and possible transformation to Hodgkin's disease. Am J Surg Pathol 16:859–867, 1992.
59. T Ohno, BN Smir, DD Weisenburger, RD Gascoyne, SD Hinrichs, WC Chan. Origin of the Hodgkin/Reed-Sternberg cells in chronic lymphocytic leukemia with ''Hodgkin's transformation.'' Blood 91:1757–1761, 1998.
60. A Matolcsy, P Casli, DM Knowles. Different clonal origin of B-cell populations of chronic lymphocytic leukemia and large cell lymphoma in Richter's syndrome. Ann NY Acad Sci 764:496–503, 1995.
61. A Matolcsy, G Inghiram, DM Knowles. Molecular genetic demonstration of the diverse evolution of Richter's syndrome (chronic lymphocytic leukemia and subsequent large cell lymphoma). Blood 83:1363–1372, 1994.
62. M Yamaguchi, T Ohno, K Oka, M Taniguchi, M Ito, K Kita, H Shiku. De novo CD5-positive diffuse large B-cell lymphomia: clinical characteristics and therapeutic outcome. Br J Haematol 105:1133–1139, 1999.
63. M Taniguchi, K Oka, A Hiasa, M Yamaguchi, T Ohno, K Kita, H Shiku. De novo CD5+ diffuse large B-cell lymphomas express VH genes with somatic mutation. Blood 91:1145–1151, 1998.
64. CE Litz, DC Arthur, KJ Gajl-Pelczalska, D Rausch, C Copenhaver, JE Coad, RD Brunning. Transformation of chronic lymphocytic leukemia to small non-cleaved cell lymphoma: a cytogenetic, immunological and molecular study. Leukemia 5:972–978, 1991.
65. E Archimbaud, C Charrin, O Gentilhomme, R Rimokh, D Guyotat, D Fiere, D Germain.

Initial clonal acute lymphoblastic transformation of chronic lymphocytic leukemia with (11; 14) and (8;12) chromosome translocations and acquired homozygosity. Acta Haematol 79: 168–173, 1988.

66. A Klepfish, L Shvide, M Shtalrid, A Tsimanis, L Guedg, K Ostrovsk, A Berrebi. Burkitt-like acute lymphoblastic leukemia (ALL-L3) transformation of B-cell chronic lymphocytic leukemia (B-CLL) (abstr). Blood 92(suppl. 1):300b, 1999.

67. V Pistoia, S Roncella, PF Di Celle, M Sessarego, G Cutrona, G Cerruti, GP Boccaccio, CE Grossi, R Foa, M Ferrarini. Emergence of a B cell lymphoblastic lymphoma in a patient with B cell chronic lymphocytic leukemia: evidence for the single cell origin of the two tumors. Blood 78:797–804, 1991.

68. CC Harland, SJ Whittaker, YL Ng, CA Holden, E Wong, NP Smith. Coexistent cutaneous T-cell lymphoma and B-cell chronic lymphocytic leukaemia. Br J Dermatol 127:519–523, 1992.

69. JG Strickler, TW Amsden, PJ Kurtin. Small B-cell lymphoid neoplasms with coexisting T-cell lymphomas. Am J Clin Pathol 98:424–429, 1992.

70. A Lee, ME Skelly, DW Kingma, LJ Medeiros. B-cell chronic lymphocytic leukemia followed by high grade T-cell lymphoma. Am J Clin Pathol 103:348–352, 1995.

71. DA Milkowski, BD Worley, MJ Morris. Richter's syndrome presenting as an obstructing endobronchial lesion. Chest 16:832–835, 1999.

72. SM Ansell, CY Li, RV Lloyd, RL Phyliky. Epstein-Barr virus infection in Richter's transformation. Am J Hematol 60:99–104, 1999.

73. JM Bennett, D Catovsky, MT Daniel, G Flandrin, DA Galton, HR Gralnick, C Sultan. Proposals for the classification of chronic (mature) B and T lymphoid leukaemias. French-American-British (FAB) Cooperative Group. J Clin Pathol 42:567–584, 1989.

74. J Williams, A Schned, JD Cotelingam, ES Jaffe. Chronic lymphocytic leukemia with coexistent Hodgkin's disease. Implications for the origin of the Reed-Sternberg cell. Am J Surg Pathol 15:33–42, 1991.

75. H Kanzier, R Kuppers, S Helmes, H Wacker, A Chott, M Hansmann, K Rajewsky. Hodgkin and Reed-Sternberg-like cells in B-cell chronic lymphocytic leukemia represent the outgrowth of single germinal-center B-cell-derived clones: potential precursors of Hodgkin and Reed-Sternberg cells in Hodgkin's disease. Blood 95:1023–1031, 2000.

76. H Choi, RH Keller. Coexistence of chronic lymphocytic leukemia and Hodgkin's disease. Cancer 48:48–57, 1981.

77. AK Gopal, SM Schuetze, DG Maloney, PL Weiden. Large cell non-Hodgkin's lymphoma and Hodgkin's disease arising synchronously in a patient with chronic lymphocytic leukemia: importance of immunocytochemistry. Blood 94:2537, 1999.

78. MH Zarrabi, F Rosner, HW Grunwald, RN Levy. Chronic lymphocytic leukemia terminating in acute leukemia. N Y State J Med 79:1072–1075, 1979.

79. BJ O'Neill, KB McCredie, E Raik, GP Tauro. Mixed leukaemia: a report of three cases. Med J Aust 2:586–591, 1970.

80. C Preudhomme, P Lepelley, V Lovi, M Zandecki, A Cosson, P Fenaux. T-cell acute lymphoblastic leukemia occurring in the course of B cell chronic lymphocytic leukemia: a case report. Leuk Lymphoma 18:361–364, 1995.

81. AN Mohamed, R Compean, ME Dan, MR Smith, A Al-Katib. Clonal evolution of chronic lymphocytic leukemia to acute lymphoblastic leukemia. Cancer Genet Cytogenet 86:143–146, 1996.

82. N Asou, M Osato, K Horikawa, K Nishikawa, O Sakitani, L Li, H Yamasaki, S Nishimura, T Okubo, H Suzushima, K Takatsuki. Burkitt's type acute lymphoblastic transformation associated with t(8;14) in a case of B cell chronic lymphocytic leukemia. Leukemia 11:1986–1988, 1997.

83. H Demiroglu, S Dundar. T-cell acute lymphoblastic leukaemic transformation of B-cell chronic lymphocytic leukaemia. Eur J Haematol 56:184–185, 1996.

84. TH Totterman, K Nilsson, C Sundstrom. Phorbol ester-induced differentiation of chronic lymphocytic leukaemia cells. Nature 288:176–178, 1980.

85. PJ Browett, BF Leber, E Coustan-Smith, JD Norton. Independent clonal origin of coexisting chronic lymphocytic leukaemia and multiple myeloma. Br J Haematol 70:126–127, 1988.

86. VP Belsito, S Iaccarino, L Liguon, C Zecca, O Villani, M De Rienzo, G De Simone, M Garcia, A Abbadessa. Chronic lymphocytic leukemia in Richter's transformation: our experience (abstr). Blood 94(suppl. 1):295b, 1999.

87. B Desablens, R Garidi, J Fernandes, JC Capiod, S Legrand, S Tabuteau. Does fludarabine increase the risk of Richter's syndrome (RS) among chronic lymphocytic leukaemia (abstr)? Haematologica 84:259, 1999.

88. S Tabuteau, J Fernandes, R Garidi, B Desablens. Richter's syndrome in B-CLL: Report of 37 cases (abstr). Blood 94(suppl. 1):306b, 1999.

89. RN Damle, T Wasil, F Fais, F Ghiotto, A Valetto, SL Allen, A Buchbinder, D Budman, K Dittmar, J Kolitz, SM Lichtman, P Schulman, VP Vinciguerra, KR Rai, M Ferrarini, N Chiorazzi. Ig V gene mutation status and CD38 expression as novel prognostic indicators in chronic lymphocytic leukemia. Blood 94:1840–1847, 1999.

90. TJ Hamblin, Z Davis, A Gardiner, DG Oscier, FK Stevenson. Unmutated Ig V(H) genes are associated with a more aggressive form of chronic lymphocytic leukemia. Blood 94:1848–1854, 1999.

91. ST Traweek, J Liu, RM Johnson, CD Winberg, H Rappaport. High-grade transformation of chronic lymphocytic leukemia and low-grade non-Hodgkin's lymphoma. Am J Clin Pathol 100:519–526, 1993.

92. W Plunkett, V Gandhi. Nucleoside analogs: cellular pharmacology, mechanisms of action, and strategies for combination therapy. In: BD Cheson, MJ Keating, W Plunkett, eds. Nucleoside Analogs in Cancer Therapy. New York: Marcel Dekker, 1997. pp 1–35.

93. HM Kantarjian, S O'Brien, TL Smith, J Cortes, FJ Giles, M Beran, S Pierce, Y Huh, M Andreeff, C Koller, CS Ha, MJ Keating, S Murphy, EJ Freireich. Results of treatment with Hyper-CVAD, a dose intensive regimen, in adult acute lymphobalstic leukemia. J Clin Oncol 18:547–561, 2000.

94. BS Dabaja, HM Kantarjian, JE Cortes, DA Thomas, A Sarris, SM O'Brien, MJ Keating, FJ Giles. Fractionated cyclophosphamide, vincristine, liposomal daunorubicin (daunoXome), dexamethasone (hyperCVXD) regimen in Richter's syndrome (abstr). Blood 94(suppl. 1): 260b, 1999.

95. K van Biesen, CS Ha, S Murphy, P McLaughlin, A Rodriguez, K Amin, A Forman, J Romaguera, F Hagemeister, A Younes, C Bachier, A Sarris, KS Sobocinski, JD Cox, F Cabanillas. Risk factors, treatment and outcome of central nervous system recurrence in adults with intermediate-grade and immunoblastic lymphoma. Blood 91:1178–1184, 1998.

96. CN Gutteridge, AC Newland. Chronic lymphocytic leukaemia complicating null cell acute lymphoblastic leukaemia. Clin Lab Haematol 8:77–79, 1986.

97. J Dierlamm, L Michaux, A Criel, I Wlodarska, H Van den Berghe, DK Hossfeld. Genetic abnormalities in chronic lymphocytic leukemia and their clinical and prognostic implications. Cancer Genet Cytogenet 94:27–35, 1997.

98. TH Que, JG Marco, J Ellis E Matutes, VB Babapulle, S Boyle, D Catovsky. Trisomy 12 in chronic lymphocytic leukemia detected by fluorescence in situ hybridization: analysis by stage, immunophenotype, and morphology. Blood 82:571–575, 1993.

99. A Criel, I Wlodarska, P Meeus, M Stul, A Louwagie, A Van Hoof, M Hidajat, C Mecucci, H Van den Berghe. Trisomy 12 is uncommon in typical chronic lymphocytic leukaemias. Br J Haematol 87:523–528, 1994.

100. E Matutes, D Oscier, J Garcia-Marco, J Ellis, A Copplestone, R Gillingham, T Hamblin, D Lens, GJ Swansbury, D Catovsky. Trisomy 12 defines a group of CLL with atypical morphology: correlation between cytogenetic, clinical and laboratory features in 544 patients. Br J Haematol 92:382–388, 1996.

101. JM Hernandez, C Mecucci, A Criel, P Meeus, I Michaux, A Van Hoof, G Verhoef, A Louwagie, JM Scheiff, JL Michaux. Cytogenetic analysis of B cell chronic lymphoid leukemias classified according to morphologic and immunophenotypic (FAB) criteria. Leukemia 9: 2140–2146, 1995.
102. A Criel, G Verhoef, R Vlietinck, C Mecucci, J Billiet, L Michaux, P Meeus, A Louwagie, A Van Orshoven, A Van Hoof, M Boogaerts, H Van den Berghe, C De Wolf-Peeters. Further characterization of morphologically defined typical and atypical CLL: a clinical, immunophenotypic, cytogenetic and prognostic study on 390 cases. Br J Haematol 97:383–391, 1997.
103. T Han, N Sadamori, H Ozer, R Gajera, GA Gomez, ES Henderson, A Bhargava, J Fitzpatrick, J Minowada, ML Bloom. Cytogenetic studies in 77 patients with chronic lymphocytic leukemia: correlations with clinical, immunologic, and phenotypic data. J Clin Oncol 2:1121–1132, 1984.
104. RK Brynes, A Mccourty, NC Sun, CH Koo. Trisomy 12 in Richter's transformation of chronic lymphocytic leukemia. Am J Clin Pathol 104:199–203, 1995.
105. J Hebert, P Jonveaux, MF d'Agay, R Berger. Cytogenetic studies in patients with Richter's syndrome. Cancer Genet Cytogenet 73:65–68, 1994.
106. A Cuneo, M Balboni, N Piva, GM Rigolin, MG Roberti, C Mejak, S Moretti, R Bigoni, R Balsamo, P Cavazzini. Atypical chronic lymphocytic leukaemia with t(11;14)(q13;q32): karyotype evolution and prolymphocytic transformation. Br J Haematol 90:409–416, 1995.
107. C Pocock, E Matutes, A Wotherspoon, D Cunningham, D Catovsky. Fludarabine therapy may precipitate large cell transformation in chronic lymphocytic leukemia but not in follicular lymphoma (abstr). Blood 92(suppl. 1):429a, 1998.
108. BD Cheson, DA Vena, J Barret, B Freidlin. Second malignancies as a consequence of nucleoside analog therapy for chronic lymphoid leukemias. J Clin Oncol 17:2454–2460, 1999.
109. G Meinhardt, CM Wendtner, M Hallek. Molecular pathogenesis of chronic lymphocytic leukemia: factors and signaling pathways regulating cell growth and survival. J Mol Med 77: 282–293, 1999.
110. I Cano, J Martinez, E Quevedo, J Pinilla, A Martin-Recio, A Rodriguez, A Castaneda, R Lopez, T Perez-Pino, F Hernandez-Navarro. Trisomy 12 and p53 deletion in chronic lymphocytic leukemia detected by fluorescence in situ hybridization: association with morphology and resistance to conventional chemotherapy. Cancer Genet Cytogenet 90:118–124, 1996.
111. D Lens, MJ Dyer, JM Garcia-Marco, PJ De Schouwer, RA Hamoudi, D Jones, N Farahat, E Matutes, D Catovsky. p53 abnormalities in CLL are associated with excess of prolymphocytes and poor prognosis. Br J Haematol 99:848–857, 1997.
112. I Cordone, S Masi, FR Mauro, S Soddu, O Morsilli, T Valentini, ML Vegna, C Guglielmi, F Mancini, S Giuliacci, A Sacchi, F Mandelli, R Foa. p53 expression in B-cell chronic lymphocytic leukemia: a marker of disease progression and poor prognosis. Blood 91:4342–4349, 1998.
113. H Dohner, K Fischer, M Bentz, K Hansen, A Benner, G Cabot, D Diehl, R Schlenk, J Coy, S Stilgenbauer. p53 gene deletion predicts for poor survival and non-response to therapy with purine analogs in chronic B-cell leukemias. Blood 85:1580–1589, 1995.
114. G Gaidano, P Ballerini, JZ Gong, G Inghirami, A Neri, EW Newcomb, IT Magrath, DM Knowles, R Dalla-Favera. p53 mutations in human lymphoid malignancies: association with Burkitt lymphoma and chronic lymphocytic leukemia. Proc Natl Acad Sci USA 88:5413–5417, 1991.
115. S Ogawa, A Hangaishi, S Miyawaki, S Hirosawa, Y Miura, K Takeyama, N Kamada, S Ohtake, N Uike, C Shimazaki. Loss of the cyclin-dependent kinase 4-inhibitor (p16; MTS1) gene is frequent in and highly specific to lymphoid tumors in primary human hematopoietic malignancies. Blood 86:1548–1556, 1995.
116. B Quesnel, C Preudhomme, N Philippe, M Vanrumbeke, I Dervite, JL Lai, F Bauters, E Wattel, P Fenaux. p16 gene homozygous deletions in acute lymphoblastic leukemia. Blood 85:657–663, 1995.

117. T Uchida, T Watanabe, T Kinoshita, T Murate, H Saito, T Hotta. Mutational analysis of the CDKN2 (MTS1/p16ink4A) gene in primary B-cell lymphomas. Blood 86:2724–2731, 1995.
118. MA Haidar, XB Cao, T Manshouri, LL Chan, A Glassman, HM Kantarjian, MJ Keating, MS Beran, M Albitar. p16INK4A and p15INK4B gene deletions in primary leukemias. Blood 86:311–315, 1995.
119. Y Yamada, Y Hatta, K Murata, K Sugawara, S Ikeda, M Mine, T Maeda, Y Hirakata, S Kamihira, K Tsukasaki, S Ogawa, H Hirai, HP Koeffler, M Tomonaga. Deletions of p15 and/or p16 genes as a poor-prognosis factor in adult T-cell leukemia. J Clin Oncol 15:1778–1785, 1997.
120. L Qian, J Gong, J Liu, JD Broome, PRK Koduru. Cyclin D2 promoter disrupted by t(12; 22)(p13;q11.2) during transformation of chronic lymphocytic leukaemia to non-Hodgkin's lymphoma. Br J Haematol 106:477–485, 1999.
121. LG Larsson, M Schena, M Carlsson, J Sallstrom, K Nilsson. Expression of the c-myc protein is down-regulated at the terminal stages during in vitro differentiation of B-type chronic lymphocytic leukemia cells. Blood 77:1025–1032, 1991.
122. R Greil, B Fasching, P Loidl, H Huber. Expression of the c-myc proto-oncogene in multiple myeloma and chronic lymphocytic leukemia: an in situ analysis. Blood 78:180–191, 1991.
123. UL Torelli, GM Torelli, G Emilia, L Selleri, D Venturelli, T Artusi, A Donelli, A Colo, C Fornieri. Simultaneously increased expression of the c-myc and mu chain genes in the acute blastic transformation of a chronic lymphocytic leukaemia. Br J Haematol 65:165–170, 1987.
124. E Arranz, B Martinez, A Richart, G Echezarreta, A Roman, C Rivas, J Benitez. Increased C-MYC oncogene copy number detected with combined modified comparative genomic hybridization and FISH analysis in a Richter syndrome case with complex karyotype. Cancer Genet Cytogenet 106:80–83, 1998.
125. SF Lyons, DN Liebowitz. The roles of human viruses in the pathogenesis of lymphoma. Semin Oncol 25:461–475, 1998.
126. D Rubin, SD Hudnall, A Aisenberg, JO Jacobson, NL Harris. Richter's transformation of chronic lymphocytic leukaemia with Hodgkin's-like cells is associated with Epstein-Barr virus infection. Mod Pathol 7:91–98, 1994.
127. H Aoki, M Taishita, M Kosaka, S Saito. Frequent mutations in D and/or J$_H$ segment of Ig gene in Waldenström's macroglobulinemia and chronic lymphocytic leukemia (CLL) with Richter's syndrome but not in common CLL. Blood 85:1913–1919, 1995.
128. FJ Giles, S O'Brien, HM Kantarjian, E Estey, C Koller, W Plunkett, LY Yang, JF Seymour, LE Robertson, S Lerner, MJ Keating. Sequential cis-platinum, fludarabine, and arabinosyl cytosine (PFA) or cyclophosphamide, fludarabine, and arabinosyl cytosine (CFA) in patients with Richter's syndrome (RS): A pilot study (abstract). Blood 88(Suppl. 1):93a, 1996.
129. J Rodriguez, MJ Keating, S O'Brien, RE Champlin, IF Khouri. Allogeneic haematopoietic transplantation for Richter's syndrome. Br J Haematol 110:897–899, 2000.

22

Supportive Care in Chronic Lymphocytic Leukemia

FARHAD RAVANDI, MICHAEL J. KEATING, and SUSAN M. O'BRIEN

The University of Texas M. D. Anderson Cancer Center, Houston, Texas

I. INTRODUCTION

Considerable advances in the understanding of the biology of chronic lymphocytic leukemia (CLL) and cellular events responsible for the pathogenesis of the disease have occurred over the past two decades (1). These have already contributed to better definition of the disease and its variants, more accurate diagnosis, and the introduction of more effective chemotherapy regimens (2,3).

In CLL, as well as other hematological malignancies, improvements in supportive care have played a major role in the observed advances. With continued progress and the increased life expectancy of patients with CLL, it can be expected that supportive measures will continue to play a significant role (4). Indeed, the introduction of some therapies, such as the nucleoside analogs and progenitor cell transplantation has been associated with an increased emphasis on supportive care.

CLL is an indolent disease with a protracted course, which spans years and is accompanied by progressive deterioration of the marrow function secondary to disease-related effects and treatment (5). Infections, which increase in incidence and severity with disease progression, are related to defects in cellular and humoral immunity associated with the disease and therapy (6). Another significant cause of morbidity is the anemia and thrombocytopenia related to marrow failure and hypersplenism and autoimmune phenomena associated with the disease (7). These cytopenias not only result in symptoms but eventually limit application of potentially effective therapies and therefore their control is of considerable interest.

Therefore, the supportive measures in therapy of CLL are attempts to improve the immune defects associated with the disease to reduce the incidence and severity of infec-

tions and to improve cytopenias, thus allowing administration of disease-specific therapy
(4). Some important supportive measures have been partially reviewed in other chapters
of this book and include strategies for prevention of infections using growth factors, replacement of immunoglobulins and immunization, and procedures such as splenectomy
to reduce the cytopenias.

In this chapter we review the various ancillary measures used in the management
of CLL, with particular emphasis on the applications of splenectomy, cytokines, and intravenous immunoglobulins.

II. SPLENECTOMY

A. Historical Aspects

References to the removal of the spleen for various medical conditions date back to ancient
Greek and Roman literature (8). Therapeutic splenectomies were recorded in the 1800s,
and the earliest reported case of splenectomy in CLL is from Guy's Hospital in London
(9). Because of the inadequacy of surgical techniques and lack of adequate transfusion
support, this patient and a significant number of other patients undergoing the procedure
died postoperatively in the early series (9–11). However, with improvements in surgical
practices the procedure has become a feasible option with an estimated perioperative mortality of 5%. In the 1980s several series of patients undergoing the procedure were reported, establishing it as an effective and reasonably safe means of correcting the hematological deficits in most patients treated (11–22). These series were unable to demonstrate
a survival benefit because of their retrospective nature, small numbers of patients, and
variable response criteria. Recent series, published in the 1990s, used more stringent response criteria and confirmed that the procedure can be performed with modest morbidity
and low mortality and results in significant hematological benefits in most patients (23–
27). These studies also involved limited patient numbers and were unable to determine
the impact of the procedure on survival (20,22,23). To date, there have been no randomized
trials examining this issue; the M. D. Anderson study used a group of matched controls
and concluded that overall survival was equivalent in splenectomized and control patients
(27).

B. Indications for Splenectomy

The term "hypersplenism" was initially introduced by Chauffard in 1907 to describe a
condition comprising any combination of anemia, thrombocytopenia, and leukopenia together with a normocellular bone marrow and splenomegaly (28–31). Although the details
of splenic function are not fully explained, it is clear that an enlarged spleen can sequester
and destroy large numbers of red cells, platelets, and white cells (32–34). Splenomegaly
can also result in an increase in the total plasma volume and lead to spurious cytopenias
(25,28,34). The role of the spleen in producing humoral factors that may suppress marrow
production has been questioned (35,36). Indeed, the ratio of total body to venous hematocrit is increased in all patients with an enlarged spleen (37). Therefore, there are a number
of mechanisms by which an enlarged spleen may contribute to the cytopenias seen in
advanced CLL.

It is clear that immunological mechanisms may also contribute to decreased blood
counts, and although the spleen is the site of destruction of these antibody-damaged cells,
the term hypersplenism is not applicable to such situations. A spleen-based immune dys-

function is seen in animals with experimental splenomegaly, and other evidence supports a direct role for the spleen in immune cytopenias (38). Thus, patients with CLL and auto-immune cytopenias may benefit from splenectomy (7,16,39–44). Historically, the indications for splenectomy in CLL were to correct steroid-refractory autoimmune hemolytic anemia and immune thrombocytopenia and to relieve the mechanical symptoms associated with a massively enlarged spleen (Table 1).

With the increased application of nucleoside analogs in the therapy of CLL, there has been a growing reluctance to use corticosteroids because of the increased risk of atypical infections associated with such combined therapy (45). This, together with the continued advances in surgical and transfusion techniques, has led to an earlier consideration of this modality for the treatment of immune cytopenias and to its examination for a broader range of indications. Multiple series have shown the safety and efficacy of splenectomy for reversing cytopenias not associated with immune mechanisms and have confirmed the applicability of this modality to improve blood counts to allow continued therapy (11–27).

It has been suggested that patients with preserved marrow hematopoiesis or documented immune cytopenias are more likely to benefit from splenectomy. In patients with an enlarged spleen and defective bone marrow function, the benefit of splenectomy has been less certain. Possible beneficial effects would include reduction in plasma volume, removal of bulky tumor, and return of red cells and platelets to the circulation (17). Although most series of patients with advanced stage disease have reported overall improvements for most patients, such benefits have not been universal (11–27). Therefore, techniques to predict which patients are unlikely to respond satisfactorily to splenectomy are of considerable interest. Such techniques have included examination of bone marrow smears to assess marrow reserve (12), as well as more complicated approaches such as estimation of erythropoietic activity of the marrow by measuring marrow iron turnover (ferrokinetics) (17), measurement of the splenic red cell volume (17), red cell mass, and plasma volume (17,25); or the establishment of hypersplenism using ^{51}Cr-labeled erythrocytes (12). In one report low preoperative values of hemoglobin and platelet count were reported to be negatively and positively correlated with the postoperative increments, respectively (23). Platelet response was also significantly associated with presplenectomy platelet count, with better responses seen in patients with higher counts. However, there was no association with presplenectomy LDH values and response (23). In a recent report the factors associated with a significantly inferior survival after splenectomy were increased marrow leukemic infiltration ($p = 0.002$) and a lower preoperative hemoglobin ($p = 0.028$) (27). Measurement of residual hematopoiesis by histological assessment of megakaryocyte numbers, percent marrow erythroid cells, or percent marrow leukemic infiltrate was not predictive of response (27). A significant correlation between splenic

Table 1 Indications for Splenectomy in CLL

Absolute "classical" indications
   Steroid-refractory immune thrombocytopenia
   Steroid-refractory autoimmune hemolytic anemia
   Symptomatic bulky splenomegaly
Relative indications
   "Hypersplenism" with refractory cytopenias
   CLL with isolated splenomegaly

weight and postoperative hemoglobin and neutrophil increments but not platelet increment was reported (p values 0.026, 0.04, and 0.44, respectively) (27). However, no accurate method of preoperative assessment of spleen weight exists. Probably because of the multi-factorial nature of the cytopenias, none of these techniques or measurements has been shown to consistently predict the likelihood of response to splenectomy. Seymour et al.(27) noted that impaired performance status (≥ 2) was predictive of greater risk of mortality.

C. Reports of Splenectomy in CLL

Several groups have published their experience with splenectomy in CLL (11–27). Because the procedure is considered standard therapy in patients with immune cytopenias, most of these series excluded such patients. Adler et al. (12) reported 20 patients with CLL together with 30 patients with other lymphoid malignancies. This series, as well as others, suffers from small numbers and variable response criteria (12–16). They reported an overall surgical mortality of 8% and a good response in all hematological parameters in 27 of 48 evaluable patients, with 80% of the group showing improvement in one or more parameters (12). The median survival after splenectomy was 14.6 months.

Several other series investigated the role of this procedure in patients with advanced disease and refractory cytopenias. Gallhofer et al. (22) reviewed their experience with 20 patients with stage C disease and marked splenomegaly and compared their outcome to a similar group of nonsplenectomized patients. Patients undergoing splenectomy showed clinical improvement, with 85% achieving stage A and 10% stage B disease after the procedure (22). Ten patients were alive 24 to 135 months after the procedure, with a better survival for the splenectomized patients compared with the control group ($p < 0.001$) (22). In the series reported by Ferrant et al. (17) 20 of 40 CLL patients evaluated for splenectomy actually underwent the procedure. All but two patients normalized their hematocrit, and all but one patient achieved a normal platelet count. However, survival measured from the time of diagnosis or the time of surgery was equivalent to the 20 nonsplenectomized patients (17). Stein et al. (19) reviewed their experience with 13 patients with stage III or IV CLL who had refractory disease unresponsive to chemotherapy. They showed an improvement in median hematocrit from 27.5% preoperatively to 35% 1 month after the procedure. The platelet count also improved from a preoperative median of 46×10^9/L to a median of 261×10^9/L postoperatively (19). The median survival after surgery was 24 months, with four patients surviving more than 30 months (19).

Three publications in the 1990s have helped better define the role of this procedure in the management of patients with CLL (23,24,27). The Roswell Park group examined their experience with splenectomy over a 17-year period in 30 patients with CLL and 3 patients with prolymphocytic leukemia (PLL) (23). By use of the response criteria previously published by Han et al., (46), they addressed one of the major weaknesses of the previously published reports. Improvements in hemoglobin of ≥ 3 g/dl were noted in 50% of anemic patients, and improvements in platelet count of $\geq 50 \times 10^9$/L were noted in all 12 thrombocytopenic patients (23). These responses were durable with a median duration of platelet response of 18 months and a median duration of hemoglobin response of 62 months (23). The response to splenectomy was not associated with the presplenectomy bone marrow pattern. The operative mortality rate of 6% was consistent with other reports. Mayo Clinic investigators reported their experience with 50 patients who underwent splenectomy over a 16-year period (24). Despite a performance status of ≥ 2 in 32% of the patients the operative mortality was only 4% (24). Most patients (94%) had Rai stage 3

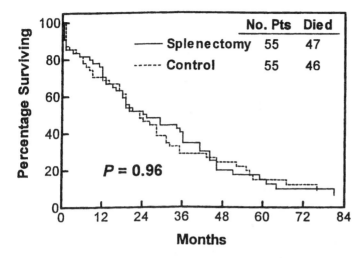

Figure 1   Overall survival of patients undergoing splenectomy (solid line) versus matched controls (dotted line). (Reprinted with permission from Ref. 27.)

or 4 disease with extensive marrow infiltration, massive splenomegaly, and cytopenias refractory to chemotherapy (24). Significant hematologic responses were noted; 77% of anemic patients improved their hemoglobin by at least 3g/dl or to >11 g/dl. Similarly, 70% of thrombocytopenic patients achieved a platelet count >100 × 10⁹/L. These responses were durable lasting greater than 1 year in more than 80% of patients (24). No association was found between spleen size or degree of marrow dysfunction and response to splenectomy. The authors concluded that splenectomy is efficacious in achieving durable remissions of refractory cytopenias and in relieving symptoms related to massive splenomegaly, but despite the increased ability to administer chemotherapy its impact on sur-

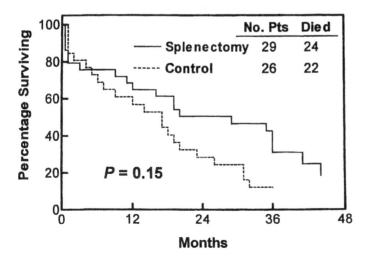

Figure 2   Overall survival of Rai stage IV patients undergoing splenectomy (solid line) and their matched controls (dotted line). (Reprinted with permission from Ref. 27.)

Table 2   Reported Series of Splenectomy in CLL

Ref.	No. total (CLL)	% Operative mortality	Preoperative (CLL only) (Patient no.)			Postoperative rise (CLL) (Patient no.)			% RR	Survival* (median, months)
			Anemia (I)	↓ Plt (I)	↓ WBC	RBC	Plt	WBC		
12	50 (20)	8	17 (3)	16	NR	NR	14	NR	80	NR
19	13	0	13	9	NR	13	9	NR	100	(24)
22	20	0	20	20	NR	19	19	NR	95	$p < 0.001$ (45)
20	9	0	8 (4)	NR	NR	9	9	NR	100	NR
21	43	9	1†	33†	NR	NR	26	NR	83	(48)
17	20	0	20	20	NR	18	19	NR	95	(17)
18	62 (44)	1.6	10.9[M]	44† 71.5[M]	123.5[M]	12.2[M]	303[M]	95.9[M]	97	5-year—43%
23	33	6	6† 17	25†	NR	14	23	NR	85	(36)
25	14	0	13	13	NR	12	11	NR	86	$p < 0.002$‡ (45)

Ref									RR	
26	19	5	3† (2)	14†	NR	NR	12	NR	100	(108)
24	50	4	9.4[M] (10)	62[M]	32.2[M]	12.6[M]	256[M]	50.9[M]	77[1] 70[2] 64[3]	(20)
27	55	9	29 (12)	30 (12)	19[N]	18	27	14	38[1] 81[2] 59[4] (p > 0.2)	(27)
11	13	8	9.4[M]	51.5[M]	2.6[M]	12.6[M]	131.7[M]	7.3[M]	76	(31)
117	20	10	11 (11)	12	5	18	18	2	90	(44)
118	18	0	9	9	4	NR	NR	NR	83	(30)
16	9	0	NR	9	NR	NR	7	NR	88	(24)
119	15	0	NR	15	NR	NR	14	NR	57	(30)
15	42	0	37	9	NR	21	9	NR	NR	NR

Ref, Reference number; ↓ Plt, decreased platelets; WBC, white blood cell count; RBC, red blood cell; RR, overall response rate (improvement in at least one cytopenia); (I), suspected or confirmed immune hemolytic anemia or thrombocytopenia; NR, Not recorded.

* When compared with nonsplenectomized controls, p values are given.

† Stage rather than presence or absence of anemia or thrombocytopenia was recorded.

‡ In calculating the p value survival from the time of developing stage C rather than from the time of surgery was measured.

[1,2,3] Response reported for patients with anemia, thrombocytopenia or both, respectively.

[4] Response rate for patients with neutropenia.

[M] Median values are given.

[N] Number of patients with neutropenia is reported.

Table 3 Selected Reports of Splenic Irradiation in CLL

Ref.	No.	Median age (range)	Radiation dose (cGy)	Indication (patients)				Toxicity	Res (%)	Duration (m)
				Size	Pain	↓ Hgb	↓ Plt			
47	14	51 (NR)	200–1750 (3–14 days)	7	7			None "serious"	87, 78, 91, 26	18 (1–51)
48	22	69 (40–82)	125–2400 (2–30 days)	31*	10*	16*	12*	↓ Plt, infection	61, 80, 25, 14	14 (3–116)
49	22	60† (31–76)	420–1080	NR	NR	NR	NR	NR	73	NR
58	22	69 (43–86)	250–2400	5	8	2	(7)‡	Mild GI ↓ Plt, ↓ WBC	77	12
59	38	70 (45–80)	1000	NR	NR	NR	NR	None	63, 78[H]	7 (1.5–>120)
60	52	61 (39–81)	200–1000	NR	NR	NR	NR	↓ Hgb, ↓ Plt, ↓ WBC, infection	82[H]	9 (3–24)

Ref, Reference; No., patient numbers; cGy, centiGrays; NR, not recorded; ↓ Hgb; anemia; ↓ Plt, thrombocytopenia; Res, response to therapy (reported for size, pain, anemia and thrombocytopenia); m, months.
* Reported as number of courses.
† Mean value reported.
‡ Patients with a combination of abnormalities.
[H] Hematological response.

vival is uncertain (24). In the largest series published to date, investigators at the University of Texas M.D. Anderson Cancer Center reported their 21-year experience with 55 patients (27). These patients were compared with a group of 55 fludarabine-treated patients matched for baseline characteristics. Perioperative mortality was 9%, with all deaths occurring in patients with a performance status $\geq$2 (27). The hematological benefits of splenectomy were substantial. Eighty-one percent of thrombocytopenic patients had an increment of at least 50×10^9/L at 1 month. Similarly, 59% of neutropenic patients achieved a neutrophil increment of 1.0×10^9/L, and 38% of anemic patients had an increase in their hemoglobin of at least 3 g/dl (27). Of the eight assessable pancytopenic patients, six had improvements in all three lineages after splenectomy. This was the first large series in which the role of the procedure in improving the neutrophil count was also examined. Most patients in this series received chemotherapy after the surgery, and this precluded an analysis of response duration. However, the authors believed that the hematological improvements affected an increased tolerance to subsequent chemotherapy. Despite this fact and using a group of matched controls, they were unable to show a benefit in the overall survival for splenectomized patients (2-year actuarial survival rate of 50% $\pm$ 7% vs 46% $\pm$ 7% in the controls) (Figure 1) (27). Because the frequency of response was higher for the thrombocytopenic patients (Rai stage 4), this group was analyzed separately. Their survival with splenectomy, although superior, was not significantly different from controls ($p = 0.15$) (Figure 2) (27). The authors concluded that splenectomy can be performed with relative safety even in patients with advanced refractory CLL and is associated with substantial hematological benefit in most patients, with the Rai stage 4 patients being most likely to gain hematological, and, potentially, survival benefit (27).

Therefore, although the experience with splenectomy in CLL is limited to single institution studies with small series of patients, there is consensus regarding the relative safety of the procedure and the likelihood of hematological benefit. Regarding a survival benefit, this question could only be answered by a large randomized trial. However, the scarcity of candidates for the procedure and ethical issues surrounding the denial of the surgery to patients who are likely to achieve symptomatic benefit are likely to prevent such a study. Therefore, splenectomy should be considered in patients with CLL who have symptomatic splenomegaly, immune cytopenias refractory to steroids, or advanced disease with cytopenias unresponsive to therapy. Table 2 is a summary of reports of splenectomy in patients with CLL.

D. Splenic Irradiation

Although splenic irradiation has been advocated by some investigators in the treatment of cytopenias and pain associated with massive splenomegaly, its application has not received widespread acceptance (47–49). Resolution of cytopenias was seen in less than 25% of patients treated by this modality, and thrombocytopenia worsened in some patients (48).

Before the introduction of effective chemotherapy, radiation therapy was frequently used in the treatment of patients with CLL (50–56). This included total body irradiation (TBI) (52,55), as well other modes of radiation including radioactive phosphorus (56) and splenic radiation (53). The earliest reference to the application of splenic irradiation in CLL dates back to 1903 (57). More recently, several groups have investigated the toxicity and beneficial effects of this modality in patients with CLL (47–49,58–60). These retrospective series have reported high response rates in relieving pain and reducing the spleen size but less consistent effects on cytopenias (Table 3). The toxicity associated with the procedure was minimal in most series with only one septicemic death directly attributed to the treatment (48). Other side effects included gastrointestinal toxicity and worsening of cytopenia, with several patients having marked thrombocytopenia and leucopenia develop in some series (58,60). In one study an unpredictable and sometimes precipitous fall in leukocyte count was seen even with small radiation doses, and the authors recommended commencing treatment with fraction sizes of 25 to 50 cGy (48). It has also been suggested that small radiation fractions are more effective in the selective destruction of the more radiosensitive suppressor T-lymphocyte population believed to be responsible for the hypogammaglobulinemia and bone marrow stem cell suppression seen in CLL (61–64).

In summary, splenic irradiation is generally reserved for patients with splenomegaly, cytopenias, and who are not candidates for splenectomy. Although adhesions associated with radiation may increase complications of surgery, some reports suggest that use of radiation therapy in this scenario may allow a rapid clinical response and thus permit surgical removal of the spleen (60). In some patients who remain poor surgical candidates, repeated courses of radiation have been used with success and long-term responses (48,58,60).

III. COLONY-STIMULATING FACTORS

A. Hematopoietic Growth Factors in CLL

Hematopoietic growth factors and cytokines are small polypeptides or glycoproteins that play a pivotal role in normal and neoplastic cell proliferation. The binding of these molecules to their cell surface receptor results in the activation of signal transduction pathways leading to gene transcription and modulation of cellular processes (65). The main role of the hematopoietic growth factors in oncology has been to shorten the period of myelosuppression associated with chemotherapy administration. Traditionally, the treatment of CLL has been mainly supportive with the use of steroids and alkylating agents at doses not likely to produce significant myelosuppression. However, newer regimens, particularly nucleoside analogs in combination with cytotoxic agents, can induce significant granulocytopenia (4).

Patients with CLL are at a higher risk of infections, both bacterial and viral in origin (66). Indeed, infections were the main cause of mortality in most published series (67,68). It is estimated that up to 80% of patients are likely to have serious infections develop during the course of their disease, and infections will be the ultimate cause of death in no less than 60% to 85% of patients (69). The risk of infections developing also rises with the progression of the disease.

The cause of infections in CLL is related to disease and therapy-associated factors, which are considered in detail in the next chapter. Defects related to the increased incidence of infection include deficiency in immunoglobulins, poor T-cell function, and neutropenia resulting from infiltration of the bone marrow (6,66). Chemotherapy may worsen cytopenias and exacerbate the immunological incompetence of the patient. These agents may also directly affect the signaling pathways governing this process. For example, fludarabine causes a profound and specific loss of signal transducer and activator of transcription (Start 1), which is important in signaling pathways of a number of cytokines such as interleukin-2. This may contribute not only to the antineoplastic properties of this agent but also to its immunosuppressive effects, which are similar to those seen in Stat1- deficient mice (70).

Therefore, hematopoietic growth factors may be used in an attempt to reverse the cytopenias resulting from disease progression or from the effects of chemotherapy. Initially, the major concern with these agents was the possibility of stimulation of proliferation of leukemic cells. A number of studies in a variety of hematological disorders investigated the use of these agents in chemotherapy-induced myelosuppresson (71–78). Heterogeneity in response was noted, but exacerbation of the underlying disease was not a significant occurrence. Recent studies have examined the specific role of these agents in the management of CLL.

B. Reports of Growth Factor Therapy in CLL

The role of hematopoietic growth factors in combating cytopenias associated with the disease, and its treatment has been examined by several investigators (79–84). Kurzrock et al. reported two patients with CLL and a patient with myelodysplastic syndrome (MDS) who were treated with subcutaneous granulocyte-macrophage stimulating factor (GM-CSF) (79). They noted an unusual response pattern with marked eosinophilia without an increase in neutrophils when the higher dose of GM-CSF (125–300 $\mu g/m^2/day$) was used. In contrast, a low-dose regimen of 10 $\mu g/m^2/day$ resulted in the rise of neutrophils to physiological levels without a significant increase in eosinophils (79). Hollander et al. reported a patient with CLL and severe persistent neutropenia who had bilateral pneumonia develop. GM-CSF, administered at a dose of 2 $\mu g/kg$ body weight every 12 hours, resulted in a sustained rise of the neutrophil count and full resolution of the pneumonia (80). Itala et al. (81) treated 12 patients with advanced CLL with COP (cyclophosphamide, vincristine, prednisone) chemotherapy together with prophylactic GM-CSF. The median neutrophil counts 2 and 3 weeks after the first cycle of COP were significantly higher in the GM-CSF–treated patients compared with those not receiving growth factor support (2.24 and 5.47 $\times$ $10^9/L$ vs 0.59 and 0.75 $\times$ $10^9/L$, $p < 0.02$ and $p < 0.002$, respectively). A similar trend for the neutrophil counts after the next two cycles also existed but did not reach statistical significance. In this small study no significant differences were found in number of febrile days, days of intravenous antibiotic therapy, or hospitalization (81). In a prospective study, the same group evaluated the effects of long-term GM-CSF in eight patients with CLL and chronic neutropenia (82). They reported an increase in the neutrophil count in all patients by a median of 6.6-fold. Significant improvements in the neutrophil count were usually noted after 2 weeks of treatment. Also of interest was enhanced granulocyte function as measured by chemiluminescence (CL), random migration, and fMLP-stimulated chemotaxis (82). In another small study, the effect of GM-CSF on peripheral blood and bone marrow granulocytes of seven patients with CLL was investigated (83). The neutrophil count in the peripheral blood rose by a median of 193% (range, 142%–980%, $p = 0.02$) and the increase persisted for more than 2 weeks after the discontinuation of the treatment. The percentage of myeloid cells also increased in the marrow (median increase 166%, range 57%–1800%) (83). Variable responses in platelets to GM-CSF have also been reported with both enhanced thrombopoiesis and thrombocytopenia (71,76,85).

A prospective study to investigate the use of granulocyte-colony stimulating factor (G-CSF) to abrogate neutropenia developing after fludarabine was performed at the University of Texas M. D. Anderson Cancer Center (84). Historical control data indicated a high incidence of granulocytopenia (79%) and infections (54%) in patients with previously treated advanced stage disease after fludarabine therapy (2,84,86–89). In an attempt to overcome this problem 25 previously treated patients with Rai stage 3 or 4 disease were treated with monthly courses of fludarabine (30 mg/m^2/day for 5 days), followed by G-CSF at a dose of 5 µg/kg/day administered subcutaneously starting day 6 and continuing until the beginning of the next treatment course or until the granulocyte count was >10 × 10^9/L. The incidence of infections and neutropenia in these patients was then compared with the matched historical control group. There was a significant reduction in the incidence of neutropenia (absolute neutrophil count [ANC] <1.0 × 10^9/L) in the G-CSF– treated group compared with controls (45% vs 79%; p = 0.002). When the level of ANC of 0.5 × 10^9/L was used, the significance of the difference in the two groups increased (15% vs 63% in the G-CSF–treated vs controls; p = 0.001). Delay in therapy occurred in only 20% of G-CSF–supported courses versus 50% of controls (p = 0.005), and incidence of pneumonia was 8% in the treated group versus 37% for the controls. The incidence of other infections (sepsis, minor infections and fever of unknown origin) was similar for the two groups (84).

Thus, growth factor therapy is effective in ameliorating the granulocytopenia associated with advanced CLL and its treatment. With the introduction of more myelotoxic regimens, such benefits are likely to become more relevant.

IV. INTRAVENOUS IMMUNOGLOBULIN (IVIG)

A. Applications of IVIG in CLL

Clinical applications of IVIG in CLL include (1) replacement therapy in hypogammaglobulinemic patients to treat and prevent infectious complications, and (2) treatment of immune cytopenias. As mentioned earlier, infectious complications are the major cause of morbidity and mortality in patients with CLL, particularly in those with advanced disease (90). Increased susceptibility to infections is multifactorial (91–95), with decreased immunoglobulin levels one of the major factors responsible for the increased susceptibility to infections in CLL (66). These infections are often caused by encapsulated bacteria and frequently involve the respiratory tract, skin, or the urinary tract (66). Although the level of serum IgG may correlate with the risk of infection, quantity of specific antibody subclasses is likely to be a better indicator of the risk of specific infections.

The incidence and severity of hypogammaglobulinemia increases with progression of disease, length of time from diagnosis, and the extent of bone marrow involvement (96). Gamm et al. reported that a high value of β$_2$-microglobulin at the time of diagnosis was associated with an increased likelihood of early immunoglobulin deficiency (96). They reported an increased likelihood of hypogammaglobulinemia with advancing Rai stage and extensive marrow infiltration (Tables 4 and 5) (96). Overall, up to 50% of patients with CLL have low serum immunoglobulin levels (97).

The use of intramuscular immunoglobulin administration was unsuccessful largely because of the volume limitations associated with this route, which precluded achievement and maintenance of meaningful elevations in immunoglobulin levels (98,99). Later, reports of IVIG in small patient series suggested an association with decreased risk of infection (100–102). In a randomized, controlled, double-blind, multicenter trial, placebo was compared with IVIG (Gammagard, Baxter Healthcare Group, Glendale, CA), 400 mg/kg body weight every 3 weeks for 1 year, in 81 patients with B-CLL and either hypogammaglobulinemia or history of prior infection (103). The patients who received IVIG had significantly less bacterial infections (23 compared with 42; p = 0.01) and a longer interval

Table 4 Patterns of Bone Marrow Involvement and Hypogammaglobulinemia

Marrow infiltration	Patient numbers	Degree of hypogammaglobulinemia, No. (%)	
		IgG < 8.0 g/L	IgG > 8.0 g/L
Nodular	21	3 (14)	18 (86)
Diffuse:			
Interstitial	28	8 (28)	20 (72)
Complete	18	15 (83)	3 (17)
		$p = 0.00002$	

Source: Adapted from Ref. 96.

to first infection ($p = 0.026$). In the 57 patients who completed 1 full year of the study (where seasonal bias could be eliminated), treatment with IVIG was associated with a 14 bacterial infections compared with 36 in controls ($p = 0.0001$). No significant difference was found in the incidence of viral and fungal infections (103). No differences in survival between the two groups was noted.

In a follow-up report, Griffiths et al. examined 12 patients from the initial group who continued the same dose and schedule of IVIG in a crossover, double-blind study (101,104). During the 191 3-week periods of IVIG therapy, no life-threatening bacterial infections were encountered compared with 9 infections during the 162 similar periods of placebo treatment. Other bacterial infections were also reduced in frequency, with 11 episodes in the IVIG-treated patients compared with 3 in the placebo group (101,104). The p value for the difference in all bacterial infections in the two groups was 0.001. Infections tended to occur when the serum immunoglobulin level was less than normal (<6.4 g/L; $p = 0.046$) (101,104). There was no effect on the incidence of viral and fungal infections.

Cost-effectiveness of the prophylactic administration of IVIG to CLL patients has been questioned (105–107). It was estimated that an expense of $6 million was required to achieve 1 quality-adjusted life-year, without an increase in life expectancy (105). Methods of improving the cost-effectiveness include administration of lower doses or limiting use to higher risk patients. In an attempt to explore the first possibility, a multicenter study compared two regimens of IVIG in 34 patients with CLL (250 mg/kg or 500 mg/kg every 4 weeks for 1 year) (96,108). No significant difference was found in the incidence of

Table 5 Association of Serum IgG Level and Rai Stage

Rai stage	Patient numbers	IgG level	
		<6.0 g/L	>6.0 g/L
0	10	0	10
I and II	55	12 (22)	43 (78)
III and IV	31	13 (42)	18 (58)
All	96	25	71
		$p = 0.016$	

Source: Adapted from Ref. 96.

infections in the two groups ($p = 0.3$). However, this study was not powered to detect even moderate differences in bacterial infection rates between the two groups.

Molica et al. conducted a crossover study in 42 patients with CLL and hypogammaglobulinemia (IgG < 600 mg/dl) and/or history of at least one severe infection in the preceding 6 months (109). Patients received IVIG, 300 mg/kg every 4 weeks for 6 months, or no therapy. They were then switched to observation or the same regimen of IVIG for a further 12 months, and finally IVIG or no treatment for another 6 months. The authors noted a protective effect against infections by IVIG with a benefit for the patients who completed either 12 or 6 months of IVIG prophylaxis. However, they concluded that even the low-dose regimen is not a cost-effective way of preventing infections in CLL patients (109).

In an attempt to improve cost-effectiveness of IVIG, Jurlander et al. (110) administered a lower dose of IVIG (10 g every 3 weeks) to 15 patients with hypogammaglobulinemia and a history of recurrent infections. Serum immunoglobulin levels were significantly higher than baseline after 3 doses ($p = 0.0002$) and stabilized within the normal range after 11 doses. The total number of infections was reduced during the therapy period compared with a similar time interval before IVIG, and the number of antibiotic prescriptions was reduced (not statistically significant) (110). The number of hospital admissions related to infection and number of febrile episodes were significantly reduced ($p = 0.047$ and $p = 0.004$, respectively).

Most studies clearly indicate the effectiveness of IVIG (in various doses) in reducing the incidence of bacterial infections in patients with CLL. Nevertheless, issues related to expense, as well as whether early use of antibiotics might be a less expensive way of obtaining the same effect, are ongoing concerns. Our approach is to use IVIG in patients with hypogammaglobulinemia and repeated sino/pulmonary infections poorly controlled with or recurrent after antibiotic therapy.

B. Role of IVIG in the Management of Immune Cytopenias

As elaborated in Chapter 21 of this book, a common complication of CLL is the development of autoimmune cytopenias. Autoimmune hemolytic anemia (AIHA) occurs in 5% to 37% of patients with CLL, autoimmune thrombocytopenia (AIT) in 1% to 3% of patients, and pure red cell aplasia (PRCA) is a less common but probably an underreported complication of the disease (7,111). Both splenectomy and IVIG have a significant role in the management of immune complications of CLL, in particular AIHA (7). The role of IVIG in the treatment of AIHA was examined in a meta-analysis comprising several small series (112). This analysis included 18 patients with CLL and AIHA and 55 patients with other causes. Overall, a greater than 2 g/dl increase in hemoglobin was seen in 40% of patients. Doses of IVIG of 400 mg/kg/day for 5 days or 1 g/kg/day for 5 to 7 days produced a similar response rate (112). In the 18 patients with CLL, therapy with IVIG was also associated with a decrease in spleen and lymph node size (100). Improvements were, however, transient, and IVIG was needed every 3 to 4 weeks (113). Almost all patients received concomitant steroid treatment (113). Therefore, IVIG is indicated in the treatment of AIHA associated with CLL when a rapid response is necessary, when a limited response is adequate, and when the patient is already receiving steroid therapy (7).

The association of PRCA and CLL has been reported infrequently (114). It is likely that the condition is underreported as multiple other causes of anemia limit its diagnosis.

Steroids and cyclosporin are the mainstay of therapy, and use of IVIG has rarely been reported (114). Similarly, the application of IVIG in the treatment of AIT in CLL is limited to a few case reports (115,116).

V. CONCLUDING REMARKS

With more effective treatments for cancers and prolongation of life expectancy, supportive care has become increasingly important in the management of patients. This is particularly important in patients with CLL who have an indolent disease, amenable to effective long-term control. Supportive care measures in CLL are likely to involve the amelioration of cytopenias associated with the disease and its treatment to reduce the complications of the disease, particularly infection. Although splenectomy, growth factors, and IVIG have not been extensively applied in the management of CLL patients, better understanding of their role and mechanisms of action is likely to lead to their increased application or more targeted use.

REFERENCES

1. JC Reed. Molecular biology of chronic lymphocytic leukemia: implications for therapy. Semin Hematol 35:3–13, 1998.
2. BD Cheson. Therapy for previously untreated chronic lymphocytic leukemia: a reevaluation. Semin Hematol 35:14–21, 1998.
3. MJ Keating. Chronic lymphocytic leukemia. Semin Oncol 26:107–114, 1999.
4. S O'Brien. Clinical challenges in chronic lymphocytic leukemia. Semin Hematol 35:22–26, 1998.
5. KR Rai, T Han. Prognostic factors and clinical staging in chronic lymphocytic leukemia. Hematol Oncol Clin North Am 4:447–456, 1990.
6. VA Morrison. The infectious complications of chronic lymphocytic leukemia. Semin Oncol 25:98–106, 1998.
7. LF Diehl, LH Ketchum. Autoimmune disease and chronic lymphocytic leukemia: autoimmune hemolytic anemia, pure red cell aplasia, and autoimmune thrombocytopenia. Semin Oncol 25:80–97, 1998.
8. EL Eliason, J Johnson. Splenectomy. Surgery 13:177, 1943.
9. T Bryant. Case of excision of the spleen for an enlargement of the organ, attended with leucocythemia. In a patient under the care of Dr. Wiks, with remarks. Guy's Hosp Rep 13: 411–418, 1868.
10. WJ Mayo. Review of 500 splenectomies with special reference to mortality and end results. Ann Surg 88:409–415, 1928.
11. MM Strumia, PV Strumia, D Bassert. Splenectomy in leukemia: hematologic and clinical effects on 34 patients and review of 299 published cases. Cancer Res 26:519–528, 1966.
12. S Adler, L Stutzman, J Sokal, et al. Splenectomy for hematologic depression in lymphocytic lymphoma and leukemia. Cancer 35:521–528, 1975.
13. LT Yam, WH Crosby. Early splenectomy in lymphoproliferative disorders. Arch Intern Med 133:270–274, 1974.
14. PJ Morris, IA Cooper, JP Madigan. Splenectomy for haematological cytopenias in patients with malignant lymphomas. Lancet 2:250–253, 1975.
15. BE Christensen, MM Hansen, A Videbaek. Splenectomy in chronic lymphocytic leukaemia. Scand J Haematol 18:279–287, 1977.
16. SA Merl, ME Theodorakis, J Goldberg, et al. Splenectomy for thrombocytopenia in chronic lymphocytic leukemia. Am J Hematol 15:253–259, 1983.

17. A Ferrant, JL Michaux, G Sokal. Splenectomy in advanced chronic lymphocytic leukemia. Cancer 58:2130–2135, 1986.
18. JR Delpero, G Houvenaeghel, JA Gastaut, et al. Splenectomy for hypersplenism in chronic lymphocytic leukaemia and malignant non-Hodgkin's lymphoma (published erratum appears in Br J Surg 1990 Aug; 77[8]:957). Br J Surg 77:443–449, 1990.
19. RS Stein, D Weikert, V Reynolds, et al. Splenectomy for end-stage chronic lymphocytic leukemia. Cancer 59:1815–1818, 1987.
20. SJ Mentzer, RT Osteen, H Fletcher Starnes, et al. Splenic enlargement and hyperfunction as indications for splenectomy in chronic leukemia. Ann Surg 205:13–17, 1986.
21. B Pegourie, JJ Sotto, D Hollard, et al. Splenectomy during chronic lymphocytic leukemia. Cancer 59:1626–1630, 1987.
22. G Gallhofer, JV Melo, J Spencer, et al. Splenectomy in advanced chronic lymphocytic leukaemia. Acta Haematol 77:78–82, 1987.
23. R Thiruvengadam, M Piedmonte, M Barcos, et al. Splenectomy in advanced chronic lymphocytic leukemia. Leukemia 4:758–760, 1990.
24. TF Neal Jr, A Tefferi, TE Witzig, et al. Splenectomy in advanced chronic lymphocytic leukemia: a single institution experience with 50 patients. Am J Med 93:435–440, 1992.
25. G Majumdar, AK Singh. Role of splenectomy in chronic lymphocytic leukaemia with massive splenomegaly and cytopenia. Leuk Lymphoma 7:131–134, 1992.
26. JE Coad, E Matutes, D Catovsky. Splenectomy in lymphoproliferative disorders: a report on 70 cases and review of the literature. Leuk Lymphoma 10:245–264, 1993.
27. JF Seymour, JD Cusack, SA Lerner, et al. Case/control study of the role of splenectomy in chronic lymphocytic leukemia. J Clin Oncol 15:52–60, 1997.
28. JW Athens. Disorders primarily involving the spleen. In: GR Lee, TC Bithell, J Foerster, et al., eds. Wintrobe's Clinical Hematology. 9th ed. Philadelphia, London: Lea & Febiger, 1993. pp 1704–1722.
29. EL Amorosi. Hypersplenism. Semin Hematol 2:249, 1965.
30. W Dameshek, S Estren. Hypersplenism. Med Clin North Am 34, 1950.
31. JW Duckett. Splenectomy in treatment of secondary hypersplenism. Ann Surg 157:737, 1963.
32. GW Donaldson, M McArthur, AI Macpherson, et al. Blood volume changes in splenomegaly. Br J Haematol 18:45–55, 1970.
33. CS Wright. Direct splenic arterial and venous blood studies in the hypersplenic syndromes before and after epinephrine. Blood 6:195, 1951.
34. RH Aster. Pooling of platelets in the spleen: role in the pathogenesis of "hypersplenic" thrombocytopenia. J Clin Invest 45:645–657, 1966.
35. WH Crosby. Is hypersplenism a dead issue? Blood 20:94, 1962.
36. G Ruhrenstroth-Bauer. The role of humoral splenic factors in the formation and release of blood cells. Semin Hematol 2:229, 1965.
37. H Fudenberg. The body hematocrit/venous hematocrit ratio and the splenic reservoir. Blood 17:71, 1961.
38. JH Jandl, NM Files, SB Barnett, et al. Proliferative response of the spleen and liver to hemolysis. J Exp Med 122:299–326, 1966.
39. K Rai, DP Patel. Chronic lymphocytic leukemia. In: R Hoffman, EJ Benz, SJ Shattil, et al., eds. Hematology: Basic Principles and Practice, 2nd ed. New York, Edinburgh, London, Madrid, Melbourne, Milan, Tokyo: Churchill Livingstone, 1995, pp 1308–1322.
40. KA Foon, KR Rai, RP Gale. Chronic lymphocytic leukemia: new insights into biology and therapy. Ann Intern Med 113:525–539, 1990.
41. TJ Hamblin, DG Oscier, BJ Young. Autoimmunity in chronic lymphocytic leukaemia. J Clin Pathol 39:713–716, 1986.
42. WW Coon. Splenectomy in the treatment of hemolytic anemia. Arch Surg 120:625–628, 1985.

43. AJ Bowdler. The role of the spleen and splenectomy in autoimmune hemolytic disease. Semin Hematol 13:335–348, 1976.
44. G Cherrkow. Results of splenectomy in autoimmune haemolytic anemia. Br J Haematol 2: 237–249, 1956.
45. S O'Brien, H Kantarjian, M Beran, et al. Results of fludarabine and prednisone therapy in 264 patients with chronic lymphocytic leukemia with multivariate analysis-derived prognostic model for response to treatment [see comments]. Blood 82:1695–1700, 1993.
46. T Han, EZ Ezdinli, K Shimaoka, et al. Chlorambucil vs. combined chlorambucil-corticosteroid therapy in chronic lymphocytic leukemia. Cancer 31:502–508, 1973.
47. RW Byhardt, KC Brace, PH Wiernik. The role of splenic irradiation in chronic lymphocytic leukemia. Cancer 35:1621–1625, 1975.
48. MJ Guiney, KH Liew, GG Quong, et al. A study of splenic irradiation in chronic lymphocytic leukemia. Int J Radiat Oncol Biol Phys 16:225–229, 1989.
49. G De Rossi, C Biagini, M Lopez, et al. Treatment by splenic irradiation in 22 chronic lymphocytic leukemia patients. Tumori 68:511–514, 1982.
50. RE Johnson. Role of radiation therapy in management of adult leukemia. Cancer 39:852–855, 1977.
51. RE Johnson, AR Kagan, HR Gralnick, et al. Radiation-induced remissions in chronic lymphocytic leukemia. Cancer 20:1382–1387, 1967.
52. RE Johnson. Total body irradiation of chronic lymphocytic leukemia: incidence and duration of remission. Cancer 25:523–530, 1970.
53. H Awwad. The effects of splenic irradiation on the ferrokinetics of chronic leukemia with a clinical study. Blood 29:242–256, 1967.
54. JC Cook, W Romano. Chronic lymphocytic leukemia and radiation therapy. Am J Roentgenol 88:892–901, 1962.
55. JA del Regato. Total body irradiation in the treatment of chronic lymphogenous leukemia. Am J Roentgenol 120:504–520, 1974.
56. EE Osgood, AJ Seaman. Treatment of chronic leukemias-Results of therapy by titrated, regularly spaced, radioactive phosphorus or roentgen irradiation. JAMA 150:1372–1379, 1952.
57. N Senn. Case of spleno-medullary leukemia successfully treated by use of roentgen ray. Med Rec NY 63:281, 1903.
58. K Aabo, S Walbom-Jorgensen. Spleen irradiation in chronic lymphocytic leukemia (CLL): palliation in patients unfit for splenectomy. Am J Hematol 19:177–180, 1985.
59. M Roncadin, M Arcicasa, MG Trovo, et al. Splenic irradiation in chronic lymphocytic leukemia. A 10-year experience at a single institution. Cancer 60:2624–2628, 1987.
60. T Chisesi, G Capnist, S Dal Fior. Splenic irradiation in chronic lymphocytic leukemia. Eur J Haematol 46:202–204, 1991.
61. D Catovsky, F Lauria, E Matutes, et al. Increase in T gamma lymphocytes in B-cell chronic lymphocytic leukaemia. II. Correlation with clinical stage and findings in B-prolymphocytic leukaemia. Br J Haematol 47:539–544, 1981.
62. P Hersey, J Wotherspoon, G Reid, et al. Hypogammaglobulinaemia associated with abnormalities of both B and T lymphocytes in patients with chronic lymphatic leukaemia. Clin Exp Immunol 39:698–707, 1980.
63. SK Durum, N Gengozian. The comparative radiosensitivity of T and B lymphocytes. Int J Radiat Biol 34:1–15, 1978.
64. AER Thomson, S Vaughn-Smith, WE Peel, et al. The intrinsic radiosensitivity of lymphocytes in chronic lymphocytic leukaemia, quantitatively determined independently of cell death factors. Int J Radiat Biol 6:943–961, 1985.
65. SC Clark, R Kamen. The human hematopoietic colony-stimulating factors. Science 236: 1229–1237, 1987.
66. HM Chapel, C Bunch. Mechanisms of infection in chronic lymphocytic leukemia. Semin Hematol 24:291–296, 1987.

67. S Molica. Infections in chronic lymphocytic leukemia: risk factors, and impact on survival, and treatment. Leuk Lymphoma 13:203–214, 1994.
68. BD Cheson. Infectious and immunosuppressive complications of purine analog therapy. J Clin Oncol 13:2431–2448, 1995.
69. M Itala, H Helenius, J Nikoskelainen, et al. Infections and serum IgG levels in patients with chronic lymphocytic leukemia. Eur J Haematol 48:266–270, 1992.
70. DA Frank, S Mahajan, J Ritz. Fludarabine-induced immunosuppression is associated with inhibition of STAT1 signaling. Nat Med 5:444–447, 1999.
71. S Vadhan-Raj, M Keating, A LeMaistre, et al. Effects of recombinant human granulocyte-macrophage colony-stimulating factor in patients with myelodysplastic syndromes. N Engl J Med 317:1545–1552, 1987.
72. S Vadhan-Raj, S Buescher, HE Broxmeyer, et al. Stimulation of myelopoiesis in patients with aplastic anemia by recombinant human granulocyte-macrophage colony-stimulating factor [published erratum appears in N Engl J Med 1989 Feb 2;320(5):329]. N Engl J Med 319: 1628–1634, 1988.
73. JE Groopman, RT Mitsuyasu, MJ DeLeo, et al. Effect of recombinant human granulocyte-macrophage colony-stimulating factor on myelopoiesis in the acquired immunodeficiency syndrome. N Engl J Med 317:593–598, 1987.
74. JH Antin, BR Smith, W Holmes, et al. Phase I/II study of recombinant human granulocyte-macrophage colony-stimulating factor in aplastic anemia and myelodysplastic syndrome. Blood 72:705–713, 1988.
75. F Herrmann, G Schulz, A Lindemann, et al. Hematopoietic responses in patients with advanced malignancy treated with recombinant human granulocyte-macrophage colony-stimulating factor. J Clin Oncol 7:159–167, 1989.
76. A Ganser, B Volkers, J Greher, et al. Recombinant human granulocyte-macrophage colony-stimulating factor in patients with myelodysplastic syndromes—a phase I/II trial. Blood 73: 31–37, 1989.
77. JA Thompson, DJ Lee, P Kidd, et al. Subcutaneous granulocyte-macrophage colony-stimulating factor in patients with myelodysplastic syndrome: toxicity, pharmacokinetics, and hematological effects. J Clin Oncol 7:629–637, 1989.
78. RE Champlin, SD Nimer, P Ireland, et al. Treatment of refractory aplastic anemia with recombinant human granulocyte-macrophage-colony-stimulating factor. Blood 73:694–699, 1989.
79. R Kurzrock, M Talpaz, JA Gomez, et al. Differential dose-related haematological effects of GM-CSF in pancytopenia: evidence supporting the advantage of low-over high-dose administration in selected patients. Br J Haematol 78:352–358, 1991.
80. AA Hollander, HC Kluin-Nelemans, HR Haak, et al. Correction of neutropenia associated with chronic lymphocytic leukaemia following treatment with granulocyte-macrophage colony-stimulating factor. Ann Hematol 62:32–34, 1991.
81. M Itala, S Vanhatalo, K Remes. Effect of recombinant human granulocyte-macrophage colony-stimulating factor (GM-CSF) on chemotherapy-induced myelosuppression in patients with chronic lymphocytic leukemia: a crossover study. Leuk Lymphoma 25:503–508, 1997.
82. M Itala, TT Pelliniemi, K Remes, et al. Long-term treatment with GM-CSF in patients with chronic lymphocytic leukemia and recurrent neutropenic infections. Leuk Lymphoma 32: 165–174, 1998.
83. P de Nully Brown, MM Hansen. GM-CSF treatment in patients with B-chronic lymphocytic leukemia. Leuk Lymphoma 32:365–368, 1999.
84. S O'Brien, H Kantarjian, M Beran, et al. Fludarabine and granulocyte colony-stimulating factor (G-CSF) in patients with chronic lymphocytic leukemia. Leukemia 11:1631–1635, 1997.
85. EH Estey, R Kurzrock, M Talpaz, et al. Effects of low doses of recombinant human granulo-

cyte-macrophage colony stimulating factor (GM-CSF) in patients with myelodysplastic syndromes. Br J Haematol 77:291–295, 1991.

86. MJ Keating, S O'Brien, H Kantarjian, et al. Long-term follow-up of patients with chronic lymphocytic leukemia treated with fludarabine as a single agent. Blood 81:2878–2884, 1993.

87. S O'Brien, H Kantarjian, M Beran. Fludarabine (FAMP) and cyclophosphamide (CTX) therapy in chronic lymphocytic leukemia (CLL). Blood 88:480a, 1996.

88. S O'Brien, H Kantarjian, M Beran. Fludarabine (FAMP) and mitoxantrone therapy in chronic lymphocytic leukemia (CLL0). Blood 88:588a, 1996.

89. MJ Keating, S O'Brien, S Lerner, et al. Long-term follow-up of patients with chronic lymphocytic leukemia (CLL) receiving fludarabine regimens as initial therapy. Blood 92:1165–1171, 1998.

90. JS Lee, DO Dixon, HM Kantarjian, et al. Prognosis of chronic lymphocytic leukemia: a multivariate regression analysis of 325 untreated patients. Blood 69:929–936, 1987.

91. EC Besa. Recent advances in the treatment of chronic lymphocytic leukemia: defining the role of intravenous immunoglobulin. Semin Hematol 29:14–23, 1992.

92. RT Jim, EH Reinhard. Agammaglobulinemia in chronic lymphocytic leukemia. Ann Intern Med 44:790–796, 1956.

93. E Kansu, E Akalin, C Civelek, et al. Serum bactericidal and opsonic activities in chronic lymphocytic leukemia and multiple myeloma. Am J Hematol 23:191–196, 1986.

94. N Chioazzi, SM Fu, G Moutagen. T cell helper defect in patients with chronic lymphocytic leukemia. J Immunol 122:1087–1090, 1979.

95. DG Miller. Patterns of immunological deficiency in lymphomas and leukemias. Ann Intern Med 57:703–716, 1962.

96. H Gamm, C Huber, H Chapel, et al. Intravenous immune globulin in chronic lymphocytic leukaemia. Clin Exp Immunol 97 (suppl 1):17–20, 1994.

97. P Fiddes, R Penny, JV Wells. Clinical correlations with immunoglobulin levels in chronic lymphocytic leukemia. Aus NZ J Med 4:346–350, 1972.

98. GH Fairley, RB Scott. Hypogammaglobulinemia in chronic lymphocytic leukemia. Br Med J 4:920–924, 1961.

99. D Miller, DA Karnofsky. Immunologic factors and resistance to infection in chronic lymphocytic leukemia. Am J Med 31:748–757, 1961.

100. EC Besa. Use of intravenous immunoglobulin in chronic lymphocytic leukemia. Am J Med 76:209–218, 1984.

101. H Griffiths, V Brennan, J Lea, et al. Crossover study of immunoglobulin replacement therapy in patients with low-grade B-cell tumors. Blood 73:366–368, 1989.

102. C Bunch, H Chapel, K Raj. Intravenous immune globulin reduces bacterial infections in chronic lymphocytic leukemia: a controlled, randomized clinical trial. Blood 70:224a, 1987.

103. leukemia. Cgftsoiicl: Intravenous immunoglobulin for the prevention of infection in chronic lymphocytic leukemia- a randomized, controlled clinical trial. N Engl J Med 319:902–907, 1988.

104. M Dicato, H Chapel, H Gamm, et al. Use of intravenous immunoglobulin in chronic lymphocytic leukemia. A brief review. Cancer 68:1437–1439, 1991.

105. JC Weeks, MR Tierney, MC Weinstein. Cost effectiveness of prophylactic intravenous immune globulin in chronic lymphocytic leukemia [see comments]. N Engl J Med 325:81–86, 1991.

106. EC Besa, D Klumpe. Prophylactic immune globulin in chronic lymphocytic leukemia [letter; comment]. N Engl J Med 326:139, 1992.

107. HM Chapel, M Lee. Immunoglobulin replacement in patients with chronic lymphocytic leukemia (CLL): kinetics of immunoglobulin metabolism. J Clin Immunol 12:17–20, 1992.

108. H Chapel, M Dicato, H Gamm, et al. Immunoglobulin replacement in patients with chronic lymphocytic leukaemia: a comparison of two dose regimes. Br J Haematol 88:209–212, 1994.

109. S Molica, P Musto, F Chiurazzi, et al. Prophylaxis against infections with low-dose intravenous immunoglobulins (IVIG) in chronic lymphocytic leukemia. Results of a crossover study. Haematologica 81:121–126, 1996.

110. J Jurlander, CH Geisler, MM Hansen. Treatment of hypogammaglobulinaemia in chronic lymphocytic leukaemia by low-dose intravenous gammaglobulin. Eur J Haematol 53:114–118, 1994.

111. FR Mauro, R Foa, R Cerretti, et al. Autoimmune hemolytic anemia in chronic lymphocytic leukemia: clinical, therapeutic, and prognostic features. Blood 95:2786–2792, 2000.

112. G Flores, C Cunningham-Rundles, AC Newland, et al. Efficacy of intravenous immunoglobulin in the treatment of autoimmune hemolytic anemia: results in 73 patients. Am J Hematol 44:237–242, 1993.

113. EC Besa. Rapid transient reversal of anemia and long-term effects of maintenance intravenous immunoglobulin for autoimmune hemolytic anemia in patients with lymphoproliferative disorders. Am J Med 84:691–698, 1988.

114. G Chikkappa, MH Zarrabi, MF Tsan. Pure red-cell aplasia in patients with chronic lymphocytic leukemia. Medicine (Baltimore) 65:339–351, 1986.

115. E Fiorentino, L Coppotelli, M Pergolini, et al. [The efficacy of i.v. immunoglobulins at high doses in a case of thrombocytopenia with an immune pathogenesis in chronic lymphocytic leukemia]. Clin Ter 140:17–23, 1992.

116. M Montillo, A Tedeschi, P Leoni. Recurrence of autoimmune thrombocytopenia after treatment with fludarabine in a patient with chronic lymphocytic leukemia [letter; comment]. Leuk Lymphoma 15:187–188, 1994.

117. JM Holt, LJ Witts. Splenectomy in leukaemia and the reticuloses. Q J Med 35:369–384, 1966.

118. PG Gill, RG Souter, PJ Morris. Splenectomy for hypersplenism in malignant lymphomas. Br J Surg 68:29–33, 1981.

119. SI Schwartz. Splenectomy for thrombocytopenia. World J Surg 9:416–421, 1985.

23

Infections in Patients with Chronic Lymphocytic Leukemia

Pathogenesis, Spectrum, and Therapeutic Approaches

VICKI A. MORRISON

Veterans Affairs Medical Center, Minneapolis, Minnesota

I. INTRODUCTION

Infectious complications continue to be of great significance in the disease course of patients with chronic lymphocytic leukemia (CLL), being a major contributor to morbidity and mortality (1–6). These patients are predisposed to infections both because of the immune compromise, predominantly hypogammaglobulinemia, inherent to the primary disease process, and additional immunosuppression related to therapy with agents such as corticosteroids, purine analogs, and other cytotoxic drugs. It has been estimated that up to 80% of CLL patients will have their disease course complicated by infections, which range from moderate to life-threatening in severity (1–3). Infection is the leading cause of death in most series, accounting for mortality in 30% to 60% of CLL patients (1–4,7,8). Despite advances in therapeutics and antimicrobial support over the past five decades, the incidence of infection has nonetheless remained relatively constant (3,4,9). The introduction of purine analogs into the therapeutic armamentarium for this disease process in the past two decades had an impact on the spectrum of infectious complications seen in this population. Although bacterial infections, especially of the respiratory tract, remain most common (1–3), the occurrence of opportunistic infections, such as those caused by *Candida* species and herpesviruses, has increased, related to the prolonged T-cell immunosuppression induced by this group of agents (10–14). In this chapter we will discuss the pathogenesis of infection in this population, the spectrum of infections seen, risk factors for infection, and potential approaches for infection prophylaxis.

II. PATHOGENESIS

The pathogenesis of infection in patients with CLL is multifactorial. Inherent immune defects are influenced by the stage of disease, in addition to therapy administered. Although humoral immune dysfunction, specifically hypogammaglobulinemia, is the predominant immune defect (1–3,5,15), abnormalities in cell-mediated immunity, complement activity, and neutrophil function have also been described (1,2,16–21). However, the relationship between hypogammaglobulinemia and subsequent infection has been more clearly defined than the risk of infection with defects in other aspects of immunity.

A. Hypogammaglobulinemia

The prevalence of hypogammaglobulinemia, which is persistent and often profound, approaches 100% in patients with CLL (6,22,23). The development of hypogammaglobulinemia may be related to functional abnormalities of the T cells and to dysfunction of the nonclonal CD5- B cells, which may decreased because of progressive dilution or inhibition (24,25). The occurrence of hypogammaglobulinemia correlates with the duration and stage of disease and approaches 70% by 7 years after diagnosis (5,26,27). This immune defect is not reversed by therapy with conventional agents, despite a hematological improvement in the disease process (28). Reports of improvement in the hypogammaglobulinemia with fludarabine therapy are only preliminary (29). The hypogammaglobulinemia primarily involves immunoglobulin (Ig) subtypes IgG3 and IgG4.

Hypogammaglobulinemia has been associated with the frequency (or number) of infections in these patients (1,5,9,15,28,30–34). In Fairley's series, low serum immunoglobulin levels were present in 67% of the patients, and correlated with the number of infections and disease duration (5). The relationship between hypogammaglobulinemia and recurrent infections was also noted by Ultmann (15). The relationship between immunoglobulin levels at presentation and survival has been examined in several studies. An initial deficiency of either IgG, IgA, or IgM was not found to influence survival in Ben-Bassat's series (27). However, Rozman et al. (26) reported that the presence of hypogammaglobulinemia at diagnosis, specifically an IgG level of less than 700 mg/dl, was prognostic for shortened survival among a series of 247 patients. Low levels of IgM did not have an impact on survival in their series. They also noted that the frequency of low IgG and IgA levels increased with more advanced stage disease; however, this relationship was not seen with IgM levels.

Likewise, the impact of specific immunoglobulin class deficiencies has also been examined. In Montserrat's series, the most common immunoglobulin class deficiency was IgM, followed by IgA, and lastly by IgG (35). This observation is in contrast to Foa's series, in which IgA was the most common immunoglobulin deficiency (36). Although the correlation between hypogammaglobulinemia and infection risk is well recognized in these patients, the relationship between a deficiency in a specific immunoglobulin class and the risk of infection is not as clearly established. Chapel & Bunch (1) reported an association between low serum IgG levels and recurrent infections. Itala also found a significant association between low serum IgG levels, disease stage, and infection (30). Multiple infections were more common in patients with low levels of either IgG, IgA, or

IgM in North's series (1). This association was most marked in patients with a low IgG; the relationship between infection and low IgA or IgM levels was less marked. In a more recent report, patients with a low serum IgA level had a significantly higher infection rate compared with patients with a normal IgA level (37–39). In this series, 69% of patients with a low serum IgA had at least four infections compared with 27% of patients with a normal serum IgA. The impact of a low serum IgA remained significant when major infections were examined. No major infections occurred in 85% of patients with a normal serum IgA. Among patients with a low serum IgA, 46% had no major infections, whereas the remaining 54% sustained at least one major infection. A marginal association ($p <$ .06) was found between a low serum IgG and infection rate; however, this association disappeared after stratification for the IgA level. The association between a high infection rate and low serum IgA level persisted, however, after stratification by serum IgM level. No association was found between a low serum IgM and infection rate in this series. The increased frequency of respiratory tract infections in this population may be related to deficiencies in serum IgA and IgG4 (26,40). Likewise, because IgG3 is important in immunity against herpesvirus infections, deficiencies in this immunoglobulin may predispose to these infections (1,41).

Aittoniemi et al. (42) examined the influence of serum immunoglobulins and mannan-binding lectin on the risk of infection in a series of 28 CLL patients. Mannan-binding lectin is an acute phase reactant that is a component of the lectin pathway of complement. It functions to opsonize microbes for phagocytic cells, and deficiency of this substance is associated with increased susceptibility to infection. Nine of the 28 patients (32%) sustained either severe or moderate infections. The presence of hypogammaglobulinemia and of low levels of the IgG2 and IgG4 subtypes was associated with an increased risk of infection. The levels of IgG2 and IgG4 in these patients correlated with the IgA levels. However, in subsequent multivariate analysis, only a low IgA level was found to be an independent risk factor for infection. Last, the mean concentration of mannan-binding lectin was significantly higher in patients with infection than in those patients without infection.

B. Complement

Complement (C) has a crucial role in the control of infections caused by encapsulated organisms, because opsonization with complement is necessary for subsequent neutrophil interactions. Deficiencies of C1, C4, and C2 have been associated with pneumococcal infections; likewise, deficiencies in C3, C5, C6, C7, or C8 may predispose to neisserial infections. Serum concentrations of C2, C3, C4, properdin, and total hemolytic complement have been found to be normal to increased in CLL patients in some series (18,28). However, in a recently reported series, reduced levels of complement were found in 100% of advanced stage CLL patients, and in 40% of patients with early stage disease (43). Nonetheless, defects in complement activation and binding have been found in CLL patients (18,28). Health examined the binding of C3b to *Staphylococcus aureus*, *Streptococcus pneumoniae*, and *Escherichia coli* in a series of CLL patients and found that low amounts of C3b were bound to bacteria (18). Variable defects in opsonization were also present among the bacterial isolates tested. The addition of normal serum to the CLL serum resulted in normalization of the C3b binding activity, implying that an inhibitor of complement activity was not present. The authors concluded that a defect was present in either the activation or the activity of C3 in the CLL patients' sera and postulated that a deficiency in a heat-labile factor in the sera resulted in decreased activation and binding of C3. In addition, it was found that less C3b was bound in the sera of patients with a prior history of bacterial infections than in the sera of patients who had no prior infections. In contrast to these findings, Miller and Karnofsky (28) found no relationship between complement levels and past infections in this series of CLL patients. Despite these findings of complement abnormalities in CLL patients, no relationship has been consistently established between serum complement levels and the risk of infectious complications.

C. Neutropenia and Phagocytic Cell Defects

Although a relative neutropenia is present in untreated CLL patients, the absolute neutrophil count is usually normal to only slightly decreased (33). However, with disease progression, leukemic infiltration of the bone marrow and suppression of granulopoiesis by cellular or humoral mediators may result in neutropenia. The use of aggressive myelosuppressive chemotherapy regimens may also result in neutropenia, thus predisposing these patients to common bacterial and fungal infections.

Neutrophil function is generally normal in untreated CLL patients (19). Although normal neutrophil phagocytosis is reported in some series (44–46), others have found that sera of CLL patients will inhibit neutrophil phagocytic and bactericidal activity (47). Concentrations of neutrophil alkaline phosphatase and neutral protease in the monocytes of a series of untreated CLL patients were found to be normal, although deficiencies in β-glucuronidase, lysozyme, and myeloperoxidase were present (20). Similar enzyme deficiencies were also present in the neutrophils of some patients. These defects may resolve with hematological remission.

D. Cell-mediated Immunity

Although cell-mediated immune function is also abnormal in CLL patients, no relationship has been clearly established between cellular immune dysfunction and subsequent infectious complications. Although the absolute T-lymphocyte count is generally normal to slightly increased, these cells display abnormalities in their antigen receptors (48). Abnormalities in T-cell subsets, as an increase in the percentage of T-suppressor lymphocytes, resulting in a decreased CD4/CD8 ratio, are also seen (16,49,50). Excessive T-suppressor and deficient T-helper cell function with regard to B-cell proliferation has also been found (17). Reduced T-cell colony-forming capacity, defective spontaneous and antibody-dependent cytotoxicity mediated by E-rosette–positive and E-rosette–negative cells, and defects in NK cell activity have been reported (16,50). CLL-derived NK cells have defects in activation and lysis of appropriate targets, which may potentially contribute to the occurrence of hypogammaglobulinemia, because CD16+ CLL-derived NK cells inhibit mitogen-induced immunoglobulin secretion by normal B cells (51,52). As with the B-lymphocyte defects, the T-cell defects become more pronounced in patients with advanced stage disease.

Impaired cell-mediated immunity to recall antigens, resulting in poor delayed hypersensitivity responses to a variety of skin test antigens, has also been found (21,28,33,48). B-CLL cells secrete TGF-β, which inhibits B-cell proliferation and also releases circulating IL-2 receptors, which potentially bind endogenous IL-2, with a resultant downregulation of T-cell function (41). CD8+ B-CLL T-cells may secrete IL-4, which can induce the expression of the bcl-2 protein, which may contribute to the pathogenesis and progression of CLL (41). In addition, unlike normal B cells, the B-CLL cells are ineffective antigen-presenting cells caused by membrane defects of the CD5+ B-cells. This defect may be related to the low levels of surface immunoglobulin on the B-CLL cells, and their suboptimal expression of costimulatory molecules CD80 and CD86, in addition to CD79b.

E. Mucosal Immunity

The systemic humoral immune defects in CLL patients are well recognized. However, little data exist regarding the integrity of mucosal immunity in these patients, and the relationship between systemic immune dysfunction and mucosal immune defects. In a preliminary study, levels of serum and mucosal (salivary) IgA, IgG, and IgM were measured in a series of CLL patients and control subjects (37–39). Systemic hypogammaglobulinemia was common, with deficiencies present in at least one immunoglobulin class in 74% of the patients. The most frequent serum immunoglobulin deficiency was IgM, which was low in 74% of patients; serum IgG and IgA levels were low in 36% and 33% of patients, respectively. Despite these consistent serum immunoglobulin deficiencies, variable changes were seen in mucosal immunoglobulin levels. As in serum, salivary IgM levels were profoundly decreased in the CLL patients compared with controls. However, there were no differences in salivary IgG or IgA between CLL patients and control subjects. Those patients with a low serum IgA had a significantly higher infection rate compared with patients with a normal IgA level. However, there was no correlation between serum IgG or IgM levels or salivary immunoglobulin levels and infection rate.

Questions thus remain in the understanding of mucosal immunity in CLL patients. Our preliminary data of low mucosal IgM levels in saliva suggest that the mucosal B cells of these patients, in addition to systemic B cells, may also have defects in immune function. Preservation of the salivary IgA and IgG levels may simply reflect transudation of these immunoglobulins from serum to mucosal surfaces. Alternatively, the lack of perturbation of mucosal IgA and IgG levels in saliva may support a differential regulation of systemic and mucosal immunity in these patients. Examination of the immunoglobulin genes, specifically those that participate in forming the antigen-binding sites (as the variable region of the heavy chain [V_H genes], may provide more information on the status of the mucosal immunity in these patients and will aid in determining whether the mucosal immune system is regulated independently of its systemic counterpart and if the mucosal B cells are part of the malignant B-cell clone.

F. Splenectomy

Indications for splenectomy in CLL patients include autoimmune hemolytic anemia, immune thrombocytopenia, splenomegaly, and cytopenia caused by hypersplenism. These patients are subsequently predisposed to infections with encapsulated bacteria. Seymour et al. reported on the outcome of 55 patients who underwent splenectomy for CLL at the M.D. Anderson Cancer Center from 1971 to 1993 (53). In the perioperative period, minor wound or urinary tract infections occurred in 18% of the patients and pneumonia/basilar atelectasis for which antibiotics were administered in 25%. The perioperative mortality was 9%, with deaths related to septic complications in all cases. A preoperative performance status of 2 or greater was identified as a risk factor for this complication ($p <$ 0.05). The authors did not comment on long-term infectious complications seen among the splenectomized patients.

III. SPECTRUM OF INFECTIONS

A. Spectrum of Infection in Patients Treated with Conventional Cytotoxic Agents

Most infections complicating the course of CLL patients treated with agents as alkylators and corticosteroids are bacterial in origin (1–3,6,15,33). Recurrent bacterial infections are also a hallmark of these patients. A variety of common bacterial isolates have been reported in these patients. The attack rate of pneumococcal bacteremia in CLL patients has been estimated at 10.8/1000 (54). Infections caused by *S. aureus* have been more common in hypogammaglobulinemic patients in some series (15,55). Infections with enteric gram-negative organisms, especially as bacteremic isolates, have been frequent in other series (56,57). This spectrum of infection reflects the more profound immunosuppression seen in heavily pretreated patients or those with advanced stage disease. The most common pathogens in these patients (*S. aureus*, *S. pneumoniae*, *Hemophilus influenzae*, and gram-negative enteric organisms such as *E. coli*, *Klebsiella pneumoniae*, and *Pseudomonas aeruginosa*) are also common in patients with hypogammaglobulinemia of other causes, suggesting the importance of immunoglobulin in control of these infections. Pathogen-specific antibodies are critical for killing and clearing these organisms, whether it be anti-body-mediated lysis of gram-negative organisms by complement or antibody plus complement-mediated opsonization and killing of gram-positive organisms by phagocytic cells. In contrast to these bacterial infections, mycobacterial infections (either *Mycobacterium tuberculosis* or the atypical mycobacteria) are infrequently reported in this population.

Another consistent feature of bacterial infections in CLL patients is a predilection to originate at mucosal sites. The respiratory tract is the most common site of infection in these patients and also of fatal infections (1–3,6,15,33,58). Although pneumonia is most common, upper respiratory tract infections such as sinusitis are also frequent. Other common sites of infection include the urinary tract, skin and soft tissue, and the bloodstream, the latter being common in patients with profound neutropenia (59).

Fungal infections are considerably less common than bacterial infections in these patients, generally occurring in patients with advanced stage disease and with chemotherapy-induced neutropenia (60–62). The incidence of cryptococcosis in a large, single-institution series of CLL patients was 2.4% (61). The cryptococcal infections were disseminated at the diagnosis, and mortality was high. Histoplasmosis may occur in both treated and chemotherapy-naive patients (62). Although mortality is high with disseminated infection, localized *Histoplasma* infections may be successfully eradicated. Opportunistic fungal infections, such as those caused by *Candida* and *Aspergillus* species, most often occur in patients with prolonged periods of therapy-related neutropenia. *Pneumocystis carinii* infections are rarely reported in patients treated with conventional chemotherapy agents (60).

Viral infections are likewise much less common than bacterial infections in CLL patients and also tend to occur in heavily pretreated patients (1,3,6,15,56,57). Although these infections may result in substantial morbidity, they are not a significant cause of mortality. Herpesvirus infections, especially herpes simplex and varicella zoster, are most common and are more often localized than disseminated (57). A syndrome of chronic indolent orofacial herpes simplex virus infection has also been described in CLL patients (63).

B. Spectrum of Infection in Patients Treated with Purine Analogs

In the 1980s, the purine analog chemotherapy agents (fludarabine, deoxycoformycin [DCF], chlorodeoxyadenosine [2-CDA] were introduced into clinical use for the therapy of hematological malignancies. Fludarabine has been the most widely used of these agents for the treatment of CLL. Initial results from a multicenter intergroup trial have shown an improved response rate to fludarabine compared with that seen with conventional alkylator therapy (64). However, the introduction of these agents was accompanied by a different spectrum of infectious complications than those seen with the use of traditional alkylating agents, including opportunistic infections with *Pneumocystis*, *Listeria*, *Mycobacterium tuberculosis*, *Nocardia*, and herpesviruses. The pathogenesis of infection in fludarabine-treated patients is related to the selective quantitative and qualitative (or functional) T-cell abnormalities induced by this agent (10–14,65). A severe decline in the total T-cell count is seen early in therapy. Profound, prolonged suppression of the CD4 count occurs, with median CD4 counts of 150 to 200 cells/µl, resulting in a decreased CD4/CD8 ratio. A lesser effect is seen on the CD8 and natural killer cells. Although the CD4 count improves considerably within 3 months after discontinuation of therapy, quantitative abnormalities may persist for up to 1 to 2 years. Fludarabine also causes a decrease in the B-cell count in addition to a transient monocytopenia; effects on the immunoglobulin levels may be variable.

The major dose-limiting toxicities in the initial fludarabine trials in CLL patients were neutropenia, infections, and fever (29,66–68). Infections were seen in up to 50% of patients in some series and were more common in certain patient subsets. A significantly higher incidence of severe infections such as bacteremia and pneumonia occurs in heavily pretreated patients and in those with advanced Rai stage disease (12,13,29,67,69). In one series, the incidence of infection was 12% in previously untreated patients with Rai stage 0 to II disease and 54% in previously treated patients with Rai stage III to IV disease (12). In another series of CLL patients treated with fludarabine, either alone or in combination, the incidence of severe infections was 3% to 4%, and that of moderate infections was 1% to 2% (70). The experience with fludarabine therapy in 724 patients with refractory CLL who obtained the drug by means of the group C protocol mechanism of the National Cancer Institute was reported by Sorenson et al. (71). Of the 705 patients evaluable for toxicity, grade 1 or 2 infectious toxicities were sustained in 26% of cases and grade 3 toxicities in 22%. Grade 4 or 3 febrile neutropenia was seen in 4.8% and 8.7% of patients, respectively. Response to therapy was also related to risk of infection, because patients with a biopsy-documented complete remission had a lower incidence of infection than patients with persistent nodular or interstitial aggregates in the bone marrow or partial responders (29,69,72). Most infections occurred early in the treatment course, usually during the first three cycles of therapy (12,72,73). Infections are generally uncommon in responding patients after discontinuation of initial fludarabine therapy. In a follow-up of a large cohort of patients treated at the M. D. Anderson Cancer Center, the incidence of infections for patients in remission was one episode for every 3.3 patient-year at risk and decreased with time-off therapy (74). In this series, infections were less common in complete responders than in partial responders. However, opportunistic infections, such as a case of listeriosis reported 2 years after completion of therapy in a patient with a normal CD4 count, may still occur (75). The risk of infection may increase after disease recurrence (69). The increased risk of these various opportunistic infections may be related to more than the low CD4 counts. Concomitant steroid therapy may act synergistically, with steroid-induced suppression of mononuclear phagocyte function (12,29,76,77). In addition, opportunistic infections may be more common in patients with low levels of IgG, IgA, or IgM (65).

The spectrum of infections that occurs in fludarabine-treated patients includes the bacterial infections common to patients with CLL, in addition to a spectrum of opportunistic infections (11,12,19,69–85). In a preliminary report of a series of patients with refractory CLL who received fludarabine as second-line therapy, a 20% incidence of severe opportunistic infections was seen (86). Bacterial pathogens reported include *Listeria* (2,12,75,76,84), *Nocardia* (84), *Mycobacterium tuberculosis* (69,84), atypical mycobacteria (84), and *Legionella* (84). Fungal infections may be localized or disseminated and are caused most often by *Candida* (11,83), *Aspergillus* (11,79,84), *Cryptococcus* (84), and *Torulopsis* (2). *Pneumocystis carinii* infections have also been reported (2,11,12,73,77–79). *Listeria* and *Pneumocystis* infections appear to be more frequent in patients receiving concomitant corticosteroids (12). Herpesvirus infections reported include pulmonary (77,84), hepatic (11), and disseminated (11,84) cytomegalovirus infections; dermatomal (11,29,69,72,81) or disseminated varicella zoster (2,11,66); and oral herpes simplex reactivation (29). Influenza (69) and hepatitis A infections (11,84) have also been described. However, despite many anecdotal reports of opportunistic infections occurring in fludarabine-treated patients, data regarding the actual incidence of these infections are less clear.

Data regarding the relative risk and spectrum of infections in fludarabine-treated patients compared with patients treated with conventional alkylator-based therapy are now emerging. In a recent EORTC trial, patients with previously untreated B-cell CLL with advanced stage disease were randomly assigned to therapy with either fludarabine or high-dose chlorambucil (10 mg/m^2/d) (87). In a preliminary report, with a median follow-up of 32 months, moderate to major infections were more common in the fludarabine-treated patients (37%) compared with those receiving chlorambucil (12%) ($p = 0.043$).

The infectious complications among a series of 544 previously untreated CLL patients who were randomly assigned to therapy with chlorambucil, fludarabine, or fludarabine plus chlorambucil on an intergroup trial have been recently reported (88). The infection follow-up period was the interval from study entry until either reinstitution of initial therapy, therapy with a second agent, or death. Patients treated with fludarabine plus chlorambucil had more infections than those patients receiving either single agent ($p < 0.0001$). Comparing the two single-agent therapy arms, there were more infections on the fludarabine arm per month of follow-up than on the chlorambucil arm ($p = 0.055$). Fludarabine therapy was associated with more major infections and more herpesvirus infections compared with chlorambucil ($p = 0.008$, 0.004, respectively). *Pneumocystis* infections were distinctly unusual in this series.

Preliminary efficacy and toxicity results of the use of fludarabine in combination with other agents have been reported. Fludarabine plus cyclophosphamide has been used for the therapy of CLL patients in several trials (89–91). Patients with previously untreated CLL with progressive disease received this combination in addition to granulocyte-colony stimulating factor (G-CSF) in an Eastern Cooperative Oncology Group trial (90). *Pneumocystis* prophylaxis was begun with initiation of therapy and continued for at least 6 months after the last chemotherapy dose. In a preliminary report of 36 patients, there were 28% grade 3 and 17% grade 4 nonhematological toxicities, primarily infections. Likewise, in a preliminary report in which this combination was used in refractory CLL patients, a 37% incidence of pneumonia was seen, including one case each caused by *Pneumocystis* and *Aspergillus* (91). Last, the combination of fludarabine plus cyclophosphamide is being compared with dose-intensified chlorambucil by the German CLL Study Group (92). In a preliminary report, severe (grade 3 or 4) infections were seen in only one patient on the chlorambucil arm and in no patients receiving fludarabine plus cyclophosphamide. Fludarabine has also been used in combination with cytarabine, mitoxantrone, and dexa-methasone (FAND) in a small series of younger, previously treated CLL patients (93). Prophylaxis with acyclovir, fluconazole, and trimethoprim-sulfamethoxazole was used. No severe or atypical infections have yet been seen.

Infectious toxicities reported with the other purine analogs have been similar to the experience with fludarabine. In Dillman's phase II trial in which CLL patients received therapy with deoxycoformycin, opportunistic infections caused by agents such as herpes simplex, herpes zoster, *Candida* and *Pneumocystis* occurred in 26% of patients (94). The infections occurred in the first 6 weeks of therapy and were more common in patients with advanced stage disease. Robak et al (95) reported on a series of 113 patients 55 year of age or younger who received therapy with 2-CDA. Sixty-seven patients were previously treated, and 46 received the agent as initial therapy. Severe infections, such as sepsis and pneumonia, occurred more commonly in pretreated patients (45%) than in those who received the drug as initial therapy (26%) ($p < 0.05$). Infection-related mortality approached 10% in this series. In another series of 43 elderly patients who received 2-CDA, either as initial therapy (33 patients) or for treatment of relapsed or refractory disease (10 patients), infections occurred in 16% of patients (96). Cases of disseminated herpes zoster and pulmonary aspergillosis were reported from a series of CLL patients with advanced stage refractory disease treated with chlorodeoxyadenosine (97). In another study, previously untreated patients with progressive or symptomatic CLL were randomly assigned to therapy with either 2-chlorodeoxyadenosine or chlorambucil, both in combination with prednisone (98). The rates of infectious complications were similar in both groups (33% with 2-CDA, 27% with chlorambucil, $p > 0.05$).

C. Spectrum of Infection in Patients Treated with Newer Agents

Campath-1H, an IgG1 monoclonal antibody that recognizes CD52, is also being used in CLL treatment trials. Prolonged lymphopenia, especially of the CD4 and CD8 T-cells, is a common consequence of therapy with this agent. Because of the increased risk of opportunistic infections, patients commonly receive prophylaxis with acyclovir, fluconazole, and trimethoprim-sulfamethoxazole. In a small series in which CLL patients who failed prior fludarabine therapy were treated with Campath-1H, opportunistic infections were common, occurring in 10 of 13 patients (99,100). This included four episodes of *Pneumocystis* pneumonia, three cases of herpes zoster, one case of invasive aspergillosis and CMV pneumonitis, one patient with orbital candidal infection, and one *Pseudomonas* abscess. In a multicenter phase II study of Campath-1H therapy in 29 patients with either relapsed or refractory CLL, infections were the main toxicity (101). Localized herpes simplex virus reactivation was seen in 11 patients (38%), oral candidiasis in five, and *Pneumocystis* pneumonia in two patients. Pneumonia caused by other organisms occurred in four patients. Three cases of bacteremia, one with *Klebsiella pneumoniae*, and two with *Staphylococcus aureus*, were seen.

Infections may be less common in previously untreated patients who receive initial therapy with Campath-1H. Österborg et al. reported on nine previously untreated patients who received Campath-1H therapy, of whom only one had opportunistic infections develop, specifically cytomegalovirus pneumonitis and oral candidiasis (102). In a preliminary report of a subsequent phase II trial of this agent in 15 previously untreated CLL patients, two cases of cytomegalovirus reactivation causing fever without pneumonitis, which responded promptly to ganciclovir, were reported (103). One explanation for this agent being better tolerated in previously untreated patients may be related to their better overall clinical condition and performance status compared with those CLL patients who are heavily pretreated.

Reports of therapy with rituximab in CLL patients are now emerging. In a preliminary report of 31 patients with relapsed CLL or prolymphocytic leukemia who received rituximab, 15 of whom were evaluable for toxicity, eight infections were noted (104). Preliminary findings of a recently completed cooperative group trial of therapy with rituximab plus fludarabine in previously untreated CLL patients have shown only a small number of opportunistic infections with agents such as herpesviruses and *Pneumocystis carinii* (Morrison, personal communication).

IV. RISK FACTORS FOR INFECTION

A variety of clinical factors have been identified that enhance the risk of infection in patients with CLL (105). Morra et al. (106). reported a significant correlation between disease stage and the risk of infection. In their series of 83 patients, they found that not only were infections more frequent, but they were also more severe with more advanced stage disease. Similar findings were reported by Itala et al. (30) in which 82% of patients with Binet stage C disease sustained severe infections compared with only 33% of Binet stage A patients. The response to therapy may also be of importance in the development of infections. In a series of 174 patients who received initial therapy with fludarabine, either alone or in combination with corticosteroids, Keating et al. (74) reported a significant association between the quality of the remission and the probability of infectious complications. Patients achieving a complete remission had the lowest likelihood of infections or febrile episodes developing compared with patients with a partial remission.

Anaissie et al. (107) reported on risk factors for infection identified among a series of 402 CLL patients who received therapy with fludarabine, alone (113 patients) or in combination with corticosteroids (289 patients). This series included both previously treated and chemotherapy, naive patients. In univariate analysis, prior chemotherapy, advanced stage disease, failure to respond to fludarabine, elevated serum β_2-microglobulin level, low serum albumin level, elevated serum creatinine level, and low granulocyte count were found to be risk factors for infection. However, in subsequent multivariate analysis, only advanced stage disease, prior therapy for CLL, and an elevated serum creatinine level were identified as independent risk factors for major infection.

Risk factors for infections were also examined in the recently reported intergroup trial of patients who received therapy with either fludarabine, chlorambucil, or the combination of the two agents (88). Neutropenia was more common in patients with infection on the combination therapy arm than in either of the two single-agent therapy arms, in which the incidence of neutropenia was similarly infrequent. Advanced age and an elevated creatinine clearance were risk factors for infection only among those patients who received fludarabine plus chlorambucil. Although a low serum IgG level (<500 mg/dl) was a risk factor for infection, advanced stage disease was not associated with infection in this series. In contrast to Keating's single institution findings, there was no association between the best response to therapy and the occurrence of major infections among these patients.

Last, infections seem to be more common in patients who have received therapy for their disease process, whether this be chemotherapy or corticosteroids, compared with previously untreated patients. This is likely related to the therapy-related neutropenia seen with some of these agents and resultant defects in cell-mediated immunity occurring with corticosteroid or purine analog therapy.

V.   STRATEGIES FOR PROPHYLAXIS OF INFECTION

A.   Infection Prophylaxis

No strict guidelines for infection prophylaxis have been formulated for this population. Because the use of concomitant corticosteroids with fludarabine increases the risk for *Pneumocystis* infections, the use of prophylaxis should be considered in this setting. Therapy with Campath-1H has also been found to increase the risk for opportunistic infections, especially with *Pneumocystis*, herpesviruses, and *Candida* spp. Prophylaxic therapy for these organisms is often incorporated into treatment schedules with this agent. In a preliminary report of the infectious complications among a large series of CLL patients enrolled in an intergroup treatment trial, herpesvirus infections, especially those caused by varicella zoster, were more common among patients who received fludarabine than those treated with chlorambucil (88). Most of these infections were cases of localized dermatomal zoster without dissemination. However, the issue of routine antiviral prophylaxis in patients receiving fludarabine therapy needs to be examined in a randomized prospective manner before firm recommendations for routine antiviral prophylaxis can be made.

The use of more intensive antimicrobial prophylaxis may be required for CLL patients who undergo allogeneic or autologous blood or marrow transplantation. In a small series reported from the United Kingdom, infections caused by cytomegalovirus, *Toxoplasma*, and *Listeria* complicated the course of patients undergoing allogeneic transplantation for CLL (108,109). Similar infections have been reported from other institutions (110). These opportunistic infections may be especially problematic in the setting of steroid therapy for graft-versus-host disease and extensive prior therapy with purine analogs such as fludarabine.

B.   Growth Factors

The use of fludarabine plus (G-CSF) was examined in a series of CLL patients from the M. D. Anderson Cancer Center (111). In previously treated patients with Rai stage II to IV CLL, the use of G-CSF after fludarabine therapy resulted in a decreased incidence of myelosuppression and of pneumonia compared with a historical control group of patients receiving fludarabine alone. The incidence of pneumonia was 8% in the group receiving G-CSF compared with 37% in the historical control group. The use of growth factors such as G-CSF has also been incorporated into myelosuppressive combination therapy regimens, such as fludarabine plus cyclophosphamide, in an effort to preserve dose intensity.

C.   Immunoglobulin Replacement

The benefit of prophylactic intravenous immunoglobulin (IVIG) was examined in a randomized placebo-controlled multicenter study of 81 CLL patients who were either hypogammaglobulinemic or had a prior history of infection (58). Those patients who received

IVIG (400 mg/kg every 3 weeks) had significantly fewer bacterial infections than patients who received placebo. Specifically, infections caused by *Streptococcus pneumoniae* and *Haemophilus influenzae*, but not gram-negative organisms, were less common in the patients who received IVIG. In addition, patients who received IVIG remained free of serious bacterial infection for a longer time than the control patients. However, this benefit was limited to moderate or minor infections; there was no decrease in major or life-threatening infections. Nor was there a difference in the incidence of viral or fungal infections in the two groups. Interestingly, the risk for bacterial infection did not correlate with the IgG level. In a subsequent cost-effectiveness analysis of this study, it was found that the decrease in bacterial infections related to prophylactic IVIG administration may not result in improved quality or length of life, and that this treatment was not cost-effective (112,113).

The use of low-dose prophylactic immunoglobulin has also been examined. A series of 34 CLL patients who had either a low IgG level or at least one serious infection were randomly assigned to receive 250 or 500 mg/kg IVIG monthly for a year; no placebo control group was included in this trial (114–116). The incidence of infection was comparable in the two groups. In Jurlander's series, 15 CLL patients with hypogammaglobulinemia and a history of recurrent infections given 10 g of IVIG every 3 weeks for a mean period of 12 months had a significant reduction in febrile episodes and hospital admissions for infection (117). Last, Molica et al. (118). reported on a series of 42 CLL patients who had an IgG level of <600 mg/dl and/or a history of at least one severe infection in the preceding 6 months. Patients were initially randomly assigned to therapy with 300 mg/kg IVIG every 4 weeks for 6 months or observation. After this, they were switched to observation or IVIG for another 12 months, and, last, to IVIG or observation for an additional 6 months. A lower incidence of infection was found in patients who received either 6 or 12 months of prophylactic IVIG compared with patients only observed. Of note in this study was that restoration of the IgG levels (seen in 17 of 25 patients) did not correlate with a decrease in the number of infections. The authors also concluded that this low-dose treatment approach was not cost-effective.

A potential difficulty with prophylactic IVIG therapy is that although IgG is replaced by these infusions, low levels of IgM or IgA are not replaced. The normal catabolic rate of IgG does not appear to be altered by IVIG administration (119). At present, many questions remain regarding the optimal dose and schedule of IVIG administration, and, more importantly, which subset of patients will benefit from such an approach. Some will consider this approach for the subset of patients with a low IgG level in the setting of severe recurrent bacterial infections, especially with encapsulated organisms.

D. Immunization

The response of CLL patients to a variety of immunizations has been examined in several series. Suboptimal response to vaccination in these patients may be related not only to impaired antibody production but also to defects in antigen presentation. Shaw examined a series of CLL patients who received typhoid, diphtheria, influenza, and mumps vaccines and found antibody responses to be poor whether the patients had normal or decreased immunoglobulin levels (33). Response to immunization with diphtheria toxoid was likewise impaired in Cone's series (21). Larson reported that immunization with a pneumococcal polysaccharide vaccine elicited little to no antibody response in eight of nine CLL patients (120). In a more recent report, Jacobson found that antibody titers following pneumococcal immunization were lower in CLL patients than in patients with multiple myeloma or normal controls (121).

The response of CLL patients to influenza vaccine has also been studied. Mean antibody titers after influenza vaccination were low in a small series of CLL patients (122). Patients who were hypogammaglobulinemic or were receiving chemotherapy had a significantly depressed response to vaccination. In a more recent study, Gribabis reported the results of influenza vaccination in 43 CLL patients (123). Approximately half of the patients were hypogammaglobulinemic, and two thirds had early stage disease. An antibody response to the vaccine occurred in 81% of patients; hypogammaglobulinemic patients responded less often than patients with normal immunoglobulin levels. Reimmunization with influenza vaccine at 1 month may potentially be necessary in this population because of a decline in antibody titers.

VI. FUTURE ENDEAVORS/CONCLUSION AREAS OF FUTURE ENDEAVORS

Despite many advances in therapy and supportive care of patients with CLL over the past five decades, infections continue to have a significant impact on the course and outcome of patients with CLL. Delineation of the effects of new chemotherapeutic and immune modulating agents not only on the outcome parameters of the primary disease but also on immune function and infectious complications will remain an important element in decisions regarding therapeutic options for these patients. Further examination of mucosal immune function in these patients may add to the understanding of the pathogenesis of infection in this population. Last, subsets of CLL patients identified to be at increased risk for infection may be used for future prospective studies of both prophylactic and therapeutic interventions to reduce the incidence and impact of infection in this patient population.

REFERENCES

1. HM Chapel, C Bunch. Mechanisms of infection in chronic lymphocytic leukemia. Semin Hematol 24:291–296, 1987.
2. DP Kontoyianis, EJ Anaissie, GP Bodey. Infection in chronic lymphocytic leukemia: A reappraisal. In: BD Cheson, ed. Chronic Lymphocytic Leukemia: Scientific Advances and Clinical Developments. New York: Marcel Dekker, Inc., 1993. pp 399–417.
3. JT Twomey. Infections complicating multiple myeloma and chronic lymphocytic leukemia. Arch Intern Med 132:562–565, 1973.
4. MM Hansen. Chronic lymphocytic leukaemia: clinical studies based on 189 cases followed for a long time. Scand J Haematol (Suppl) 18:3–286, 1973.
5. GH Fairley, RB Scott. Hypogammaglobulinaemia in chronic lymphatic leukaemia. BMJ 4: 920–924, 1961.
6. VA Morrison. The infectious complications of chronic lymphocytic leukemia. Semin Oncol 25:98–106, 1998.
7. S Molica. Infections in chronic lymphocytic leukemia: risk factors and impact on survival and treatment. Leuk Lymphoma 13:203–214, 1994.
8. T Sudhoff, M Arning, W Schneider. Prophylactic strategies to meet infectious complications in fludarabine-treated CLL. Leukemia 11 (suppl 2):S38–S41, 1997.
9. RP Hudson, SL Wilson. Hypogammaglobulinemia and chronic lymphatic leukemia. Cancer 13:200–204, 1960.

10. G Juliusson. Immunological and genetic abnormalities in chronic lymphocytic leukaemia: Impact of the purine analogues. Drugs 47 (suppl 6):19–29, 1994.

11. PW Wijermans, WBJ Gerrits, HL Haak. Severe immunodeficiency in patients treated with fludarabine monophosphate. Eur J Haematol 50:292–296, 1993.

12. S O'Brien, H Kantarjian, M Beran, T Smith, C Koller, E Estey, LE Robertson, S Lerner, M Keating. Results of fludarabine and prednisone therapy in 264 patients with chronic lymphocytic leukemia with multivariate analysis-derived prognostic model for response to treatment. Blood 2:1695–1700, 1993.

13. MJ Keating, S O'Brien, LE Robertson, H Kantarjian, M Dimopoulos, P McLaughlin, F Cabanillas, V Gregoire, LY Yang, V Gandhi. New initiatives with fludarabine monophosphate in hematologic malignancies. Semin Oncol 20 (suppl 7):13–20, 1993.

14. MJ Keating, S O'Brien, H Kantarjian, LB Robertson, C Koller, M Beran, E Estey. Nucleoside analogs in treatment of chronic lymphocytic leukemia. Leuk Lymphoma 10:139–45, 1993.

15. JE Ultmann, W Fish, E Osserman, A Gellhorn. Clinical implications of hypogammaglobulinemia in patients with chronic lymphocytic leukaemia and lymphocytic lymphosarcoma. Ann Intern Med 51:501–516, 1959.

16. R Foa, D Catovsky, F Lauria, DA Galton. Reduced T-colony forming capacity by T-lymphocytes from B-chronic lymphocytic leukemia. B J Haematol 46:623–632, 1980.

17. NE Kay. Abnormal T-cell subpopulation function in CLL: Excessive suppressor (T-gamma) and deficient helper (T-mu) activity with respect to B-cell proliferation. Blood 57:418–420, 1987.

18. ME Heath, BD Cheson. Defective complement activity in chronic lymphocytic leukemia. Am J Haematol 19:63–73, 1985.

19. DR Boggs. Cellular composition of inflammatory exudates in human leukaemia. Blood 15:466–475, 1960.

20. HI Zeya, E Keku, F Richards, CL Spurr. Monocyte and granulocyte defect in chronic lymphocytic leukemia. Am J Pathol 95:43–54, 1979.

21. L Cone, JW Uhr. Immunological deficiency disorders associated with chronic lymphocytic leukemia and multiple myeloma. J Clin Invest 43:2241–2248, 1964.

22. TH Brem, ME Morton. Defective serum gamma globulin formation. Ann Intern Med 43:465–479, 1955.

23. RTS Jim, EH Reinhard. Agammaglobulinemia and chronic lymphocytic leukemia. Ann Intern Med 44:790–796, 1956.

24. A Apostopoulos, A Simeonidis, N Zoumbos. Prognostic significance of immune function parameters in patients with chronic lymphocytic leukemia. Eur J Haematol 44:39–44, 1990.

25. G Dighiero. Hypogammaglobulineremia and disordered immunity in CLL. In: BD Cheson, ed. Chronic Lymphocytic Leukemia: Scientific Advances and Clinical Developments. New York: Marcel Dekker, Inc., 1993. pp 147–166.

26. C Rozman, E Montserrat, N Viñolas. Serum immunoglobulins in B-chronic lymphocytic leukemia. Cancer 61:279–283, 1988.

27. I Ben-Bassat, A Many, M Modan, C Peretz, B Ramot. Serum immunoglobulins in chronic lymphocytic leukemia. Am J Med Sci 278:4–9, 1979.

28. DG Miller, DA Karnofsky. Immunologic factors and resistance to infection in chronic lymphatic leukemia. Am J Med 31:748–757, 1961.

29. MJ Keating. Fludarabine phosphate in the treatment of chronic lymphocytic leukemia. Semin Oncol 17:49–62, 1990.

30. M Itala, H Helenius, J Nikoskelainen, K Remes. Infections and serum IgG levels in patients with chronic lymphocyic leukemia. Eur J Haematol 48:266–270, 1992.

31. A Videbaek. Some clinical aspects of leukemia. Acta Haematol 24:54–58, 1960.

32. R Creyssal, R Morel, M Pellet, et al. Deficit en gamma-globulines et complications infectieuses des leucemies lymphoides chroniques. Sang 29:383–398, 1958.

33. RK Shaw, C Szwed, DR Boggs, JL Fahey, E Frei, E Morrison, JP Utz. Infection and immunity in chronic lymphocytic leukaemia. Arch Intern Med 106:467–478, 1960.

34. MB Van Scoy-Mosher, M Bick, V Capostagno, RL Walford, RA Gatti. A clinicopathologic analysis of chronic lymphocytic leukemia. Am J Hematol 10:9–18, 1981.

35. E Montserrat, JP Marques-Pereira, MT Gallart, C Rozman. Bone marrow histopathologic patterns and immunologic findings in B-chronic lymphocytic leukemia. Cancer 54:447–451, 1984.

36. R Foa, D Catovsky, M Brozovic, G Marsh, T Ooyirilangkumaran, M Cherchi, DAG Galton. Clinical staging and immunological findings in chronic lymphocytic leukemia. Cancer 44: 483–487, 1979.

37. VA Morrison, NL Opstad, EN Janoff. Mucosal immunoglobulin levels in patients with chronic lymphocytic leukemia and multiple myeloma (abstr 1075). Proc Am Soc Clin Oncol 15:364, 1996.

38. VA Morrison, NL Opstad, EN Janoff. Correlation of systemic and mucosal immunoglobulin (Ig) levels in patients (pts) with chronic lymphocytic leukemia (CLL) and multiple myeloma (MM) (abstr 92). Thirty-fourth Proceedings of the Infectious Diseases Society of America, 1996.

39. VA Morrison, JR Hibbs, EN Janoff. Systemic and mucosal immunoglobulin levels and risk of infection in patients with chronic lymphocytic leukemia and multiple myeloma (abstr 948). Blood 88 (suppl 1):240a, 1996.

40. TI Robertson. Complications and causes of death in B-cell chronic lymphocytic leukemia. Aust NZ J Med 20:44–50, 1990.

41. MM Bartik, D Welker, NE Kay. Impairments in immune cell function in B cell chronic lymphocytic leukemia. Semin Oncol 25:27–33, 1998.

42. J Aittoniemi, A Miettinen, S Laine, M Sinisalo, P Laippala, L Vilpo, J Vilpo. Opsonising immunoglobulins and mannan-binding lectin in chronic lymphocytic leukemia. Leuk Lymphoma 34:381–385, 1999.

43. M Schlesinger, I Broman, G Lugassy. The complement system is defective in chronic lymphatic leukemia patients and in their healthy relatives. Leukemia 10:1509–1513, 1996.

44. MM Strumia, F Boerner. Phagocytic activity of circulating cells in the various types of leukemia. Am J Pathol 13:335–350, 1937.

45. AI Braude, J Feltes, M Brooks. Differences between the activities of mature granulocytes in leukemic and normal blood. J Clin Invest 33:1036–1046, 1954.

46. K Tornyos. Phagocytic activity of cells of the inflammatory exudate in human leukemia. Cancer Res 27:1756–1759, 1967.

47. AJ Sbarra, W Shirley, RJ Selvaraj, E Ouchi, E Rosenbaum. The role of the phagocyte in host-parasite interactions. I. The phagocytic capabilities of leukocytes from lymphoproliferative disorders. Cancer Res 24:1958–1968, 1964.

48. F Caligaris-Cappio, TJ Hamblin. B-cell chronic lymphocytic leukemia: A bird of a different feather. J Clin Oncol 17:399–408, 1999.

49. CD Platsoucas, M Galinski, S Kempin, L Reich, B Clarkson, RA Good. Abnormal T-lymphocyte subpopulations in patients with B cell chronic lymphocytic leukemia: An analysis by monoclonal antibodies. J Immunol 129:2305–2312, 1982.

50. CD Platsoucas, G Hernandes, SL Gupta, S Kempin, B Clarkson, RA Good, S Gupta. Defective spontaneous and antibody-dependent cytotoxicity mediated by E-rosette-positive and E-rosette-negative cells in untreated patients with chronic lymphocytic leukemia: Augmentation by in vitro treatment with interferon. J Immunol 125:1216–1223, 1980.

51. N Kay, RT Perri. Immunobiology of malignant B cells and immunoregulatory cells in B-chronic lymphocytic leukemia. Clin Lab Med 8:163–177, 1988.

52. SL Zaknoen, NE Kay. Immunoregulatory cell dysfunction in chronic B-cell leukemias. Blood Rev 4:165–174, 1990.

53. JF Seymour, JD Cusack, SA Lerner, RE Pollock, MJ Keating. Case/control study of the role of splenectomy in chronic lymphocytic leukemia. J Clin Oncol 15:52–60, 1997.

54. M Chou, AE Brown, A Blevins, A Armstrong. Severe pneumococcal infection in patients with neoplastic disease. Cancer 51:1546–1550, 1983.

55. GP Bodey. Infection in cancer patients. A continuing association. Am J Med 81(suppl 1A): 11–26, 1986.

56. E Monserrat-Costa, E Matutes, C Rozman, E Feliu, A Granena, L Hernandez-Nieto, B Nomdedeu, A Urbano-Marquez. Infecciones en la leukemia linfoide cronica. Sangre 22: 968–975, 1977.

57. P Travade, JD Dusart, M Cavaroc, J Beytout, M Rey. Les infections graves associées à la leucémie lymphoide chronique. 159 épisodes infectieux observés chex 60 malades. La Presse Méd 15:1715–1718, 1986.

58. Cooperative Group for the Study of Immunoglobulin in Chronic Lymphocytic Leukemia. Intravenous immunoglobulin for the prevention of infection in chronic lymphocytic leukemia. N Engl J Med 319:902–907, 1988.

59. JW Mayo, RP Wenzel. Rates of hospital-acquired bloodstream infections in patients with specific malignancy. Cancer 50:187–190, 1982.

60. AE Reed, BA Body, MB Austin, HF Frierson. Cunninghamella bertholletiae and Pneumocystis carinii pneumonia as a fatal complication of chronic lymphocytic leukemia. Hum Pathol 19:1470–1472, 1988.

61. MH Kaplan, PP Rosen, D Armstrong. Cryptococcosis in a cancer hospital. Cancer 39:2265–2274, 1977.

62. CA Kaufmann, KS Israel, JW Smith, AC White, J Schwartz, GF Brooks. Histoplasmosis in immunosuppressed patients. Am J Med 64:923–932, 1978.

63. AP Barrett. Chronic indolent orofacial herpes simplex virus infection in chronic leukemia: A report of three cases. Oral Surg 66:387–390, 1988.

64. KR Rai, B Peterson, J Kolitz, L Elias, L Shepherd, J Hines, B Cheson, C Schiffer. A randomized comparison of fludarabine and chlorambucil for patients with previously untreated chronic lymphocytic leukemia. A CALGB, SWOG, CTG/NCI-C and ECOG inter-group study (abstr 2414). Blood 88 (suppl 1):141a, 1996.

65. JC Byrd, NS Dow, RS Howard, SL Greenfield, CK Williams, LF Diehl. Marked depletion of natural killer cells in chronic lymphocytic leukemia patients receiving fludarabine: A consideration for future immune-based therapy (abstr 96). Proc Am Soc Oncol 16:28a, 1997.

66. P McLaughlin, FB Hagemeister, F Swan Jr, F Cabanillas, O Pate, JE Romaguera, MA Rodriguez, JR Redman, M Keating. Phase I study of the combination of fludarabine, mitoxantrone, and dexamethasone in low-grade lymphoma. J Clin Oncol 12:575–579, 1994.

67. MJ Keating, E Estey, S O'Brien, H Kantarjian, LE Robertson, W Plunkett. Clinical experience with fludarabine in leukaemia. Drugs 47 (suppl 6):39–49, 1994.

68. SR Ross, D McTavish, D Faulds. Fludarabine: A review of its pharmacological properties and therapeutic potential in malignancy. Drugs 45:737–759, 1993.

69. MJ Keating, S O'Brien, H Kantarjian, W Plunkett, E Estey, C Koller, M Beran, EJ Freireich. Long-term follow-up of patients with chronic lymphocytic leukemia treated with fludarabine as a single agent. Blood 81:2878–2884, 1993.

70. M Montillo, A Tedeschi, E Orlandi, et al. Infectious events in indolent lymphoproliferative disorders treated with regimens including fludarabine. Blood 90 (suppl 1):195a, 1997.

71. JM Sorensen, DA Vena, A Fallavollita, HG Chun, BD Cheson. Treatment of refractory chronic lymphocytic leukemia with fludarabine phosphate via the group C protocol mechanism of the National Cancer Institute: Five-year follow-up report. J Clin Oncol 15:458–465, 1997.

72. MJ Keating, H Kantarjian, M Talpaz, J Redman, C Koller, B Barlogie, W Velasquez, W Plunkett, EJ Freireich, KB McCredie. Fludarabine: A new agent with major activity against chronic lymphocytic leukemia. Blood 74:19–25, 1989.

73. CA Puccio, A Mittelman, SM Lichtman, RT Silver, DR Budman, T Ahmed, EJ Feldman, M Coleman, PM Arnold, ZA Arlin. A loading dose/continuous infusion schedule of fludarabine phosphate in chronic lymphocytic leukemia. J Clin Oncol 9:1562–1569, 1991.

74. MJ Keating, SO O'Brien, S Lerner, C Koller, M Beran, LE Robertson, EJ Freireich, E Estey, H Kantarjian. Long-term followup of patients with chronic lymphocytic leukemia (CLL) receiving fludarabine regimens as initial therapy. Blood 92:1165–1171, 1998.

75. C Girmenia, FR Mauro, S Rahimi. Late listeriosis after fludarabine plus prednisone treatment. Br J Haematol 87:407–408, 1994.

76. E Anaissie, DP Kontoyiannis, H Kantarjian, L Elting, LE Robertson, M Keating. Listeriosis in patients with chronic lymphocytic leukemia who were treated with fludarabine and prednisone. Ann Intern Med 117:466–469, 1992.

77. PJ Schilling, S Vadhan-Raj. Concurrent cytomegalovirus and pneumocystis pneumonia after fludarabine therapy for chronic lymphocytic leukemia. N Engl J Med 323:833–834, 1990.

78. Y Bastion, B Coiffier, JD Tigaud, D Espinouse, PA Bryon. Pneumocystis pneumonia in a patient treated with fludarabine for chronic lymphocytic leukemia. Eur J Cancer 27:671, 1991.

79. L Bergmann, K Fenchel, B Jahn, PS Mitrou, D Hoelzer. Immunosuppressive effects and clinical response of fludarabine in refractory chronic lymphocytic leukemia. Ann Oncol 4: 371–375, 1993.

80. A Kemena, S O'Brien, H Kantarjian, L Robertson, C Koller, M Beran, E Estey, W Plunkett, S Lerner, MJ Keating. Phase II clinical trial of fludarabine in chronic lymphocytic leukemia on a weekly low-dose schedule. Leuk Lymphoma 10:187–193, 1993.

81. LE Robertson, S O'Brien, C Koller, et al. A three-day schedule of fludarabine in chronic lymphocytic leukemia (CLL). Blood 80 (suppl 1):47a, 1992.

82. W Hiddemann, R Rottmann, B Wormann, A Thiel, M Essink, C Ottensmeier, M Freund, T Buchner, J Van De Loo. Treatment of advanced chronic lymphocytic leukemia by fludarabine: Results of a clinical phase-II study. Ann Hematol 63:1–4, 1991.

83. MJ Keating, H Kantarjian, S O'Brien, C Koller, M Talpaz, J Schachner, CC Childs, EJ Freireich, KB McCredie. Fludarabine: A new agent with marked cytoreductive activity in untreated chronic lymphocytic leukemia. J Clin Oncol 9:44–49, 1991.

84. JC Byrd, JB Hargis, KE Kester, DR Hospenthal, SW Knutson, LF Diehl. Opportunistic pulmonary infections with fludarabine in previously treated patients with low-grade lymphoid malignancies: A role for Pneumocystis carinii pneumonia prophylaxis. Am J Hematol 49: 135–142, 1995.

85. C Sanders, EA Perez, HJ Lawrence. Opportunistic infections in patients with chronic lymphocytic leukemia following treatment with fludarabine. Am J Hematol 39:314–315, 1992.

86. P Giraldo, L Palomera, P Mayayo, JJ Moneva, P Diego, M Pardo, P Rabasa, D Rubio-Felix. Fludarabine as single therapy for advanced stage of refractory chronic lymphocytic leukemia (abstr 4192). Blood 92 (suppl 1):276b, 1998.

87. B Jaksic, M Brugiatelli, S Suciu, E Baumelou, PW Wijermans, A Delmer, KJ Roozendaal, A Teixeira, U Jehn, W Feremans, A Belhabri, A Venditti, K Indrak, P Rodts, G Solbu, R Willemze. Randomized phase II study in untreated B-cell chronic lymphocytic leukemia (B-CLL) comparing fludarabine (FAMP) vs. high dose continuous chlorambucil (HD-CLB) (abstr 421). Blood 92 (suppl 1):103a, 1998.

88. VA Morrison, KR Rai, B Peterson, JE Kolitz, L Elias, JD Hines, L Shepherd, RA Larson, CA Schiffer. The impact of therapy with chlorambucil (C), fludarabine (F), or chlorambucil + fludarabine (F+C) on infections in patients with chronic lymphocytic leukemia (CLL): An intergroup study (CALGB 9011) (abstr 2020). Blood 92 (suppl 1):490a, 1998.

89. IW Flinn, JC Byrd, C Morrison, J Jamison, C Miller, RJ Christie, S Gore, P Burke, G Vogelsang, MR Grever. Fludarabine and cyclophosphamide: A highly active and well tolerated regimen for patients with previously untreated chronic lymphocytic leukemia (CLL) (abstr 424). Blood 92 (suppl 1):104a, 1998.

90. IW Flinn, S Lee, JM Bennett, CI Falkson, P Flynn, S Pundaleeka, E Stadtmauer, F Schnell, M Tallman, JM Rowe. Phase II trial of fludarabine and cyclophosphamide (Flu/Cy) in patients with previously untreated chronic lymphocytic leukemia: An Eastern Cooperative Oncology Group study (abstr 4610). Blood 94(suppl 1):309b, 1999.

91. H Gonzalez, B Cazin, G Dighiero, H Merle-Beral, JP Vernant, JL Binet, K Maloum. Fludarabine (FAMP) and cyclophosphamide (CTX) combination in chronic lymphocytic leukemia (CLL) (abstr 4193). Blood 92 (suppl 1):277b, 1998.

92. M Hallek, M Wilhelm, B Emmerich, H Dohner, HP Fostisch, O Sezer, M Herold, W Knauf, R Busch, B Schmitt, CM Wendtner, R Kuse, M Freund, A Franke, F Schriever, C Nerl, E Thiel, W Hiddemann, G Brittinger, and the GCLLSG. Fludarabine plus cyclophosphamide (FC) and dose intensified chlorambucil (DIC) for the treatment of chronic lymphocytic leukemia (CLL): Results of two phase II studies (CLL-2-Protocol) of the German CLL Study Group (GCLLSG) (abstr 4613). Blood 94(suppl 1):310b, 1999.

93. FR Mauro, R Foa, I Cordone, D Traisci, MC Rapanotti, A Proia, R Cerretti, F Mandelli. Combination of fludarabine, ara-C, novantrone® and dexamethasone (FAND) in young patients with previously treated CLL (abstr 4209). Blood 92(suppl 1):280b, 1998.

94. RO Dillman, R Mick, OR McIntyre. Pentostatin in chronic lymphocytic leukemia: A phase II trial of Cancer and Leukemia Group B. J Clin Oncol 7:433–438, 1989.

95. T Robak, JZ Blonski, H Urbanska-Rys, M Blasinska-Morawiec, AB Skotnicki 2-Chlorodeoxyadenosine (cladribine) in the treatment of patients with chronic lymphocytic leukemia 55 years old and younger. Leukemia 13:518–523, 1999.

96. T Robak, M Blasinska-Morawiec, JZ Blonski, A Dmoszynska. 2-Chlorodeoxyadenosine (cladribine) in the treatment of elderly patients with B-cell chronic lymphocytic leukemia. Leuk Lymphoma 34:151–157, 1999.

97. LD Piro, CJ Carrera, E Beutler, DA Carson. 2-Chlorodeoxyadenosine: An effective new agent for the treatment of chronic lymphocytic leukemia. Blood 72:1069–1073, 1988.

98. T Robak, M Blasinka-Morawiec, JZ Blonski, E Krykowski, A Dmoszynska, AB Skotnicki, L Konopka, A Hellmann, J Dwilewicz-Trojaczek, B Zdziarska, S Kotlarek-Haus, S Maj. Randomized multicenter study of the effectiveness of 2-chlorodeoxyadenosine with prednisone versus chlorambucil with prednisone in previously untreated chronic lymphocytic leukemia (CLL) (abstr 2021). Blood 92 (suppl 1):490a, 1998.

99. D Janson, S Nissel-Horowitz, M Sattler, KR Rai. Complete and partial response (CR, PR) in treatment of advanced refractory B-cell chronic lymphomytic leukemia (B-CLL) using Campath-1H (abstr 541). Blood 82(suppl 1):139a, 1993.

100. KR Rai, M Hoffman, D Janson, A Fuchs, N Shevde, P Kollipara, A Sawitsky. Immunosuppression and opportunistic infections (OI) in patients with chronic lymphocytic leukemia (CLL) following Campath I-H therapy (abstr 1381). Blood 86(suppl 1):348a, 1995.

101. A Österborg, MJS Dyer, D Bunjes, GA Pangalis, Y Bastion, D Catovsky, H Mellstedt. Phase II multicenter study of human CD52 antibody in previously treated chronic lymphocytic leukemia. J Clin Oncol 15:1567–1574, 1997.

102. A Österborg, AS Fassas, A Anagnostopoulos, MJS Dyer, D Catovsky, H Mellstedt. Humanized CD52 monoclonal antibody Campath-1H as first-line treatment in chronic lymphocytic leukemia. Br J Haematol 93:151–153, 1996.

103. H Mellstedt, A Osterborg, J Lundin, M Bjorkholm, F Celsing, H Hagberg, R Hast, V Hjalmar, E Kimby, M Luthman, O Tullgren, B Werner. Campath-1H therapy of patients with previously untreated chronic lymphocytic leukemia (CLL) (abstr 2019). Blood 92 (suppl 1):490a, 1998.

104. B Emmerich, D Huhn, C Peschel, M Wilhelm, C von Schilling, M Bentz, M Hallek, B Knauf, R Kuse, AD Ho. Treatment of chronic lymphocytic leukemia (CLL) with the anti-CD20 antibody rituximab (abstr 4608). Blood 94 (suppl 1):309b, 1999.

105. G Juliusson. Complications in the treatment of CLL with purine analogues. Hematol Cell Ther 39:S41–S44, 1997.

106. E Morra, A Nosari, M Montillo. Infectious complications in chronic lymphocytic leukemia. Hematol Cell Ther 41:145–151, 1999.
107. EJ Anaissie, DP Kontoyiannis, SO O'Brien, H Kantarjian, L Robertson, S Lerner, MJ Keating. Infections in patients with chronic lymphocytic leukemia treated with fludarabine. Ann Intern Med 129:559–566, 1998.
108. J Mehta, R Powles, S Singhal, U Riley, J Treleaven, D Catovsky. Antimicrobial prophylaxis to prevent opportunistic infections in patients with chronic lymphocytic leukemia after allogenic blood or marrow transplantation. Leuk Lymphoma 26:83–88, 1997.
109. A Zomas, J Mehta, R Powles, J Treleaven, T Iveson, S Singhal, B Jameson, B Paul, S Brincat, D Catovsky. Unusual infections following allogenic bone marrow transplantation for chronic lymphocytic leukemia. Bone Marrow Transplant 14:799–803, 1994.
110. SN Rabinowe, RJ Soiffer, JG Gribben, H Daley, AS Freedman, J Daley, K Pesek, D Neuberg, G Pinkus, PR Leavitt. Autologous and allogenic bone marrow transplantation for poor prognosis patients with B-cell chronic lymphocytic leukemia. Blood 82:1366–1376, 1993.
111. S O'Brien, H Kantarjian, M Beran, C Koller, M Talpaz, S Lerner, MJ Keating. Fludarabine and granulocyte colony-stimulating factor (G-CSF) in patients with chronic lymphocytic leukemia. Leukemia 11:1631–1635, 1997.
112. JC Weeks, MR Tierney, MC Weinstein. Cost effectiveness of prophylactic intravenous immune globulin in chronic lymphocytic leukemia. N Engl J Med 325:81–86, 1991.
113. ER Stiehm. New uses for intravenous immune globulin. N Engl J Med 325:123–125, 1991.
114. M Dicato, H Chapel, H Gamm, M Lee, F Ries, S Marichal, C Wirth, H Griffith, V Brennan. Use of intravenous immunoglobulin in chronic lymphocytic leukemia. A brief review. Cancer 68:1437–1439, 1991.
115. H Gamm, H Huber, H Chapel, M Lee, F Ries, MA Dicato. Intravenous immune globulin in chronic lymphocytic leukaemia. Clin Exp Immunol 97(suppl 1):17–20, 1994.
116. H Chapel, M Dicato, H Gamm, V Brennan, F Ries, C Bunch, M Lee. Immunoglobulin replacement in patients with chronic lymphocytic leukemia: a comparison of two dose regimens. Br J Haematol 88:209–212, 1994.
117. J Jurlander, GC Hartmann, MM Hansen. Treatment of hypogammaglobulinaemia in chronic lymphocytic leukaemia by low-dose intravenous gammaglobulin. Eur J Haematol 53:114–118, 1994.
118. S Molica, P Musto, F Chiurazzu, G Specchia, M Brugiatelli, L Cicoira, D Levato, F Nobile, M Carotenuto, V Liso, B Rotoli. Prophylaxis against infections with low-dose intravenous immunoglobulins (IVIG) in chronic lymphocytic leukemia. Results of a crossover study. Haematologica 81:121–126, 1996.
119. HM Chapel, M Lee. Immunoglobulin replacement in patients with chronic lymphocytic leukemia (CLL): Kinetics of immunoglobulin metabolism. J Clin Immunol 12:17–20, 1992.
120. DL Larson, LJ Tomlinson. Quantitative antibody studies in man, III: Antibody response in leukemia and other malignant lymphomata. J Clin Invest 32:317–321, 1953.
121. DR Jacobson, HS Ballard, R Silber, et al. Antibody response in pneumococcal immunization in patients with chronic lymphocytic leukemia. Blood 72(suppl 1):205a, 1988.
122. AI Schafer, WH Churchill, P Ames, L Weinstein. The influence of chemotherapy on response of patients with hematologic malignancies to influenza vaccine. Cancer 43:25–30, 1979.
123. DA Gribabis, GA Pangalis, PG Panayiotidis, VA Boussiotis, C Hannoun. Influenza vaccine in B-chronic lymphocytic leukemia patients. Blood 80 (suppl 1):48a, 1992.

24

Prolymphocytic Leukemia of B- and T-Cell Types

Biology and Therapy

ESTELLA MATUTES, VASANTHA BRITO-BABAPULLE, M. R. YULLIE, and DANIEL CATOVSKY

Royal Marsden Hospital, London, England

CLAIRE DEARDEN

St. George's Hospital Medical School, London, England

I. INTRODUCTION

Prolymphocytic leukemia (PLL) was first described by Galton and colleagues (1974) (1) as a variant form of chronic lymphocytic leukemia (CLL). The disease is characterized by its distinct clinical and laboratory features, namely splenomegaly and high white blood cell (WBC) counts, with the circulating lymphoid cells being medium size lymphocytes with a prominent nucleolus designated "prolymphocyte." The B-cell nature of the leukemic cells was demonstrated in some of these cases when immunological markers first become available. Almost simultaneously, a case of T-PLL was reported in a patient with similar clinical characteristics and morphology but in whom the neoplastic circulating cells were shown to form rosettes with sheep erythrocytes (2). We have subsequently studied a large series of patients with T-PLL (3), and it has become apparent that this disease is probably as frequent as B-PLL. However, both B- and T-cell PLL are rare and only account for approximately 2% among disorders seen with $>10 \times 10^9$/L lymphocytosis. B- and T-PLL have some clinical features and cell morphology in common, and this together with historical reasons justifies retention of the term "PLL" for both diseases. However, their biology and pathogenesis are very different and, thus, they are in fact distinct clinicopathological entities.

　　We summarize here the clinical and laboratory characteristics of PLL on the basis of data in 210 cases (150 T-cell and 60 B-cell) investigated at our institution.

A. B-Prolymphocytic Leukemia

1. Clinical Features

B-PLL exclusively affects adults, with 85% of patients older than 50 years of age. In our series, the median age in B-PLL was 70 years (range, 41–92 years). Men are equally affected as women (M/F: 1). Main presenting features are abdominal discomfort, sweating, weight loss, and anemia, whereas lymphadenopathy is rare and, if present, is usually of low volume. In rare cases, the disease is discovered by chance on a routine examination, and the clinical course is indolent but ultimately the disease progresses (4; our data).

Table 1 summarizes the main physical and laboratory findings of B-PLL. Splenomegaly is almost invariably present, whereas lymphadenopathy is detected in one third of the patients; pleural effusions and ascites, unlike T-PLL, are rare and central nervous system (CNS) involvement is infrequent but may develop during the course of the disease.

Laboratory findings show a high WBC count with one third of patients running counts greater than 200×10^9/L. Anemia and thrombocytopenia are seen in close to two thirds of the patients. Serum immunoglobulins, as a rule, are normal except in a small number of cases in which a small monoclonal band is detected; hypogammaglobulinemia unlike in B-CLL is rare. Hyperuricemia and a mildly raised lactate dehydrogenase (LDH) are frequent, and there may be abnormalities of the liver function tests. In contrast to CLL, autoimmune hemolytic anemia or autoimmune thrombocytopenia are infrequent in B-PLL

2. Morphology

Examination of May-Grumwald-Giemsa–stained peripheral blood films is the key diagnostic test in B-PLL. The blood picture is homogeneous, with most (>55%) of cells being prolymphocytes. These cells are of medium size, have relatively condensed but not clumped nuclear chromatin, and a single central vesicular nucleolus (Figure 1). The nuclear outline is usually regular. In approximately 50% of B-PLL cases, there is a minority of large cells, sometimes with bilobed nucleus, fine dispersed chromatin, and two or more nucleoli resembling immunoblasts. Electron microscopic analysis further confirms the characteristics seen at light microscopy, with cells having a nucleus with the heterochromatin distributed at the periphery and a prominent single nucleolus.

Bone marrow aspirates in PLL usually show heavy infiltration by prolymphocytes with variable residual hemopoiesis. This test, however, is not essential for diagnosis, because the morphology is better appreciated on peripheral blood films.

Table 1 Clinical and Laboratory Features of B-PLL*

Feature	Proportion of cases
Splenomegaly	87%
Lymphadenopathy	38%
WBC $\times 10^9$/L (range)	15–700
>200×10^9/L	38%
Hb <10 g/dl	64%
Platelets <100×10^9/L	36%

* Out of a series of 50 patients.

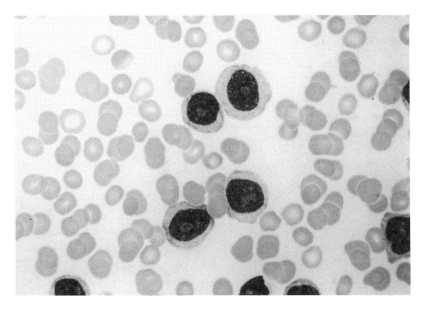

Figure 1   Peripheral blood film from a patient with B-PLL shows medium size lymphocytes with prominent single nucleolus.

3. Histology

The pattern of bone marrow infiltration in trephine biopsy specimens is similar in B- and T-PLL, but it is not specific to these diseases and may be similar to that of CLL or B-cell lymphomas. The lymphoid infiltration is often dense, with the most frequent patterns being mixed (interstitial plus diffuse) and diffuse. Residual hemopoietic reserve is variable, and reticulin is always increased (5). The cell morphology in the sections shows a predominant population with the features of prolymphocytes and the absence of small cells.

Spleen histology in B-PLL shows involvement of both white and red pulp. The white pulp shows large nodules composed by prolymphocytes and larger cells. This pattern of involvement is similar to CLL but different from hairy cell leukemia (HCL) and HCL-variant, both diseases that involve predominantly the splenic red pulp. Rarely, lymph node histological findings are available in B-PLL, with material usually obtained during splenectomy. The pattern of lymph node involvement is diffuse with obliteration of the follicular centers. The predominant cells are prolymphocytes with prominent nucleolus. Liver histological study shows infiltration of the portal tracts and sinuses.

4. Immunological Markers

B-prolymphocytes are mature B-cells but with an immunophenotype different from that of CLL. The cells are positive with the pan-B-cell markers CD19, CD20, and CD24, express strongly membrane CD22, surface immunoglobulins (SmIg) with light chain restriction, and FMC7 (6) (Figure 2). The predominant Ig heavy chains expressed are IgM and IgD, but a minority of cases are IgG or IgA positive. Of 37 cases we tested for heavy chains, 31 were IgM+, with 20 of them coexpressing IgD; three cases were IgG+, and the three others IgA+. Unlike CLL, B-prolymphocytes are strongly positive with monoclonal antibodies (McAb) that recognize the β-chain of the B-cell receptor complex clustered

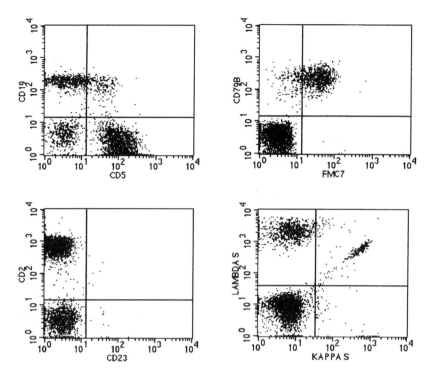

Figure 2 Flow cytometry profile from a B-PLL case shows that most cells express strongly lambda light chain and are CD79b+, FMC7+, CD23−, CD5−.

under CD79b [e.g., SN8 (7,8)]; CD5 and CD23 may be weakly expressed in one third of the cases (Table 2), but both antigens are coexpressed in cells from a single case in only 13% of patients. Quantitative flow cytometry analysis has shown a significantly stronger expression of CD79b and weaker CD5 in B-PLL compared with CLL (9). According to the scoring system for the diagnosis of CLL based on the expression of five markers (CD5, CD23, FMC7, intensity of CD22, and SmIg), scores in B-PLL range from 0 to 2 in contrast to CLL, in which scores are 4 or 5 in >85% of cases (6). The immunophenotype of PLL is also different from that of HCL and HCL-variant (10). Unlike HCL-variant, close to a third of B-PLL cases express weakly CD25 (Table 2) and unlike HCL, B-prolymphocytes are consistently negative with HC2 and CD103, and only a few cases are CD11c+. The McAb CD38 is positive in a third of B-PLL cases and CD10 is, as a rule, negative (5% positive cases).

5. Chromosome Abnormalities and Molecular Genetics

Chromosome abnormalities in B-PLL are usually complex, involving different chromosomes such as 1, 3, 6q, and 14 (11). The most common abnormalities involve chromosome 14 at band q32 documented in about half of the cases and t(11;14)(q13;q32), leading to the rearrangement of the BCL-1 gene with breakpoints as in mantle-cell lymphoma in 25% of cases (11,12). Other abnormalities in B-PLL are del6q21, t(3;8)(p13;q13), and del(12)(p12–13). In contrast to CLL, trisomy 12 is rare (13). Recent data from our laboratory applying fluorescence in situ hybridization (FISH) have demonstrated the presence

Table 2 Immunological Markers in
B-PLL*

Marker	Proportion of positive cases (%)
Kappa+	74
Lambda+	26
FMC7+	66
CD22+ (strong)	70
CD79b+	76
CD5+	31
CD23+	30
CD25+ (weak)	39
CD11c+	27
CD38+	37

* All cases were CD2 negative and CD19 or
CD37 positive.

of 11q23 deletions in more than one third of B-PLL and deletions of the retinoblastoma
(RB1) gene at 13q14 in half of the cases (14). Abnormalities of chromosome 17p are
present in some B-PLL, but deletion of p53 or missense mutations are frequent (15). In
our experience, p53 abnormalities are found in 75% of B-PLL (16) (Figure 3 see color
plate [noted as Figure 24.3]). This is the highest incidence reported so far in lymphoid
malignancies and, to some extent, it may account for the resistance to therapy in B-PLL.
A t(8;24)(q24;q32) involving the *c-myc* oncogene is rare in B-PLL but has been described
in a few cases (17), and we have documented a case with concurrent abnormalities of
p53 and the *c-myc* oncogene, the latter resulting from a t(2;8) (18).

6. Differential Diagnosis (Table 3)

B-PLL needs to be distinguished from CLL with increased (>10%) prolymphocytes or
CLL/PL and lymphomas in leukemic phase, particularly mantle-cell lymphoma. The distinction between CLL/PL and B-PLL is made on morphology, immunological markers,
and molecular genetics. In CLL/PL, there is a mixture of small CLL lymphocytes with
larger cells (e.g., prolymphocytes and immunoblast-like cells) whereas, in B-PLL, the
picture is more uniform without the small cellular component. By definition, B-PLL has
greater than 55% circulating prolymphocytes, whereas in CLL/PL the proportion of such
cells ranges from 11% to 55%, and the prolymphocytes are more pleomorphic. Immunological markers are useful in cases that offer diagnostic problems. The immunophenotype
in CLL/PL is similar or identical to CLL with "CLL" scores ranging from 4 to 5, whereas
in B-PLL the scores are low (see earlier). Although some CLL/PL cases may progress
during the disease course to a PLL-like picture, they can be distinguished from B-PLL,
because the blood morphology is pleomorphic and cells retain the immunophenotypical
and genetic characteristics of CLL.

The differential diagnosis of B-PLL with non-Hodgkins lymphomas in leukemic
phase arises mainly with mantle-cell lymphoma, particularly with those cases with blastoid
morphology and with follicular lymphoma with circulating centroblasts. In general, but
not always, the WBC count in the lymphoma cases is not as high as in B-PLL, and there
is pleomorphism in the morphology of the circulating cells. In follicular lymphoma, there

Table 3 Differential Features Between B-PLL and Other B-Cell Disorders

Feature	B-PLL	CLL/PL	MCL*	HCL-variant
Splenomegaly	+++	++	++	+++
Response to purine analogs†	+	+	−/+	−/+
Prognosis	Poor	Intermediate	Poor	Intermediate
Morphology	>55% PL cells	11–55% PL and small cells	Cleaved nucleus and speckled chromatin	Hairy cytoplasm nucleolated
CLL "score"	0–2	4–5	1–2	0–1
Histology	W&R pulp	W&R pulp	Mantle-zone	R pulp
Molecular genetics	t(11;14) and others	Trisomy 12 del13q	t(11;14)	Complex; various

* Leukemic phase of MCL.
† Fludarabine, deoxycoformycin, and/or cladribine.
CLL/PL, chronic lymphocytic leukemia with increased prolymphocytes; B-PLL, B-prolymphocytic leukemia; MCL, mantle-cell lymphoma; HCL-variant, hairy cell leukemia variant; W&R, white and red; −/+, <25% cases; +, 25–50% cases; ++, 50–75% cases; +++, >75% of cases.

is usually a mixed population of small centrocytes with scanty cytoplasm and centroblasts that may have a nucleolus but located at the nuclear periphery. In mantle-cell lymphoma, the cells have variable size, an irregular or slightly indented nuclear outline, speckled chromatin, and rarely a prominent nucleolus; the latter, however, may be a feature of the blastoid forms of mantle-cell lymphoma. Because molecular genetics may be identical in mantle-cell lymphoma and B-PLL, histology together with cell morphology are important tools for the differential diagnosis between the two conditions.

B-PLL may be also confused with the rare HCL-variant. Spleen and bone marrow histology and immunological markers will help distinguish between these two diseases. In contrast to B-PLL, in both the HCL-variant and the typical HCL, the spleen histology shows predominantly or exclusively red pulp involvement and the pattern of bone marrow infiltration is interstitial with spacing among the cells. Cells from HCL-variant are larger in size and have more abundant and irregular cytoplasm than the prolymphocytes. The immunophenotype of HCL-variant using markers of HCL (10) is, on the other hand, not very different from B-PLL except for the CD103 expression.

7. Clinical Course, Prognosis, and Therapy

Although in some patients the disease may be discovered by chance and can remain stable for months or even years with gradually increasing spleen size and prolymphocyte counts, there is always progression. Three of our B-PLL had "smouldering" disease with WBC ranging from 10 to 16, but progressively they had splenomegaly and developed a rising WBC up to 500 × 10⁹/L over a period of up to 2 years. A retrospective survey of 35 B-PLL patients has shown a median survival of 65 months, with anemia and lymphocytosis greater than 100 × 10⁹/L being predictors of a shorter survival (4).

Responses to a single alkylating agent (e.g., chlorambucil) are usually poor or transient. Therefore, this drug is not recommended as initial therapy. In a retrospective study, 8 of 17 B-PLL patients achieved a partial response (PR) to COP (cyclophosphamide, vincristine, and prednisolone) or chlorambucil and prednisolone (4). Responses to CHOP

(COP plus adriamicin) seem to be of better quality. Some patients have been treated with purine analogs with encouraging results, and one patient achieved a complete response (CR) with subcutaneous treatment with Campath-1H (19). Saven et al. (20) have documented CR lasting from 1 to 55+ months in five of eight B-PLL patients treated with claridribine and a PR in the remaining three patients with a median duration of 3 months; another report documented three responders to claridribine (4). Ten of our patients received purine analoges (6 fludarabine, 2 claridribine, and 4 pentostatin), and six of them achieved PR to fludarabine ($n = 2$), claridribine ($n = 2$), and pentostatin ($n = 2$), but we have not seen CRs. Splenectomy can be useful as a debulking procedure sometimes combined with leukapheresis to control very high counts. This may allow effective palliation for many months.

II. T-PROLYMPHOCYTIC LEUKEMIA

A. Clinical Features (Table 4)

T-PLL affects adults and is slightly more common in men. The median age in our series was 63 years (range, 33–91 years), and the male/female ratio was 1.3. Patients often are seen with widespread disease with organomegaly and raised lymphocyte counts. Lymphadenopathy and skin lesions may be initial manifestations in T-PLL. A few patients are asymptomatic at presentation, and the disease is discovered on a routine examination (21; our data). Main physical and laboratory findings are shown in Table 3. Splenomegaly, lymphadenopathy, and skin lesions, usually nodules or a disseminated maculopapular rash, are the most frequent findings. Pleural effusions and ascites are common, and central nervous system involvement, either meningeal or brain deposits, is rare.

Laboratory findings show a high lymphocyte count with half of the patients having counts greater than 200×10^9/L. Anemia and thrombocytopenia are less common than in B-PLL, detected in less than half of the patients.

Serology for the human T-cell leukemia virus (HTLV) types I and II is always negative in T-PLL, including the rare T-PLL seen in patients of Afro-Caribbean origin (3); thus, these retroviruses are not etiologically involved in T-PLL. These findings have been more recently confirmed by DNA analysis by means of the polymerase chain reaction

Table 4 Clinical and Laboratory Features of T-PLL*

Feature	Proportion of cases
Splenomegaly	79%
Lymphadenopathy	46%
Skin lesions	23%
Effusions†	12%
WBC $\times 10^9$/L (range)	10–1000
$>200 \times 10^9$/L	45%
Hb <10 g/dl	25%
Platelets $< 100 \times 10^9$/L	44%

* From a series of 150 patients.
† Pleural effusions, ascites, and/or pericarditis.

(PCR), using a set of primers specific to HTLV-I/II sequences. All T-PLL cases tested were negative (22).

B. Morphology

Most circulating cells in T-PLL are prolymphocytes. T-prolymphocytes usually are smaller than B-prolymphocytes, have less abundant and more often irregular cytoplasm with protrusions or blebs, and a more marked cytoplasmic basophilia (Figure 4). The nuclear outline in half of the T-PLL cases is regular as in B-prolymphocytes, whereas in the remainder is irregular. In 20% of T-PLL cases, the cells are small, have condensed chromatin, and the nucleolus is small and only visible in a proportion of cells by light microscopy but is always visible by electron microscopy (23). This variant form of T-PLL is designated small-cell variant (Figure 5); the cell phenotype and cytogenetics are those of typical T-PLL, supporting the view that they are different forms of the same disease (3). Another morphological variant of T-PLL is the cerebriform form, previously described as Sezary-like cell leukemia (24). In the latter condition, the cells have a highly convoluted or cerebriform nucleus identical to Sezary cells by light and electron microscopy. However, the clinical features, high WBC counts, rapidly progressive course and rare skin involvement, and cytogenetics with the presence of inv(14) support the view that Sezary-like cell leukemia is a variant of T-PLL (25,26). This and the small-cell T-PLL variant are now being incorporated into the forthcoming WHO classification of lymphoid malignancies.

   Bone marrow aspirates always show a variable degree of lymphoid infiltration, but they are not essential for diagnosis, because estimation of the hemopoietic reserve and degree of infiltration is better shown on trephine biopsy specimens.

C. Histology

The pattern of bone marrow infiltration in the core biopsy specimens in T-PLL shows, like in B-PLL, a heavy interstitial and/or diffuse infiltration with increased reticulin (5).

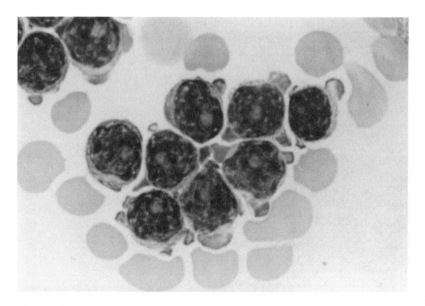

Figure 4   Peripheral blood film from a T-PLL shows that most cells have an irregular nucleus, prominent nucleolus and basophilic cytoplasm with protrusions.

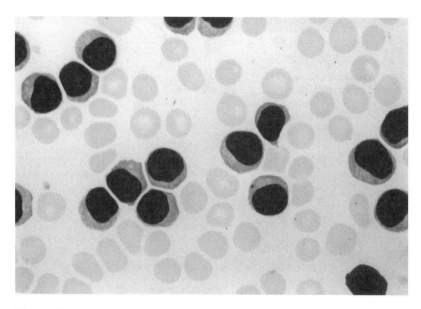

Figure 5   Circulating cells from a small cell variant T-PLL. The picture is monomorphic and most of the cells have small size, relatively condensed chromatin, deeply basophilic cytoplasm; a small nucleolus can be seen in a few cells.

Spleen histology shows infiltration of both the white and red pulp by small and medium size cells with morphological features of prolymphocytes. This pattern of infiltration is different from that seen in T-cell large granular lymphocyte leukemia in which the red pulp is predominantly involved with or without reactive hyperplasia of the follicular centers.

Rarely, lymph node histology is available for diagnosis. The pattern of lymphoid involvement is either diffuse or there is a predominant expansion of the paracortical zone with residual follicular centers. The lymphocytes are small or medium size, often with irregular nucleus and a small nucleolus. Histology of the liver is similar to B-PLL with lymphoid infiltrates in the portal tracts and sinuses. The skin histology shows a distinct pattern of infiltration. Most cases have dermal lymphoid infiltration without evidence of epidermotropism, the pattern seen in Sezary syndrome, even in the few patients in whom skin lesions manifest with erythroderma. The lymphoid infiltrates in the skin usually arrange around the skin appendages, a pattern rarely seen in other T-cell diseases (27). In some cases, the dermal infiltrates are heavy and extend to the subcutaneous fat.

D.   Immunological Markers (Table 5)

T-prolymphocytes have a mature/postthymic phenotype and thus the cells are negative with antibodies against the enzyme terminal deoxynucleotidyl transferase (TdT) and the cortical CD1a marker. Most cases are CD2, CD5, and CD7 positive. CD7 is expressed particularly with bright intensity in contrast to other T-cell disorders in which CD7 is weakly expressed or negative (28,29). The most common phenotype of T-prolymphocytes is CD4+, CD8− found in two thirds of cases; cells coexpress CD4 and CD8 in approximately 25% of cases (Figure 6), whereas a CD8+ CD4− phenotype is rare (Table 4). The CD4+ CD8+ phenotype with negative CD1a and TdT is rarely found in other mature T-cell disorders and suggests that T-prolymphocytes are at a stage of differentiation inter-

Table 5 Immunological Markers in T-PLL*

Marker	Proportion of positive cases (%)
Membrane CD3+	84
CD7+	99
CD4+CD8−	63
CD4+CD8+	23
CD4−CD8+	13
CD4−CD8−	1
Anti-TCR α/β	66
CD25+	22
CD38+	42
HLA−DR+	2

* All cases were CD2+, CD5+, CD52+ and negative with TdT, CD1a, and natural killer associated markers (CD16, CD56, CD57).

mediate between thymic and post-thymic T-cells. This is also suggested by the absence or weak expression of CD3 in a proportion of cases and the strong CD7 reactivity, a pattern more characteristic of cells from thymic malignancies (29). Approximately 20% or 25% of T-PLL cases are negative with McAb against the T-cell receptor (TCR) α/β complex; however, the beta and gamma chain genes of the TCR are rearranged in all cases (30). Natural killer–associated markers, as a rule, are negative. T-prolymphocytes express CD52 in the membrane with bright intensity compared with normal T-lymphocytes (31). Although CD52 is a marker of little diagnostic value, the strong reactivity seen in T-prolymphocytes might relate in part to the high rate of clinical responses of T-PLL to the humanized monoclonal antibody Campath-1H (CD52).

E. Chromosome Abnormalities and Molecular Genetics

T-PLL is characterized by recurrent chromosome abnormalities specially involving the 14q32.1 breakpoint (3,32,33). The most frequent abnormality, seen in 75% of cases, is inv(14)(q11;q32.1) or t(14;14)(q11;q32.1) (Figure 7), leading to the juxtaposition of the *TCL1* locus at 14q32.1 to the TCR-alpha chain gene locus at 14q11 (34). Another abnormality is t(X;14)(q28;q21) that also juxtaposes the TCR-alpha chain gene locus to a *TCL1* gene homolog, *MTCP1*, at Xq28 (35).

A second recurrent abnormality that occurs in more than half of the cases is i(8q), trisomy 8 and/or occasionally t(8;8)(p11;q12) or add(8)(p11) (3,32). FISH studies have shown that the i(8q) is dicentric and should be described as idic(8)(p11) with a loss of sequences distal to 8p11–12 (36). Thus, these abnormalities not only result in the amplification of the q arm but consistently involve 8p. Although rearrangement of *c-myc* mapped to 8q24 has not been demonstrated in T-PLL, we have documented overexpression of the *c-myc* oncoprotein in the cases with iso8q and trisomy 8 (37).

More recently, abnormalities of chromosome 12p have been described that suggest the presence of one or more suppressor genes involved in the pathogenesis of T-PLL (38,39).

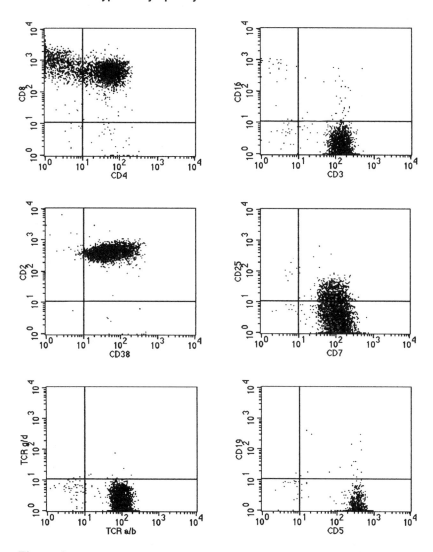

Figure 6   Flow cytometry analysis in a T-PLL case illustrating that most of the cells are positive with CD3, CD2, CD38, CD7, anti-TCR and coexpress CD4 and CD8.

Abnormalities involving 11q23 may be detected by chromosome analysis in a few cases but are more often demonstrated by molecular methods as discussed later. Progress has been made recently in our understanding of the molecular pathology of T-PLL by the demonstration of the frequent involvement of the *ATM* gene, which maps to 11q23.

Germline mutation of both alleles of this gene causes ataxia telangiectasia (AT), a severe multisystem disorder. *ATM* protein recognizes DNA damage signals (e.g., because of γ-irradiation) and causes arrest of cell cycle progression at the G1-S checkpoint (through phosphorylation at ser15 of p53) and at G2-M checkpoint (through phosphorylation of Chk2). AT is associated with the early onset and increased prevalence of a wide range of both solid and hematological tumors. One of these is a mature T-cell leukemia with a striking cytogenetic and immunophenotypical similarity to T-PLL (33,40). However, AT-

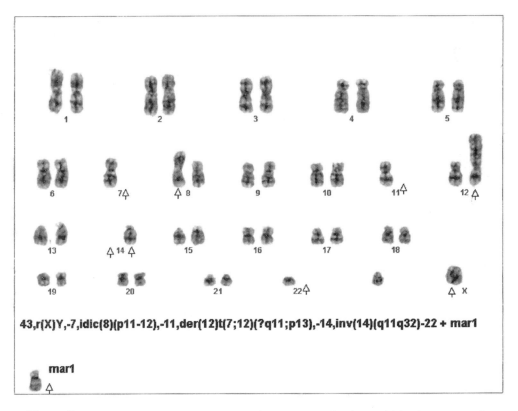

43,r(X)Y,-7,idic(8)(p11-12),-11,der(12)t(7;12)(?q11;p13),-14,inv(14)(q11q32)-22 + mar1

mar1

Figure 7   G-banded karyotype of a metaphase from a T-PLL showing multiple chromosome abnormalities.

related T-PLL has no reported karyotypic abnormalities at 11q23, and it has a higher
prevalence and lower age of onset. This suggests that *ATM* might be involved in non-
AT-related T-PLL.

Rearrangements that disrupt the *ATM* gene were detected by Southern blotting and
by staining single DNA fibers with labeled cosmids spanning the gene (41). Nucleotide
changes causing amino-acid substitution or premature chain termination were detected in
about half of the cases. Missense mutations cluster in the 3′ end of the gene in or close
to the kinase domain that phosphorylates p53 (42). Although deletions of p53 detected
by FISH and overexpression of the p53 protein are present in T-PLL, no p53 mutations
have been detected in T-PLL by DNA sequencing covering exons 1 to 11 (42,43). Thus,
impairment of p53 phosphorylation rather than loss of function may be a step in T-PLL
tumorigenesis. Mutational analysis indicated that there was a reduction to homozygosity,
and so this biallelic inactivation provided strong evidence that *ATM* is a tumor suppressor
gene. However, it is an unusual tumor suppressor gene. This is because risk of T-PLL is
not elevated in AT heterozygotes, and no sporadic T-PLL patient tested has been found
to be an AT heterozygote. This suggests that acquired mutation of *ATM* can contribute
to development of T-PLL, whereas inherited mutation at one *ATM* allele apparently does
not. Moreover, loss of *ATM* function confers no immediately apparent growth advantage.

Indeed, AT lymphocytes display elevated spontaneous apoptosis. Furthermore, loss of *ATM* function lays the basis for the appearance of mutated T-cell clones in AT patients that can persist for extended periods. The characteristic karyotypic abnormality in these lymphocytes is inv(14) or t(14;14) (44). This suggests that activation of the *TCL1* locus may counteract the elevated rate of spontaneous apoptosis normally seen in AT lymphocytes and that acquisition of a 14q32.1 breakpoint is an early event in the pathogenesis of sporadic T-PLL.

Because reciprocal translocations in T-PLL recur at chromosome 14q32, the region was proposed to harbor an oncogene locus. Cloning of translocation breakpoints defined a 350-kb region of 14q32.1 in which several CpG islands were detected. Near one of these islands, a gene was identified encoding a novel 14-kDa protein that was expressed in T-PLL and in immature T- and B-cells. The gene was considered a target of the translocations and so was called *TCL1* (T-cell leukemia 1) (34). Direct evidence that *TCL1* is an oncogene is provided by observations that transgenic mice expressing human *TCL1* in the T-cell compartment develop late-onset mature T-cell leukemias (45). Recently, a *TCL1* homolog called *TCL1b* has been identified adjacent to *TCL1*, and it has been shown to form fusion transcripts with its neighbors *TNG1* and *TNG2* (46,47). Of four T-PLL samples expressing *TCL1*, one expressed *TCL1b*, two expressed *TNG1* plus *TNG2*, and one did not express any of these genes. Because all four genes lie within the minimum breakpoint region in 14q32.1, it appears that translocation alone is not sufficient to activate all four genes. Furthermore, because expression of *TCL1* is also seen in some B-cell acute lymphoblastic leukemias, Burkitt's lymphoma, and AIDS-related lymphoma, where inv(14) or t(14;14) are not recurrent, it is possible that there are other mechanisms of activation of these genes.

A third *TCL1* homolog has been identified from the small proportion of T-PLL cases with reciprocal translocations between 14q11 and Xq28 rather than 14q32.1 (35,48). Translocation breakpoints in Xq28 lie within or immediately upstream of *MTCP1* (mature T-cell proliferation 1). This translocation permits expression of an alternate transcript of *MTCP1* called *MTCP1B1*, whose product is oncogenic and homologous to *TCL1* protein. *TCL1* and *MTCP1B1* have a similar intron-exon structure, indicating a common ancestral gene.

F. Differential Diagnosis

The differential diagnosis of T-PLL arises with other post-thymic T-cell leukemias and rarely with immature or thymic-derived leukemias or lymphomas. Immunological markers, TdT and CD1a, will distinguish T-PLL from thymic malignancies, because these are only expressed by cells in the latter conditions and negative in T-PLL. Morphology of the circulating cells is the main test to distinguish T-PLL from other post-thymic leukemias, particularly T-cell large granular lymphocyte leukemia in which the predominant population are granular lymphocytes or the peripheral T-cell lymphomas and ATLL that show a pleomorphic picture. HTLV-I serology is important to rule out ATLL. The cerebriform variant of T-PLL needs to be distinguished from Sezary syndrome. Unlike Sezary syndrome, in T-PLL, skin lesions do not show epidermotropism, and the lymphocyte counts are often significantly more elevated. Cytogenetic analysis will demonstrate in the cerebriform variant, chromosome abnormalities [e.g., inv(14)] characteristic of T-PLL. The small cell T-PLL variant can be confused with CLL in those cases in which immunological markers are not performed. The latter are essential to confirm the diagnosis of T-PLL.

G. Clinical Course, Prognosis, and Therapy

The clinical course of T-PLL is aggressive, with a median survival time of 7 months in our historical series of T-PLL (3). This outcome of T-PLL patients has improved in the last few years with the use of new drugs, particularly pentostatin (2'-deoxycoformycin) and antibodies such as Campath-1H (49–51). In T-PLL, prognosis does not correlate with the WBC, but bulky disease (e.g., hepatomegaly and lymphadenopathy) is a less favorable feature. Few T-PLL patients may have apparently low-grade disease. Twelve patients in our series had mild stable and/or slowly progressive lymphocytosis for up to 3 years without need of treatment or were well controlled with short pulses of steroids or chlorambucil, but ultimately all 12 patients progressed.

T-PLL does not usually respond to alkylating agents. Responses to combination chemotherapy such as CHOP are achieved in close to a third of the patients, but they are usually partial (3). The disease responds well to pentostatin when given as a single agent on a weekly schedule at a dose of 4 mg/m^2. With this schedule, more than half of the cases respond to pentostatin, most with partial responses and 9% with complete responses maintained for up to 1 year (49). Cases with a CD4+ CD8− phenotype appear to respond better than those with a CD8+ phenotype. The outcome of T-PLL has further improved with the use of the humanized monoclonal antibody Campath1H. We have treated 22 T-PLL patients with Campath1H administered as a 2-hour infusion three times a week at a dose of 30 mg until maximal response. Most patients were resistant or relapsed after pentostatin and some were in a PR. The overall response rate was 77%, with 59% CR. These responses were durable with a median disease-free survival of 9 months (range, 5–37 months). Clearance of malignant cells from blood and bone marrow was generally rapid, and resolution of skin infiltration, lymphadenopathy, and/or splenomegaly occurred in half the affected patients. However, patients with serous effusions, hepatic, and/or CNS involvement were resistant to therapy. There was no correlation between response and other disease features such as WBC, immunophenotype, cytogenetics, or previous treatments. Three patients who relapsed achieved a second CR, lasting for 5 to 6 months after a further course of Campath1H. Median survival was significantly prolonged in patients achieving a CR (13.5 months) compared with those achieving a PR (6 months) or the nonresponders (2.5 months), including a patient that survived more than 4 years (51). This has allowed collection of uncontaminated peripheral blood stem cells in some patients followed with high-dose therapy and autologous transplantation. This procedure has been carried out in three patients who survived for 12 to 19 months after autograft but have all relapsed and died. Campath1H should currently be considered as first-line therapy in T-PLL, with the use of high-dose therapy with autologous transplantation to consolidate responses.

REFERENCES

1. DAG Galton, JM Goldman, E Wiltshaw, D Catovsky, K Henry, GJ Goldenberg. Prolymphocytic leukaemia. Br J Haematol 27:7–23, 1974.
2. D Catovsky, J Galetto, A Okos, DAG Galton, E Wiltshaw, G Stathopoulos. Prolymphocytic leukaemia of B and T cell type. Lancet 11:232–234, 1973.
3. E Matutes, V Brito-Babapulle, J Swansbury, J Ellis, R Morilla, C Dearden, A Sempere, D Catovsky. T-prolymphocytic leukemia is a disease entity. Clinical and laboratory features of 78 cases. Blood 78:3269–3274, 1991.

4. L Shvidel, M Shatalrid, L Bassous, A Klepfish, E Vorst, A Berrebi. B-cell prolymphocytic leukemia: a survey of 35 patients emphasizing heterogeneity, prognostic factors and evidence for a group with an indolent course. Leuk Lymphoma, 33:169–179, 1999.

5. L Hernandez-Nieto, IA Lampert, D Catovsky. Bone marrow histological patterns of B-cell and T-cell prolymphocytic leukemia. Hematol Pathol 3:79–84, 1989.

6. E Matutes, K Owusu-Ankomah, R Morilla, J Garcia Marco, A Houlihan, TH Que, D Catovsky. The immunological profile of B-cell disorders and proposal of a scoring system for the diagnosis of CLL. Leukemia 8:1640–1645, 1994.

7. M Okazaki, Y Luo, T Han, M Yoshida, BK Seon. Three new monoclonal antibodies that define a unique antigen associated with prolymphocytic leukemia/non-Hodgkin's lymphoma and are effectively internalized after binding to the cell surface antigen. Blood 81:84–94, 1993.

8. AP Zomas, E Matutes, R Morilla, K Owusu-Ankomah, BK Seon, D Catovsky. Expression of the immunoglobulin-associated protein B29 in B-cell disorders with the monoclonal antibody SN8 (CD79b). Leukemia 10:1966–1970, 1996.

9. E Cabezudo, P Carrara, R Morilla, E Matutes. Quantitative analysis of CD79b, CD5 and CD19 in mature B-cell lymphoproliferative disorders. Haematologica 84:413–418, 1999.

10. E Matutes, R Morilla, K Owusu-Ankomah, A Houliham, P Meeus, D Catovsky. The immunophenotype of hairy cell leukemia (HCL). Proposal for a scoring system to distinguish HCL from B-cell disorders with hairy or villous lymphocytes. Leukemia Lymphoma 14(suppl 1): 57–61, 1994.

11. V Brito-Babapulle, S Pittman, JV Melo, M Pomfret, D Catovsky. Cytogenetic studies on prolymphocytic leukemia. 1. B-cell prolymphocytic leukemia. Hematol Pathol 1:27–33, 1987.

12. V Brito-Babapulle, J Ellis, E Matutes, D Oscier, T Khokhar, K MacLennan, D Catovsky. Translocation t(11;14)(q13;q32) in chronic lymphoid disorders. Genes Chromosomes Cancer 5:158–165, 1992.

13. H Dohner, S Pohl, M Bulgay-Morschel, S Stilgenbauer, M Bentz, P Lichter. Trisomy 12 in chronic lymphoid leukemias-a metaphase and interphase cytogenetic analysis. Leukemia 7: 516–520, 1993.

14. D Lens, E Matutes, D Catovsky, LJA Coignet. Frequent deletions at 11q23 and 13q14 in B-cell prolymphocytic leukemia (B-PLL). Leukemia 14:427–430, 2000.

15. H Dohner, K Fischer, M Bentz, K Hansen, A Benner, G Cabot, D Diehl, R Schlenk, J Coy, S Stilgenbauer. p53 gene deletion predicts for poor survival and non-response to therapy with purine analogs in chronic B-cell leukemias. Blood 85:1580–1589, 1995.

16. D Lens, PJ de Schouwer, RA Hamoudi, M Abdul-Rauf, N Farahat, E Matutes, T Crook, MJ Dyer, D Catovsky. p53 abnormalities in B-cell prolymphocytic leukemia. Blood 89:2015–2023, 1997.

17. D Feneux, D Choquet, C de Almeida, F Davi, R Garand, F Valensi, C Leonard, H Merle-Beral. Cytogenetic studies by FISH on B cell prolymphocytic leukemia. Blood 88(suppl 1): 155b, 1996.

18. D Lens, LJA Coignet, V Brito-Babapulle, CSP Lima, E Matutes, MJS Dyer, D Catovsky. B cell prolymphocytic leukemia (B-PLL) with complex karyotype and concurrent abnormalities of the p53 and c-myc gene. Leukemia 13:873–876, 1999.

19. AL Bowen, A Zomas, E Emmett, E Matutes, MJ Dyer, D Catovsky. Subcutaneous Campath 1H in fludarabine-resistant/relapsed chronic lymphocytic and B-prolymphocytic leukaemia. Br J Haematol 96:617–619, 1997.

20. A Saven, T Lee, M Schultz, A Jacobs, D Ellison, R Longmire, L Piro. Major activity of cladribine in patients with de novo B-cell prolymphocytic leukemia. J Clin Oncol 15:37–43, 1997.

21. R Garand, J Goasguen, A Brizard, J Buisine, A Charpentier, JF Claisse, E Duchayne, M Lagrange, C Segonds, X Trousard, G Flandrin. Indolent course as a relative frequent presentation in T prolymphocytic leukaemia. Br J Haematol 103:488–494, 1998.

22. R Pawson, TF Schulz, E Matutes, D Catovsky. The human T-cell lymphotropic viruses type

I/II are not involved in T-prolymphocytic leukemia and large granular lymphocytic leukemia. Leukemia 11:1305–1311, 1997.

23. E Matutes, J Garcia-Talavera, M O'Brien, D Catovsky. The morphological spectrum of T-prolymphocytic leukaemia. Br J Haematol 64:111–124, 1986.

24. E Matutes, DM Keeling, AC Newland, CS Scott, D Mitchell, N Traub, DG Wardle, D Catovsky. Sezary cell-like leukemia: a distinct type of mature T-cell malignancy. Leukemia 4:262–266, 1990.

25. R Pawson, E Matutes, V Brito-Babapulle, H Maljaie, M Hedges, J Mercieca, M Dyer, D Catovsky. Sezary cell leukemia: a distinct T-cell disorder or a variant form of T-prolymphocytic leukaemia? Leukemia 11:1009–1013, 1977.

26. V Brito-Babapulle, SH Maljaie, E Matutes, M Hedges, M Yullie, D Catovsky. Relationship of T leukaemias with cerebriform nuclei to T-prolymphocytic leukaemia: a cytogenetic analysis with in situ hybridization. Br J Haematol 96:724–732, 1997.

27. RB Mallet, E Matutes, D Catovsky, K MacLennan, PS Mortimer, CA Holden. Cutaneous infiltration in T-cell prolymphocytic leukaemia. Br J Dermatol 132:263–266, 1994.

28. E Matutes, D Catovsky. Mature T-cell leukemias and leukemia/lymphoma syndromes. Review of our experience in 175 cases. Leukemia Lymphoma 4:81–91, 1991.

29. L Ginaldi, E Matutes, N Farahat, M de Martinis, R Morilla, D Catovsky. Differential expression of CD3 and CD7 in T-cell malignancies: a quantitative study by flow cytometry. Br J Haematol 93:921–927, 1996.

30. L Foroni, J Foldi, E Matutes, D Catovsky, N O'Connor, R Baer, A Forster, TH Rabbitts, L Luzzatto. Alpha and beta T cell receptor genes: rearrangements correlate with haematological phenotype in T-cell leukemias. Br J Haematol 67:307–318, 1987.

31. L Ginaldi, M de Martinis, E Matutes, N Farahat, R Morilla, MJS Dyer, D Catovsky. Levels of expression of CD52 in normal and leukemic B and T cells: correlation with in vivo therapeutic responses to Campath 1H. Leukemia Res 22:185–191, 1998.

32. V Brito-Babapulle, M Pomfret, E Matutes, D Catovsky. Cytogenetic studies on prolymphocytic leukemia. II. T-cell prolymphocytic leukemia. Blood 70:926–931, 1987.

33. V Brito-Babapulle, D Catovsky. Inversions and tandem translocations involving chromosome 14q11 and 14q32 in T-prolymphocytic leukemia and T-cell leukemias in patients with ataxia telangiectasia. Cancer Genet Cytogenet 55:1–9, 1991.

34. L Virgilio, MG Narducci, M Isobe, LG Billips, MD Cooper, CM Croce, G Russo. Identification of the TCL1 gene involved in T-cell malignancies. Proc Natl Acad Sci USA 91:12530–12534, 1994.

35. M-H Stern, J Soulier, M Rosenzwajg, K Nakahara, N Canki-Klaim, A Aurias, F Sigaux, IR Kirsch. MTCP-1 a novel gene on the human chromosome Xq28 translocated to the T cell receptor alpha locus in mature T cell proliferations. Oncogene 8:2475–2483, 1993.

36. SH Maljaie, V Brito-Babapulle, L Hiorns, D Catovsky. Abnormalities of chromosome 8, 11, 14 and X in T-prolymphocytic leukemia studied by fluorescence in situ hybridization. Cancer Genet Cytogenet 103:110–116, 1998.

37. HS Maljaie, V Brito-Babapulle, E Matutes, LR Hiorns, PJJC de Schouwer, D Catovsky. Expression of c-myc oncoprotein in chronic T cell leukemias. Leukemia 9:1694–1699, 1995.

38. F Salomon-Nguyen, F Brizard, M Le Coniat, I Radford, R Berger, A Brizard. Abnormalities of the short arm of chromosome 12 in T-cell prolymphocytic leukemia. Leukemia 12:972–975, 1998.

39. V Brito-Babapulle, A Sorour, E Matutes, D Catovsky. Chromosome 12p abnormalities in T-prolymphocytic leukemia. A study by fluorescence in situ hybridization. Blood 94(suppl): 275a, 1999.

40. AMR Taylor, JA Metcalfe, J Thick, YF Mak. Leukemia and lymphoma in Ataxia Telangiectasia. Blood 87:423–438, 1996.

41. MR Yullie, LJA Coignet, SM Abraham, F Yaqub, L Luo, E Matutes, V Brito-Babapulle, I

Vorechovsky, MJS Dyer, D Catovsky. ATM is usually rearranged in T-cell prolymphocytic leukemia. Oncogene 16:789–796, 1998.

42. I Vorechovsky, L Luo, MJS Dyer, D Catovsky, PL Amlot, JC Yaxley, L Foroni, L Hammarstrom, ADB Webster, MAR Yullie. Clustering of missense mutations in the ataxia-telangiectasia gene in a sporadic T-cell leukaemia. Na Gen 17:96–99, 1997.

43. V Brito-Babapulle, H Maljaie, R Hamoudi, S Watson, E Matutes, P de Schouwer, M Yullie, M Dyer, D Catovsky. Studies of the p53 gene and protein expression in Sezary syndrome (SS) and T-prolymphocytic leukaemia (T-PLL). Br J Haematol 101:87, 1998.

44. MH Stern, FR Zhang, C Griscelli, G Thomas, A Aurias. Molecular characterization of different ataxia telangiectasia T-cell clones. I. A common breakpoint at the 14q11.2 band splits the T-cell receptor alpha-chain gene. Human Genetics 78:33–36, 1988.

45. L Virgilio, C Lazzeri, R Bichi, K Nibu, MG Narducci, G Russo, JL Rothstein, CM Croce. Deregulated expression of TCL1 causes T cell leukemia in mice. Proc Natl Acad Sci USA 95:3885–3889, 1998.

46. Y Pekarsky, C Hallas, M Isobe, G Russo, CM Croce. Abnormalities at 14q32.1 in T-cell malignancies involve two oncogenes. Proc Natl Acad Sci USA 96:2949–2951, 1999.

47. C Hallas, Y Pekarsky, T Itoyama, J Varnum, R Bichi, JL Rothstein, CM Croce. Genomic analysis of human and mouse TCL1 loci reveals a complex of tightly clustered genes. Proc Natl Acad Sci USA 96:14418–14423, 1999.

48. J Thick, JA Metcalfe, YF Mak, D Beatty, M Minegishi, MJ Dyer, G Lucas, AM Taylor. Expression of either the TCL1 oncogene or transcripts from its homologue MTCP1/c6.1B in leukaemic and non-leukaemic T cells from ataxia telangiectasia patients. Oncogene 12:379–386, 1996.

49. J Mercieca, E Matutes, C Dearden, K MacLennan, D Catovsky. The role of pentostatin in the treatment of T-cell malignancies: analysis of response rate in 145 patients according to disease subtype. J Clin Oncol 12:2588–2593, 1994.

50. R Pawson, MJS Dyer, R Barge, E Matutes, PD Thornton, E Emmett, JC Kluin-Nelemans, WE Fibbe, R Willenze, D Catovsky. Treatment of T-cell prolymphocytic leukemia with human CDw52 antibody. J Clin Oncol 15:2667–2672, 1997.

51. CE Dearden, E Matutes, MJS Dyer, P Leoni, A Pareira, M Lima, GF Tjonnifjord, B Nomededeu, D Catovsky. Campath-1H treatment of T-prolymphocytic leukaemia (T-PLL). Blood, (suppl 94), 1999.

25

Chronic T-Cell and NK-Cell Leukemias

EDGAR G. MIRANDA and THOMAS P. LOUGHRAN, Jr.

H. Lee Moffitt Cancer Center and Research Institute, Tampa, Florida

The French-American-British Cooperative Group proposed a classification for chronic T-cell leukemias and designated four subgroups: (1) LGL Leukemia, (2) T-prolymphocytic leukemia, (3) Adult T-cell leukemia/lymphoma, and (4) Cutaneous T-cell Lymphoma/Sezary syndrome (1). The clinicopathological features of chronic T-cell leukemias will be discussed in this chapter, except for the category of T-prolymphocytic leukemia which is described in Chapter 24. Other less common chronic T-cell lymphoproliferative disorders not included in the FAB classification will also be discussed (Table 1).

I. LARGE GRANULAR LYMPHOCYTE LEUKEMIA

A syndrome of increased number of circulating large granular lymphocytes (LGL) associated with chronic neutropenia was recognized as a distinct clinical entity in 1977 (2). A major question was whether this LGL proliferation represented a reactive process or a clonal malignant expansion. Clonal cytogenetic abnormalities found in unstimulated cultures of peripheral blood and/or splenic mononuclear cells from two patients were the first evidence that supported the theory of clonal expansion (3).

Several terms have been used to describe this disorder: chronic T-cell lymphocytosis with neutropenia (4,5), T8 chronic lymphocytic leukemia (CLL) (6), granulated T-cell lymphocytosis with neutropenia (7), T-suppressor cell CLL (8), neutropenia with T lymphocytosis (9), NK and suppressor T-cell CLL (10), T-cell CLL (11–13), T-gamma lymphocytosis or T-gamma lymphoproliferative disorder (14–16), and lymphoproliferative disorder of granular lymphocytes (17,18). In 1985, LGL leukemia was the proposed term for this disorder based on the demonstration of clonality and tissue invasion of marrow,

Table 1 Clinical and Phenotypic Characteristics of T-Cell and NK-Cell Leukemias

Disease	Clinical characteristics	Phenotype
Large granular lymphocyte, T-cell	Recurrent bacterial infections, neutropenia, rheumatoid arthritis, splenomegaly	CD3(+), CD8(+), CD16(+) CD57(+), Rarely CD56(+)
Large granular lymphocyte, NK-cell	Mild neutropenia, severe anemia and hepatosplenomegaly, jaundice; aggressive clinical course	CD3(−), CD56(+), CD57(−)
Adult T-cell leukemia/ lymphoma (ATL)	Lymphadenopathy, hepatosplenomegaly, skin rash, hypercalcemia	CD3(+), CD4(+), CD25(+)
Cutaneous T-cell lymphoma (CTCL)	Indolent skin disease; leukemic phase with erythodema	CD3(+), CD4(+), CD7(−)
T-cell CLL/PLL	Generalized lymphadenopathy, hepatosplenomegaly, bone marrow involvement, B symptoms	CD3(+), CD4(+), CD7(+)
NK-cell lymphoma	Symptoms depend on site of involvement, nasopharynx predominant site, initially not with bone marrow involvement; leukemic phase has aggressive course	CD3(−), CD56(+)
NK-like T-cell lymphoma	B symptoms, marked hepatosplenomegaly, usually without lymphadenopathy or bone marrow involvement	CD3(+), CD56(+)
Gamma-delta T-cell lymphoma	Mostly extranodal disease, with involvement of liver, spleen, skin, GI track, and thyroid gland, B symptoms	CD3(+), CD8(−/+) CD16(+), CD56(+), TCR gamma/delta(+)
Posttransplant T-cell lymphoproliferative disorder	Usually after solid organ transplantation, with aggressive behavior similar to NK and NK-like lymphoma	CD3(+), CD8(+) and variable expression of CD56
S-100 Lymphoproliferative disorder	Aggressive clinical course, splenomegaly without prominent lymphadenopathy, leukocytosis; CNS involvement reported in leukemic phase	CD3(+), CD8(−/+), CD56(+), S-100(+)

spleen, and liver. In 1990, the Morphologic, Immunologic, Cytogenetic (MIC) Cooperative Study Group agreed with the term LGL leukemia as the preferable terminology (19). The term LGL leukemia has also been accepted by the REAL classification (20).

On the basis of evidence that clonal LGL proliferations could either be of CD3+ (T-cell) or CD3− (NK cell) origin, it was proposed that LGL leukemia could be subclassified in T-LGL leukemia and NK-LGL leukemia. T-LGL is characterized by clonal CD3+ LGL proliferation, and NK-LGL leukemia is characterized by CD3− LGL proliferation (21).

A. T-LGL Leukemia (Clonal CD3+)

1. Clinical Features

This type of LGL disorder represents 85% of the cases of LGL leukemia. The incidence is the same for men and women and affects primarily patients at a median age of 55 years. Only 10% of the patients with LGL leukemia are younger than 40 years of age. Approximately one third of the patients are asymptomatic at the time of diagnosis. The other two thirds usually have a recurrent history of bacterial infections typically involving sinuses, perirectal area, skin, and sometimes more life-threatening diseases like pneumonia or sepsis. Other opportunistic infections, like fungal viral or parasitic infections, are rare.

Rheumatoid arthritis (RA) is a common clinical manifestation associated with T-LGL leukemia, occurring in approximately 25% of these patients (21–23). These patients resemble those patients with Felty's syndrome, with the clinical triad of neutropenia, splenomegaly, and rheumatoid arthritis. The presence of severe erosive arthritis and the extra-articular manifestations of RA are commonly seen in patients with Felty's syndrome but are rarely seen in patients with T-LGL leukemia (23,24). Small series have shown that 11% to 35% of patients with Felty's syndrome have a clonal LGL disorder (4,5,7). The true prevalence of LGL proliferation in RA is not well characterized and is probably underestimated.

Clonal CD3+ LGL populations have been identified in small series of patients with Felty's syndrome. Loughran et al. found 4 of 12 patients with clonal CD3+ proliferation (23), and Gonzalez-Chambers et al. found clonal disease in 8 of 23 patients (25). Patients with Felty's syndrome and patients with LGL leukemia and RA have a similar high frequency of inheritance of HLA-DR haplotype (26,27). These data suggest that LGL leukemia and Felty's syndrome are part of the same disease spectrum. Increased numbers of cells with a phenotype similar to leukemic LGL have been observed in the blood and synovial fluid from patients with RA (23). These observations raised the possibility of a common pathogenic link between LGL leukemia and RA.

B symptoms (fever, night sweats, and weight loss) occur in approximately 20% to 30% of patients with LGL leukemia. Splenomegaly occurs in 20% to 50% of patients and hepatomegaly in 20%. Lymphadenopathy is a rare physical finding in T-LGL leukemia (21,22).

2. Hematological Features

Hematological findings in patients with T-LGL leukemia include neutropenia (<2,000/uL), which is usually severe (48%); anemia (49%); thrombocytopenia (19%); and lymphocytosis (74%), usually greater than 4000/uL. Examination of the peripheral blood smear is essential for the diagnosis of LGL leukemia. The presence of an increased number of large lymphocytes with abundant pale cytoplasm and prominent azurophilic granules is characteristic of LGL leukemia. Clonally expanded lymphocytes with the typical CD3+, CD57+ phenotype sometimes may not have LGL morphological features on peripheral smear. The normal LGL count is 200 to 400 cells/uL, whereas in patients with LGL leukemia the median is 4200/uL (28), although clonal disease has been documented in patients with LGL count within the normal range. Most of the patients have a modest lymphocytosis, with median lymphocyte count of 7800/μL.

The mechanism of neutropenia is not completely understood. Maturation arrest of the myeloid series has been observed and also lymphocytic infiltration. In contrast to CLL in which further deterioration of hematological features is secondary to increased lymphocytic infiltration and marrow replacement, in T-LGL leukemia the infiltration is not sufficiently severe to account for the neutropenia. Antineutrophil antibodies are common (2,24,29,30), and decreased survival of neutrophils has been demonstrated, supporting an autoimmune mechanism for the neutropenia. These antibodies may represent immune complex deposition rather than specific neutrophil antibodies. Recently Fas ligand has been implicated in the development of neutropenia in these patients (31), and a disregulated apoptotic pathway is a central feature of this disease (32–34).

Other hematological findings in patients with T-LGL leukemia include anemia and less frequently thrombocytopenia. Cases of both Coombs'-positive and Coombs'-negative hemolytic anemia have been reported in patients with T-LGL leukemia (35–38).

3. Immune Abnormalities

Serological abnormalities are common, including polyclonal hypergammaglobulinemia, hypogammaglobulinemia (less frequently), circulating immune complexes, and a positive test for rheumatoid factor or antinuclear antibody. Occasionally cases with monoclonal gammopathy of undetermined significance or myeloma have been associated with LGL leukemia (39). Antiplatelet antibodies are also common.

Defects in cellular immunity have also been observed in patients with T-LGL. Natural killer cell numbers and functional activity are decreased (28). Antibody-dependent cellular cytotoxic activity is usually preserved, but diminished proliferative responses to mitogens and impairment in formation of high affinity IL-2 receptors are often observed in leukemic cells (40–42).

4. Phenotype of T-LGL

Most T-LGL express CD3, TCR alpha-beta, CD8, CD16, CD57, and rarely CD56. Variable expression of CD16 has been observed in CD3+ leukemic LGL, and this discrepancy may be due to the anti-CD16 monoclonal antibodies used for staining. It is likely that CD16 is expressed on leukemic LGL from all patients.

T-LGL can be subclassified on the basis of the expression of CD4, CD8, and TCR markers, but the clinical significance is unknown. More than 95% of the cases have a CD3+, TCR alpha-beta+, CD4−, and CD8+ phenotype. Other variants of leukemic LGL have been reported such as CD3+, TCR gamma-delta+, either CD4−, CD8+, or CD4−, CD8−. Few patients with CD3+, TCR alpha-beta, CD4+, CD8− have been observed, but interestingly these patients usually have normal or only moderately low neutrophil counts (29,36,43).

Molecular studies of the T-cell receptor gene rearrangement are the best way to demonstrate that this disorder constitutes a clonal process. Clonal chromosomal abnormalities have also been detected in some patients (2).

5. Etiology

The etiology for the clonal expansion of LGL is not known. It has been suggested that antigen activation and lymphokine secretion, like IL-12 and IL-15 (44), could lead to leukemic LGL proliferation (45). Clonal evolution is another alternative explanation but could depend on additional genetic abnormalities and environmental factors.

The role of a retroviral infection may represent a pathway for antigen activation. Initially, 6 of 12 patients with T-LGL leukemia were found to have serological reactivity to human T-cell leukemia virus antigens (46). European studies concurred with these findings, but no seropositivity was observed in Japanese patients with leukemic LGL (47). HTLV-II sequences were cloned from marrow mononuclear cell DNA using PCR in a patient with T-LGL leukemia who never received a blood transfusion and was not an intravenous drug abuser (48). HTLV-I was also found in another patient, but this patient had received multiple blood transfusions. However, most patients are not infected with either HTLV-1 or HTLV-II. Most patients with LGL leukemia have antibodies directed at the BA 21 epitope of the p21 envelope protein of HTLV-I (49). Familial transmission of retroviral infections has been observed, and cases of LGL proliferation have been found in a father and his children and a mother and her son (50). These findings suggest the possibility of an infectious agent as a cause for LGL leukemia.

6. Diagnosis

The presence of chronic neutropenia, pure red cell aplasia, adult-onset cyclic neutropenia, or RA are clinical characteristics that make one suspicious of the diagnosis of T-LGL leukemia. Initial workup should include a careful examination of the peripheral smear. Although absolute lymphocytosis is not always present, most of the patients have an increased number of LGL cells.

Phenotypical characteristics are essential for the diagnosis, so flow cytometry is required. Another important diagnostic test for the diagnosis of T-LGL leukemia is the demonstration of clonal T-cell gene rearrangement. Lymphocytosis is a clinical presentation of other entities, so one needs to differentiate LGL leukemia from other disorders causing lymphocytosis. Viral infections like Epstein-Barr virus, CMV, and HIV can also produce lymphocytosis, but the presence of clonal LGL proliferation and TCR gene rearrangement is distinctive of LGL leukemia.

7. Prognosis and Therapy

Large granular lymphocyte leukemia is an uncommon chronic disorder. Long-term follow-up studies of these patients have been reported, demonstrating a variable life expectancy. A large series of patients with LGL were followed for a mean period of 23 months, and 26 deaths were reported among 151 patients (18). Another study reported a median survival longer than 10 years (22). One prospective study reported a 20% mortality rate over a 4-year period, but the study included patients without documented clonal disease and patients with CD3− LGL leukemia. Definitive data regarding the natural history of T-LGL leukemia are lacking. An LGL leukemia registry has been established in the United States to resolve this issue (www.moffitt.usf.edu/lgl-leukemia/registry.htm).

Although T-LGL is considered a chronic disease, most of the patients will require treatment. The most common indication for treatment is recurrent infection in the presence of severe neutropenia. The optimal treatment for the neutropenia is unknown. In a small series of patients, four of the five patients treated with cyclosporine (CSA) attained normal neutrophil counts ($>1.5 \times 10(9)/L$) within 21 to 75 days. The fifth patient required growth factor to improve neutropenia. Despite resolution of neutropenia, the clonal T-LGL population persisted, and neutropenia recurred with attempts to taper the CSA dose (51). Myeloid growth factors have been used with limited success. GM-CSF seems to be ineffective (52,53), and few patients have responded to G-CSF (54,55). Low-dose oral methotrexate (10 mg/m² weekly) was used in 10 patients with T-LGL leukemia, and 5 of these patients achieved complete clinical remission (normal CBC) and 1 patient had partial response (sustained neutrophil count $>500/\mu L$). Molecular analysis of T-cell receptor gene rearrangement failed to demonstrate abnormal clone in three of the five patients achieving complete clinical remission (21). Prednisone has also shown effectiveness in the treatment of some patients but not in others (55–57). Splenectomy has limited effectiveness (58).

T-LGL leukemia has been associated with pure red cell aplasia (59). Various treatments including chemotherapy or immunosuppressive drugs have shown effectiveness (35–38). Rarely there appears to be progression to a more aggressive disease. The use of combination chemotherapy has not been successful in this type of patient (20).

B. NK-LGL Leukemia (Clonal CD3−)

1.   Clinical and Hematological Features

Patients with NK-LGL leukemia tend to be younger than those with T-LGL with a median age of 39 years. The gender distribution is equal as in T-LGL leukemia.

This type of clonal LGL proliferation usually has an acute clinical course. Neutropenia is usually mild, and severe neutropenia is uncommon. The anemia and thrombocytopenia are generally more severe. Most of the patients have an absolute lymphocytosis at presentation and often a rapid increase in LGL counts in only a few weeks ($50,000/\mu L$) (60–65).

NK-LGL leukemia is usually characterized by hepatoslenomegaly, jaundice, and ascites (61,63,65,66). The analysis of the peritoneal fluid usually reveals LGL cells. Lymph node involvement has been observed more commonly in NK-LGL type than CD3+ LGL. Infiltration of the bone marrow is as frequently seen as in T-LGL leukemia. CNS involvement has been documented by the presence of LGL cells on spinal fluid examination (60). Coagulopathy has also been reported (62,63,65). Immune abnormalities have not been studied extensively in NK-LGL.

2.   Phenotype of NK-LGL Leukemia

NK-LGL leukemia is characterized by expansion of cells with a CD3−, CD4−, CD8−, CD56+, and CD57− phenotype. The examination of peripheral smears under the light microscope is essential but cannot differentiate it from T-LGL leukemia. Ultrastructural features may differ from the CD3+ to the CD3− LGL leukemia. The T-LGL type is characterized by parallel tubular arrays, whereas the NK type do not contain these structures (67).

3.   Etiology

Epstein-Barr virus has been implicated as a possible etiological factor for the development of NK-LGL leukemia (65). Most of the positive findings come from Japanese studies. American and European researchers have generally not been able to detect the EVB virus genome in chronic cases of LGL proliferation.

4. Prognosis and Therapy

NK-LGL leukemia has an acute presentation with dramatic systemic symptoms. In a series of 11 patients with documented NK-LGL leukemia, nine died within the first 2 months after the diagnosis. The most common cause of death is disseminated disease with associated coagulopathy and multiorgan failure (61–64). At the time of autopsy LGL infiltration was found in most of the organs (spleen, marrow, liver, lymph nodes, small bowel, and kidneys) (61,62).

Aggressive treatment is required, and one option is to use combination chemotherapy. ProMACE-CytaBOM was used in one patient with NK-LGL leukemia. Other chemotherapeutic agents used included cyclophosphamide, vincristine, and prednisone (65). It is not confirmed whether there is a preexisting chronic phase before acute proliferation. Peripheral blood stem cell allogenic transplant was performed in one patient with NK-LGL leukemia, with a reported duration of remission of 10 months (68).

II. ADULT T-CELL LEUKEMIA

Human T-lymphotrophic virus I (HTLV-I) is the etiological agent involved in the pathogenesis of adult T-cell leukemia/lymphoma (ATL) (69–71). HTLV-I was isolated first from a patient with suspected cutaneous T-cell lymphoma. Subsequently, it was recognized that the patient had ATL, a clinical syndrome first described in Japan (72). The clinical features and natural history of the disease vary. HTLV-I is endemic in Central Africa, certain Caribbean islands, the southeastern United States, and the southwest region of Japan. Different modes of transmission have been postulated, including mother to newborn by means of breast feeding and during sexual intercourse (72). HTLV-I has also been implicated in diseases other than ATL, including a degenerative neurological disease termed HTLV-I associated myelopathy (73).

A. Clinical Features

The median age of onset of ATL is 55 years of age. Clinical manifestations vary according to stage of disease, but usually patients are first seen with lymphadenopathy and hepatosplenomegaly (72). Other areas of involvement include skin, CNS, bone marrow, lung, and intestinal tract. In 28% of the cases serum calcium is elevated with or without lytic bone lesions. The white blood cell count is variable. Thrombocytopenia or anemia is uncommon.

Diversity in clinical presentations exists in ATL and is classified according to the patterns of clinical manifestations. In 1991, the Japanese Lymphoma Study Group (74) classified ATL according to serum LDH levels, serum calcium levels, lymphocyte count, and tumor lesions (70). Patients with chronic ATL (71) are characterized by increased ATL cells ($4 \times 10(9)$/L or more), occasional skin involvement, mild lymphadenopathy, and elevated serum LDH. A smoldering subtype (74–76) is associated with a small number of ATL cells (less than $4 \times 10(9)$/L), occasional skin lesions, and no other clinical abnormalities. The lymphoma type usually presents with lymphadenopathy, without lymphocytosis, 1% or less abnormal T cells, and no extranodal manifestations. The acute type is characterized by more aggressive disease with leukemic manifestations and tumor lesions (74). One of the criticisms of this classification was the lack of correlation with prognosis. A new classification of adult T-cell leukemia based on prognosis was proposed by the Takatsuki group in 1994 (77). The use of Ki-67 antigen was demonstrated to be a valuable prognostic factor for this disease. If Ki-67 expression is found on greater than 18% of peripheral blood T-cells, the prognosis is poor and is classified as aggressive ATL. These patients have a poor survival, regardless of the clinical stage developed by JLSG. Patients with low numbers of Ki-67–positive cells usually have a better prognosis (77). These criteria are used in treatment decisions.

B. Diagnosis

The diagnosis of ATL is based on histology, cellular markers, and genetic testing. ATL cells are characterized by a CD2+, CD3+, CD4+, CD25+ phenotype. The presence of anti-HTLV-I antibodies and clonality of proviral DNA is also required for the diagnosis. One of the proposed mechanisms for the expression of the IL-2 receptor involves the expression of the *tax* gene of HTLV-I (72).

Chromosomal abnormalities in chromosome 3 (21% of the cases), 21 (9%), monosomy of chromosome X (38%), and loss of a Y chromosome (17%) have been reported. Structural chromosomal abnormalities have also been found, 14q11 and 14q32 being the most frequently involved in such translocations (78).

C. Treatment

Several treatment modalities have been tested in ATL, including single agents and combination chemotherapy. A Japanese study showed improvement in survival and quality of life in a small series of patients treated with combination chemotherapy (79). Retinoids have shown biological activity in inducing apoptosis of ATL cells (80), but no clinical trial has been reported. Two patients have received bone marrow transplants. One of the patients had acute ATL and relapsed 3 months later, whereas the second patient had chronic ATL and became free of disease within 18 months of follow-up after transplant (81). ATL is usually resistant to conventional chemotherapy, and one of the possible explanations includes the expression of multidrug resistance protein. Inhibition of the expression of MDR genes could represent an alternative modality for the treatment of ATL in addition to combination chemotherapy (82). Newer treatment interventions have been tested in ATL, including antiretrovirals alone or in combination with interferon alpha (83), as well as arsenic trioxide and interferon alpha (84). A case report of a patient with ATL showed complete remission for about 249 days after treatment with 2-chlorodeoxyadenosine follow by a period of partial response of 10 weeks until the progression of ATL with clinical evidence of lymphadenopathy (85).

III. CUTANEOUS T-CELL LYMPHOMA

Cutaneous T-cell lymphoma (CTCL) is an uncommon lymphoma characterized pathologically by epidermotrophic infiltrates of clonal malignant T lymphocytes (86–88). It was described initially in the nineteenth century by a French dermatologist and given the name mycosis fungoides because of the mycotic-like plaques or tumors seen in early phases of the disease. The annual incidence is 0.29 per 100,000 and accounts for less than 0.5% of the new cases of non-Hodgkin's lymphomas diagnosed in the United States each year (89). However, it is the most common of the primary lymphomas of the skin. CTCL is usually a disease of older patients, with a peak age of 55 to 60 years old at presentation and a male/female ratio of 2:1. This disease has also been described in a younger population with similar clinical characteristics.

The clinical course is usually indolent, and long-term survival is common. CTCL is usually preceded by several years of persistent scaly patches or plaques, which could resemble psoriasis or eczematous dermatitis. The pathological diagnosis in early stages is very difficult and may take several years and visits to the dermatologist before establishing the diagnosis.

An erythrodermic leukemic variant characterized by generalized erythroderma, lymphadenopathy, splenomegaly, and circulating atypical T cells is known as Sezary syndrome. The prognosis and management is different compared with more limited forms of cutaneous disease.

A. Etiology

The cause of CTCL is not known. There are two main hypotheses for CTCL pathogenesis. First, the lymphocytic infiltration may be clonal or malignant from the beginning. There may be resistance mechanisms that suppress disease manifestations, but, eventually, these are overcome and CTCL develops. A second hypothesis is that CTCL may develop from a benign reactive process in which chronic antigenic stimulation eventually results in neoplastic transformation (90). Several case report series support the role of chronic antigenic stimulation from environmental chemicals (91,92). A large case-control study to investigate the relationship between chemical exposure and CTCL showed an increased relative risk of 4.3 for patients in manufacturing and construction industries (93). However, these data conflict with another case-controlled study (94). Therefore the role of chemical exposure in the development of CTCL is not defined.

Viral infection has been implicated in the origin of CTCL. Human T-lymphotropic virus-I (HTLV-I) was first isolated from a patient with manifestations of CTCL (94). Other investigations have suggested a role for HTLV-like retrovirus in CTCL pathogenesis (95,96).

B. Clinical Manifestations

Clinical features of CTCL are nonspecific during initial stages of the disease. Scaly skin lesions are similar to eczematous, atopic, or contact dermatitis and psoriasis. In the early phases of the disease, these patchy erythematous lesions tend to have a "bathing trunk" distribution, although any part of the body can be involved. Some of these patients respond to local treatment with a topical steroid, which in some cases may delay the diagnosis of CTCL. Not all patients with this initial presentation progress to CTCL, but many will have pathological changes consistent with CTCL develop. The median duration from the onset of skin manifestations to the clinical and pathological diagnosis of CTCL is approximately 6 years (96). Multiple biopsies sometimes are required before establishing the diagnosis.

Patches evolve to plaques, which are characterized by palpable, erythematous, and well-demarcated lesions. In some patients, the palms and/or sole are involved with fissuring of the skin, but in other patients these areas are spared despite more extensive involvement in other parts of the body. Without treatment these lesions can become ulcerated and develop into tumors. Ulcerated lesions are a source for infection, which is a common cause of significant morbidity in these patients. CTCL can also be seen as generalized erythroderma, the so called "l'homme rouge" (Red man syndrome). This presentation is usually associated with intermittent periods of intense pruritus. The time of progression of patch to plaque phase is unknown and variable. A small percentage of patients may have tumors without any preexisting lesions. This is known as "D'emblee presentation."

The presence of generalized erythroderma, pruritus, and circulating malignant cells is known as Sezary syndrome. This variant of CTCL is associated with splenomegaly, lymphadenopathy, and peripheral blood findings of more than 15% to 20% circulating atypical hyperconvoluted lymphocytes. There is a correlation between the extent of skin involvement and extracutaneous manifestations (87). Patients with generalized erythroderma or with numerous skin tumors are more likely to develop extracutaneous disease. The organs more frequently affected are lungs, spleen, liver, and gastrointestinal track.

C. Diagnosis

The most challenging dilemma is the differentiation of CTCL from inflammatory dermatoses at early stages of presentation. The classic histopathological description of CTCL is a dense bandlike infiltrate within the upper dermis of lymphoid cells with hyperchromatic, convoluted nuclei and scant cytoplasm (97). These mononuclear cell intraepidermal aggregates are known as Pautrier microabsceses or microaggregates. The epidermis is usually acanthotic but typically lacks significant intercellular edema (spongiosis). The deep dermis and subcutis are usually histologically normal (97).

Initially, the patchy lesions are flat because of less tumor density and minimal or no epidermal hyperplasia. In progression to a tumor state, the cell infiltration at the dermis becomes more prominent, making these lesions nodular and palpable on physical examination. The epidermal layer may be free of tumor cell infiltration. The architectural features may resemble other cutaneous lymphomas, but the cytological characteristics of hyperchromatic, convoluted nuclei and scant cytoplasm allow the pathologist to establish the diagnosis of CTCL.

Histopathological criteria for the diagnosis of CTCL have been developed (97), which take into consideration the level of epidermal and dermal involvement. These diagnostic categories include "diagnostic for CTCL," "consistent with CTCL," and "suggestive of CTCL." Another important clinical characteristic is that CTCL occurs de novo (tumor D'emblee), whereas other types of cutaneous tumors usually have had no primary skin lesions.

Immunophenotyping is another useful diagnostic tool. CTCL cells typically retain the expression of pan-T-cell markers, such as CD2, CD3, CD5, until progression to tumor stage or lymph node involvement (98,99). At these more advanced stages, the immunophenotype of CTCL resembles that of other types of T-cell lymphoma. In most of the cases CD4 (helper/inducer) is expressed, although occasionally CD8 (cytotoxic/suppressor) may be expressed. Phenotypical characteristics have also been used as a prognostic indicator. Tumors cells that are CD2(−)/CD7(+) usually have a poor prognosis (100). It is very uncommon to find CD1 expression, a CD4(−)/CD8(−), or CD4(+)/CD8(+) immunophenotype (98). More than two thirds of cases do not express CD7 (97), which is suggestive but not diagnostic for skin involvement by CTCL. Absence of CD7 in lymph nodes is usually diagnostic for neoplastic T-cell involvement (97).

In cases in which histology and immunophenotype are not diagnostic for CTCL, gene rearrangement studies are a useful tool to try to resolve the diagnostic dilemma. Methods used to detect clonal T-cell receptor gene rearrangement are either Southern blot or polymerase chain reaction (PCR) analysis (101,102).

The percentage of circulating tumor cells needed to establish the diagnosis of Sezary syndrome is controversial. The National Cancer Institute established specific criteria in terms of the number of circulating tumor cells (103). The presence of more than 5% of lymphocytes is considered significant for blood involvement. In general practice and in several referral centers a percentage of 20% or more of circulating lymphocytes or an absolute Sezary cell count of at least $1000/mm^3$ is required to establish blood involvement (104).

D. Staging and Prognosis

In 1978 the National Cancer Institute sponsored a workshop to establish a staging system for cutaneous T-cell lymphomas. The system proposed was based on the TNMB staging system. These include descriptions of skin (T), lymph nodes (N), visceral (M), and blood (B) involvement.

The T1 classification includes those patients with limited plaques, papules, or eczematous lesions covering less than 10% of the skin surface. The T2 lesions are those patients with generalized plaques, papules, or eczematous lesions covering more than 10% of the skin surface. The T3 lesions are tumors, and T4 is consider generalized erythroderma.

In terms of nodal status, N0 designates those patients with no lymph node involvement or lymphadenopathy. The N1 classification is subdivided into N1 to N3. The N1 category contains those patients with lymphadenopathy on clinical examination. This N1 category is subdivided as follows: ''o'' when a biopsy was not performed; ''n'' for normal histopathological finding on lymph node biopsy; ''r'' for a reactive lymph node; ''d'' for dermathopathic lymphadenitis. Patients who have no clinical evidence of lymphadenopathy but do have evidence of CTCL on lymph node biopsy are classified as N2. Those with both peripheral lymphadenopathy and positive biopsy are N3.

The presence or absence of visceral involvement differentiates the M0 from the M1 category. Determination of M1 status requires documentation by biopsy. Regarding blood findings the B0 category means atypical circulating cells are not present in peripheral blood or are less than 5%, whereas B1 category are those patients with more than 5% circulating atypical cells.

In the classic staging system, stage I includes patients with disease limited to the skin without node, visceral, or blood involvement. Patients with limited plaques are considered stage IA and IB and are those patients with generalized plaque. Patients with plaque disease but no palpable lymphadenopathy are stage IIA. Stage IIB are patients who have cutaneous tumors with or without lymphadenopathy. Stage IIIA is defined as a patient with erythroderma and no palpable lymphadenopathy, whereas stage IIIB includes erythrodermic patients with palpable lymphadenopathy. In the group with stage IV, those with extracutaneous involvement limited to lymph nodes are classified as stage IVA and those with visceral involvement are considered stage IVB. Blood involvement does not affect the stage designation.

The extent and the type of skin involvement and the presence of extracutaneous manifestations are the most important predictive factors for survival in patients with CTCL. Early-stage disease (T1, stage IA) has a life expectancy similar to an age-, sex-, and race-matched control population (105). Only 9% of these patients will progress to a more advanced stage of disease. Patients with stage IB or IIA have a median survival of more than 11 years (106). The likelihood of progression of patients with T2 disease is

24%. Tumor stage (T3, stage III) median survival with extracutaneous manifestations is 3.2 years compared with 4.6 years for those with no extracutaneous disease. The long-term outcome of patients with T4 disease is variable. Major predictive factors are age, overall stage, and peripheral blood involvement. Patients with generalized erythroderma (T4) usually have a poor prognosis, with an estimated median survival of less than 1.5 years Progression to a more advanced form of lymphoma (e.g., large cell lymphoma) has an impact on survival.

In one study 115 patients with CTCL were followed for a period of 2 years (107). Twenty-six patients transformed to an aggressive form of lymphoma. The stage of skin disease (T stage) at the time of transformation was an important prognostic indicator for survival. Pathologically proven stages IA, IB, and IIA patients had a 2-year survival of 86% (95% CI, 60% to 100%) from time of transformation. Patients with stage IIIB presentation had a 10-month median survival, and only 30% of these patients were alive at 2 years (95% CI, 1% to 59%). Patients with stage IV disease had a survival of 15 months from time of transformation. Factors found not to affect median survival included LDH, $beta_2$-microglobulin, and depth of invasion of the lymphoid infiltrate (107).

E. Treatment

Several therapeutic interventions are available for the treatment of CTCL. The modality of treatment will be dictated by the clinical stage. Also the patient's overall clinical condition, accessibility of treatment, and socioeconomic factors all need to be considered before deciding on therapeutic intervention. In this section we are going to emphasize the treatment for advanced stages of the disease.

1.   Stages I and II

Topical chemotherapy agents, phototherapy (PUVA), or total skin electron beam therapy (EBT) are considered initial treatment modalities for patients with early stages of the disease.

Phototherapy with ultraviolet-B (UVB) and ultraviolet-A (UVA) are modalities available for treatment for psoriasis and CTCL. UVA may produce additional beneficial effect because of greater penetration to the upper dermal infiltrate of CTCL. In 1974, a new treatment for psoriasis was introduced (108). This treatment was adopted for the management of CTCL. It consists of using a photosensitizing drug psoralen in combination with high-intensity long-wave UVA irradiation. The acronym PUVA has been used to describe this treatment. One proposed mechanism of action of PUVA is that psoralen intercalates with DNA, and exposure to UVA produces cross-links between opposite strands of DNA (96). Other mechanisms of action have also been proposed, (e.g., inhibition of DNA synthesis, direct cytotoxic effect, immunomodulation, and inhibition of mediators of inflammation).

Topical chemotherapeutic agents like mechlorethamine hydrochloride are another option for the management of limited patch/plaque T1 lesions. The standard duration of treatment is 6 months with a response rate of about 70% to 80% (105,109,110). Twenty-five percent of the patients have a durable CR 10 years later. Fifty percent of the patients had recurrent disease develop when treatment was discontinued. One of the complications of mechlorethamine hydrochloride is acute and delayed hypersensitivity reaction. Secondary skin malignancies are another possible complication from treatment, like squamoproliferative lesions on the skin (111,112).

BCNU is another topical chemotherapeutic agent with similar effectiveness to mechlorethamine hydrochloride, but its systemic absorption increases the chances of secondary hemalotogical complications (113). Patients can also have telangiectasias develop where the drug is applied. Aggressive treatment with either chemotherapeutic agent has not shown any improvement in survival.

2. Stages III and IV

The erythrodermic stage of CTCL is usually difficult to treat with total-skin EBT because of the presence of preexistent skin irritation. A minimal dose of electron beam treatment could be more futile than beneficial. One possible initial treatment for this stage of the disease is low-dose PUVA followed by gently increasing doses, or a combination treatment of PUVA and interferon. Combined modality treatment may be preferable for patients who have had single therapy with either PUVA or interferon alone fail (114).

Extracorporeal photochemotherapy is probably the preferred primary treatment for erythrodermic CTCL. The treatment consists of providing a photosensitizing drug like psoralen and then collecting patients' white blood cells through a pheresis procedure. The collected cells are exposed to UVA, and then these irradiated cells are returned to the patient. This treatment is best given in patients with no extracutaneous disease or with only limited lymph node involvement. The frequency of the treatment will vary, depending on the severity of the disease. The estimated CR rate is 21%, but 41% of the patients experience at least a 50% improvement of skin lesions. One of the proposed mechanisms of action of photopheresis is that it acts as an immunomodulator triggering an antitumor response against CTCL cells. Photopheresis can also be combined with interferon or retinoic acids, with variable response rates reported.

Systemic chemotherapy has been shown to be appropriate treatment in patients with extracutaneous disease. Various combination chemotherapy regimens have been used (115,116). The CR rate ranges from 11% to 57%, with a PR rate from 22% to 86% (96). The most common combination chemotherapy regimen used is CHOP. Some agents have been used as a single modality, including methotrexate, fludarabine, etoposide, vinblastine, and gencitabine (117). In a phase II study, 13 pretreated patients with peripheral T-cell lymphoma were treated with gemcitabine at on days 1, 8, and 15 of a 28-day schedule. After completing three courses, one patient achieved complete remission and eight partial responses. Toxicity was minimal and the treatment was well tolerated (117). Pentostatin has been reported as an active agent in previously treated patients with CTCL. Partial and complete response was achieved in 71% and 25% of the patients, respectively (118). A phase II trial of 2-chlorodeoxyadenosine was used in patients with refractory and/or relapse CTCL. The CR rate was 14%, with a median duration of 4.5 months, and the PR rate was 14%, with a median duration of 2 months (119). A small group of patients with CTCL were treated with continuous infusion of methotrexate after fluorouracil and leucovorin rescue. Patients were treated for an average of 33 months. The median survival was 6 years (120). The overall clinical response rate of combination chemotherapy appears better when compared with use of single agents. The median duration of response is less than 1 year.

Immunotherapy has been one of the new treatment modalities implemented in CTCL. Chimeric anti-CD4 monoclonal antibody was administered intravenously as a single dose in a small series of eight patients with CTCL. The dose was escalated during the study. The treatment was well tolerated, and no clinical evidence of immunosuppression was found. Seven of the eight patients responded to treatment with a progression-free survival of 25 weeks (range, 6–52 weeks) (130).

Other modalities are being tested to assess the effectiveness in CTCL. A case report of a 22-year-old patient with Sezary syndrome who underwent 6/6 matched unrelated donor bone marrow transplants was the first successful allogeneic transplant patient reported in the literature (121). More studies are needed to establish the effectiveness of transplant in patients with CTCL.

New and emerging therapeutic modalities are being evaluated for the treatment of CTCL. One recent development is the production of humanized anti-helper T-cell antibody (122). In small series the estimated clinical response was moderate and short-lived. An IL-2-diphtheria toxin fusion protein has also been developed and tested in a multicenter phase III trial for patients with CD25(+) CTCL (103). The overall response rate was 30%, with a CR of 10% and a PR of 20%. This drug has recently been approved by the FDA for use in CTCL patients. The median survival was 6 years (121). At this point no therapeutic intervention has been shown to be effective in improving survival in patients with CTCL. More studies are required to assess the effectiveness of present treatment regimen modalities and to determine which combinations of treatment are optimal in this disease.

IV. MISCELLANEOUS

A. NK-Cell Lymphoma

Variants of non-Hodgkin's lymphomas include those of natural killer (NK) cell origin, a distinct clinicopathological entity (123,124). The phenotypical features of these tumor cells are characterized by lack of CD3 and presence of CD2 and CD56 expression. The nasopharynx is one of the predominant sites of involvement in this lymphoid malignancy, but other organs like skin, testis, gastrointestinal tract (small intestine, stomach) have been reported (125). Epstein-Barr virus infection has been considered as a possible etiological agent for the development of this disease. Pathologically, tumor cells have variable cytological appearances, with frequent angiocentricity and angioinvasion associated with zonal necrosis (angiocentric lymphoma). Cells size is also variable with intermediate and large cells.

The clinical manifestations and behavior of NK lymphoma are determined by the degree of involvement of the disease (124). In early stages, symptoms are confined to the area of involvement, usually the nasopharynx, and rarely is there marrow involvement. In the presence of multiorgan involvement, most of patients have pancytopenia, hepatosplenomegaly, and marrow involvement with hemophagocytosis. A leukemic phase has been described with an aggressive behavior and fulminant presentation of disseminated disease.

The median survival of patients with localized disease is approximately 11 to 12 months compared with 2 months for those patients with advanced disease (multiorgan involvement) (124).

Conventional chemotherapy appeared ineffective in most cases. Anthracycline-containing regimens produced a 75% remission in patients with early stage (localized) disease and 25% in cases with advanced disease. Radiation therapy is an alternative modality for patients with localized disease. High-dose chemotherapy followed by autologous bone marrow transplant has been reported in the literature and recommended as an alternative for relapsed primary nasal lymphoma after failure of conventional therapy and radiotherapy (126).

B. NK-like T-Cell Lymphoma

Natural killer cell–like lymphoma is an aggressive form of non-Hodgkin's lymphoma characterized by the coexpression of CD3 NK-cell markers, also with clonal T-cell receptor gene rearrangement (127). Clinical manifestations include weight loss, night sweats and fever (B symptoms), and marked hepatosplenomegaly, usually without lymphadenopathy. Bone marrow is almost always involved with neoplastic T cells. The prognosis is poor because of the aggressiveness of the disease. A small series of patients with NK-like lymphoma has reported a short survival (128). Two of the untreated patients died within 20 days after the diagnosis. After combination chemotherapy, three patients were able to survive 5 months after initial presentation. One patient was reported to stay in remission for 22 months at the time of the report.

C. Gamma Delta T-Cell Lymphoma

Gamma delta T-cell lymphoma is a distinct clinical entity that is characterized by aggressive behavior (129). A small case series has described typical clinical features seen in this disorder. Most of the patients exhibit extranodal disease, which may include involvement of liver, spleen, skin, gastrointestinal tract, and thyroid gland (130). Other clinical features are the presence of B symptoms and hepatosplenomegaly at the time of presentation. The median age of this disease is 34 years. The phenotype of the malignant cells is CD3+, gamma-delta+, CD4−, CD8−/+, CD16+, CD56+. Clonality can be demonstrated using T-cell receptor gene rearrangement studies (130). Gamma-delta T-cell lymphoma has been associated with viral infection by herpesvirus-6 (131) and EBV (132). This disease carries a poor prognosis despite the use of combination chemotherapy.

D. Posttransplant T-Cell Lymphoproliferative Disorders

Most posttransplant lymphoproliferative disorders (PTLD) occurring after solid organ transplantation are associated with EBV and have a B-cell origin. A small number a cases of T-cell posttransplant lymphoproliferative disorder have been reported in the literature. Phenotypical characteristics consist of CD3 and CD8 expression with variable expression of CD56 (2 of 6 were positive). Similar to NK type, NK-like, and gamma-delta T-cell lymphoma, this disease has an aggressive course.

E. S-100+ Lymphoproliferative Disorder

The S-100-positive lymphoproliferative disorder is a rare entity and is characterized by an aggressive clinical course (133). Patients usually have splenomegaly, without prominent lymphadenopathy, and an elevated white cell count. Few cases of CNS involvement have been reported at the leukemic phase. The phenotypical characteristics consist of CD4−, CD8−/+, CD56+, S-100beta+ cells. Southern blot studies have demonstrated clonal TCR gene rearrangement. The life expectancy in these patients is short. Despite treatment, most of the patients died within 8 months after the diagnosis.

REFERENCES

1. JM Bennett, D Catovsky, M-T Daniel, G Flandrin, DAG Galton, HR Gralnick, C Sultan. Proposals for the classification of chronic (mature) B and T lymphoid leukemia: French-American-British (FAB) Cooperative Group. J Clin Pathol 42:567–584, 1989.
2. RW McKenna, J Parkin, JH Kersey, KJ Gajl-Peczalska, L Peterson, RD Brunning. Chronic lymphoproliferative disorder with unusual clinical, morphologic, and ultrastructural and membrane surface markers characteristics. Am J Med 62:588–596, 1977.
3. TP Jr Loughran, ME Kadin, G Starkebaum, JL Abkowitz, EA Clark, C Disteche, LG Lum, SJ Slichter. Leukemia of large granular lymphocytes: Association with clonal chromosomal abnormalities and auto-immune neutropenia, thrombocytopenia and hemolytic anemia. Ann Intern Med 102:169–175, 1985.
4. AC Aisenberg, BM Wilkes, NL Harris, KA Ault, RW Carey. Chronic T-cell lymphocytosis with neutropenia. Report of a case studied with monoclonal antibody. Blood 58:818–822, 1981.
5. HG Herrod, WC Wang, JL Sullivan. Chronic T-cell lymphocytosis with neutropenia. Its associated with Epstein-Barr virus infection. Am J Dis Child 139:405–407, 1985.
6. JU Brisbane, LD Berman, ME Osband, RS Neiman. T8 chronic lymphocytic leukemia. A distinctive disorder related to T8 lymphocytosis. Am J Clin Pathol 80:391–396, 1983.
7. RW McKenna, DC Arthur, KJ Gajl-Peczalska, P Flynn, RD Brunning. Granulated T-cell lymphocytosis with neutropenia: Malignant or benign chronic lymphoproliferative disorder? Blood 66:259–266, 1985.
8. K Bakri, EZ Ezdinli, LP Wasser, T Han, T Sinclair, S Singh, H Ozer, J Minowada. T-suppressor cell chronic lymphocytic leukemia. Phenotypic characterization by monoclonal antibodies. Cancer 54:284–292, 1984.
9. WC Chan, I Check, C Schick, RK Brynes, J Kateley, EF Winton. A morphologic and Immunologic study of the large granular lymphocyte in neutropenia with T lymphocytosis. Blood 63:1133–1140, 1984.
10. M Palutke, L Eisenberg, J Kaplan, M Hussain, K Kithier, P Tabaczka, I Mirchandani, D Tenebaum. Natural killer and suppressor T-cell chronic lymphocytic leukemia. Blood 62: 627–634, 1983.
11. RL Phyliky, C-Y Li, LT Yam. T-cell chronic lymphocytic leukemia with morphologic and imunologic characteristics of cytotoxic/suppressor phenotype. Mayo Clin Proc 58:709–720, 1983.
12. S Tagawa, I Konishi, H Kuratune, S Katagiri, N Taniguchi, T Tamaki, R Inoue, Y Kanayama, T Tsubakio, T Machii, T Yonezawa, T Kitani. A case of T-cell chronic lymphocytic leukemia (T-CLL) expressing a peculiar phenotype (E+, OKM1+, Leu1+, OKT3−, and IgG EA−). Cancer 52:1378–1384, 1983.
13. SL Thien, D Catovsky, D Oscier, JM Goldman, HJ Van Der Reijden, CJM Melief, HC Rumke, RJM Ten Berge, AEGKR Von Dem Borne. T-chronic lymphocytic leukemia presenting as primary hypogammaglobulinemia-evidence of a proliferation of T-suppressor cells. Clin Exp Immunol 47:670–676, 1982.
14. AA Bom van Noorloos, HG Pegels, RHJ Van Oers, J Silverbusch, TM Feltkamp-Vroom, R Goudsmit, WP Zeijlemaker, AEGK von dem Borne, CJM Melief. Proliferation of t-gamma cells with killer-cell activity in two patients with neutropenia and recurrent infections. N Engl J Med 302:933–937, 1980.
15. JJ Hoks, BF Haynes, B Detrick-Hooks, LF Diehl, TL Gerrard, AS Fauci. Gamma (immune) interferon production by leukocytes from a patient with a T-gamma cell proliferative disease. Blood 59:198–201, 1982.
16. F Miedema, FG Tepstra, JW Smit, JPW Van Der Veen, CJM Melief. T-gamma lymphocytosis is clinically non-progressive but immunologically heterogeneous. Clin Exp Immunol 61: 440–449, 1985.

17. G Semenzato, F Pandolfi, T Chisesi, G De Rossi, G Pizzolo, R Zambello, L Tretin, C Agostini, E Dini, M Vespignani, A Cafaro, D Paqualetti, MC Guibellino, N Migone, R Foa. The lymphoproliferative disease of granular lymphocytes. A Heterogeneous disorder ranging from indolent to aggressive conditions. Cancer 60:2971–2978, 1987.

18. F Pandolfi, TP Loughran, G Starkebaum, T Chisesi, T Barbui, WC Chan, JC Brouet, G De Rossi, RW McKenna, F Salsano, FV Herrmann, JW Oostveen, G Schlimok, A Cafaro, R Zambello, MC Garcia-Rodriguez, CH Geisler, G Pizzolo, RG Steis, JU Brisbane, ME Kadin, A Mantovani, S Tagawa, AS Fauci, G Gastl, M Palutke, SJ Proctor, HF Pross, P Mancini, F Aiuti, G Semenzato. Clinical course and prognosis of the lymphoproliferative disease of granular lymphocytes. A multicenter study. Cancer 65:341–348, 1990.

19. JM Bennett, G Juliusson, C Mecucci. Morphologic, Immunologic, and cytogenetic classification of chronic (mature) B and T lymphoid leukemias: Fourth meeting of the MIC Cooperative group. Cancer Res 50:2212, 1990.

20. NL Harris, ES Jaffe, H Stein, PM Banks, JKC Chan, ML Cleary, G Delsol, C De wolf-Peeters, B Falini, KC Gatter, TM Grogan, PG Isaacson, DM Knowles, DY Mason, H-K Muller-Hermelink, SA Pileri, MA Piris, E Ralfkiaer, RA Warnke. A Revised European-American Classification of Lymphoid Neoplasms: A Proposal From The International Lymphoma Study Group. Blood 84:1361–1392, 1994.

21. TP Jr Loughran. Clonal diseases of large granular lymphocytes. Blood 82:1–14, 1993.

22. MV Dhodapkar, CY Li, JA Lust, A Teferi, RL Phyliky. Clinical spectrum of clonal proliferation of T-large granular lymphocytes: A T-cell clonopathy of undetermined significance? Blood 84:1620–1627, 1994.

23. TP Jr Loughran, G Starkebaum, P Kidd, P Neiman. Clonal proliferation of large granular ymphocytes in rheumatoid arthritis. Arthritis Rheum 31:31–36, 1988.

24. WJ Wallis, TP Jr Loughran, ME Kadin, EA Clark, GA Starkebaum. Polyarthritis and neutropenia associated with circulating large granular lymphocytes. Ann Intern Med 103:357–361, 1985.

25. R Gonzales-Chambers, D Przepiorka, A Winkelstein, A Agarwal, TW Starz, WE Kline, H Hawk. Lymphocyte subsets associated with T-cell receptor B-chain gene rearrangement in patients with rheumatoid arthritis and neutropenia. Arthritis Rheum 35:516–520, 1992.

26. SJ Bowmann, M Sivakumaran, N Snowden, M Bhavnani, MA Hall, GS Panayi, JS Lanchbury. The large granular lymphocyte syndrome and rheumatoid arthritis. Immunogenic evidence for a broader definition of Felty's syndrome. Artritis Rheum 37:1326–1330, 1994.

27. G Starkebaum, TP Jr Loughran, LK Gaur, P Davis, BS Nepon. Immunogenetic similarities between patients with Felty's syndrome and those with clonal expression of large granular lymphocytes in rheumatoid arthritis. Arthritis Rheum 40:624–626, 1997.

28. TP Jr Loughran, KE Draves, G Starkebaum, P Kidd, CA Clark. Induction of NK Activity in large granular lymphocyte leukemia: Activation with anti-CD3 monoclonal antibody and interleukin 2. Blood 69:72–78, 1987.

29. TP Jr Loughran, G Starkebaum. Large granular lymphocyte leukemia: Report of 38 cases and review of the literature. Medicine 66:397–405, 1987.

30. PK Rustagi, T Han, L Ziolkowski, DL Farolino, MS Curie, GL Logue. Granulocyte antibodies in leukemic chronic lymphoproliferative disorders. Br J Haematol 66:461–465, 1987.

31. R Perzova, TP Jr Loughran. Constitutive expression of Fas ligand in large granular lymphocyte leukaemia. Br J Haematology 97:123–126, 1997.

32. T Lamy, JH Liu, TH Landowski, WS Dalton, TP Jr Loughran. Dysregulation of CD95/CD95 ligand-apoptotic pathway in CD3+ large granular lymphocyte leukemia. Blood 92:4771–4777, 1998.

33. N Itoh, M Yonehara, S Mizushima, M Samashima, A Hase, Y Seto, S Nagata. The polypeptide encoded by cDNA for human cell surface antigen Fas can mediate apoptosis. Cell 66: 233–243, 1991.

34. S Nagata. Apoptosis by death factor. Cell 88:355, 1997.

35. LJ Levitt, GR Reyes, DK Moonka, K Besch, RA Miller, EG Engleman. Human T cell leuke- mia virus-I-associated T-suppressor cell inhibition of erythropoiesis in a patient with pure rd cell aplasia and cronic T-gamma lymphoproliferative disease. J Clin Invest 81:538–548, 1988.

36. K Oshimi. Granular lymphocyte proliferative disorders: Report of 12 cases and review of the literature. Leukemia 2:617–627, 1988.

37. K Oshimi, S Hoshino, M Takahashi, M Akahoshi, H Satio, Y Kobayashi, H Hirai, F Takaku, N Yahagi, Y Oshimi, Y Horie, H Mizoguchi. Ti(WT31)-negative, CD3− positive, large granular lymphocyte leukemia with nonspecific cytotoxicity. Blood 71:923–931, 1988.

38. T Motoji, O Yamada, M Takahashi, K Oshimi, H Mizogushi. A case of granular lymphocyte leukemia with pure red cell aplasia. The usefulness of gene analysis in assessing therapeutic effect. Am J Hematol 39:212–219, 1992.

39. R Bassan, M Pronesti, M Buzzetti, P Allavena, A Rambaldi, A Mantovani, T Barbui. Autoim- munity and B-cell dysfunction in chronic proliferative disorders of large granular lympocyte/ natural killer cells. Cancer 63:90–95, 1989.

40. TP Jr Loughran, G Starkebaum, FW Ruscetti. Similar rearrangements of T cell receptor beta gene in cell lines and uncultured cells from patients with large granular lymphocyte leukemia. Blood 72:613–615, 1988.

41. TP Jr Loughran, JA Aprile, FW Ruscetti. Anti-CD3 monoclonal antibody-mediated cytotox- icity occurs through an interleukin-2 independent pathway in CD3+ large granular lympho- cytes. Blood 75:935–940, 1990.

42. V Pistoia, AJ Carroll, EF Prasthofer, AB Tilden, KS Zuckerman, M Ferrarini, CE Grossi. Establishment of Tac-negative, interleukin-2-dependent cytotoxic cell lines from large granu- lar lymphocytes (LGL) of patients with expanded LGL populations. J Clin Immunol 6:457– 466, 1986.

43. L Foroni, E Matutes, J Foldi, R Morilla, TH Rabbitts, L Luzzatto, D Catovsky. T-cell leuke- mias with rearrangement of the gamma but not beta T-cell receptor genes. Blood 71:356– 362, 1988.

44. R Zambello, M Facco, L Trentin, MA Cassatella, R Raimondir, A Cerutti, C Enthammer, M Facco, C Agosti, G Semenzato. IL-12 involved in the activation of CD3+ granular lym- phocytes in patients with lymphoproliferative disease of granular lymphocytes. Br J Haematol 92:308–314, 1996.

45. AJ Aprile, M Russo, MS Pepe, TP Jr Loughran. Activation signals leading to proliferation of normal and leukemic CD3+ large granular lymphocytes. Blood 78:1282–1285, 1991.

46. G Starkebaum, TP Jr Loughran, VS Kalyanaraman, ME Kadin, PG Kidd, JW Singer, FW Ruscetti. Serum reactivity to Human T-cell leukemia/lymphoma virus type I proteins in pa- tients with large granular lymphocyte leukemia. Lancet 1:596–599, 1987.

47. N Imamura, A Kuramoto, K Kawa-Ha, H Fujii, T Takiguchi. Negative association between the human T-cell leukaemia virus type 1 and a large granular lymphocyte leukaemia in Japan. Lancet 2:962, 1988.

48. TP Jr Loughran, T Coyle, MP Sherman, G Starkebaum, GD Ehrlich, FW Ruscetti, BJ Poiesz. Detection of human T-cell leukemia/lymphoma virus, type II in a patient with LGL leukemia. Blood 80:1116–1119, 1992.

49. TP Jr Loughran, KG Hadlock, R Perzova, TC Gentile, Q Yang, SK Foung, BJ Poiesz. Epitope mapping of HTLV envelope seroreactivity in LGL Leukemia. Br J Haematol 101:318–324, 1998.

50. F Le Deist, G De Saint Basile, J Coulombel, Breton-Gorius, M Maier-Redelsperger, K Belj- orde, C Bremard, C Griscelli. A familial occurrence of natural killer cell-T-lymphocyte pro- liferation disease in two children. Cancer 67:2610–2617, 1991.

51. R Sood, CC Stewart, PD Aplan, H Murai, P Ward, M Barco, MR Baer. Neutropenia associ- ated with T-cell large granular lymphocyte leukemia: Long-term response to cyclosporin therapy despite persistence of abnormal cells. Blood 91:3372–3378, 1998.

52. C Thomassen, C Nissen, A Gratwohl, A Tichelli, A Stern. Agranulocytosis associated with T-gamma-lymphocytosis: No improvement of peripheral blood granulocyte count with human-recombinant granulocyte-macrophage colony-stimulating factor (GM-CSF). Br J Haematol 71:157–158, 1989.

53. R Gonzalez-Chambers, C Rosefeld, A Winkelstein, L Dameshek. Eosinophilia resulting from administration of recombinant granulocyte-macrophage colony-stimulating factor (rhGM-CSF) in a patient with T-gamma-lymphoproliferative disease: Am J Hematol 36:157–159, 1991.

54. T Kaneko, Y Ogawa, Y Hirata, S Hoshino, M Takahashi, K Oshimi, H Mizogichi. Agranulocytosis associated with granular lymphocyte leukaemia. Improvement of peripheral blood granulocytes colony-stimulating factor (G-CSF). Br J Haematol 74:121–122, 1990.

55. DF Lang, CS Rosenfeld, HS Diamond, RK Shadduck, ZR Zeigler. Successful treatment of T-gamma-lymphoproliferative disease with human-recombinant granulocyte colony stimulating factor. Am J Hematol 40:66–68, 1992.

56. B Freimark, L Lanier, J Phillips, T Quertermous, R Fox. Comparison of T-cell Receptor gene rearrangements in patients with large granular and Felty's syndrome. J Immunol 138:1724–1729, 1987.

57. H Vie, S Chavalier, R Garand, J-P Moisan, V Praloran, M-C Devilder, JF Moreau, J-P Souillou. Clonal expansion of lymphocytes bearing the T-cell receptor in a patient with large granular lymphocyte disorder. Blood 74:285–290, 1989.

58. TP Jr Loughran, G Starkebaum, E Clark, P Wallace, ME Kadin. Evaluation of splenomegaly in large granular lymphocyte leukemia. Br J Haematol 67:135–140, 1987.

59. M Masuda, Y Arai, H Nishina, S Fuchinoue, H Mizoguchi. Large granular lymphocyte leukemia with pure red cell aplasia in a renal transplant recipient. Am J Hematol 57:72–76, 1998.

60. LA Fernandez, B Pope, C Lee, E Zayed. Aggressive natural killer cell leukemia in an adult with establishment of a NK cell line. Blood 67:925–930, 1986.

61. DNJ Hart, BW Baker, MJ Inglis, JC Nimmo, GC Starling, E Deacon, M Rome, MEJ Beard. Epstein-Barr viral DNA in acute large granular lymphocyte (natural killer) leukemic cells. Blood 79:2116–2123, 1992.

62. S Koizumi, H Seki, T Tachinami, M Taniguchi, A Matsuda, K Taga, T Nakarai, E Kato, N Taniguchi, H Nakamura. Malignant clonal expansion of large granular lymphocytes with a Leu-11+, Leu-7-surface phenotype: In vitro responsiveness of malignant cells to recombinant human interleukin 2. Blood 68:1065–1073, 1986.

63. T Ohno, T Kanoh, Y Arita, H Fujii, K Kuribayashi, T Masuda, Y Horiguchi, M Taniwaki, T Nosaka, M Hatanaka, H Uchino. Fulminant clonal expansion of large granular lymphocytes. Characterization of their morphology, phenotype, and function. Cancer 62:1918–1927, 1988.

64. Y Ohno, R Amakawa, S Fukuhara, C-R Huang, H Kamesaki, H Amano, T Imanaka, Y Takahashi, Y Arita, T Uchiyama, K Kita, H Miwa. Acute transformation of chronic large granular lymphocyte leukemia associated with additional chromosome abnormality Cancer 64:63–67, 1989.

65. W Sheridan, EF Winton, WC Chan, DS Gordon, WR Vogler, C Phillips, KF Bongiovanni, TA Waldmann. Leukemia of non-T lineage natural killer cells. Blood 72:1701–1707, 1988.

66. M Taniwaki, S Tagawa, H Nishigaki, S Horiike, S Misawa, C Shimazaki, T Maekawa, H Fujii, T Kitani, T Abe. Chromosomal abnormalities define clonal proliferation in CD3– large granular lymphocyte leukemia. Am J Hematol 33:32–38, 1990.

67. EF Prasthofer, JC Barton, D Zarcone, CE Grossi. Ultrastructural morphology of granular lymphocyte (GL) from patients with immunophenotypically homogeneous expansions of GL population (GLE). J Submicrosc Cytol 19:345–354, 1987.

68. HA K Kawa, S Ishihara, T Ninomiya, K Yamura-Yagi, J Hara, F Murayama, A Tawa, K Hirai. CD3-negative lymphoproliferative disease of granular lymphocytes containing Epstein-Barr viral DNA. J Clin Invest 84:51–55, 1992.

69. I Miyoshi, I Kubonishi, S Yoshimoto, T Akagi, Y Ohtsuki, Y Shiraishi, K Nagata, Y Hinuma.

Type C virus particles in a cord T-cell line derived by co-cultivating normal human cord leukocytes and human leukemic T cells. Nature 294:770–771, 1981.

70. BJ Poiesz, FW Ruscetti, AF Gazdar, PA Bunn, JD Minna, RC Gallo. Detection and isolation of type C retrovirus particles from fresh and cultured lymphocytes of a patient with cutaneous T cell lymphoma. Proc Natl Acad Sci USA 77:7415–7419, 1980.

71. Y Himana, K Nagata, M Misaka, M Nakai, T Matsumoto, K Kinoshita, S Shirakawa, I Miyoshi. Adult T cell leukemia. Antigen in an ATL cell line and detection of antibodies to the antigen in human sera. Proc Natl Acad Sci USA 78:6476–6480, 1981.

72. K Takatsuki, ed. Adult T-Cell leukaemia. New York: Oxford University Press, 1994.

73. TC Gentile, TP, Jr. Loughran. Potential role of human T-cell leukemia/lymphoma viruses (HTLV) in diseases other than acute T-cell leuekemia/lymphoma (ATL). In: KE Ugen, M Bendinelli, H Friedman, eds. Human Retroviral Infection. New York: Kluwer Academic/ Plenum Publishers, pp 17–28, 2000.

74. M Shimoyama, Members of The Lymphoma Study Group (1984–87). Diagnostic criteria and classification of clinical subtypes of adult T-cell leukemia-lymphoma. Br J Haematol 79:428–437, 1991.

75. F Kawano, K Yamaguchi, H Nishimura, H Tsuda, K Takatsuk. Variation in the clinical courses of adult T-cell leukemia. Cancer 55:851–856, 1985.

76. K Yamaguchi, H Nishimura, H Kohrogi, M Jono, Y Miyamoto, K Takatsuki. A proposal for smoldering adult T-cell leukemia: A clinicopathologic study of five cases. Blood 62:758–766, 1983.

77. K Shirono, T Hattori, K Takatsuki. A new classification of clinical stages of adult T-cell leukemia based on prognosis of the disease. Leukemia 8:1834–1837, 1994.

78. N Kamada, M Sakurai, K Miyamoto, I Sanada, N Sadamori, S Fukuhara, S Abe, Y Shiraishi, T Abe, Y Kaneko, M Shimoyama. Chromosome Abnormalities in adult T-cell leukemia/ lymphoma: A Karyotype Review Committee Report. Cancer Res 52:1481–1493, 1992.

79. K Matsushita, T Matsumoto, H Ohtsubo, H Fujiwara, N Imamura, S Hidaka, T Kukita, C Tei, M Matsumoto, N Arima. Long-term maintenance combination chemotherapy with OPEC/MPEC (vincristine or methotrexate, prednisolone, Etoposite and cyclophosphamide) or with daily daily oral Etoposite and prednisolone can improve survival and quality of life in adult T-cell leukemia/lymphoma. Leuk Lymphoma 36:67–75, 1999.

80. J Dierov, BE Sawaya, M Prosniak, RB Gartenhaus. Retinoic acid modulates a bimodal effect on the cell cycle progression in human adult T-cell leukemia cells. Clin Cancer Res 5:2540–2547, 1999.

81. K Obama, M Tara, H Sao, H Taji, Y Morishima, H Mougi, Y Maruyama, M Osame. Allogenic bone marrow transplantation as a treatment for adult T-cell leukemia. Int J Hematol 69: 203–205, 1999.

82. K Ikeda, M Oka, Y Yamada, H Soda, M Fukuda, A Kinohira, K Tsukamoto, Y Noguchi, H Isomoto, F Takesshima, K Murase, S Kamihira, M Tomonaga, S Kohno. Adult T-cell leukemia cell over-express the multidrug-resistance-protein (MRP) and lung-resistance-protein genes. Int J Cancer 82:599–604, 1999.

83. EF Chan, YG Dowdy, B Lee, WG McKenna, KR Fox, RJ Levy, MA Wasik, AH Rook. A novel chemotherapeutic regimen (interferon alfa, zidovudine, and etretinate) for adult T-cell lymphoma resulting in rapid tumor destruction. J Am Acad Dermatol 40:116–121, 1999.

84. A Bazarbachi, ME El-Sabban, R Nasr, F Quignon, C Awarajil, J Kersual, L Dianooux, Y Zermati, JH Haidar, O Hermine, H de The. Arsenic trioxide and interferon-alpha synergize to induce cell cycle arrest and apoptosis in human T-cell lymphotropic virus type I-transformed cells. Blood 93:278–283, 1999.

85. N Uike, I Choi, A Tokoro, T Goto, Y Yufu, M Kozuru, K Tobini. Adult T-cell leukemia-lymphoma successfully treated with 2-chlorodeoxyadenosine. Int Med 37:411–413, 1998.

86. H Rappaport, LB Thomas. Mycosis fungoides. The pathology of extracutaneous involvement. Cancer 34:1198–1229, 1974.

87. MA Lutzner, RL Edelson, P Schien, I Green, C Kirkpatrick, A Ahmed. Cutaneous T cell lymphomas. The Sezary syndrome, mycosis fungoides, and related disorders. Ann Intern Med 83:534–552, 1975.

88. R Willemze, H Kerl, W Sterry, E Berti, L Cerroni, S Chimenti, JL Diaz-Perez, ML Geerts, M Goos, R Knobler, E Ralfkiaer, M Snatucci, N Smith, J Wechsler, WA Van Vloten, CJL Meijer. EORTC classification of primary cutaneous lymphomas. A proposal from the cutaneous lymphoma study group of the European organization for research and treatment of cancer. Blood 90:354–371, 1997.

89. M Weinstock, J Horm. Mycosis fungoides in the United States: Increasing incidence and descriptive epidemiology. JAMA 260:42–46, 1988.

90. RSH Tan, CM Butterworth, H McLaughlin, S Malka, PD Samman. Mycosis fungoides: A disease of antigen persistence. Br J Dermatol 91:607–616, 1974.

91. MH Green, NA Dalager, SI Lamberg, CE Argyropoulos, JF Jr Fraumeni. Mycosis funoides. Epidemiologic observations. Cancer Treat Rep 63:597–606, 1979.

92. AB Fischman, PA Jr Bunn, JG Guccion, MJ Mathews, JD Minna. Exposure to chemicals, physical agents and biologic agents in mycosis fungoides and the Sezary syndrome. Cancer Treat Rep 63:591–596, 1979.

93. SR Cohen, SS Kurt, IM Braverman, GJ Beck. Mycosis fungoides: Clinicopathologic relationships, survival and therapy in 59 patients with observations on occupation as a new prognostic factor. Cancer 46:2654–2666, 1980.

94. E Tyup, A Burgoyne, T Aichitson, R Mackie. A case-control study of possible causatve factors in mycosis fungoides. Arch Dermatol 123:196–200, 1987.

95. BJ Poiesz, FW Ruscetti, AF Gazdar, PA Bunn, JD Minna, RC Gallo. Detection and isolation of type c retrovirus particles from fresh and cultures lymphocytes of a patient with cutaneous T-cell lymphoma. Proc Natl Acad Sci USA 77:7415–7419, 1980.

96. D Zucker-Franklin, BA Pancake. The role of human T-cell lymphotropic viruses (HTLV-I and II) in cutaneous T-cell lymphomas. Semin Dermatol 13:160–165, 1994.

97. R Hoppe, G Wood, EA Abel. Mycosis fungoides and Sezary syndrome: Pathology, staging and treatment. Curr Probl Cancer 14:295–371, 1990.

98. GS Woods, LM Weis, RA Warnke, J Sklar. The immunopathology of of cutaneous lymphomas: Immunophenotypic and immunogenotypic characteristics. Semin Dermatol 5:334–345, 1986.

99. SA Michie, EA Abel, RT Hoppe, RA Warnke, GS Woods. Expression of T-cell receptor antigens in mycosis fungoides and inflammatory skin lesions. J Invest Dermatol 93:116–120, 1989.

100. BA Agnarsson, EC Vonderheid, ME Kadin. Cutaneous T-cell lymphoma with suppressor/cytotoxic (CD8) phenotype: Identification of rapidly progressive and chronic subtypes. J Am Dermatol 22:569–577, 1990.

101. LM Weiss, E Hu, GS Wood, C Moulds, ML Cleary, R Warnke, J Skar. Clonal rearrangement of T-cell receptor genes in mycosis fungoides and dermatopathic lymphadenopathy. N Engl J Med 313:539–544, 1985.

102. M Ashton-Key, M Du, N Kirkmaham, A Wotherspoon, PG Isaacson. The value of the polymerase chain reaction in the diagnosis of cutaneous T-cell infiltrates. Am J Surg Pathol 21: 743–747, 1997.

103. PJ Bunn, S Lambert. Report of the Committee on Staging and Classification of Cutaneous T-cell Lymphomas. Cancer Treat Rep 63:725–728, 1979.

104. H Youn, Y Kim, RT Hoppe. Mycosis fungoides and Sezary syndrome. Semin Oncol 26: 276–289, 1999.

105. Y Kim, R Jensen, G Watanabe, A Varghese, RT Hoppe. Clinical stage IA (limited patch and plaque) Mycosis fungoides. Arch Dermatol 132:1309–1313, 1996.

106. Y Kim, S Chow, A Varghese, RT Hoppe. Clinical characteristics and long-term outcome of

patients with generalized patch and/or plaque (T2) mycosis fungoides. Arch Dermatol 135: 26–32, 1999.

107.   E Diamandidou, M Colome-Grimmer, L Fayad, M Duvic, R Kurzrock. Transformation of mycosis fungoides/Sezary syndrome: Clinical characteristics and prognosis. Blood 92:1150–1159, 1998.

108.   JA Parrish, TB Fitzpatrick, L Tanenbaum, MA Pathak. Phototherapy of psoriasis with oral methoxsalen and long wave ultraviolet light. N Engl J Med 291:1207–1211, 1974.

109.   D Ramsay, P Halperin, A Zeleniuch-Jacquotte. Topical mechlorethamine therapy for early stage mycosis fungoides. J Am Acad Dermatol 19:684–691, 1988.

110.   E Vonderheid, E Tan, AF Kantor, L Sharger, B Micaily, EJ Van Scott. Long-term efficacy curative potential and carcinogenicity of topical mechlorethamine in cutaneous T cell lymphoma. J Am Acad Dermatol 20:416–428, 1989.

111.   EA Abel, E Sendagorta, RT Hoppe. Cutaneous malignancies and metastatic squamous cell carcinoma following topical therapies for mycosis fungoides. J Am Acad Dermatol 14:1006–1013, 1986.

112.   B Smoller, R Marcus. Risk of secondary cutaneous malignancies in patients with long-standing mycosis Fungoides. J Am Acad Dermatol 30:201–204, 1994.

113.   H Zachkeim, E Epstein, W Crain. Topical carmustine (BCNU) for cutaneous T cell lymphoma: A 15-year experience 1n 143. J Am Acad Dermatol 22:802–810, 1990.

114.   S Gottlieb, J Wolfe, F Fox, FE Fox, BJ Denarda, WH Macey, PG Bromley, SR Lessin, AH Rook. Treatment of cutaneous T-cell lymphoma with extracorporeal photopheresis monotherapy and in combination with recombinant interferon alfa: A 10 year experience at a single institution. J Am Acad Dermatol 35:946–957, 1996.

115.   PJ Bunn, S Hoffman, D Norris, LE Golitz, JL Aeling. Systemic therapy of cutaneous T-cell lymphoma (mycosis fungoides and the Sezary syndrome). Ann Intern Med 121:592–602, 1994.

116.   S Rosen, F Foss. Chemotherapy for mycosis fungoides and the Sezary syndrome. Hematol Oncol Clin North Am 9:1109–1116, 1995.

117.   PL Zinzani, M Magagnoli, M Bendandi, GF Orcioni, F Gherlinzoni, P Albertim, SA Pileri, S Tura. Therapy with Gemcitabine in pretreated peripheral T-cell lymphoma patients. Ann Oncol 9:1351–1353, 1998.

118.   R Kurzrock, S Pilat, M Duvic. Pentostatin therapy of T-cell lymphomas with cutaneous manifestations. J Clin Oncol 17:3117–3121, 1999.

119.   TM Kuzel, A Hurria, E Samuelson, MS Tallman, HH Jr., Roenigk, AW Rademaker, ST Rosen. Phase II trial of 2-chlorodeoxyadenosine for the treatment of cutaneous T-cell lymphoma. Blood 87:901–911, 1996.

120.   DL Schappell, JC Alper, CJ McDonald. Treatment of advanced mycosis fungoides and Sezary syndrome with continuous infusions of methotrexate followed by fluorouracil and leucovorin recue. Arch Dermatol 131:307–313, 1995.

121.   A Molina, A Nademanee, DA Arber, SJ Forman. Remission of refractory Sezary syndrome after bone marrow transplantation from a matched unrelated donor. Biol Blood Marrow Transplant 5:400–404, 1999.

122.   S Knox, RT Hoppe, D Maloney, I Gibbs, S Fowler, C Marquez, PJ Cornbleet, R Levy. Treatment of cutaneous T-cell lymphoma with chimeric anti_CD4 monoclonal antibody. Blood 87:893–899, 1996.

123.   NL Harris, ES Jaffe, H Stein, PM Banks, JK Chan, ML Cleary, G Delson, C De Wolf-Peeters, B Falini, KC Gotter. A revised European-American classification of lymphoid neoplasms: a proposal from the International Lymphoma Study Group. Blood 84:1361–1392, 1994.

124.   YL Kwong YL, AC Chan, R Liang, AK Chiang, CS Chim, TK Chan, D Todd, FC Ho. CD56+ NK Lymphomas: clinicopathological features and prognosis. Br J Haemato 97:821–829, 1997.

125. CH. Dunphy. Natural killer cell lymphoma of the small intestine: diagnosis by flow cytometric immunophenotyping of paracentesis. Diagn Cytopathol 20:246–248, 1999.

126. R Liang, F Chen, CK Lee, YL Kwong, CS Chim, CC Yau, E Chiu. Autologous bone marrow transplantation for primary nasal T/NK cell lymphoma. Bone Marrow Transplant 19:91–93, 1997.

127. TC Gentile, AH Uner, RE Hutchinson, TC Wright, J Ben-Ezra, EC Russel, TP Jr. Loughran. CD3+, CD56+ aggressive variant of large granular lymphocyte leukemia. Blood 23:2321, 1994.

128. WR Macon, ME Williams, JP Greer, RD Hammer, AD Glick, RD Collins, JB Cousar. Natural killer-like T cell lymphomas: aggressive lymphomas of T-large granular lymphocytes. Blood 87:1474–1483, 1996.

129. CB Cooke, L Krenacs, M Stetler-Stevenson, TC Greiner, M Raffeld, DW Kingma, L Abruzzo, C Frantz. Hepatosplenic T-cell lymphoma: a distinct clinopathological entity of cytotoxic gamma delta T-cell origin. Blood 88:4265–4274, 1996.

130. M Yamaguchi, T Ohno, H Nakamine, K Oka, F Matsuzuka, H Miwa, H Shiku, N Kimura, K Nanba, K Kita. Gamma delta T-cell lymphoma: a clinicopathologic study of 6 cases including extrahepatosplenic type. Int J Hematol 69:186–195, 1999.

131. WC Lin, JO Moore, KP Mann, ST Traweek, C Smith. Post transplant CD8+ gamma delta T-cell lymphoma associated with human herpes virus-6 infection. Leuk Lymphoma 33:377–384, 1999.

132. B Arnulf, C Copie-Bergman, MH Delfau-Largue, A Lavergne-Slove, J Bosq, J Wechsler, M Wassef, C Matuchansky, B Epardeau, M Stern, M Bagot, F Reyes, P Gaulard. Nonhepatosplenic gammadelta T-cell lymphoma: a subset of cytotoxic lymphomas with mucosal or skin localization. Blood 91:1723–1731, 1998.

133. A Zarate-Osorno, M Raffeld, EL Berman, MM Ferguson, R Andrade, ES Jaffe. S-100 Positive T-cell lymphoproliferative disorder: a case report and review of the literature. Am J Clin Pathol 102:478–480, 1994.

26

Current Concepts in the Management of Hairy Cell Leukemia

MARTIN S. TALLMAN

Northwestern University Medical School, and Robert H. Lurie Comprehensive Cancer Center, Chicago, Illinois

MARK A. HOFFMAN

Long Island Jewish Medical Center, New Hyde Park, New York

LOANN C. PETERSON

Northwestern University Medical School, Chicago, Illinois

Hairy cell leukemia (HCL) is an uncommon chronic B-cell lymphoproliferative disorder that has become one of the most effectively treated hematological malignancies. Remarkable progress has been made in the treatment of patients with this disease since the clinical development of the purine analogs 2′-deoxycoformycin (2′-DCF) and 2-chlorodeoxyadenosine (2-CdA). These agents either inhibit or resist the action of the enzyme adenosine deaminase (ADA), which mediates the degradation of deoxyadenosine. Lymphocytes are abundant in deoxyadenosine, and the accumulation of deoxyadenosine is toxic to lymphocytes and results in lymphopenia, analogous to the lack of lymphocyte development in ADA-deficient children with severe combined immunodeficiency syndrome. Remarkably, equally high rates of durable complete remission (CR) are achieved in both untreated and previously treated patients, a phenomenon not typically observed in the treatment of malignant disease with cytotoxic chemotherapy. Furthermore, patients with large tumor burdens, identified by marked infiltration of the bone marrow and massive splenomegaly, have as favorable an outcome as those with minimal disease. Therefore, these agents are now the treatments of choice for all patients with HCL and have supplanted earlier approaches such as splenectomy and interferon-α. Because a single 7-day cycle of 2-CdA induces a high rate of durable CR and is associated with few toxicities other than culture-negative fever, this agent is particularly attractive. However, it is not known if one purine analog offers a survival advantage over the other. Long-term follow-up will be necessary to identify such an advantage given the indolent natural history of the disease.

I. INTRODUCTION

Hairy cell leukemia is an uncommon chronic B-cell lymphoproliferative disorder first reported by Ewald in 1923 as leukemic reticuloendotheliosis (1), but described as a distinct clinical entity by Bouroncle and colleagues in 1958 (2). The disease occurs most frequently in middle-aged men and is characterized by splenomegaly, pancytopenia, and infiltration of the bone marrow with lymphocytes that have irregular cytoplasmic projections (3–7). Immunoglobulin gene rearrangement studies have confirmed that HCL is a clonal B-cell malignancy (8–10). Most patients have an indolent course (5,6). However, eventually many patients have life-threatening pancytopenia, symptomatic splenomegaly, or constitutional symptoms develop, which necessitate treatment.

The treatment of HCL has undergone major evolution since the first reports of the success of splenectomy (11–20), to the purine analogs 2'-deoxycoformycin (2'-DCF) (21–43) and 2-chlorodeoxyadenosine (2-CdA) (44–56). These agents have become the treatments of choice, because most patients with both previously treated and untreated disease achieve durable CR with either drug. The activity of interferon-α was first reported in patients with HCL by Quesada et al. in 1984 (57), and although a high overall response rate is achieved, most responses are partial and patients eventually relapse when the drug is discontinued (58–76). Currently no role exists for interferon-α in the primary treatment of HCL except possibly in the unusual patient unresponsive to or relapsing after a purine analog. The success of the purine analogs represents one of the triumphs in the treatment of malignant diseases.

II. PATHOLOGY OF HAIRY CELL LEUKEMIA

Cytopenias involving one or more cell lines dominate the peripheral blood findings in patients with HCL. Leukopenia is the most common and is characterized by both an absolute neutropenia and monocytopenia. Hairy cells can be identified on Wright's-stained peripheral blood smears from most patients, although they may be rare and found only after a prolonged search. The cells are about one to two times the size of a small lymphocyte (Figure 1, see color plate [Fig. 26.1]). They are usually round, oval, or indented but may be monocytoid or convoluted. Their nuclei are positioned in a central or eccentric location. The chromatin pattern is reticular or netlike in appearance, and nucleoli are indistinct or absent. The cytoplasm is moderate to abundant in amount and pale blue-gray in color with cytoplasmic borders that are irregular with fine ruffles or hairlike projections. These hairy projections are more readily evident on ultrastructural examination (77) and/or scanning electron microscopy, although the latter is not routinely carried out (78).

Examination of the bone marrow (BM) trephine biopsy is essential in establishing the diagnosis of HCL (79–83). The bone marrow is often inaspirable because of extensive reticulin fibrosis. When aspirable, hairy cells are often observed in the smear. The BM is hypercellular in most patients, and hairy cell infiltration may be diffuse, focal, or interstitial (Figure 2, see color plate [Fig. 26.2]). In patients with diffuse involvement, replacement of large areas of the BM may completely efface the normal bone marrow. When the BM is focally involved, the infiltrates are not clearly demarcated but rather subtle and patchy, and the hairy cells merge with the surrounding hematopoietic tissue. The hairy cell nuclei are widely separated from each other by abundant, clear, or lightly eosinophilic cytoplasm. In occasional cases the hairy cell nuclei are elongated, giving a spindle cell appearance. Mitoses are inconspicuous. Mast cells may be numerous. Extravasated red cells are frequently seen and blood lakes, similar to those observed in the spleen, may also be present. The extent of involvement of the BM by HCL may be difficult to appreciate in routinely stained sections and is usually more apparent when examined by immunohistochemistry with antibodies to B-cell–associated antigens such as CD20 or DBA.44 (Figure 3, see color plate [Fig. 26.3]). Approximately 10% to 20% of patients have a hypocellular BM. Occasionally, the hypocellularity may be profound with small numbers of hairy cells infiltrating around fat cells (79–85). Reticulin stains of the BM trephine biopsy usually document moderate to marked increase in reticulin fibers. In some cases, the reticulin fibers appear to surround individual hairy cells, with the fibrosis extending into the adjacent, more normal-appearing BM tissue.

Demonstration of tartrate-resistant acid phosphatase (TRAP) activity has been used to confirm the diagnosis of HCL (86). Cells positive for TRAP are found in almost all cases at diagnosis. The TRAP reaction can be performed on peripheral blood films, marrow aspirate smear, or touch preparations of BM. Although TRAP positivity is not specific for HCL, a positive TRAP stain together with a morphologically characteristic BM biopsy is essentially diagnostic of HCL. Immunophenotyping of the malignant cells by flow cytometry is now common and has become the standard method for confirming the diagnosis.

III. IMMUNOPHENOTYPIC FINDINGS

Hairy cells exhibit a mature B-cell phenotype and express strong monoclonal surface immunoglobulin and pan-B-cell antigens, including CD19, CD20, and CD22, and lack CD5 expression (87). Hairy cells also strongly express CD11c, a marker associated with myelomonocytic cells, CD103, an antigen also present on mucosal-associated T-cells and some activated B lymphocytes, and CD25, the interleukin-2 receptor (87–89). The interleukin-2 receptor undergoes cleavage, and the soluble IL-2 receptors circulate in the peripheral blood. Detection of high levels is typical for HCL as opposed to other lymphoproliferative disorders, which may mimic HCL (89).

Antibodies against B-cell–associated antigen, including L26(anti-CD20) and DBA.44, react with hairy cells in fixed, routinely processed tissue sections. These antibodies are not specific for HCL; however, immunohistochemical studies that use the antibodies can document the proliferation of B-cells and highlight the extent of BM infiltration by hairy cells at the time of diagnosis and after therapy (90–95).

IV. MOLECULAR FINDINGS

Two preliminary reports suggest that overexpression of cyclin D1, involved in cell cycle regulation, may be involved in the pathogenesis of HCL (96,97). In one study, cyclin D1 was overexpressed, but without evidence of the 11q13 chromosomal abnormality, the location to which the BCI-1 gene encoding cyclin D1 has been mapped (96).

V. DIFFERENTIAL DIAGNOSIS

The differential diagnosis of HCL includes other small B-cell lymphoproliferative disorders associated with splenomegaly (98), such as prolymphocytic leukemia (99–101), splenic marginal zone B-cell lymphoma (splenic lymphoma with villous lymphocytes) (102–105), and HCL variant (106–110). Patients with B-cell prolymphocytic leukemia characteristically have splenomegaly, but this disorder can usually be distinguished from HCL by the marked lymphocytosis, the morphology of the prolymphocytes, and differences in immunophenotypic profile, including negativity for CD11c and CD103. Splenic marginal zone lymphoma shares some clinical and morphological features with HCL; however, in contrast, the cells usually do not exhibit strong TRAP positivity, and the BM infiltrates, when found, are sharply demarcated and frequently intrasinusoidal (111). The immunophenotype profile differs from HCL in that the cells are usually negative for CD103 and CD25 (102). HCL variant exhibits morphological features intermediate between hairy cells and prolymphocytes and is associated with prominent leukocytosis, lack of monocytopenia, and expression of the interleukin-2 receptor β chain, but not the α chain (CD25) (112). Systemic mast-cell disease may resemble HCL in the trephine biopsy sections. However, immunohistochemical studies show that the mast cells, unlike hairy cells, are negative for B-cell–associated antigen and positive for lysozyme and tryptase (113).

VI. TREATMENT

A. Indications

Patients are often asymptomatic at diagnosis and can be observed for many months or years before treatment is required. There is no clear benefit to early treatment. It is routine practice to initiate therapy when the patient has one or more of the following develop: significant cytopenias; symptomatic splenomegaly or adenopathy; repeated infections; or constitutional symptoms such as fever, night sweats, or fatigue. Typical peripheral blood counts that warrant treatment include an absolute neutrophil count of $<1000/\mu L$, a hemoglobin <11.0 g/dl, or a platelet count $<100,000/\mu L$.

B. Role of Splenectomy

Splenectomy was the first effective therapy for HCL (11–20). Although splenectomy does not induce remission in the BM, the peripheral blood counts return to normal in approximately 40% to 70% of patients, particularly in patients with a low hairy cell index (12). Coad and colleagues reported that among 22 patients hematological CR and PR was achieved in 86% of patients (19). Furthermore, the four patients achieving hematological CR have not required additional treatment after a lead follow-up time of 16 years from splenectomy. This response was maintained for a median of 25 months with an overall survival (OS) at 5 years as approximately 60% to 100% (16,19). The mechanism(s) by which splenectomy improves the peripheral blood counts is not completely understood. Splenectomy likely relieves hypersplenism, because blood cells pool in the spleen, and spleens are usually enlarged in patients with HCL. However, this procedure may also remove a source of cytokine production with consequent influence on the marrow microenvironment. Currently, there is no role for splenectomy as initial therapy except in the very rare instance of splenic rupture (114,115). Anecdotal reports suggest that splenectomy may be useful if symptomatic splenomegaly and pancytopenia persist after interferon or purine analog therapy (116,117).

C. Cytotoxic Chemotherapy

Various single chemotherapeutic agents or combination chemotherapy regimens had been used with some success in patients in whom splenectomy failed before the clinical development of interferon-α or purine analogs (118–121). However, historically, infectious complications have limited this approach. Given the success with purine analogs, there is no role for chemotherapy in the treatment of HCL.

1. Interferon-α

(a) Mechanism(s) of Action

Quesada and colleagues reported interferon-α (IFN-α) to be an effective therapy in patients with HCL in 1984 (57), and since then, numerous studies have confirmed its activity (58–76). The precise mechanism of action of IFN-α is not known. Hairy cell leukemia may involve a deficiency in the production of cytokines such as granulocyte colony-stimulating factor, granulocyte-macrophage colony-stimulating factor, interleukin-3 (IL-3), interleukin-6 (IL-6), and tumor necrosis factor, perhaps related to the characteristic monocytopenia (122). IFN-α increases intracellular IL-6 in HCL and induces secretion of IL-6 from peripheral blood mononuclear cells from HCL patients, but not healthy donors. Interferon induces natural killer cell activity, expression of HLA class II antigens, integrin expression on hairy cells, and tumor necrosis factor-alpha (TNF-α) secretion by hairy cells (61,123–125). Therefore, the benefits of IFN-α may result in part from the induction of hematopoietic growth factors within the leukemic cell population. An alternative hypothesis suggests induction of differentiation such that the hairy cells are less responsive to the influence of growth factors (126).

(b) Clinical Results

Although purine analogs have replaced IFN-α as initial treatment, some historical perspective regarding the benefits of IFN-α is important. Despite a high overall response rate of 75% to 90%, most patients treated with IFN-α achieve only partial remission (defined as normalization of all peripheral blood counts) (58–76). Only approximately 4% of patients achieve CR (defined as normalization of the peripheral blood counts and achieving a normocellular bone marrow with less than 5% hairy cells). Interferon-α is commonly administered at a dose of 2×10^6 IU/m^2 subcutaneously three times a week for 12 to 18 months. During the first 2 months of treatment, the white blood cell count and hemoglobin often decrease. The platelets normalize first, followed by the hemoglobin and the white blood cell count. The absolute neutrophil count rises to greater than 1500/μL after a median of 5 months of therapy. Common toxicities include flulike symptoms, anorexia and fatigue, nausea and vomiting, diarrhea, dry skin, peripheral neuropathies, and central nervous system dysfunction including depression or memory loss. Elevated hepatic transaminase is the most common laboratory abnormality other than myelosuppression. The median failure-free survival after discontinuing IFN-α ranges from 6 to 25 months in different series (73–76). Patients with greater than 30% hairy cells in the BM or a platelet count of less than 160,000/μL at the end of treatment have a higher risk of early relapse. One report suggests that patients can be maintained on long-term IFN-α, although the benefits are not clear. After an induction at a dose of 3×10^6 IU subcutaneously given three times a week, investigators in France gave maintenance therapy at a dose of 1×10^6 IV three times a week to responders or no maintenance (20). Only 13% stopped therapy because of progressive disease. None of the patients receiving maintenance therapy relapsed after a follow-up of 2 to 65 months compared with 37 of 56 patients not receiving maintenance for a median of 33 months (18–74). Maintenance human lymphoblastoid interferon at a dose of 3×10^6 IV per week improved failure-free survival in another randomized trial (127).

Therefore, treatment of HCL with IFN-α is effective, resulting in normalization of the peripheral blood counts in most patients. However, CR in the bone marrow is uncommon. In addition, residual disease can be demonstrated in splenic tissue after splenectomy in apparent complete responders (116). Although IFN-α is no longer administered as primary therapy, it may play a role in the therapeutic strategy for patients who have purine analogs fail (128).

2. Purine Analogs

(a) 2'-Deoxycoformycin

Mechanism(s) of action. 2'-Deoxycoformycin (2'-DCF) was the first treatment to induce a high-rate of CR in HCL (22–43). Almost 30 years ago it was recognized that inherited deficiency of the enzyme ADA was associated with severe combined immunodeficiency in children, manifested by lymphopenia and repeated infections (129,130). The lymphopenia was attributed to the accumulation of deoxynucleotide triphosphate (131, 132). 2'-Deoxycoformycin is an irreversible inhibitor of ADA, the enzyme found in all lymphoid cells critical to purine metabolism. Deoxyadenosine triphosphate metabolites accumulate and are thought to be responsible for cytotoxicity in HCL.

Clinical results. It was logical to attempt to deliberately inhibit ADA to induce lymphopenia in patients with malignant lymphoproliferative disease. Early trials were conducted in patients with leukemia (133,134). Although cytotoxicity was seen, systemic toxicity was severe. Grever and colleagues paved the way for further studies in 1981 by demonstrating that the maximal tolerated dose was less than that required to inhibit ADA (135).

A number of studies have been reported in which 2'-DCF has been administered in a variety of different doses and schedules (Table 1). Spiers and colleagues initially reported remarkable activity of 2'-DCF in two patients (21). Subsequently, Kraut and colleagues at Ohio State University reported CR in 9 of 10 patients with a lower dose of pentostatin (4 mg/m² every 2–4 weeks) (23). Spiers and coinvestigators from the Eastern Cooperative Oncology Group (ECOG) subsequently reported a CR rate of 59% and a PR rate of 37% among 27 patients (24). In this trial, 2'-DCF was given at a dose of 5 mg/m² on 2 consecutive days every 2 weeks until maximum response. In an expanded ECOG study, 50 patients with HCL were treated with the same dose and schedule (32). The overall response rate was 84%, and CR was achieved in 64% of patients. Most patients achieved maximal response within 6 months. Toxicities included nausea, vomiting, skin rash, and conjunctivitis, as well as significant neurological toxicities in four patients. Neutropenia was "life-threatening" in 70% of patients; however, this was limited to the first two to three cycles of therapy. Mortality was attributable to infection in 6% of patients. Grever and colleagues subsequently reported that a lower dose of 2'-DCF (4 mg/m²) was potentially less toxic and equally effective, because both normal and malignant lymphocytes have low levels of ADA activity, and low doses of 2'-DCF are sufficient to inhibit the enzyme (28).

Table 1 Activity of 2′-Deoxycoformycin in Hairy Cell Leukemia

Reference	No. of pts.	Prior therapy	Response (%)		
			Complete	Partial	None
Johnston (26)	28	18	25 (89)	3 (11)	0
Ho (27)	33	30	11 (33)	15 (45)	4 (13)
Kraut (28)	23	13	20 (87)	1 (04)	2 (9)
Grem (29)	66	66	37 (56)	15 (23)	10 (15)
Blick (31)	10	10	10 (91)	1 (09)	0
Cassileth (32)	50	31	32 (64)	10 (20)	8 (16)
Catovsky (33)	148	23	110 (74)	33 (22)	5 (3)
Golomb (34)	85	85	36 (42)	35 (42)	14 (15)
Grever (38)	154	0	117 (76)	4 (3)	0
Seymour (41)	15	15	14 (93)	0	1 (17)
Ribeiro (42)	49	31	22 (44)	26 (52)	2 (4)
Rafel (43)	80	43	56 (72)	13 (16)	1 (1)

Other investigators have administered a lower dose of 2′-DCF (usually 4 mg/m^2 every 2 weeks) and generally have produced similar results with less toxicity (26,28, 31,33,38,41–43). In one study sponsored by the National Cancer Institute of Canada, patients were treated with 2′-DCF at a dose of 4 mg/m^2 IV every 2 weeks, and CR was attained in 20 of 23 patients (87%) (21). In this study, infections were infrequent, and there were no deaths. CD4-positive cells were found to be significantly decreased after treatment. However, this finding was reversible, and no opportunistic infections or second malignancies were noted after 2 years of follow-up. In an additional study, patients were treated with 2′-DCF at a dose of 4 mg/m^2 IV weekly for 3 consecutive weeks, with therapy repeated every 8 weeks (23). Complete remission was achieved in 25 of 28 patients (89%) after completing two cycles of therapy. Transient neutropenia occurred during the first cycle only, and 12 patients had fever and/or infection develop; however, no deaths occurred. In the National Cancer Institute experience of patients treated with 2′-DCF by the special exemption mechanism, the CR rate among patients who had received multiple previous therapies was 56%, and the PR rate was 22% (29). No relapses were observed after a median of 7 months of follow-up. Catovsky and colleagues reported results of a large experience of 148 patients previously treated with splenectomy, IFN-α, or both, given 2′-DCF at what has become a standard dose of 4 mg/m^2 every 2 weeks (33). The CR rate was 76%, and the PR rate was 22%. At 6 years, 76% of patients remain in continuous CR (40).

2′-Deoxycoformycin proved to be a very effective treatment for HCL, inducing a high rate of CR and, therefore, a comparison of IFN-α with the previous standard approach with 2′-DCF was undertaken. A large prospective randomized intergroup study demonstrated that the CR rate and relapse-free survival (approximately 88% at 4 years for patients randomly assigned to 2′-DCF at 4 mg/m^2 IV every 2 weeks compared with 30% for patients randomly assigned to IFN-α, 3.0 × 10^6 U SQ three times a week (2 tailed $p <$ 0.001, log-rank test) were significantly better with 2′-DCF than IFN-α (38). However, no improvement was seen in overall survival with 2′-DCF, in part attributable to the ability to salvage patients failing interferon with the purine analog, because patients not responding to or progressed after the initial assigned treatment were permitted to cross over and receive the other drug.

3. 2′-Deoxycoformycin Plus Interferon-α

Two studies have reported results of the combination of 2′-DCF and IFN-α (136,137). Martin and colleagues treated 15 patients with 2′-DCF at 4 mg/m²/week for 3 weeks followed by IFN-α at 3×10^6 units SQ daily for 4 weeks for a total of 14 months with alternating 28-day cycles (136). In contrast to all other trials of 2′-DCF in HCL, the definition of CR required the absence of HCL in sequential required bilateral bone marrow biopsies 2 months apart. No patients achieved CR with this strict criterion, but all patients achieved PR, and at a median of 27 months of follow-up no patients had progressive disease. Habermann et al. in an ECOG trial administered IFN-α at 3×10^6 units SQ three times a week for 3 months followed by 2′-DCF, 4 mg/m² IV every 2 weeks for a maximum of 12 months (137). The overall response rate was 94% with a CR rate of 70%. Fewer infections occurred in this trial than in the previous ECOG trial (32); however, the dose of 2′-DCF was lower in this trial with sequential treatment. There is no apparent benefit to the combination of 2′-DCF plus IFN-α compared with 2′-DCF alone.

4. 2-Chlorodeoxyadenosine

(a) Mechanism(s) of Action

2-chlorodeoxyadenosine is a purine analog that does not inhibit ADA, as does 2′-deoxycoformycin but is resistant to the enzyme. This agent accumulates in the lymphoid cells presumably because they are rich in the enzyme deoxycytidine kinase (138). This enzyme phosphorylates 2-CdA, creating a deoxynucleotide that cannot readily exit the cell, causing lymphotoxicity analogous to the lack of lymphocyte development in ADA-deficient children (129,130). This results in induction of the DNA strand breaks and depletion of NAD and ATP by poly(ADP) ribosylation of nuclear proteins and apoptosis (138). The DNA strand breaks may result from the inhibition of DNA polymerases and subsequent repair (139,140). The purine analogs appear to kill lymphocytes by both p53-dependent and p53-independent mechanisms (141).

(b) Clinical Results

A summary of studies regarding 2-CdA in HCL is provided in Table 2. 2-CdA was first reported to be effective for HCL by Piro and colleagues in 1990 (44). Twelve patients were treated with a single cycle of 2-CdA at a dose of 0.1 mg/kg/day by continuous infusion for 7 days, and a complete pathological remission was obtained in 11 of the 12 patients within 8 weeks of treatment. None of the patients had relapsed at a median of 15.5 months of follow-up. No patients experienced the usual toxicities of cytotoxic chemotherapy, including nausea, emesis, alopecia, or other constitutional symptoms. Fever was common, generally between days 5 and 7, and coincided with a rapid decline in the number of circulating hairy cells. Remarkably, no infections were documented, and the fever was attributed to cytokine release from hairy cells. In an updated report by the same investigators, 144 patients were treated and 85% achieved a CR (48). Even those patients with residual disease evident by routine light microscopic evaluation had complete normalization of their peripheral blood counts. Estey and colleagues reported similar results in 46 patients with a CR rate of 78% and a PR rate of 11% (45). Febrile episodes occurred in 40% of patients of whom two had pneumonia, one had catheter-related phlebitis, and one

Table 2   Activity of 2-Chlorodeoxyadenosine in Hairy Cell Leukemia

Reference	No. of pts.	Prior therapy	Response (%)		
			Complete	Partial	None
Estey (45)	46	27	36 (78)	5 (11)	5 (11)
Juliusson (46)	16	3	12 (75)	0	4 (25)
Tallman (47)	50	15	40 (80)	19 (20)	0
Piro (48)	144	75	123 (85)	17 (12)	3 (02)
Lauria (50)	37	12	29 (78)	8 (22)	0
Hoffman (51)	49	28	37 (76)	12 (24)	0
Cheson (54)	861	513	431 (50)	318 (37)	111 (13)
Saven (55)	349	176	319 (91)	22 (07)	8 (02)
Bastie (56)	29	14	25 (86)	3 (10)	

had fatal candida sepsis. The only series with a significant number of infectious complications is that by Juliusson and Liliemark (46). In this report, two patients with advanced disease died early of invasive mycosis and another three patients recovered from cytomegalovirus and candidal infections. However, one of these patients had received prior 2′-DCF relatively recently before 2′-CdA, which may have contributed to profound immunosuppression. In an initial study at Northwestern University, 16 (80%) of 20 patients assessable at 3 months achieved CR and 4 (20%) achieved PR with minimal toxicity (47). The most frequent toxicities were myelosuppression and culture-negative fever. Myelosuppression (neutrophils <1000/μL or >50% decreased from a baseline or platelet count <100,000/μL or >50% decrease from baseline) occurred in 66% of patients; however, 63% of these patients were neutropenic before therapy. A temperature >101°F was observed in 48% of patients, most often during the last 2 to 3 days of the 7-day cycle and generally lasted 2 to 10 days. The only infectious complication in this series was a community-acquired pneumonia 2 weeks after treatment in an older patient. Hoffman and colleagues reported that 37 (76%) of 49 patients achieved CR (4). No viral, fungal, or other opportunistic infections were observed other than a single case of dermatomal herpes zoster 16 months after treatment. The largest group of patients treated at a single institution was reported by Saven and colleagues (55). Of 349 evaluable patients, 319 (91%) achieved CR and 22 (7%) achieved PR. The relapse rate was 26% at a median duration of 52 months follow-up. The time-to-treatment failure rate for the 341 responding patients was 19% at 48 months, 10% of CRs and 54% of PRs. In the aggregate experience, the CR rate is approximately 75% to 85%. The largest collection of patients has been reported by Cheson and colleagues, who have provided outcome data on 861 evaluable patients receiving 2-CdA through the Group C Protocol Mechanism from the National Cancer Institute (54). The CR rate of 50% is considerably less, and the PR rate of 37% is higher than in other reports; however, there was no central pathology review, and it is possible that some patients had other indolent lymphoproliferative disorders. The 4-year disease free survival and overall survival were 84% and 86%, respectively.

Fludarabine monophosphate is a third purine analog that is resistant to ADA. Two brief case reports suggest that fludarabine can produce normalization of the peripheral blood counts in previously treated patients with HCL (142,143). Given the success of the other two purine analogs, there appears to be no role for fludarabine in the treatment of HCL.

Table 3 Alternative Doses, Schedules, and Routes of Administration of 2-CdA in HCL

Reference	Dose	Route	Schedule	No. of pts.	Response (%) Complete	Partial	None
Juliusson (146)	3.4 mg/m^2	SQ	Daily × 7 days	73	59 (81)*	11 (15)	3 (4)
Robak (52)	0.1 mg/kg	IV	Over 2 hr each day × 5 days	23	19 (83)	4 (1)	0
Lauria (147)	0.15 m/kg	IV	Weekly × 6 wk	25	19 (76)	6 (24)	0
Chacko (148)	0.15 mg/kg	IV	Weekly × 6 wk	7	7 (100)†	0	0
Juliusson (149)	2 mg/m^2	SQ	Daily × 7 days	8	5 (63)	3 (38)	0

* 5 of 59 patients (75%) achieving CR did so after 1 cycle and 4 required 2 cycles (5%).
† Complete hematologic remission. Three of 7 patients had residual disease by bone marrow immunohistochemistry 6 months after treatment. Three of 6 patients treated with 0.09 μg/kg/day by IV infusion for 7 days also had residual disease detected.

D. Alternative Routes and Schedules

Alternative routes and schedules of administration to the standard 7-day continuous intravenous infusion have included a 5-day 2-hour bolus infusion (52,144), subcutaneous administration (145,146), and oral administration (144,145) (Table 3). The experience with a 2-hour bolus infusion is limited, but preliminary data suggest that the response rate (82%) is similar to that achieved with the standard 7-day continuous infusion schedule (52). Juliusson and coinvestigators have tested subcutaneous injections of 2-CdA at a dose of 3.4 mg/m^2 in 73 patients administered daily for 7 days (146). The CR rate was 81% after either one (55 patients) or two courses (4 patients) of therapy. Pharmacokinetic studies showed that plasma 2-CdA levels were similar to those observed after the intravenous infusion schedule. A weekly schedule of a single 3-hour infusion each week for 6 weeks has been tested in a small number of patients (147,148). All patients achieved CR. Furthermore, no patient had fever develop, and only 14 required red cell transfusions. Juliusson et al. treated eight patients with a low dose of 2 mg/m^2 each day subcutaneously for 7 days and reported a CR rate of 63% and a PR rate of 38% (149). In this report, 38% of patients had febrile neutropenia develop, requiring hospitalization and/or intravenous antibiotics. Whether these alternative schedules of administration are as effective as the conventional 7-day continuous infusion schedule is not yet clear. Further studies comparing these different schedules will be needed.

The concept of administering a single cycle of an antineoplastic agent with the achievement of a higher rate of CR is treatment of malignant disease. It is not known whether additional cycles of 2-CdA for patients with residual disease (either identified on routine morphological evaluation only by immunostains in flow cytometry) is beneficial. Similarly, it is not known whether consolidation with one or more cycles of 2-CdA for patients in CR will decrease the relapse rate.

VII. COMPARISON OF PURINE ANALOGS

Because extremely high CR rates are achievable with 2'-DCF and 2-CdA in HCL and the incidence of toxicity is low, these agents are now the treatment of choice for all patients with both newly diagnosed HCL and those with relapsed disease not previously treated with a purine analog.

There have been no prospective randomized trials comparing 2'-DCF and 2-CdA. Because both purine analogs induce high rates of durable CR, the disease is uncommon and has a long natural history; a long time and extensive resources would be required to detect even large differences. However, the degree of minimal residual disease (MRD), as determined by immunostaining with anti-B-cell monoclonal antibodies, has been compared in a retrospective analysis, and there seems to be no significant difference in the extent of MRD in patients who achieve CR with either agent (150). Dearden and colleagues have reported results of patients treated with either purine analog and suggest that the disease-free interval may be shorter after treatment with 2-CdA (151). However, the groups of patients are not directly comparable, because those receiving 2'-DCF have routinely received more prolonged treatment, and it has been routine to administer several courses after the achievement of CR compared with 2-CdA with which no patients have been treated with more than one cycle as initial therapy.

VIII. IMMUNOSUPPRESSION WITH PURINE ANALOGS

Both 2'-DCF and 2-CdA are associated with prolonged immunosuppression (46,152–154). With 2'-DCF, a decrease in the total lymphocyte count occurs, with a reduction in T cells greater than B cells or NK cells. The levels of CD4+ and CD8+ cells decrease to less than 200 cells/μL for at least 6 months after 2'-DCF treatment is discontinued. In a series of 15 patients treated with 2'-DCF with long follow-up, the median time to recovery of CD4+ lymphocyte counts to normal was 54 months. Treatment with 2-CdA induces similar suppression of CD4+ lymphocyte counts. The median time to recovery of CD4+ lymphocyte counts to normal after 2-CdA was 40 months. Despite such immunosuppression, opportunistic infections, other than an occasional case of herpes zoster, are distinctly uncommon unless purine analog treatment is associated with corticosteroid exposure. Raspadori and colleagues have provided insight into the possible reasons that infections are surprisingly uncommon (155). Although 2-CdA induces profound reduction in CD4+/CD55RA+ T-cells, recovery of another subset, CD4+/Cd45RO+ T-cells, may be protective enough to prevent the development of infections.

IX. BONE MARROW HYPOPLASIA AFTER PURINE ANALOG THERAPY

Another finding of interest in patients who have received 2-CdA is the presence of unexpected foci of hypoplasia and even aplasia in trephine BM biopsies performed as part of evaluation. These foci may be present in patients otherwise in CR with normal peripheral blood counts (156). In some cases, the areas of hypoplasia and aplasia show regeneration of hematopoiesis over time. The long-term significance of these areas of hypoplasia is unclear.

X. LONG-TERM OUTCOME WITH PURINE ANALOGS

Several studies have addressed the relapse rate, progression-free survival (PFS) and overall survival for patients with HCL treated with 2'-deoxycoformycin and 2-CdA. Most patients with either previously treated or untreated HCL achieve durable remissions with either multiple cycles of 2'-deoxycoformycin or a single cycle of 2-CdA. The relapse rates appear low. In the report from Northwestern University, 7 of 52 patients (14%) had relapsed at

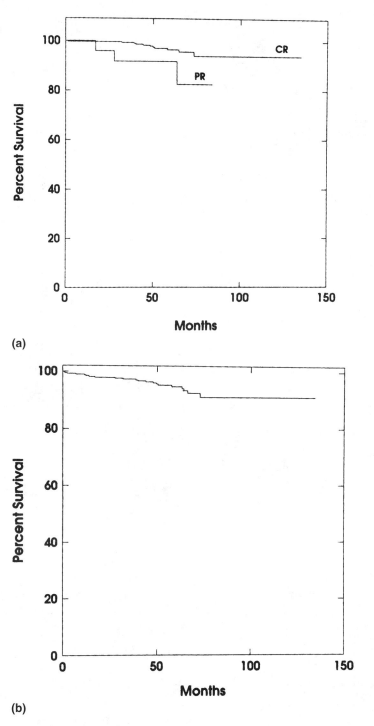

(a)

(b)

Figure 4   (a) Overall survival of patients treated with 2-CdA achieving a CR or PR. (From Ref. 51.) (b) Overall survival of all patients treated with 2-CdA. (From Ref. 51.)

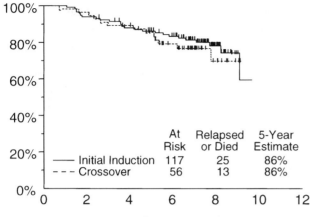

(a) Years After Complete Response

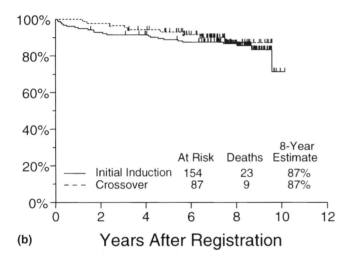

(b) Years After Registration

Figure 5 (a) Relapse-free survival of patients treated with 2'-DCF by age, initial. (From Ref. 150.) (b) Overall survival of patients treated with interferon-α or 2'-DCF (p = 0.086). (From Ref. 150.)

a median duration of 24 months (range, 12–44 months) (157). The PFS is 72% at 4 years and 83% for those patients achieving CR. The overall survival is 86% at 4 years. Seymour and colleagues from the M. D. Anderson Cancer Center reported that 8 of 40 patients (20%) relapsed at a median of 30 months (154). In the report by Saven and colleagues of 349 patients with either previously treated or untreated disease, 91% achieved CR and 70% achieved PR (55). The relapse rate for 341 patients responding to 2-CdA was 19% at 48 months and overall survival was 96% (Figures 4a and b). Investigators at the M. D. Anderson Cancer Center reported an EFS of 54% and an overall survival rate at 7 years of 87% among 99 patients treated (158).

Excellent long-term outcome after treatment with 2′-DCF also has been consistently reported. Kraut and colleagues reported that 11 of 24 patients (45%) had relapsed from CR after treatment with 2′-DCF at a median of 30 months (36). Grever and colleagues reported a relapse-free survival (RFS) rate of 91% at 7 years among 117 patients achieving CR on the 2′-DCF arm of a prospective randomized study comparing 2′-DCF to interferon (39). A recent update of the long-term outcome of these patients indicated that 76% $\pm$ 4% of patients remain alive and disease-free at 8 years and the overall survival was 87% $+$ 2% (159). (Figures 5a and b). A similar excellent outcome was reported by Catovsky (34). These investigators observed a 5-year overall survival rate of 88% among 110 patients treated with 2′-DCF.

The outcomes with both 2′-DCF and 2-CdA are excellent. The ease of administration of a single cycle of 2-CdA and the scarcity of toxicities are attractive advantages. However, long-term follow-up will be needed to determine whether one agent provides a substantially longer remission duration or survival.

XI. EVALUATION OF MINIMAL RESIDUAL DISEASE

The remarkable activity of the purine analogs has led to the examination of posttreatment bone marrow biopsies to detect MRD in patients otherwise in CR. Immunohistochemistry using anti-CD20 antibodies in paraffin-embedded biopsy specimens is a useful technique to identify MRD (87–91) (Figures 6a and b, see color plate [Figs. 26.6a and b]). Depending on the criteria used, 13% to 51% of patients in apparent CR have evidence of MRD, the presence of which may predict relapse (93). Molecular studies also suggest that the malignant clone may be present in patients in apparent remission (161). Flow cytometry also can be used to date at MRD. Because of the unique immunophenotype of HCL, flow cytometry is both a sensitive and specific method (160).

XII. APPROACH TO PATIENTS WHO RELAPSE AFTER A PURINE ANALOG

It is unclear whether treating patients at early relapse with only MRD is beneficial as opposed to waiting until signs or symptoms develop. Now that it is apparent that a small number of patients are relapsing after purine analog treatment, developing a salvage treatment approach is important. Retreatment with a second cycle of 2-CdA at relapse after a successful first cycle leads to a second CR in approximately 40% to 60% of patients (53,55,157,162) (Table 4). Patients may also respond to IFN-α (128). However, no series of patients receiving 2′-DCF after treatment with 2-CdA has been reported. In contrast, the initial reports of patients treated with 2-CdA included small numbers of patients who had relapsed after treatment with 2-DCF. Many of these patients achieved complete and durable remission (163).

A. Immunotoxin Therapy

Kreitman and colleagues recently reported four patients with resistant HCL treated with the immunotoxin LMB-2, which is composed of the FV portion of the anti-TAC (anti-CD25) antibody linked to a 38-kD truncated form of pseudomonas exotoxin A (164). One

Table 4   Outcome of Retreatment with 2-CdA for Relapsed HCL

Reference	No. of pts.	Med remission duration after initial cycle of 2-CdA (mo) (range)	Response (%)			Response duration (mo)
			Complete	Partial	None	
Saven (55)	53	30 (7–85)*	33 (62)	14 (26)	6 (11)	NA
Hoffman (51)	6	29 (12–55)	3 (50)	3 (50)	0	CR: 6+, 14+, 20+ PR: 2+, 9+, 10
Tallman (157)	5	24 (12–45)	2 (40)	3 (60)	0	CR: 6+, 24+ PR: 9, 9+, 15+
Lauria (50)†	10	23 (11–26)	6 (60)	3 (30)	1 (10)	NA
Thomas (158)	10	NA	9 (90)	1 (10)	0	NA

* Refers to all patients treated with a cycle of 2-CdA.
† Eight of the 10 patients had achieved PR after the first cycle of 2-CdA.
NA = not available.

patient achieved a CR after two cycles, and the other three patients achieved partial remission with >98% reduction in circulating cells.

B.   Rituximab (Chimeric anti-CD20 Antibody)

Rituximab is a monoclonal antibody targeting the B-cell antigen CD20. This agent has significant activity against a variety of B-cell lymphoproliferative disorders. There is now preliminary experience with rituximab in relapsed or recurrent HCL, indicating that it is an effective agent in the salvage setting (165–167). However, follow-up of these initial reports is short.

XIII.   RISK OF SECOND MALIGNANCIES

An early report suggested that patients with HCL have an increased incidence of second malignancies (168). Kampmeier and colleagues reported a significantly increased incidence of second malignancies in HCL patients treated with IFN-α (169). Among 69 patients treated with IFN-α2b followed for a median of 91 months, 13 (19%) had a second malignancy develop, half of which were of hematological origin. However, this association has not been uniformly observed. Given the fact that the purine analogs are immunosuppressive, it will be important to determine whether patients treated with either 2′-DCF or 2-CdA are at risk for second malignancies. Kurzrock and colleagues reported no excess of second malignancies among 350 patients treated with either interferon, 2-CdA, or 2′-DCF (170). Au and co-investigators recently reported an apparently inherent significant risk of second malignancies in patients with HCL that was more related to tumor burden than to a specific treatment effect (171). Cheson and colleagues reviewed long-term follow-up data on National Cancer Institute Group C Protocols with 2′-DCF (362 treated patients) and 2-CdA (928 treated patients) for patients with HCL and found 27 and 61 second malignancies, respectively (172). Nucleoside analogs were not associated with a significantly increased risk of second malignancies beyond that already associated with the undergoing disease.

XIV. FUTURE DIRECTIONS

The purine analogs have supplanted splenectomy and IFN-α as the treatment of choice for all patients with HCL. The long-term outcomes appear equivalent with either 2'-DCF or 2-CdA, but very long-term follow-up will be necessary to determine whether one or the other agent offers a significant survival advantage. Future directions will include clinical testing of an oral formulation of 2-CdA or 2'-DCF and exploring approaches for patients with MRD who appear at risk to recur. Patients who relapse after 2'-DCF usually respond well to 2-CdA, but determination of whether the reverse is true will require further study. Finally, although patients who have purine analogs fail may respond to interferon, it is not likely to be curative. Novel strategies such as the LMB-2 immunotoxin or rituximab are needed for this subset of patients.

REFERENCES

1. O Ewald. Die leukamische reticuloendothelioses. Deutsches Arch Kin Med 142:222–228, 1923.
2. BA Bouroncle, BK Wiseman, CA Doan. Leukemic reticuloendotheliosis. Blood 13:609, 1958.
3. R Schrek, WJ Donnelly. "Hairy" cells in blood in lymphoreticular neoplastic disease and "flagellated" cells of normal lymph nodes. Blood 27:199–211, 1966.
4. D Catovsky. Hairy cell leukemia and prolymphocytic leukemia. Clin Haematol 6:245–268, 1977.
5. HM Golomb, D Catovsky, DW Golde. Hairy cell leukemia: A clinical review based on 71 cases. Ann Intern Med 89:677–683, 1978.
6. G Flandrin, F Sigaux, G Sebahoun, P Boufette. Hairy cell leukemia: Clinical presentation and follow-up of 211 patients. Semin Oncol 11:458–471, 1984.
7. CA Westbrook, JE Groopman, DW Golde. Hairy cell leukemia: Disease pattern and prognosis. Cancer 54:500–506, 1984.
8. SJ Korsmeyer, WC Greene, J Cossman, SM Hsu, JP Jensen, LM Neckers, SL Marshall, A Bakhshi, JM Depper, WJ Leonard, ES Jaffe, TA Waldman. Rearrangement and expression of immunoglobulin genes and expression of Tac antigen in hairy cell leukemia. Proc Natl Acad Sci USA 80:4522–4526, 1983.
9. ML Cleary, GS Wood, R Warnke, J Chao, J Sklar. Immunoglobulin gene rearrangements in hairy cell leukemia. Blood 64:99–104, 1984.
10. L Foroni, D Catovsky, L Luzzatto. Immunoglobulin gene rearrangements in hairy cell leukemia and other chronic B-cell lymphoproliferative disorders. Leukemia 1:389–392, 1987.
11. J Jansen, J Hermans, J Remme, GJ den Ottolander, PL Cardozo. Hairy cell leukemia. Clinical features and effect of splenectomy. Scand J Haematol 21:60–67, 1978.
12. U Mintz, HM Golomb. Splenectomy as initial therapy in 26 patients with leukemic reticuloendotheliosis (hairy cell leukemia). Cancer Res 39:2366–2370, 1979.
13. J Jansen, J Hermans. Splenectomy in hairy cell leukemia: A retrospective multicenter analysis. Cancer 47:2066–2076, 1981.
14. HM Golomb, JW Vardiman. Response to splenectomy in 65 patients with hairy cell leukemia: An evaluation of spleen weight and bone marrow involvement. Blood 61:349–352, 1983.
15. MJ Magee, S McKenzie, DA Filippa, ZA Arlin, TS Gee, BD Clarkson. Hairy cell leukemia:

durability of response to splenectomy in 26 patients and treatment of relapse with androgens in six patients. Cancer 56:2557–2562, 1985.

16. AS Van Norman, DM Nagorney, JK Martin, RL Philoky, DM Ilstrup. Splenectomy for hairy cell leukemia: A clinical review of 63 patients. Cancer 57:644–648, 1986.

17. MJ Ratain, JW Vardiman, CM Barker, HM Golomb. Prognostic variables in hairy cell leukemia after splenectomy as initial therapy. Cancer 62:2420–2424, 1988.

18. RV Smalley, J Connors, RL Tuttle, S Anderson, W Robinson, JK Whisnant. Splenectomy vs alpha interferon: A randomized study in patients with previously untreated hairy cell leukemia. Am J Hematol 41:13–18, 1992.

19. JE Coad, E Matutes, D Catovsky. Splenectomy in lymphoproliferative disorders: A report on 70 cases and review of the literature. Leuk Lymph 10:245–264, 1993.

20. X Troussard, G Flandrin. Hairy cell leukemia. An update on a cohort of 93 patients treated at a single institution. Effects of interferon in patients relapsing after splenectomy and in patients with or without maintenance treatment. Leuk Lymphoma 14:99–105, 1994.

21. AS Spiers, SJ Parekh, MB Bishop. Hairy cell leukemia: induction of complete remission with pentostatin (2′-deoxycoformycin). J Clin Oncol 2:1336–1342, 1984.

22. JB Johnston, RI Glazer, L Pugh, LG Israels. The treatment of hairy cell leukemia with 2-deoxycoformycin. Br J Haematol 63:525–534, 1986.

23. EH Kraut, BA Bouroncle, MR Grever. Low-dose deoxycoformycin in the treatment of hairy cell leukemia. Blood 68:1119–1122, 1986.

24. ASD Spiers, D Moore, PA Cassileth, DP Harrington, FJ Cummings, RS Neiman, JM Bennett, M O'Connell. Remissions in hairy cell leukemia with pentostatin (2′-deoxycoformycin). N Engl J Med 316:825–830, 1987.

25. MR Grever, JM Leiby, EH Kraut, et al. Low-dose deoxycoformycin in the treatment of hairy cell leukemia. Blood 68:1196–1201, 1986.

26. JB Johnston, E Eisenhauer, WE Corbett, JG Scott, SD Zaentz. Efficacy of 2-deoxycoformycin in hairy cell leukemia: A study of the National Cancer Institute of Canada Clinical Trials Group. J Natl Cancer Inst 80:765–769, 1988.

27. AD Ho, J Thaler, F Mandelli, F Lauria, F Zittoun, R Willemze, G McVie, AM Marmontl, O Prummer, P Stryckmans. Response to pentostatin in hairy cell leukemia refractory to interferon-alpha. The European Organization for Research and Treatment of Cancer. J Clin Oncol 7:1533–1538, 1989.

28. EH Kraut, BA Bouroncle, MR Grever. Pentostatin in the treatment of advanced hairy cell leukemia. J Clin Oncol 7:168–172, 1989.

29. J Grem, SA King, BD Cheson. Pentostatin in hairy cell leukemia. Treatment by the special exemption mechanism. J Natl Cancer Inst 81:448–453, 1989.

30. C Dearden, D Catovsky. Treatment of hairy cell leukemia with 2-deoxycoformycin. Leuk Lymphoma 1:179–185, 1990.

31. M Blick, JL Lepe-Zuniga, R Doig, JR Quesada. Durable complete remissions after 2′-deoxycoformycin treatment in patients with hairy cell leukemia resistant to interferon alpha. Am J Hematol 33:205–209, 1990.

32. PA Cassileth, B Cheuvart, ASD Spiers, DP Harrington, FJ Cummings, RS Neiman, JM Bennett, M O'Connell. Pentostatin induces durable remissions in hairy cell leukemia. J Clin Oncol 9:243–246, 1991.

33. D Catovsky, E Matutes, JG Talavera, NTJ O'Connor, SAN Johnson, E Emmett, L Corbett, J Swansbury. Long-term results with 2-deoxycoformycin in hairy cell leukemia. Leuk Lymphoma 14(suppl 1):109–113, 1994.

34. HM Golomb, R Dodge, R Mick, D Budman, R Hutchison, SJ Horning, CA Schiffer. Pentostatin treatment of hairy cell leukemia patients who fail initial therapy with recombinant alpha-interferon: A report of CALGB study 8515. Leukemia 8:2037–2040, 1994.

35. EH Kraut, MR Grever, BA Bouroncle. Long-term follow-up of patients with hairy cell leukemia after treatment with 2′-deoxycoformycin. Blood 84:4061–4063, 1994.

36. KR Rai. Comparison of pentostatin and alpha-interferon in splenectomized patients with active hairy cell leukemia: An intergroup study. Cancer and Leukemia Group B and Southwest Oncology Group. Leuk Lymphoma 14:107–108, 1994.

37. L Annino, A Ferrai, F Giona, G Cimino, S Crescenzi, MC Cava, A Pacchiarotti, F Mandelli. Deoxycoformycin induces long-lasting remission in hairy cell leukemia: Clinical and biological results of two different regimens. Leuk Lymph 14:115–119, 1994.

38. M Grever, K Kopecky, MK Foucar, D Head, JM Bennett, RE Hutchinson, WE Corbett, PA Cassileth, T Habermann, H Golomb. A randomized comparison of pentostatin vs. alpha-interferon in previously untreated patients with hairy cell leukemia: An intergroup study. J Clin Oncol 13:974–982, 1995.

39. JB Johnston, RI Glazer, L Pugh. The treatment of hairy cell leukemia with 2′-deoxycoformycin. Br J Haematol 63:525–534, 1996.

40. D Catovsky. Clinical experience with 2′-deoxycoformycin. Hematol Cell Ther 38:103–107, 1996.

41. JF Seymour, M Talpaz, R Kurzrock. Response duration and recovery of CD4+ lymphocytes following deoxycoformycin in interferon-α-resistant hairy cell leukemia: 7-year follow-up. Leukemia 11:42–47, 1997.

42. P Ribeiro, F Bouaffia, PY Peaud, M Blanc, B Salles, G Salles, B Coiffier. Long term outcome of patients with hairy cell leukemia treated with pentostatin. Cancer 85:65–71, 1999.

43. M Rafel, F Cervantes, JM Beltran, F Zuazu, LH Nieto, C Rayon, JG Talavera, E Montserrat. Deoxycoformycin in the treatment of patients with hairy cell leukemia. Cancer 88:352–357, 2000.

44. LD Piro, CJ Carrera, DA Carson. Lasting remissions in hairy cell leukemia induced by a single infusion of 2-chlorodeoxyadenosine. N Engl J Med 332:1117–1120, 1990.

45. EM Estey, R Kurzrock, HM Kantarjian, SM O'Brien, KB McCredie, M Beran, C Koller, MJ Keating, C Hirsch-Ginsberg, YO Huh. Treatment of hairy cell leukemia with 2-chlorodeoxyadenosine (2-CdA). Blood 79:882–887, 1992.

46. G Juliusson, J Liliemark. Rapid recovery from cytopenia in hairy cell leukemia after treatment with 2-chloro-2-deoxyadenosine (CdA): Relationship to opportunistic infections. Blood 79:888–894, 1992.

47. MS Tallman, D Hakimian, D Variakojis, D Koslow, GA Sisney, AW Rademaker, E Rose, K Kaul. A single cycle of 2-chlorodeoxyadenosine results in complete remission in the majority of patients with hairy cell leukemia. Blood 9:2203–2209, 1992.

48. LD Piro, JD Ellison, A Saven. The Scripps Clinic experience with 2-chlorodeoxyadenosine in the treatment of hairy cell leukemia. Leuk Lymphoma 14:121–125, 1994.

49. E Dann, S Gillis, EA Rachmilewitz, A Barak, R Ruchlemer, A Polliack. Hairy cell leukemia: Results of therapy with 2-CdA in Jerusalem. Leuk Lymphoma 14(1):127–131, 1994.

50. F Lauria, D Rondelli, PL Zinzani, M Bocchia, G Marotta, M Salvucci, D Raspadori, MA Ventura, S Birtolo, F Forconi, S Tura. Long-lasting complete remission in patients treated with 2-CdA: A 5-year survey. Leukemia 11:629–632, 1997.

51. MA Hoffman, D Janson, E Rose, KR Rai. Treatment of hairy cell leukemia with cladribine: Response, toxicity, and long-term follow-up. J Clin Oncol 15:1138–1142, 1997.

52. T Robak, M Blasinska-Morawiec, E Krykowski, J Hansz, M Komarnick, M Kazimierczak, L Konopka, S Maj, A Hellmann, JM Zaucha, L Urasinski, B Zdziarska, S Kotlarek-Haus, L Usnarska-Zubkiewicz. 2-Chlorodeoxyadenosine (2-CdA) in 2-hour versus 24-hour intravenous infusion in the treatment of patients with hairy cell leukemia. Leuk Lymphoma 22: 107–111, 1996.

53. L Fayad, R Kurzrock, M Keating, S O'Brien, H Kantarjian, M Andreiff, S Pierce, M Talpaz, E Freireich, E Estey. Treatment of hair cell leukemia (HCL) with 2-CdA: Long-term follow at M. D. Andersen Cancer Center (abstr). Blood 90:2363, 1997.

54. BD Cheson, JM Sorensen, DA Vena, MJ Montello, JA Barrett, E Damasio, M Tallman, L Annino, J Connors, B Coiffer, F Lauria. Treatment of hairy cell leukemia with 2-chlorode-

oxyadenosine via the Group C protocol mechanism of the National Cancer Institute: A report of 979 patients. J Clin Oncol 16:3007–3015, 1998.

55. A Saven, C Burian, JA Koziol, LD Piro. Long-term follow-up of patients with hairy cell leukemia after cladribine treatment. Blood 92:1918–1926, 1998.

56. JN Bastie, D Cazals-Hatem, M-T Daniel, MF D'agay, CL Rabian, S Glaisner, MP Noel-Walter, D Dabout, G Flandrin, H Dombret, D Poisson, L Degos, S Castaigne. Five years follow-up after 2-chlorodeoxyadenosine treatment in thirty patients with hairy cell leukemia: Evaluation of minimal residual disease and CD4+ lymphopenia after treatment. Leuk Lymphoma 35:555–565, 1999.

57. JR Quesada, J Ruben, JT Manning, EM Hersh, JU Gutterman. Alpha interferon for induction of remission in hairy cell leukemia. N Engl Med 310:15–18, 1984.

58. J Quesada, E Hersh, M Manning, J Ruben, M Keating, E Schnipper, L Itri, JU Gutterman. Treatment of hairy cell leukemia with recombinant alpha-interferon. Blood 68:493–497, 1986.

59. HM Golomb, A Jacobs, A Fefer, H Ozer, J Thompson, C Portlock, M Ratain, D Golde, J Vardiman, JS Burke. Alpha-2 interferon therapy for hairy-cell leukemia: A multicenter study of 64 patients. J Clin Oncol 4:900–905, 1986.

60. G Flandrin, F Sigaux, S Castaigne, C Billard, M Aguet, M Boiron, E Falcoff, L Degos. Treatment of hairy cell leukemia with recombinant alpha interferon. I. Quantitative study of bone marrow changes during the first months of treatment. Blood 67:817–820, 1986.

61. KA Foon, AE Maloish, PG Abrams, S Wrighting, HC Stevenson, A Alarif, MF Fer, WR Overton, M Poole, EF Schipper, ES Jaffe, RB Herberman. Recombinant leukocyte A interferon therapy for advanced hairy cell leukemia. Am J Med 80:351–356, 1986.

62. H Golomb, A Fefer, D Golde, H Ozer, C Portlock, R Silber, J Rappeport, MJ Ratain, MJ Thompson, EM Bonnem. Sequential evaluation of alpha-2b interferon treatment in 128 patients with hairy cell leukemia. Semin Oncol 14:13–17, 1987.

63. M Ratain, H Golomb, R Bardawil, JW Vardiman, CA Westbrook, LS Kaminer, BC Lembersky, MA Bitter, K Daly. Durability of responses to interferon alfa-2b in advanced hairy cell leukemia. Blood 69:872–878, 1987.

64. HM Golomb, MJ Ratain, A Fefer, J Thompson, DW Golde, H Ozer, C Portlock, R Silber, J Rappeport, MJ Ratain, J Thompson, EM Bonnem. A randomized study of the duration of treatment with interferon alpha-2B in hairy cell leukemia patients. J Natl Cancer Inst 80:369–373, 1988.

65. HM Golomb, A Fefer, DW Golde, H Ozer, C Portlock, R Silber, J Rappaport, MJ Ratain, J Thompson, E Bonnem, R Spiegel, L Tensen, JS Burke, JW Vardiman. Report of a multi-institutional study of 193 patients with hairy cell leukemia treated with interferon-alpha2b. Semin Oncol 15:7–9, 1988.

66. S Castaigne, F Sigaux, L Degos, G Flandrin. Hairy cell leukemia: Follow-up after alpha interferon treatment. Nouv Rev Fr Hematol 31:321–325, 1989.

67. J Thompson, P Kidd, E Rubin, A Fefer. Very low dose alpha-2b interferon for the treatment of hairy cell leukemia. Blood 73:1440–1443, 1989.

68. J Moormeier, M Ratain, C Westbrook, J Vardiman, K Daly, H Golomb. Low-dose interferon alpha-2b in the treatment of hairy cell leukemia. J Natl Cancer Inst 81:1172–1174, 1989.

69. E Berman, G Heller, S Kempin, T Gee, LL Tran, B Clarkson. Incidence of response and long-term follow-up in patients with hairy cell leukemia treated with recombinant interferon α-2-β. Blood 75:839–845, 1990.

70. JR Quesada, EM Hersh, J Manning, J Reuben, M Keating, E Schnipper, L Itri, JU Gutterman. Treatment of hairy cell leukemia with recombinant alpha-interferon. Blood 68:493–497, 1986.

71. MJ Ratain, HM Golomb, JW Vardiman, CA Westbrook, C Barker, A Hooberman, MA Bitter, K Daly. Relapse after interferon-2β therapy for hairy cell leukemia: Analysis of prognostic variables. J Clin Oncol 6:1714–1721, 1988.

72. JW Smith, DL Longo, WJ Urba, JW Clark, T Watson, J Beveridge, KC Conlon, M Sznol, SP Creekmore, WG Alvord. Prolonged subcutaneous treatment of hairy cell leukemia patients with recombinant interferon-α 2a. Blood 78:1664–1671, 1991.

73. RV Smalley, SA Anderson, RL Tuttle, J Connors, LM Thurmond, A Huang, K Castle, C Magers, JK Whishant. A randomized comparison of two doses of human lymphoblastoid interferon-α in hairy cell leukemia. Blood 78:3133–3141, 1991.

74. HM Golomb, MJ Ratain, R Mick, K Daly. Interferon treatment for hairy cell leukemia: An update on a cohort of 69 patients treated from 1983–1986. Leukemia 6:1177–1180, 1992.

75. R Spielberger, R Mick, M Ratain, H Golomb. Interferon treatment of hairy cell leukemia: An update on a cohort of 69 patients treated from 1983 to 1986. Leuk Lymphoma 14:89–93, 1994.

76. K Rai, F Davey, B Peterson, C Schiffer, RT Silver, H Ozer, H Golomb, CD Bloomfield. Recombinant alpha-2b interferon in therapy of previously untreated hairy cell leukemia: Long-term results of a study by the Cancer and Leukemia Group B. Leukemia 9:1116–1120, 1995.

77. MT Daniel, G Flandrin. Fine structure of abnormal cells in hairy cell (tricholeukocytic) leukemia, with special reference to their in vitro phagocytic capacity. Lab Invest 30(1):1–8, 1974.

78. HM Golomb, A Braylor, A Polliack. Hairy cell leukemia (leukemia reticuloendoteliosis): A scanning electron microscopic study of eight cases. Br J Haematol 28:455–460, 1975.

79. JS Burke. The value of the bone-marrow biopsy in the diagnosis of hairy cell leukemia. Am J Clin Pathol 70:876–884, 1978.

80. R Bartl, B Frisch, W Hill, R Burkhardt, W Sommerfeld, M Sund. Bone marrow histology in hairy cell leukemia. Identification of subtypes and their prognostic significance. Am J Clin Pathol 79:531–545, 1983.

81. JS Burke, H Rappaport. The diagnosis and differential diagnosis of hairy cell leukemia in bone marrow and spleen. Semin Oncol 11:334–346, 1984.

82. RD Brunning, RW McKenna. Small lymphocytic leukemias and related disorders. In: Tumors of the bone marrow, Atlas of Tumor Pathology, Third Series, Fascile 9, Washington, DC: Armed Forces Institute of Pathology, 1994. pp 254–322.

83. MA Bitter. Hairy-cell leukemia. In: DM Knowles, ed. Neoplastic Hematopathology. Baltimore: Williams & Wilkins, 1992. pp 1209–1234.

84. WM Lee, JH Beckstead. Hairy cell leukemia with bone marrow hypoplasia. Cancer 50:2207–2210, 1982.

85. I Katayama. Bone marrow in hairy cell leukemia. Hematol Oncol Clin North Am 2:585–602, 1988.

86. LT Yam, CY Li, KW Lam. Tartrate-resistant and phosphatase isoenzyme in the reticulum cells of leukemic reticuloendotheliosis. N Engl J Med 284:357–360, 1971.

87. BA Robbins, DJ Ellison, JC Spinosa, CA Carey, RJ Lukes, S Poppema, A Saven, LD Piro. Diagnostic application of two-color flow cytometry in 161 cases. Blood 82:1277–1287, 1993.

88. P Möller, B Mielke, G Moldenhauer. Monoclonal antibody HM2-1, a marker for intraepithelial T-cells and lymphomas derived thereof, also recognizes hairy cell leukemia and some B-cell lymphomas. Am J Pathol 136:509–512, 1990.

89. V Barak, I Kalichmann, A Polliack. Serum soluble IL-2 receptor levels are associated with clinical disease status and grade in lymphoma and lymphocytic leukemia. Leuk Lymphoma 8:405–408, 1992.

90. H Hounieu, SM Chittal, T al Saati, A de Mascarel, E Sabattini, S Pileri, B Falini, E Ralfkiaer, A Le Tourneau, J Selves. Hairy cell leukemia. Diagnosis of bone marrow involvement in paraffin-embedded sections with monoclonal antibody DBA.44. Am J Clin Pathol 98:26–33, 1992.

91. DJ Ellison, RW Sharpe, BA Robbins, JC Spinosa, JD Leopard, A Saven, LD Piro. Immunomorphologic analysis of bone marrow biopsies after treatment with 2-chlorodeoxyadenosine for hairy cell leukemia. Blood 84:4310–4315, 1994.

92. D Hakimian, MS Tallman, L Peterson. Detection of minimal residual disease by immuno-staining of bone marrow biopsies after 2-chlorodeoxyadenosine for hairy cell leukemia. Blood 82:1798–1802, 1993.

93. S Wheaton, MS Tallman, D Hakimian, L Peterson. Minimal residual disease may predict bone marrow relapse in patients with hairy cell leukemia treated with 2-chlorodeoxyadenosine. Blood 87:1556–1560, 1995.

94. G Konwalinka, M Schirmer, W Hilbe, F Fend, F Geisen, A Knoblechner, A Petzer, J Thaler. Minimal residual disease in hairy cell leukemia after treatment with 2-chlorodeoxyadenosine. Blood Cells, Mol Dis 21:142–151, 1995.

95. E Matutes, P Meeus, K Melennan, D Catovsky. The significance of minimal residual disease in hairy cell leukemia treated with deoxycoformycin: A long-term follow-up study. Br J Hematol 98:375–383, 1997.

96. CJ de Boer, JC Kluin-Nelemans, E Dreef, MGD Kester, DM Kluin, E Schuuring, JHJM van Krieken. Involvement of the CCND1 genes in hairy cell leukemia. Ann Oncol 7:251–256, 1996.

97. F Ishida, K Kitano, N Ichikawa, T Ito, Y Kohara, T Taniguchi, T Motokura, K Kiyosawa. Hairy cell leukemia with translocation (11;20) (q13;q11) and overexpression of cyclin D1. Leukemia Res 23:763–765, 1999.

98. SH Kroft, WG Finn, LC Peterson. The pathology of the chronic lymphoid leukemias. Blood Rev 9:234–250, 1995.

99. DA Galton, JM Goldman, E Wiltshaw, D Catovsky, K Henry, GJ Goldenberg. Prolymphocytic leukemia. Br J Haematol 27:7–23, 1974.

100. JV Melo, D Catovsky, DA Galton. The relationship between chronic lymphocytic leukemia and prolymphocytic leukemia. I. Clinical and laboratory features of 300 patients and characterization of an intermediate group. Br J Haematol 63:377–387, 1986.

101. JV Melo, D Catovsky, WT Gregory, DA Galton. The relationship between chronic lymphocytic leukemia and prolymphocytic leukemia. IV. Analysis of survival and prognostic features. Br J Haematol 65:23–29, 1987.

102. SP Mulligan, E Matutes, C Dearden, D Catovsky. Splenic lymphoma with villous lymphocytes. Br J Haematol 78:206–209, 1991.

103. PG Isaacson, E Matutes, M Burke, D Catovsky. The histopathology of splenic lymphoma with villous lymphocytes. Blood 84:3828–3824, 1994.

104. E Matutes, R Morilla, K Owusu-Ankomah, A Houlihan, D Catovsky. The immunophenotype of splenic lymphoma with villous lymphocytes and its relevance to the differential diagnosis with other B-cell disorders. Blood 83:1558–1562, 1994.

105. X Troussard, F Valensi, E Duchayne, R Garand, P Felman, M Tulliez, M Henry-Amar, PA Bryon, G Flandrin. Splenic lymphoma with villous lymphocytes: Clinical presentation, biology and prognostic factors in a series of 100 patients. Groupe Francais d'Hematologie Cellulaire (GFHC). Br J Haematol 93:731–736, 1996.

106. JC Cawley, GF Burns, FJ Hayhoe. A chronic lymphoproliferative disorder with distinctive features: A distinct variant of hairy cell leukemia. Leuk Res 4:547–559, 1980.

107. D Catovsky, M O'Brien, JV Melo, J Wardle, M Brozovic. Hairy cell leukemia (HCL) variant: A intermediate disease between HCL and B prolymphocytic leukemia. Semin Oncol 11:362–369, 1984.

108. P Zinzani, F Lauria, M Buzzi, D Raspadori, L Gugliotta, M Bocchia, S Macchi, R Algeri, S Tura. Hairy cell leukemia variant: A morphologic and clinical study of 7 cases. Haematologica 75:54–57, 1990.

109. L Sainati, F Lauria, M Buzzi, D Raspadori, L Gugliotta, M Bocchia, S Macchi, R Algeri, S Tura. A variant form of hairy cell leukemia resistant to alpha-interferon: Clinical and phenotypic characteristics of 17 patients. Blood 76:157–162, 1990.

110. SA Tetreault, B Robbins, A Saven. Treatment of hairy cell leukemia-variant with cladribine. Leuk Lymphoma 35:347–354, 1999.

111. E Labouyrie, G Marit, JP Vial, F Lacombe, P Fialon, P Bernard, A de Mascarel, JP Merlio. Intrasinusoidal bone marrow involvement by splenic lymphoma with villous lymphocytes: A helpful immunohistologic feature. Mod Pathol 10:1015–1020, 1997.

112. D de Totero, PL Tazzari, F Lauria, D Raspadori, PF di Celle, A Carbone, M Gobbi, R Foa. Phenotypic analysis of hairy cell leukemia: "Variant" cases express the interleukin-2 receptor β chain, but not the α chain (CD25). Blood 82:528–535, 1993.

113. HP Horny, C Sillaber, D Menke, E Kaiserling, M Wehrmann, B Stehberger, A Chotl, K Leckner, K Lennert, P Valent. Diagnostic value of immunostaining for tryptase in patients with mastocytosis. Am J Surg Pathol 22:1132–1141, 1998.

114. LT Yam, WH Crosby. Early splenectomy in lymphoproliferative disorders. Arch Int Med 133:270–274, 1974.

115. BA Bouroncle. Unusual presentations and complications of hairy cell leukemia. Leukemia 1:288–293, 1987.

116. GA Pangalis, VA Boussiotis, C Kittas, PG Panaiotidis, C Mitsoulis-Mentzikoff, P Loukpoulos, P Fessas. Hairy cell leukemia: Residual splenic disease after successful interferon therapy. Leuk Lymphoma 6:145–153, 1992.

117. A Polliack, E Dann. Rapid massive relapse of hairy cell leukemia during bone marrow remission after 2-CdA therapy: The spleen as a sanctuary site in hairy cell leukemia. Blood 84(6): 2057–2058, 1994.

118. TE Davis, L Waterbury, M Abeloff, PJ Burke. Leukemia reticuloendotheliosis: Report of a case with prolonged remission following intensive chemotherapy. Arch Intern Med 136:620–622, 1976.

119. HM Golomb. Progress report on chlorambucil therapy in postsplenectomy patients with aggressive hairy cell leukemia. Blood 57:464–467, 1981.

120. F Calvo, S Castaigne, F Sigaux, M Marty, L Degos, M Boiron, G Flandrin. Intensive chemotherapy of hairy cell leukemia in patients with progressive disease. Blood 65:115–119, 1985.

121. S Cold, H Brincker. Chemotherapy of progressive hairy cell leukemia. Eur J Haematol 30: 251–255, 1987.

122. JD Schwarzmeier, M Hilgarth, ST Nguyen, M Shehata, G Gruber, A Spittler, M Willheim, G Boltz-Nitulescu, P Hocker, R Berger. Inadequate production of hematopoietic growth factors in hairy cell leukemia: Up-Regulation of interleukin 6 by recombinant IFN-α in vitro. Cancer Res 56:4679–4685, 1996.

123. L Baldini, A Cortelezzi, N Polli, A Neri, L Nobili, AT Maiolo, G Lambertenghi-Deliliers, EE Polli. Human recombinant leukocyte interferon alpha-2c enhances the expression of class II HLA antigens on hairy cells. Blood 67:458–464, 1986.

124. J Burthem, A Vincent, J Cawley. Integrin receptors and hairy cell leukemia. Leuk Lymphoma 21:211–215, 1996.

125. J Jansen, G Wietnjenn, R Willemze, J Kluin-Nelemans. Production of tumor necrosis factor-alpha by normal and malignant B lymphocytes in response to interferon-alpha, interferon gamma and interleukin-4. Leukemia 6:116–119, 1992.

126. S Vecanthan, H Gamliel, HM Golomb. Mechanism of interferon action in hairy cell leukemia: A model of effective cancer biotherapy. Cancer Res 52:1056–1066, 1992.

127. G Capnist, M Federico, T Chisesi, L Resegotti, T Lamparelli, P Fabris, G Rossi, R Invernizzi, C Guarnaccia, P Leoni. Long term results of interferon treatment in hairy cell leukemia. Italian Cooperative Group of Hairy Cell Leukemia (ICGHCL). Leuk Lymphoma 14:457–464, 1994.

128. JF Seymour, EH Estey, MJ Keating, R Kurzrock. Response to interferon-α in patients with hairy cell leukemia relapsing after treatment with 2-chlorodeoxyadenosine. Leukemia 9:929–932, 1999.

129. ER Giblett, JE Anderson, F Cohen, B Pollara, HJ Meuwissen. Adenosine-deaminase deficiency in two patients with severe impaired cellular immunity. Lancet 2:1067–1068, 1972.

130. J Dissing, B Knudsen. Adenosine-deaminase deficiency and combined immunodeficiency syndrome. Lancet 16:1316, 1972.

131. A Cohen, R Hirschorn, SD Horowitz, A Rubenstein, SH Polmar, R Hong, DW Martin. De-oxyadenosine triphosphate as a potentially toxic metabolite in adenosine deaminase deficiency. Proc Natl Acad Sci USA 75:472–476, 1978.

132. RL Wortmann, BS Mitchell, NL Edward, IH Fox. Biochemical basis for differential deoxyadenosine toxicity to T and B lymphoblasts: role for 5′-nucleotidase. Proc Natl Acad Sci 76: 2434–2437, 1979.

133. JF Smyth, DG Poplack, BJ Holiman, BG Leventhal, G Yarbro. Correlation of adenosine deaminase activity with cell surface markers in acute lymphoblastic leukemia. J Clin Invest 62:710–712, 1978.

134. DG Poplack, SE Sullan, G Rivera, J Holcenberg, SB Murphy, J Blatt, JM Lipton, P Venner, DL Glaubiger, R Ungerleider, D Johns. Phase I study of 2′-deoxyco-formycin in acute lymphoblastic leukemia. Cancer Res 41:3343–3346, 1981.

135. MR Grever, MF Siaw, WF Jacob, JA Niedhart, JS Miser, MS Coleman, JJ Hutton. The biochemical and clinical consequences of 2′-deoxycoformycin in refractory lymphoproliferative malignancy. Blood 57:406–417, 1981.

136. A Martin, S Nerenstone, WJ Urba, DL Longo, JB Lawrence, JW Clark, MJ Hawkins, SP Creekmore, JW 2d Smith, RG Steis. Treatment of hairy cell leukemia with alternating cycles of pentostatin and recombinant leukocyte A interferon: results of a phase II study. J Clin Oncol 8(4):721–730, 1990.

137. TM Habermann, JW Andersen, PA Cassileth, JM Bennett, MM Oken. Sequential administration of recombinant interferon-alpha and deoxycoformycin in the treatment of hairy cell leukemia. Br J Haematol 80:466–471, 1992.

138. S Seto, CJ Carrera, M Kubota, B Wasson, DA Carson. Mechanism of deoxyadenosine and 2-chlorodeoxyadenosine toxicity to nondividing human lymphocytes. J Clin Invest 75:377–383, 1985.

139. S Seto, CJ Carrera, DB Wasson, DA Carson. Inhibition of DNA repair by deoxyadenosine in resting human lymphocytes. J Immunol 136:2839–2843, 1986.

140. P Hentosh, R Koob, RL Blakley. Incorporation of 2-halogeno-2′-deoxyadenosine 5-triphosphates into DNA during replication by human polymerases alpha and beta. J Biol Chem 2655:4033–4040, 1990.

141. AR Pettit, AR Clarke, J Cawley, SD Griffiths. Purine analogues kill resting lymphocytes by p53-dependent and -independent mechanisms. Br J Haematol 105:986–988, 1999.

142. HM Kantarjian, J Schachner, MJ Keating. Fludarabine therapy in hairy cell leukemia. Cancer 67:1291–1293, 1991.

143. EH Kraut, HG Chou. Fludarabine phosphate in refractory hairy cell leukemia. Am J Hematol 37:59–60, 1991.

144. A Saven, WK Cheung, I Smith, M Moyer, T Johannsen, E Rose, R Gollard, M Kosty, WE Miller, LD Piro. Pharmacokinetic study of oral and bolus intravenous 2-chlorodeoxyadenosine in patients with malignancy. J Clin Oncol 14:978–983, 1996.

145. J Liliemark, F Albertioni, M Hassan, G Juliusson. On the bioavailability of oral and subcutaneous 2-chloro-2′-deoxyadenosine in humans: Alternative routes of administration. J Clin Oncol 10(10):1514–1518, 1995.

146. G Juliusson, D Heldal, E Hippe, M Hedenus, C Malm, K Wallman, CM Stolt, SA Evensen, F Albertioni, G Tjonnfjord, R Lenkei, J Liliemark. Subcutaneous injections of 2-chlorodeoxyadenosine for symptomatic hairy cell leukemia. J Clin Oncol 13:989–995, 1995.

147. F Lauria, M Bocchia, D Raspadori, PL Zinzani, D Rondelli. Weekly administration of 2-CdA in patients with hairy cell leukemia: A new treatment schedule effective and safer in preventing infectious complications. Blood 89:1838–1839, 1997.

148. J Chacko, C Murphy, C Duggan, DS O'Brian, PV Browne, SR McCann. Weekly intermittent

2-CdA is less toxic and equally efficacious when compared to continuous infusion in hairy cell leukemia (Corres). Br J Haematol 105:1145–1146, 1999.

149. G Juliusson, R Lenkei, G Tjonn-fjord, D Heidol, J Liliemark. Low-dose cladribine for symptomatic hairy cell leukemia. Br J Haematol 89:637–639, 1995.

150. MS Tallman, D Hakimian, KJ Kopecky, S Wheaton, E Wollins, K Foucar, PA Cassileth, T Habermann, MR Grever, JM Rowe, LC Peterson. Minimal residual disease in patients with hairy cell leukemia in complete remission treated with 2-chlorodeoxyadenosine or 2′-deoxycoformycin and prediction of early relapse. Clin Cancer Res 5:1665–1670, 1999.

151. CE Dearden, E Matutes, BL Hilditch, GJ Swansbury, D Catovsky. Long-term follow-up of patients with hairy cell leukemia after treatment with pentostatin or cladribine. Br J Haematol 106:515–519, 1999.

152. WJ Urba, MW Baseler, WC Kopp, RC Steis, JW Clark, JW Smith, DL Coggin, DL Longo. Deoxycoformycin induced immunosuppression in patients with hairy cell leukemia. Blood 73:38–46, 1989.

153. EH Kraut, JC Neff, BA Bouroncle, D Gochnour, MR Grever. Immunosuppressive effects of pentostatin. J Clin Oncol 8:848–855, 1990.

154. JF Seymour, R Kurzrock, EJ Freireich, EH Estey. 2-Chlorodeoxyadenosine induces durable remission and prolonged suppression of CD4+ lymphocyte counts in patients with hairy cell leukemia. Blood 83:2906–2911, 1994.

155. D Raspadori, D Rondelli, S Birtolo, M Lenoci, G Nardi, G Scalia, C Sestigiani, M Tozzi, G Marotta, F Lauria. Long-lasting decrease of Cd4+/CD45RA+ T-cells in HCL patients after 2-chlorodeoxyadenosine (2-CdA) treatment. Leukemia 13:1254–1257, 1999.

156. R Siegel, MS Tallman, D Hakimian, W Spies, E Wollins, LC Peterson, J Meyer. Technetium-99-m sulfur colloid scanning and correlative magnetic resonance imaging in patients with hairy cell leukemia and hypocellular bone marrow biopsies after 2-chlorodeoxyadenosine (2-CdA). Leuk Lymphoma 35:171–177, 1999.

157. MS Tallman, D Hakimian, C Zanzig, AW Rademaker, E Wollins, D Variakojis, LC Peterson. Relapse of hairy cell leukemia after 2-chlorodeoxyadenosine: Long-term follow-up of the Northwestern University experience. Blood 88:1954–1959, 1996.

158. D Thomas, L Fayad, FJ Giles, S O'Brien, K Boyer, M Keating, R Kurzrock. Relapse of hairy cell leukemia (HCL) after 2-chlorodeoxyadenosine (2-CdA) therapy (Rx): Long-term follow-up (FU) of 99 patients (Pts) (abstr). Blood 92:420, 1998.

159. IW Flinn, KJ Kopecky, MK Foucar, et al. Long-term results in hairy cell leukemia treated with pentostatin (abstr). Blood 90:578, 1997.

160. V Douglas, G Goolsby, AR Cubbon, MS Tallman, LC Peterson. Detection of hairy cell leukemia following therapy with 2-CdA: comparison of immunohistochemistry, flow cytometry and PCR (abstr). Mod Patho 13:859, 2000.

161. D Filleul, A Delannoy, A Ferrant, A Zenebergh, S Van Daele, A Bosly, C Doyen, P Mineur, P Glorieux, P Driesschaert. A single course of 2-chlorodeoxyadenosine does not eradicate leukemic cells in hairy cell leukemia patients in complete remission. Leukemia 8:1153–1156, 1994.

162. F Lauria, D Benfenati, D Raspadori, D Rondelli, MA Ventura, S Pileri, E Sabattini, S Roggi, M Benni, S Tura. Retreatment with 2-CdA of progressed HCL patients. Leuk Lymphoma 14:143–145, 1994.

163. A Saven, LD Piro. Complete remission in hairy cell leukemia with 2-chlorodeoxyadenosine after failure with 2′-deoxycoformycin. Ann Intern Med 119:278–283, 1993.

164. RJ Kreitman, WH Wilson, D Robbins, I Margulies, M Stetler-Stevenson, TA Waldman, I Pastan. Responses in refractory hairy cell leukemia to a recombinant immunotoxin. Blood 94:1–11, 1999.

165. H Hagberg. Chimeric monoclonal anti-CD20 antibody (Rituximab)-an effective treatment for a patient with relapsing hairy cell leukemia. Medical Oncology 16(3):221–222, 1999.

166. DA Thomas, S O'Brien, J Cortes, et al. Pilot study of Rituximab in refractory or relapsed hairy cell leukemia (abstr). Blood 94(10):3116, 1999.

167. M Hoffman, L Auerbach. Bone marrow remission of hairy cell leukemia induced by Rituximab (anti-CD20 antibody) in a patient refractory to cladribine. In press.

168. R Jacobs, E Volkes, H Golomb. Second malignancies in hairy cell leukemia. Cancer 56: 1462–1467, 1985.

169. P Kampmeier, R Spielberger, J Kickstein, R Mick, H Golomb, JW Vardiman. Increased incidence of second neoplasm in patients treated with interferon α for hairy cell leukemia: A clinicopathologic assessment. Blood 83:2931–2938, 1994.

170. R Kurzrock, SS Strom, E Estey, S O'Brien, MJ Keating, H Jiang, T Adams, M Talpaz. Second cancer risk in hairy cell leukemia: Analysis of 350 patients. J Clin Oncol 15:1803–1810, 1997.

171. WY Au, RJ Klasa, R Gallagher, N Le, RD Gascoyne, JM Connors. Second malignancies in patients with hairy cell leukemia in British Columbia: A 20-year experience. Blood 92:1160–1164, 1998.

172. BD Cheson, DA Vena, J Barrett, B Freidlin. Second malignancies as a consequence of nucleoside analog therapy for chronic lymphoid leukemias. J Clin Oncol 17:2454–2460, 1999.

27

Psychological Aspects of Chronic Lymphoid Leukemia

JAHANDAR SAIFOLLAHI, MARJANEH ROUHANI, ANDREW J. ROTH,
and **JIMMIE C. HOLLAND**

Memorial Sloan-Kettering Cancer Center, New York, New York

I. INTRODUCTION

Chronic lymphocytic leukemia (CLL) is the most common of all leukemias in Western countries. The National Cancer Institute's Surveillance Epidemiology and End Results (SEER) program data for the 15-year period from 1973 to 1987 indicates that CLL accounts for 31% of all leukemias in the United States (1). There is a higher incidence rate among Caucasians compared with the African-American population (1). It is estimated that more than 7000 persons are newly diagnosed with CLL in the United States every year. CLL is considered to be mainly a disease of the elderly (median age, 70 years), but it is not unusual today to make this diagnosis even in younger age groups (i.e., 30–39 years). The incidence increases rapidly after age 55. There are no clearly discernible occupational or environmental risk factors that predispose to CLL. Although there have been reports of excess risk of CLL among farmers (2–4) with benzene and heavy solvent exposure (2,3,5) and among rubber-manufacturing workers (6,7), these associations have not been proven to be causal (8). CLL and other lymphoid, hematological, and solid tumors occur with higher than expected frequency among first-degree relatives, but there is no available proof of genetic transmission of CLL. It is a generally held belief that CLL is an indolent disease associated with a prolonged chronic course and that the eventual cause of death may be unrelated to CLL for less than 30% of all cases. The natural history is heterogeneous in most patients. Some patients die rapidly, within 2 to 3 years of diagnosis and from a complication or cause directly related to CLL. Many patients live 5 to 10 years with an initial course that is relatively benign but almost always followed by a terminal phase lasting 1 to 2 years, during which there is considerable morbidity, both from the disease itself and from complications of therapy. The most frequent causes of death are severe systemic infections (e.g., pneumonia, septicemia), bleeding, and inanition with cachexia. In a small minority of patients, a diffuse large-cell immunoblastic lymphoma supervenes terminally (Reichter's transformation) associated with a rapidly progressive course, refractoriness to all chemotherapy, and death within 6 months. Patients with CLL are considered to be at higher risk of other cancers developing; usually lung or gastrointestinal cancers occur with considerably greater frequency in CLL patients than among the general population, but these do not result in higher mortality. Advances in the treatment of the hematological malignancies have led to longer survival of many patients and cure of more. Interest in how these patients cope with the newer and more technological treatment and their quality of life has increased. The psychological issues are outlined in the following, as they relate to diagnosis, treatment, and the adaptation of survivors.

As with other cancers, the diagnosis of CLL stimulates frightening thoughts of the possible course of illness, pain, fear of disfigurement and disability, and a painful death. Newer treatments, particularly bone marrow transplant, are associated with complex, aggressive treatment. They also translate into uncertainty about acute and chronic risk of side effects and second malignancies, likelihood of cure, and the significant expense with uncertain insurance coverage of treatment. Patients often experience an initial period of disbelief and denial after diagnosis. They normally go through a period of anxiety, despair, and poor sleep and appetite, which may last a few weeks. They may have difficulty with concentration carrying out daily activities and with lingering thoughts about the uncertainty of the future. In the following weeks and months, they usually begin to adjust to the new reality. This pattern of normal response is repeated as they go through crisis points: news of poor response to treatment or relapse and movement into palliative care (9). Families experience many of the same reactions. These crisis points are associated with greater distress and more difficulty in coping. In some patients, psychiatric intervention may be needed.

These expected responses are modulated by (1) medical-related factors (stage at diagnosis, pain, treatment[s], course of disease, and complications); (2) patient-related factors (ability to cope with stressful events, stage of the life cycle and emotional maturity, support of family and others), and (3) societal factors (attitudes of the public toward particular neoplasms and treatment, the stigma associated with diagnosis, and health care policies relating to insurance). This combination of medical, personal, and societal factors have an impact on the individual, leading to their unique response.

This chapter provides a brief overview of the most frequently observed psychiatric disorders associated with CLL and their management.

II. CLINICAL PICTURE OF ANXIETY

By far, the most frequent psychological problem in patients with hematological neoplasms is anxiety. Fears and distress are normal; but more severe levels of anxiety are common: reactive anxiety (adjustment disorder with anxious mood using the standard psychiatric classification of DSM-IV), a discrete anxiety disorder, and medical or procedure-related anxiety. Individuals with a preexisting anxiety disorder are at risk of its exacerbation during illness. These disorders cause severe suffering and sometimes are so severe that they compromise the ability to obtain medical care. Early recognition and treatment are essential for optimal care. Understanding the source of the anxiety is important in choosing an appropriate treatment.

Reactive anxiety is an exaggerated form of "normal" anxiety related to illness. It differs from normal fears of cancer by the greater duration and intensity of symptoms, the impairment of normal function, and the impairment of the ability to comply with treatment. Common symptoms are nervousness, tremulousness, palpitations, shortness of breath, diarrhea, diaphoresis, numbness and tingling of the extremities, feelings of imminent death, and phobias. Fearfulness, accompanied by symptoms of anxiety (e.g., restlessness, insomnia), is expected and "normal" before painful or stressful procedures (e.g., bone marrow aspiration, chemotherapy, radiation therapy), before surgery, and while awaiting test results. Many patients with mild to moderate anxiety respond to being given adequate information with reassurance and support; some require medication to control their distress. Patients who are extremely fearful are unable to absorb information or to cooperate with procedures. They require psychological support, medication, and/or behavioral interventions to reduce symptoms to a manageable level.

III. ANXIETY ASSOCIATED WITH MEDICAL CONDITIONS

Anxiety is frequently associated with medical problems: (1) uncontrolled pain, (2) abnormal metabolic states, (3) medications that produce anxiety, (4) withdrawal states (Table 1).

Patients in severe pain are often anxious and agitated; they communicate their anguish and inability to tolerate the distress. Adequate analgesia results in reduced anxiety immediately as they experience relief from pain. However, they worry and become anxious about "the next dose." Having to wait until the pain returns to request pain medication and waiting for it to come generate anxiety again, which then escalates the pain. Analgesics should be ordered around the clock (not as needed) to reach a steady state, which allows the patient to relax and feel secure that the pain will not return between doses. Rescue doses in case the standing dose is too low should also be made available (10).

The acute onset of anxiety without an obvious reason may herald a change in metabolic state or an impending catastrophic medical event. Sudden anxiety accompanied by chest pain or respiratory distress suggests a pulmonary embolus. Patients who are hypoxic are anxious and fearful that they are suffocating or dying. Sepsis and delirium can also cause anxiety symptoms. Several drugs, such as corticosteroids, antiemetics, and antiasthmatics, precipitate anxiety; corticosteroids produce motor restlessness, agitation, depression, and at times suicidal ideation. These symptoms appear usually with high doses or during rapid tapers (11). Akathisia, motor restlessness accompanied by subjective feelings of distress and hyperactivity, is an extrapyramidal side effect of prochlorperazine and metoclopramide, neuroleptic drugs often used to control emesis. Ondansetron and granisetron, as newer agents, produce few side effects of this kind.

Table 1 Anxiety Associated with Medical Conditions

1. Uncontrolled pain
2. Abnormal metabolic states
3. Medication side effects
4. Withdrawal states

Withdrawal states from alcohol, benzodiazepines, and narcotics, usually developing within 1 to 3 days after hospital admission, result in anxiety, agitation, delirium, and violent paranoid behaviors, which may be dangerous to patients and staff. Acute changes in mental status within the first 10 days of admission should lead to a careful history of medications used for sleep, pain, anxiety, nausea, or illicit substance use, and detailed information about drinking before admission. A urine toxicology screen should be ordered as early as the problem is recognized.

IV. DIAGNOSIS OF ANXIETY STATES

It is important that the physician inquire about anxiety symptoms when distress is noted, because patients may be too embarrassed to share these concerns with their oncology staff. The stress of the diagnosis of leukemia may activate a preexisting phobia, which might otherwise be quiescent. Phobias of blood tests, needle sticks, MRI scanners, doctors, hospitals, and agoraphobia are common sources of anxiety in the hospital. Panic disorder, characterized by symptoms of autonomic discharge such as heart pounding, chest pain, sweating, hyperventilation, trembling, and a sense of impending doom, will be reactivated by a cancer diagnosis or difficult treatment.

Generalized anxiety is a chronic anxiety syndrome that may also produce autonomic symptoms and be exacerbated on a cancer diagnosis and treatment. Posttraumatic stress disorder (PTSD) may be activated by isolation or conditions that recall some prior highly frightening event. Holocaust survivors and Vietnam veterans may be vulnerable. A new aspect of PTSD is the fact that both adults and children may experience PTSD after traumatic events related to cancer treatment. An exaggerated startle response, insomnia and nightmares, reliving the feelings and distressing thoughts experienced at the time of the trauma, and avoidance of anything associated with the trauma (e.g., the hospital) occurs. The anticipatory anxiety seen at follow-up visits after the cancer treatment is finished is likely PTSD-related, responding to cues that become painful reminders. Anticipatory nausea and vomiting with anxiety are conditioned responses to chemotherapy. PTSD is likely a learned response to prior trauma that explains the symptoms, which occur in cancer survivors who experience reminders of the treatment. The initial management of anxiety requires that adequate information be given to the patient in a supportive manner. An attitude of diffidence, ridicule, or impatience makes the patients' distress worse. Cognitive therapeutic techniques identify maladaptive automatic thoughts and underlying negative assumptions the patient has about himself or herself that interfere with coping. Brief supportive therapy, crisis intervention, and insight-oriented psychotherapy are also useful. Behavioral approaches of progressive passive or active relaxation, guided imagery, meditation, biofeedback, and hypnosis treat anxiety symptoms that are associated with painful procedures, pain syndromes, and anticipatory fears of chemotherapy, radiation therapy and other cancer treatments (12). A benzodiazepine is often needed in combination with the psychological support. The choice of medication depends on the severity of the anxiety, desired duration of drug action, rapidity of onset needed, the route of administration available, the presence or absence of active metabolites, and current metabolic problems that must be considered. Dosing schedules depend on patients' drug tolerance and require individual titration. The shorter acting benzodiazepines (alprazolam, lorazepam, and oxazepam) are given three to four times per day. Short-acting benzodiazepines, particularly those that can be administered by multiple routes, are widely used with good results. Clonazepam, a longer acting drug with antiseizure properties, is useful for panic symptoms and insomnia. A rapid onset of effect is achieved with lorazepam and diazepam for management of acute anxiety.

The most common side effects of benzodiazepines are dose-dependent and are controlled by titrating the dose to avoid drowsiness, confusion, motor incoordination, and sedation. All benzodiazepines can cause respiratory depression and must be used cautiously (or not at all) in the presence of respiratory impairment. Low doses of the antihistamine; hydroxyzine; or of the neuroleptics, olanzapine, chlorpromazine, or thioridazine can be used safely and relatively effectively in situations when one is concerned about depressing central respiratory mechanisms. In patients with hepatic dysfunction, it is best to use short-acting benzodiazepines that are metabolized primarily by conjugation and excreted by the kidney (e.g., oxazepam and lorazepam) or those that lack active metabolites (i.e., lorazepam). It is important to remember that discontinuation of a benzodiazepine in a patient, who has been on a standing dose for more than 2 weeks, should be done with a tapering schedule to avoid withdrawal.

Akathisia is quickly controlled by stopping the causative drug (if possible) and adding a benzodiazepine, a beta-blocker such as propranolol, or an antiparkinsonian agent such as benztropine.

Treatment of withdrawal states from alcohol, benzodiazepines, barbiturates, or opioids depends on the particular agent. Sometimes the goal is to stabilize the patient on the agent (a benzodiazepine) and sometimes a suitable substitute must be given (a benzodiazepine for ethanol or for a barbiturate). Anxiety before chemotherapy or painful procedures and dressing changes is controlled by a short-acting benzodiazepine such as lorazepam, which also provides anterograde amnesia for the event. Given intravenously, lorazepam also reduces vomiting in patients receiving emetogenic chemotherapy. Both oral lorazepam and alprazolam reduce nausea and vomiting related to chemotherapy. Patients with leukemia need to be encouraged to take antianxiety drugs and in sufficient amounts to relieve anxiety. A stigma exists on the part of both the patient and doctor about taking these medications. Medications are readily discontinued when symptoms subside, because concerns about addiction are far exaggerated in patients who have no history of drug abuse.

V. DEPRESSIVE DISORDERS

Sadness and grieving for loss of health and dreams of the future and well-being are normal responses in cancer patients (13). A continuum is seen, beginning with these normal responses, and increasing intensity reaching the level of subsyndromal symptoms, adjustment disorder with depressed mood, and major depression and mood disorder related to medical condition. These are the most common depressive disorders encountered in patients seen at our Counseling Center at Memorial Sloan-Kettering Cancer Center. A special diagnostic challenge exists in oncology. Neurovegetative symptoms of depression are similar to many physical symptoms caused by cancer or its treatment, especially fatigue, slowed psychomotor activity, insomnia, absent libido, anorexia, and weight loss. The clinician must focus on the psychological or cognitive symptoms of depression to make a diagnosis: persistent depressed or dysphoric mood, feelings of worthlessness, guilt, anhedonia, and preoccupation with hopelessness and death including suicidal ideation.

Depression, like anxiety, may be strongly associated with various medical entities such as metabolic changes (i.e., electrolyte disturbances, hypothyroidism), the cancer itself (i.e., pancreatic tumors), the cancer treatment (i.e., chemotherapeutic agents, biological moderators, hormonal therapies), and other medications (i.e., some antibiotics, antihypertensives, corticosteroids).

Patients whose cancers are in remission and who have a good prognosis should be evaluated for depression in the same way that you would evaluate physically healthy persons.

VI. SUICIDE AND PHYSICIAN-ASSISTED SUICIDE

Suicidal ideation should be a cause for concern and be promptly evaluated and treated. Patients in advanced stages of illness may express suicidal thoughts, which are viewed by others as "rational" because of their level of illness. The debate on rational physician-assisted suicide hinges in part on this issue. However, in studies of the wish for hastened death in patients with advanced cancer and AIDS, the presence of depression is the greatest predictor of experiencing a wish for hastened death, exceeding presence of pain as a factor. There is a great need to teach physicians to evaluate patients with cancer for symptoms of depression, especially teaching them that asking about suicide does not increase the risk (Table 2) (14).

The factors for suicidal risk in patients with cancer are several. They can be elicited by taking a good medical or psychiatric history. Medically, the most important problems are uncontrolled pain, delirium in which impulse control is reduced, and advanced disease with poor prognosis. Medication review is important, because steroids and interferon produce depressive symptoms. Psychiatrically, history of prior depression or suicide attempt, substance abuse, poor social support, and present depressive symptoms are predictors. In Scandinavia, the highest incidence of suicide was found in patients who were told they had no further treatment options and who lost contact with their physicians, underscoring the need for continued support (15,16). Thus physician's availability, continued support, control of symptoms, especially pain and depression, are essential.

In evaluating depression and suicide risk, neither can be adequately assessed in the presence of poorly controlled pain. The first step is to ensure pain control is achieved and then reassess mental status. Management of pain and psychiatric symptoms is intimately related, particularly in advanced cancer where both are common. The psychiatrist working in oncology must be familiar with the basics of pain management. Factors associated with increased risk of suicide are listed in Table 3 (28).

Table 2   Evaluation of Suicidal Patient

Establish rapport—empathic approach
Obtain patient's understanding of illness and present symptoms
Assess relevant mental status—delirium (internal control)
Assess vulnerability variables
Assess support system
Obtain family history
Record prior suicide threats, attempts
Assess suicidal thinking, intent, plans
Evaluate need for one-to-one observation
Formulate immediate and long term treatment plan

Source: Adapted from W Breitbart, S Krivo. Suicide. In: JC Holland, ed.
Psycho-Oncology. New York: Oxford University Press, 1998.

Table 3 Factors Influencing Suicide, Desire for Death, and Interest in Physician-Assisted Suicide among the Terminally Ill

Psychological	Biomedical	Social
Depression	Advanced illness	Lack of support
Hopelessness	Poor prognosis	Burden to other
Loss of control	Uncontrolled pain	Caregiver burnout
Helplessness	Delirium	Concurrent stress
Preexisting psychopathology	Fatigue/exhaustion	
Existential distress	Other distressing physical symptoms	
Anger		
Fear of illness		

Source: Adapted from Refs. 16 and 17.

A growing body of literature has emerged, indicating the types of physical and psychological concerns that may give rise to a desire for hastened death and requests for physician-assisted suicide (PAS). Although this literature has not always been consistent, a growing consensus has supported many of the assumptions put forth by the initial opponents of legalization. Specifically, the issues that have received the broadest empirical support are the effects of pain, depression, social support, and cognitive dysfunction on suicidal ideation. Table 3 lists the most common psychological, biomedical, and social factors suggested in the literature to influence suicide, desire for death, and interest in physician-assisted suicide (17,18). Patients with cancer report thoughts of suicide, even at early stages of illness. The incidence of suicide in patients with cancer exceeds that in the general population only slightly; however, many patients with advanced disease who commit suicide are likely not reported (19,20). In general, patients may use the suicidal thought as a way of asserting control over an uncertain, frightening future: "I will kill myself when the cancer becomes intolerable or if the pain gets too bad." That time usually does not come, but the control issue often remains.

Breitbart et al. (21) studied interest in assisted suicide among 378 ambulatory HIV-infected patients. More than half of the patients studied acknowledged considering PAS as an option for themselves. The strongest predictors of interest in PAS were levels of depressive symptoms, hopelessness, overall psychological distress, and current suicidal ideation. Other strong predictors included social support, experience with the death of a family member or friend, race, and religious practice. Interest in PAS was not related to the presence or severity of pain, physical symptoms, or extent of HIV disease. Fairclough and colleagues (22) interviewed terminally ill cancer patients and inquired as to whether patients had thoughts of suicide, assisted suicide, or euthanasia. They found, in their sample of 523 cancer patients, that 11.6% had thoughts of ending their life or asking their physician to help them end their life, and 3.7% had discussed this issue with another party. Although age, race, caregiver burden, and duration of illness were all significant predictors of interest in euthanasia or PAS, depression was the strongest predictor of interest in dying.

A growing body of research has demonstrated an important relationship between social support and desire for death (23–25).

VII. TREATMENT OF DEPRESSION

Treatment of depression in cancer patients usually consists of supportive or cognitive behavioral psychotherapy for mild depression. Support groups are widely available and helpful (26,27). For some adjustment disorders and major depression, medication will need to be added. Only on rare occasions is electroconvulsive therapy considered in cancer patients with severe, refractory depression. These patients often have a long history of refractory depression, which worsens in the context of cancer.

Medication is chosen by its side effect profile, interaction potential with other medications, and the target symptoms and route of administration. Today, cost, availability of medication, and the patient's ability to continue with drug level monitoring, if needed, are important, as well as the ability to follow the patients' progress.

The commonly used antidepressants and their starting dose are outlined in Table 4. Selective serotonin re-uptake inhibitors (SSRI's) are commonly the first line of treatment, because of their safety and low side effect profile. It is good practice "to start low and go slow" in cancer patients in order to reduce gastrointestinal side effects of nausea, transient weight loss caused by some SSRI's, anxiety, or sedation. Short-term addition initially of a benzodiazepine helps to prevent anxiety and jitteriness. The SSRI's are safe with most chemotherapeutic agents. However, they should be avoided in patients receiving procarbazine, a monoamine oxidase inhibitor.

Tricyclic antidepressants (TCAs) are effective antidepressants but require monitoring of cardiac function and drug levels in patients who are prone to toxicity and side effects. Constipation and dry mouth are undesirable in leukemia patients, especially those on opioids. The side effects of sedation and weight gain can be used to advantage for those with difficulty sleeping, anxious symptoms, or decreased appetite. The TCAs are also well proven to be good adjunct analgesic agents, especially for neuropathic pain. Although usually taken orally, they may be administered intramuscularly or by suppository to patients who cannot tolerate medication by mouth (i.e., because of mucositis). Moreover, they are more affordable compared with newer antidepressants. Several antineoplastic agents use the hepatic cytochrome P450 system, especially the 3A4 isoenzyme seems to be significant, because it is also used by several antidepressants. For example, nefazodone and fluvoxamine inhibit the 3A4 isoenzyme. Thus, their use requires careful monitoring for increased toxicity if the patient is receiving a chemotherapy regimen that is metabolized through the 3A4 isoenzyme. A few examples of chemotherapy agents that use the 3A4 isoenzyme are vinblastine, vincristine, etoposide, and cyclophosphamide. Drug interactions can also be mediated through competition for protein binding. Highly protein-bound antidepressants can displace the chemotherapeutic agent and leave patient vulnerable to serious toxicity. Venlafaxine is the least protein bound (Table 5) (28).

Psychostimulants such as pemoline and methylphenidate are effective mood enhancers in cancer patients. They have the added benefits of rapid onset of action, improved energy level, and increased appetite in low doses. They are useful in advanced disease with severe psychomotor retardation or to counter the effects of opioids. Pemoline is unique in that it does not have an abuse potential. In addition, it comes in a chewable form that is readily absorbed through the buccal mucosa and thus is useful in patients with swallowing difficulties. Pemoline is contraindicated in liver dysfunction and might cause liver enzyme elevations that will return to baseline on discontinuation.

Bupropion, nefazodone, and mirtazepine have the least sexual dysfunction side effects among the antidepressants. The dopaminergic profile of bupropion, used as an adjunct medication, may be useful to counteract the sexual dysfunction side effect caused by other antidepressants.

Trazodone is used alone or in combination with SSRIs. The sedation, when given at bedtime, and weight gain are favorable parts of its side effect profile in patients with

Table 4 Antidepressant Medications Used in Advanced Cancer Patients

Drug	Therapeutic daily dosages mg (PO)
Second-generation antidepressants	
Serotonin selective reuptake inhibitors	
Fluoxetine	10–40
Paroxetine	10–40
Citalopram	20–40
Fluvoxamine	50–300
Sertraline	50–200
Serotonin/norepinephrine reuptake inhibitor	
Venlafaxine	37.5–225
5-HT2 antagonists/serotonin and norepinephrine reuptake inhibitors	
Nefazodone	100–500
Trazodone	150–300
Norepinephrine/dopamine reuptake inhibitor	
Buproprion	200–450
α-2 antagonist/5-HT2 antagonist	
Mirtazapine	7.5–30
Tricyclic antidepressants	
Secondary amine	
Desipramine	25–125
Nortriptyline	25–125
Tertiary amine	
Amitriptyline	25–125
Doxepin	25–125
Imipramine	25–125
Clomipramine	25–125
Heterocyclic antidepressants	
Maprotiline	50–75
Amoxapine	100–150
Psychostimulants	
Dextroamphetamine	5–30
Methylphenidate	5–30
Pemoline	37.5–150

insomnia and anorexia. Lack of anticholinergic side effects with trazodone is helpful in patients prone to delirium and cognitive dysfunction. It is also the only antidepressant that will not interact with the MAOI effect of procarbazine. However, one must consider the possible side effect of priapism in men.

VIII. DELIRIUM AND COGNITIVE CHANGES

Psychiatric consultations are often requested for patients who appear angry, depressed, agitated, psychotic, or anxious, but who, after evaluation, are found to have delirium or encephalopathy rather than a major depression or anxiety disorder. These diagnostic distinctions are important because treatment recommendations are quite different for depression, anxiety, psychosis, and delirium. Untreated delirium can lead to death, because its

Table 5   Protein Binding and CP450 Isoenzyme Profile of Commonly Used Antidepressants in Cancer Patients

Drug	Protein binding	1A2 inhibition	2C9 inhibition	2D6 inhibition	3A4 inhibition
Bupropion	80				
Citalopram	80	+	+	+	
Fluoxetine	94		+++	+++	++
Fluvoxamine	77	+++	+++		+++
Mirtazapine	85				
Nefazodone	99				+++
Paroxetine	95			+++	
Sertraline	98	++			++
Venlafaxine	27				

Source: Adapted from Ref. 27.

origin is usually a sign of organ failure or drug toxicity. Delirium, dementia, and cognitive disorders caused by medical conditions occur in roughly 15% to 20% of hospitalized cancer patients and in a significant number of terminally ill cancer patients (29). Symptoms of delirium include an inability to maintain or shift attention properly; waxing and waning of consciousness; disturbance in the sleep-wake cycle; disorientation to person, place or time; abnormal perceptions such as visual or auditory (less frequent), hallucinations, and problems with memory and language (dysnomia or dysgraphia). Delirium is distinguished from a dementia by its more rapid onset, fluctuation in level and severity of symptoms, its reversibility, and lesser degree of memory impairment. Etiologically, delirium may be a direct cause of the tumor itself (i.e., CNS lymphoma) or of metastatic spread to the CNS of other tumors by means of hematogenous or lymphatic routes. Indirect effects of infection, vascular complications, metabolic changes, organ failure, treatment effects, and nutritional state are of equal importance. Failure of vital organs, especially the liver, kidneys, and lungs, or the metabolic changes that result from thyroid or adrenal failure also cause delirium. Electrolyte imbalance, especially sodium, potassium, and calcium, may constitute a metabolic cause of altered mental status. Adequate doses of narcotic analgesics to manage cancer pain may sometimes result in oversedation and hallucinations. All steroid compounds may cause psychiatric disturbances, ranging from affective changes (emotional lability) to paranoid interpretation of events, suspiciousness of others, illusions, delusions, and hallucinations. CNS symptoms are not a prominent feature of most chemotherapeutic agents used today. Those that can cause delirium are methotrexate, 5-fluorouracil, vincristine and vinblastine, bleomycin, BCNU, cisplatin, asparaginase, and procarbazine (30). Interferon, used in treatment regimens for some leukemias and lymphomas, causes depression, somnolence, confusion, and paresthesias. Interleukin-2 can also cause depression and other mental status changes. Amphotericin B, used for patients who are immunologically compromised for the treatment of fungal infections, causes neurological side effects and delirium with intrathecal administration. Often though it is difficult to distinguish CNS effects of antifungal medication from those of fever, CNS infections, or metabolic abnormalities. Acyclovir, used in the treatment of herpes simplex and varicella zoster virus, in immunologically compromised patients with leukemia or going through bone marrow transplantation, can also cause neurotoxicity, including agitation, tremor, and disorientation (31).

Environmental manipulation and a low dose of a neuroleptic are useful for a patient who has a mild delirium without agitation. If the patient is a danger to himself or to others because of a confused or disinhibited state, observation by a one-to-one companion is indicated. Frequent reminders by staff or family, of location, day, time, and outside events, help distract patients from their internal thoughts, hallucinations, or delusions, and afford them appropriate reorientation.

Haloperidol, a high-potency neuroleptic, used in low doses orally is the drug of choice for treatment of mild delirium. It can also be used safely parenterally. The usual starting dose of 0.5 mg once or twice daily (PO, IM, IV, SC) is administered initially, with doses repeated every 45 to 60 minutes and titrated against symptoms for severely agitated patients. Haloperidol provides mild sedation and amelioration of the behavioral problems. It is often administered intravenously when patients are thrombocytopenic, unable to take medications orally because of stomatitis, or agitated (and rapid sedation is needed).

It is unclear to date how problematic the potential bone marrow–suppressing effects of neuroleptics are in patients with CLL. However, our clinical experience is that risks of harm to patient or staff by delirium often outweigh the possible marrow suppression effect of these medications.

IX. BONE MARROW TRANSPLANTATION

Treatment of CLL is a challenge for hematologists. The long physical history and the indolent nature of CLL do not support the choice of aggressive treatment. The combination of chlorambucil and prednisone is often used for first-line therapy of these patients. Biological response modifiers such as interferons, interleukins, and monoclonal antibodies have not improved responses or remission duration. The use of BMT for CLL is a relatively new approach compared with other hematological malignancies. The long natural history of CLL and significant procedure-related mortality initially deterred the use of BMT for CLL. However, improvement in transplantation procedures and supportive care have paved its way for treatment of CLL (32). Addition of autologous marrow or blood stem cell transplantation as a consolidation therapy is an effective treatment for CLL, capable of inducing durable complete remissions (33).

The psychological stressors of BMT begin with the consideration of the transplant. Although often offered as a chance of cure, it also carries significant morbidity and possible mortality. One patient with lymphoma described this as a ''nondecision.'' He said, ''I may die from the BMT, but I'll surely die if I don't have it.'' A considerable amount of planning is necessary on an outpatient basis. One study of BMT candidates noted one-third appeared to be depressed and that interpersonal sources of mastery and optimistic attitude were significantly negatively correlated with psychological distress variables (34). An important part of the planning is evaluating and shoring up the patient's social support. Patients and families visit the transplant unit in advance and speak with the staff members who will care for them. This is particularly important for patients who may live far away from the transplant site. Lesko (1989, 1993) has described many psychosocial sequelae of the various stages of transplantation, from pretransplant to posttransplant phases (35,36). Studies have differed in documentation of major psychopathology and coping styles during transplantation (37–40).

604 Saifollahi et al.

Some family members of patients undergoing BMT have been found to have alterations in immune status at various phases of the transplant (41).

Early on in the transplant process, patients must cope with central vein catheter placement, high-dose chemotherapy, and irradiation. They remain in isolation to avoid infection. They often experience nausea, vomiting, and fatigue. This part of the process is highly stressful.

The transplant itself is brief and anticlimactic compared with the pretransplant regimen and recovery phases, because it is only an intravenous infusion of one or several packets of concentrated bone marrow. The patients are then faced with a period of waiting for their "counts to come back," evidence that their immune and hematological systems are recovering. Many patients keep charts of their white cell counts, anticipating the day of "probable" recovery, although the oncologist may have stated a day of "earliest possible recovery." Often patients and their families have a strong sense of anticipatory anxiety as the numbers are charted, with anger, guilt, anxiety, or disappointment if the recovery is delayed or nonexistent. Patients are susceptible to infection and fevers and require immunosuppressive medications. Some patients respond in an opposite fashion, requesting medications to "just sleep through the experience" until they are ready for discharge. This passive attitude often upsets caregivers, because this may compromise the patient's ability to participate in proper self-care behaviors.

Bone marrow transplant recipients are at increased risk for CNS toxicity developing such as neuropsychological impairment, including compromised motor and cognitive tests (42). These deficits enhance the likelihood of poorer psychological adaptation.

There may be high level of fear when patients are ready for hospital discharge and are asked to assume greater roles in self-care after a prolonged period of dependence. Persistent fatigue is a major problem when patients resume "normal" activities at home and work (43).

Chronic anxiety and depression are the most common psychiatric sequelae of the transplantation procedure. Psychological adjustment is particularly difficult for those patients who have delayed or disrupted important developmental life tasks, such as career or young parenthood. Decreased sexual desire may be related to depression and the patients altered self-image.

Although noncompliance in the transplant process has not been well studied, it may result in life-threatening complications. Noncompliance with a range of self-care behaviors can increase risk of infection or delay functional recuperation. One recent study of BMT patients found a correlation between early increased anxiety levels and subsequent development of graft versus host disease (44). Reports of pain during BMT (45) and subsequent survival may be more closely related to physical rather than psychological factors (46).

In a stressful situation like a transplant, it is useful to try to strengthen patients' usual, adaptive coping mechanisms, rather than try to have them develop new ones. In general, successful adaptation is associated with the ability to use information about illness and treatment and the ability to delegate control and authority to others temporarily, as well as the capacity to establish a close, trusting relationship with the staff (47). A study of 100 adult patients undergoing allogeneic BMT for acute leukemia found three variables that affected outcome: illness status, presence of depressed mood, and the extent of perceived social support. Those who had depressed mood, regardless of specific psychiatric diagnosis, had poorer outcomes, suggesting the potential benefit of early psychiatric intervention (48). These variables may become important at different periods after BMT

(49,50). There may be some positive sequelae of BMT that can also contribute to QOL (i.e., greater appreciation of life and enhanced interpersonal relationships that are not well measured by standard QOL indices) (51).

Interestingly, the distress generally does not reach psychopathological proportions. There is also no significant difference in sexual activity between those treated with BMT and those treated with conventional chemotherapy, although some decrease in sexual frequency and satisfaction in women is seen compared with physically healthy women (52).

X. SURVIVORSHIP

There are more survivors of leukemia and lymphoma than ever before. This leads to new psychosocial challenges and expectations for patients. In general, survivors have both medical and psychological concerns. Medically, leukemia survivors fear relapse, either in bone marrow, the CNS, testis, or ovary. Although rare, they also have the potential for occurrence of second malignancies as a result of chemotherapy or radiation. Predictors of greater emotional stress 1 year after allogeneic marrow transplant included pretransplant family conflict, nonmarried status, and development of chronic graft versus host disease (53).

There may also be delayed toxicity of peripheral neuropathy caused by vincristine therapy, cardiomyopathy caused by anthracycline therapy and pericarditis from radiotherapy, endocrine abnormalities from radiation therapy, pulmonary fibrosis, hepatic fibrosis caused by methotrexate, and antibiotic-related renal failure (54). Psychological problems of survivorship include concern about ending treatment and fear of relapse, reentry into the expected life tasks, concerns about job discrimination, social withdrawal, health insurance difficulties, and survivor's syndrome or guilt. Kornblith et al. found in a study of Hodgkin's disease survivors that 22% met criteria for a psychiatric diagnosis. The following problems were most prominent: denial of life (31%), and health (22%) insurance, sexual problems (37%) conditioned nausea in response to reminders of chemotherapy (39%), and a negative socioeconomic effect (36%) (55). Because diagnostic symptoms of hematological malignancies are often vague and systemic, there is often an inability to ignore minor aches and pains, fatigue, and a preoccupation with loss of control over their health. To date there are no similar studies in patients with CLL. Other studies of long-term survivors of Hodgkin's disease found most patients not significantly different from nonpatients; however, there are a number of problem areas with patients (55,56). Differences in findings may be related to different treatment regimens and different time intervals between treatment and follow-up. Depression affected a considerable percentage of patients, 18% (40); however, this seemed to decrease the further out from treatment a patient was. Depression seemed to be correlated with degree of energy loss and inability to resume usual activities. Family life was also affected with findings of moderately high divorce rates, inability to have children, fears of second malignancies, and changes in sexual frequency. Screening patients for depression, increasing staff sensitivity, and helping patients to cope with depression are possible areas for future interventions. Another study of psychological adjustment of Hodgkin's survivors (39) found significantly lowered intimacy motivation, increased avoidant thinking about illness, prolonged difficulty in returning to premorbid work status, and illness-related concerns.

It is important for the physician to communicate to the patient the awareness of the previous concerns during long-term follow-up of treatment. This can be done by asking about important aspects of the patient's life such as job, relationships, and other social supports, as well as physical well-being. Asking specifically about sexual and fertility issues and other intimacy problems will make discussion of important, yet hard to talk about, subjects much easier.

XI. SUMMARY

Advances in the effectiveness of therapies for CLL has led to longer survival than ever before. Some of these therapies carry acute and chronic physical morbidity. There are many factors responsible for how a patient will cope with this morbidity and ultimately regain their health as a survivor. We have discussed a number of psychiatric and psychological issues and treatments that patients may face. Hopefully, description of these issues will aid in both their prevention and earlier identification and treatment of problems when they occur.

REFERENCES

1. JA Hernandez, KJ Land, RW McKenna. Leukemias, myeloma and other lymphoreticular neoplasms. Cancer 75:381, 1995.
2. A Blair, D White. Leukemia cell types and agricultural practices in Nebraska. Arch Environ Health 40:211, 1985.
3. LF Burmeister, SF Van Lier, P Isacson. Leukemia and farm practices in Iowa. Am J Epidemiol 115–720, 1982.
4. D Waterhouse, WJ Carman, D Schottenfeld, G Gridley, S McLean. Cancer incidence in the rural community of Tecumseh, Michigan: a pattern of increase lymphopoietic neoplasms. Cancer 77(4):763–770.
5. EW Arp, PH Wolf, H Checkoway. Lymphocytic leukemia and exposures to benzene and other solvents in the rubber industry. J Occup Med 25:598, 1983.
6. AJ McMichael, R Spirtas, LL Kupper, JF Gamble. Solvent exposure and leukemia among rubber workers: an epidemiologic study. J Occup Med 17:234, 1975.
7. RR Monson, LJ Fine. Cancer mortality and morbidity among rubber workers. J Nat Cancer Inst 61:1047, 1978.
8. L Brandt. Environmental factors and leukemia. Medical Oncology Tumor Pharmacotherapy 2:7, 1985.
9. MJ Massie, E Heilgenstein, MS Lederberg, et al. Psychiatric complications in cancer patients. In: AI Holleb, DJ Fink, GP Murphy, eds. Clinical Oncology. Atlanta: ACS, 1991.
10. W Breitbart, JA Levenson, SD Passik. Terminally ill cancer patients. In: W Breitbart, JC Holland, eds. Psychiatric Aspects of Symptom Management in Cancer Patients. Washington, DC: APA Press, 1994. pp 173.
11. MJ Massie, EJ Shakin. Management of depression and anxiety. In: W Breitbart, JC Holland, eds. Psychiatric Aspects of Symptom Management in Cancer Patients. Washington, DC: APA Press, 1994. pp 1.
12. K Gorfinkle, WH Redd. Behavioral control of anxiety, distress, and learned aversions in pediatric oncology. In: W Breitbart, JC Holland, eds. Psychiatric Aspects of Symptom Management in Cancer Patients. Washington, DC: APA Press, 1994. pp 129.
13. J Bukberg, D Penman, JC Holland. Depression in hospitalized cancer patients. Psychoso Med 43:199–212, 1984.
14. C Bolund, et al. Suicide and cancer. I. Medical and care factors in suicide by cancer patients in Sweden, 1973–1976. J Psychosoc Oncol 3:17–30, 1985.

15. C Bolund, et al. Suicide and cancer. II. Demographic and social characteristics of cancer patients who committed suicide in Sweden, 1973–1976. J Psychosoc Oncol 3:31–52, 1985.

16. W Breitbart. Suicide risk and pain in cancer and AIDS patients. In: CR Chapman, KM Foley, eds. Current and emerging issues in cancer pain: Research and practice. New York: Raven Press, 1993. pp 49–65.

17. HM Chochinov, KG Wilson. The euthanasia debate: attitudes, practices and psychiatric considerations. Can J Psychiatry 40:593–602, 1995.

18. MJ Massie, MK Popkin. Depressive disorders. In: JC Holland, ed. Textbook of Psycho-Oncology. New York: Oxford University Press, 1998. pp 518–540.

19. MJ Massie, P Gagnon, JC Holland. Depression and suicide in patients with cancer. J Pain Symptom Manage 9:325–340, 1994.

20. W Breitbart, B Rosenfeld, SD Passik. Interest in physician assisted suicide among ambulatory HIV-infected patients. Am J Psychiatry 153, 238–242, 1996.

21. DL Fairclough. Quality of life, cancer investigation and clinical practice. Cancer Invest 16: 478–84, 1998.

22. PJ van der Mass, G van der Wal, I Haverkate, et al. Euthanasia, physician assisted suicide and other medical practices involving the end of life in the Netherlands, 1990–1995. N Engl J Med 335:1699–1705, 1996.

23. HM Chochinov, KG Wilson, M Enns, et al. Desire for death in the terminally ill. Am J Psychiatry 152:1185–1191, 1995.

24. B Rosenfeld, M Galietta, W Breitbart, S Krivo. Interest in physician-assisted suicide among terminally ill AIDS patients: Measuring and understanding desire for death. Paper presented at the biennial conference of the American Psychology-Law Society, Redondo Beach, CA, 1998.

25. K Beliles, A Stoudemire. Psychopharmacologic treatment of depression in the medically ill. Psychosomatics 39:2–19, 1998.

26. FI Fawzy, WW Fawzy, LA Arndt, RO Pasnau. Critical review of psychosocial intervention in cancer care. Arch Gen Psychiatry 52:100–113, 1995.

27. JD Newport, CB Nemeroff. Treatment of depression in the cancer patient. Clin Geriatr 7:40–55, 1999.

28. MJ Massie, JC Holland, E Glass. Delirium in terminally ill cancer patients. Am J Psychiatry 140:1048–1050, 1983.

29. SB Fleishman, LM Lesko, W Breitbart. Treatment of organic mental disorders in cancer patients. In: W Breitbart, JC Holland, eds. Psychiatric Aspects of Symptom Management in Cancer Patients. Washington, DC: APA Press, 1994. pp 23.

30. LM Lesko, JC Holland. Psychological issues in patients with hematological malignancies. Recent Results in Cancer Res 108:243–270, 1988.

31. IW Flinn, G Vogelsang. Bone marrow transplantation for chronic lymphocytic leukemia. Semin Oncol 25(1):60–4, 1998.

32. VA Boussiotis, AS Freedman, LM Nadler. Bone marrow transplantation for low grade lymphoma and chronic lymphocytic leukemia. Semin Hematol 36(2):209–16, 1999.

33. F Baker, D Marcellus, J Zabora, A Polland, D Jodrey. Psychological distress among adult patients being evaluated for bone marrow transplantation. Psychosomatics 38:10–19, 1997.

34. LM Lesko. Hematological malignancies. In: JC Holland, JH Rowland, eds. Handbook of Psycho-oncology. New York: Oxford University Press, 1989. pp 218.

35. LM Lesko. Psychiatric aspects of bone marrow transplantation. Parts I and II. Psychooncology 2:161, 1993.

36. PL Jenkins, A Linington, JA Whittaker. A retrospective study of psychosocial morbidity in bone marrow transplant recipients. Psychosomatics 32:65–71, 1991.

37. JR Rodrique, SR Boggs, RS Weiner, JM Behen. Mood, coping style and personality functioning among adult bone marrow transplant candidates. Psychosomatics 34:159–165, 1993.

38. L Wettergren, A Langius, M Bjorkholm, H Bjorvell. Physical and psychosocial functioning

in patients undergoing autologous bone marrow transplantation—a prospective study. Bone Marrow Transplant 20:497–502, 1997.

39. A Molassiotis. A conceptual model of adaptation to illness and quality of life for cancer patients treated with bone marrow transplants. J Adv Nurs 26:572–579, 1997.

40. AD Futterman, DK Wellisch, J Zighelboim, M Luna-Raines, H Weiner. Psychological and immunological reactions of family members to patients undergoing bone marrow transplantation. Psychosom Med 58:472–480, 1996.

41. DM Hann, PB Jacobsen, SC Martin, LE Kronish, LM Azzarello, KK Fields. Fatigue in women treated with bone marrow transplantation for breast cancer: a comparison with women with no history of cancer. Support Care Center 5:44–52, 1997.

42. R Gregurek, B Labar, M Mrsic, D Batinic, I Ladika, V Bogdanic, D Nemet, M Skerlev, J Jakic-Razumovic, E Klain. Anxiety as a possible predictor of acute GVHD. Bone Marrow Transplant 18:585–589, 1996.

43. KL Syrjala, ME Chapko. Evidence for a biopsychosocial model of cancer treatment-related pain. Pain 61:69–79, 1995.

44. KC Murphy, PL Jenkins, JA Whittaker. Psychosocial morbidity and survival in adult bone marrow transplant recipients—a follow-up study. Bone Marrow Transplant 18:199–201, 1996.

45. LM Lesko, JC Holland. Psychological issues in patients with hematological malignancies. Recent Results Cancer Res, 108:243–270, 1988.

46. EA Colon, AL Callier, MJ Popkin, PB McGlave. Depressed mood and other variables related to bone marrow transplantation survival in acute leukemia. Psychosomatics 32:420, 1991.

47. A Molassiotis, OB Van Den Akker, DW Milligan, JM Goldman. Symptom distress, coping style and biological variables as predictors of survival after bone marrow transplantation. J Psychosom Res 42:275–285, 1997.

48. A Molassiotis. Psychosocial transitions in the long-term survivors of bone marrow transplantation. Eur J Cancer Care 6:100–107, 1997.

49. K Fromm, MA Andrykowski, J Hunt. Positive and negative psychosocial sequelae of bone marrow transplantation: implications for quality of life assessment. J Behav Med 19(3):221–240, 1996.

50. GH Mumma, D Mashberg, LM Lesko. Long-term psychosexual adjustment of acute leukemia survivors: impact of marrow transplantation versus conventional chemotherapy. Gen Hosp Psychiatry 14:43–55, 1992.

51. KL Syrjala, MK Chapko, PP Vitlaiano, et al. Recovery after allogeneic marrow transplantation: prospective study of predictors of long-term physical and psychosocial functioning. Bone Marrow Transplant 11(4):319–327, 1993.

52. SM Hubbard, DL Longo. Treatment-related morbidity in patients with lymphoma. Cur Opin Oncol 3:852–862, 1991.

53. AB Kornblith, J Anderson, DF Cella, et al. Hodgkin disease survivors at increased risk for problems in psychosocial adaptation. Cancer 70:2214–2224, 1992.

Index

B-cell lymphocytes, CLL as disorder of, 3–4
B-cell prolymphocytic leukemia (B-PLL), 526–531
  chromosome abnormalities and molecular genetics, 528–529
  clinical course, prognosis, and therapy, 530–531
  clinical features, 526
  differential diagnosis, 529–530
  histology, 527
  immunological markers, 527–528
  morphology, 526
B-cell subsets (development and repertoire of CD5+ B cells), 63–67
BcL-2 gene, 23–24, 143–144
  BcL-2 antisense, 314
  Benign lymphocytosis, 210–211
  Benzene, 40
  Benzodiazepines, 596, 597
  Binet staging system, 162, 233–234, 394–395
  Biological agents, in treatment of relapsed or refractory CLL, 314–315
  Biological markers reflecting pathogenesis of disease, 246–248
  Biology of CLL relevant to drug development, 420–422
  Bladder cancer, 52
  Blood lymphocytic count, 3
  Bone marrow aspiration and biopsy in diagnosing CLL, 237–238
Bone marrow hypoplasia, after purine analog therapy for HCL, 577
Bone marrow transplantation (BMT)
  psychological stressors of, 603–605
  in treatment of relapsed or refractory CLL, 297–303
Brick mortar, 42
Bryostatin, 314, 420
Bulky lymphadenopathy, 383
Bullous pemphigoid, 436
Bupropion, 601
Burkitt's lymphomas, 9
Butadiene, 41

Caenorhabiditis elegans (*C. elegans*), 112
  CED-8 and, 114–116
Campath 1-H, 4, 309–310, 335, 339–341, 343–346, 347, 420
  infections in CLL patients treatment with, 513–514
  in treatment of T-PLL, 538

CAP (adriamycin and prednisone in combination therapy), 275
CD20 antigen, 341–342
CD20 MAbs, 341–342
CD23, 3
  serum release of soluble CD23, 241
CD30, 138–139
CD36, 241
CD38, 3
  clinical courses of B-CLL subgroups based on expression of, 99–101
CD40, 139–141
CD40+, 248
CD40-mediated antiapoptosis pathway, 74–75
CD52 antigen, 339–341
CD54, serum release of soluble CD54, 245
CD95, 248
CD154, 420
CED-3 (cysteine proteinase), 112–113
CED-4 (adenosine triphosphate-binding protein), 113–114
CED-9, 114–116
Cell-cycle regulatory molecules, 239–240
Cell-mediated immunity, 508–509
Cellular vaccines, 185–187
Chemical agents, working with, 40–42
Chemists, 42
Chemotherapy
  combination regimens, 266–268
  combination strategies with nucleoside analogs, 288–296
    2-chlorodeoxyadenosine combinations, 294–295
    deoxycoformycin combinations, 295–296
    fludarabine and alkylators, 290–293
    fludarabine and anthracyclines or mitoxantrone, 289–290
    fludarabine and corticosteroids, 289
    fludarabine combinations in alkylator-refractory patients, 293–294
  new chemotherapeutic agents, 313, 314
  oral, in treatment of relapsed or refractory CLL, 312
  single-agent, 262–263
Chinese-Americans, incidence rate for CLL among (U.S.), 35, 36
Chlorambucil (CLB), 4, 53, 261–262, 275, 418
  prednisone and, 266, 267

About the Editor

BRUCE D. CHESON, M.D., FACP, attended the University of Virginia, Charlottesville, and Tufts University Medical School, Boston, Massachusetts. He completed his internship and residency in Internal Medicine at the University of Virginia Hospitals, Charlottesville, followed by a clinical and research fellowship in Hematology at the New England Medical Center Hospital, Boston, Massachusetts. From 1977 to 1984 he was Assistant Professor of Medicine in Hematology/Oncology at the University of Utah, Salt Lake City. In 1984 he came to the National Cancer Institute (NCI), Cancer Therapy Evaluation Program (CTEP), Baltimore, Maryland, and since 1986 has been the Head, Medicine Section, CTEP at the NCI. He is also Clinical Professor of Medicine in the Division of Hematology/Oncology at Georgetown University Medical Center, Washington, D.C. and a Senior Staff Physician in the Lymphoma Clinic, NCI. Dr. Cheson is the author of over 300 publications and abstracts and a contributor to over 30 texts; an editorial board member for numerous journals; Associate Editor of the *Journal of Clinical Oncology*, *Oncology*, and *Oncology New International*; Editor-in-Chief of *Clinical Lymphoma*; and the former editor of the American College of Physician's Medical Knowledge Self-Assessment® Program in Oncology. He has served on several committees for the American Society of Clinical Oncology (ASCO), including its Board of Directors, and edits *ASCO News*. Dr. Cheson is an Honorary Board Member of the Lymphoma Research Foundation of America, as well as a Special Expert Advisor to the Food and Drug Administration. Dr. Cheson's clinical interests focus on the development and evaluation of new therapeutic approaches for hematological malignancies.